CONTENTS

Contents

Contents

CONTRIBUTORS

Dr Huda Al-Ansari, MD DTM&H
Consultant Paediatrician in Infectious
    Diseases
Department of Paediatrics
Salmaniya Hospital
Bahrain

**Dr David J Atherton, MA MB
    BChir FRCP**
Consultant Paediatric Dermatologist
Great Ormond Street Hospital for
    Children NHS Trust
London, UK

Mr C Martin Bailey, BSc FRCS
Senior Consultant ENT Surgeon
Department Of Paediatric
    Otolaryngology
Great Ormond Street Children
    Hospital for Children NHS Trust
London, UK

**Dr Michael Baraitser, BSc MBChB
    FRCP**
Previously Consultant in Clinical
    Genetics
Great Ormond Street Children
    Hospital for Children NHS Trust
London, UK

**Dr J Harry Baumer, MBChB FRCP
    FRCPCH**
Consultant Paediatrician
Derriford Hospital
Plymouth, UK

**Professor Charles GD Brook, MD
    FRCPCH FRCP**
Emeritus Professor of Paediatric
    Endocrinology
University College London Hospitals
    and Great Ormond Street Hospital
    for Children
London, UK

**Dr Rose de Bruyn, MBBCh DMRD
    FRCR**
Consultant Paediatric Radiologist
Department of Radiology
Great Ormond Street Hospital for
    Children NHS Trust
London, UK

Ms Lesley Cavalli
Specialist Speech & Language
    Therapist
ENT Team – Team Leader
Speech & Language Therapy
    Department
Great Ormond Street Children
    Hospital for Children NHS Trust
London, UK

Ms Frances M Cook
Principal Speech and Language
    Therapist
The Michael Palin Centre for
    Stammering Children
London, UK

**Dr Mehul T Dattani, MD DCH
    FRCPCH FRCP**
Reader and Honorary Consultant in
    Paediatric Endocrinology
Biochemistry, Endocrinology and
    Metabolism Unit
UCL Institute of Child Health
London, UK

Dr Robert Dinwiddie, FRCPCH
Honorary Consultant Paediatrician
Department of Respiratory Medicine
Great Ormond Street Hospital for
    Children NHS Trust
London, UK

**Dr Sally A Feather, MA MB BChir
    MRCP PhD**
Consultant Paediatric Nephrologist
Department of Paediatric Nephrology
St James's University Hospital
Leeds, UK

Mr John A Fixsen, MChir FRCS
Previously Consultant Orthopaedic
    Surgeon
Great Ormond Street Hospital for
    Children NHS Trust
London, UK

Dr Mark N Gaze, MD FRCP FRCR
Consultant Clinical Oncologist
Department of Oncology
University College Hospital and
    Great Ormond Street Hospital for
    Children NHS Trust
London, UK

Dr Bert JA Gerritsen, MD, PhD
Consultant Paediatrician
Oosterschelde Hospital
Goes, Netherlands

**Professor David Goldblatt, MBChB
    PhD MRCP FRCPCH,**
Professor of Vaccinology and
    Immunology
Honorary Consultant Paediatric
    Immunologist
UCL Institute of Child Health
London, UK

Dr Chula DA Goonasekera, PhD
Consultant Paediatric Nephrologist
Faculty of Medicine
University of Peradeniya
Peradeniya, Sri Lanka

**The late Dr David B Grant, MD
    FRCP**
Previously Consultant in Paediatric
    Endocrinology
Great Ormond Street Hospital for
    Children NHS Trust
London, UK

**Professor Richard Grundy, BSc
    MBChB MSc MRCP FRCPCH
    PhD**
Professor of Paediatric Neuro-
    Oncology and Cancer Biology
The Children's Brain Tumour Research
    Centre
University of Nottingham Medical
    School
Nottingham, UK

**Dr Magdi H El Habbal, MBChB
    MSc MD FRCPCH**
Consultant in Paediatrics and
    Cardiology
Department of Paediatrics
Hull Royal Infirmary
Hull, UK

**Professor Ian M Hann, MD
    FRCPath FRCP**
Consultant in Paediatric Haematology
Professor of Haematology / Oncology
Great Ormond Street Hospital for
    Children NHS Trust
London, UK

**Dr Paul I Hargreaves, MBBS
    FRCPCH MSc CCDS**
Consultant Paediatrician and
    Designated Doctor for Child
    Protection
Chelsea and Westminster Hospital,
London, UK

**Professor John I Harper, MD FRCP
    FRCPCH**
Professor of Paediatric Dermatology
Great Ormond Street Hospital for
    Children NHS Trust
London, UK

Mr Robert A Hill, FRCS
Consultant Orthopaedic Surgeon
Great Ormond Street Hospital for
    Children NHS Trust
London, UK

**Dr Susan M Hill, BM MRCP(UK)
    MRCPCH DM**
Consultant Paediatric
    Gastroenterologist
Department of Paediatric
    Gastroenterology,
Great Ormond Street Hospital for
    Children NHS Trust
London, UK

Mr John M Hodapp, MD
Staff Pediatric Urologist
Pediatric Urology Division
Children's Specialisits of San Diego
San Diego, California, USA

**Dr David P Inwald, MBBChir
    MRCP MRCPCH PhD**
Consultant Paediatric Intensivist
St Mary's Hospital NHS Trust
London, UK

Dr Alan D Irvine, MD FRCPI MRCP
Consultant Paediatric Dermatologist
Our Lady's Hospital for Sick Children
Dublin, Ireland

Dr Alison M Jones, MBBCh FRCPCH PhD
Consultant Paediatric Immunologist
Great Ormond Street Hospital for
  Children NHS Trust
London, UK

Mr David HA Jones, FRCS
Consultant Orthopaedic Surgeon
Great Ormond Street Hospital for
  Children NHS Trust
London, UK

Dr Fenella J Kirkham, MBBChir FRCPCH
Reader in Paediatric Neurology
Neurosciences Unit
The Wolfson Centre
UCL Institute of Child Health and
Great Ormond Street Hospital for
  Children NHS Trust
London, UK

Dr Sarah E Ledermann, MB MRCP
Associate Specialist in Paediatric
  Nephrology
Great Ormond Street Hospital for
  Children NHS Trust
London, UK

Dr Gill A Levitt, BSc MRCP DCH
Consultant Paediatric Oncologist
Great Ormond Street Hospital for
  Children NHS Trust
London, UK

Dr Debra Lomas, MA MB BChir MRCP
Associate Specialist in Paediatric
  Dermatology
Great Ormond Street Hospital for
  Children NHS Trust
London, UK

Mr Murali Mahadevan, FRACS
Clinical Director and Consultant
  Surgeon
Department of Paediatric
  Otolaryngology, Head & Neck
  Surgery
Starship Children's Hospital
Auckland, New Zealand

Dr Katie M Mallam, MBChB MRCPCH
Specialist Registrar in Paediatric
  Endocrinology
Bristol Royal Hospital for Children
Bristol, UK

Dr Stephen D Marks, MBChB MSc MRCP DCH FRCPCH
Consultant Paediatric Nephrologist
Great Ormond Street Hospital for
  Children NHS Trust
London, UK

Dr Michael Mars, PhD BDS FDS DoOrth
Consultant Orthodontist
Great Ormond Street Children
  Hospital for Children NHS Trust
London, UK

Dr Anthea G Masarei, BAppSc PhD MRCSLT
Previously Specialist Speech and
  Language Therapist
Great Ormond Street Children
  Hospital for Children NHS Trust
London, UK

Dr Antony J Michalski, FRCPCH PhD
Consultant Paediatric Oncologist
Great Ormond Street Hospital for
  Children NHS Trust
London, UK

Professor Pierre DE Mouriquand, MD, FRCS
Professor of Pediatric Surgery
  (Urology)
Department of Paediatric Urology
Debrousse Hospital
Lyon, France

Dr Kevin J Murray, MBBS FRACP
Consultant Paediatric Rheumatologist
Department of Rheumatology
Princess Margaret Hospital for
  Children
Perth, Australia

Dr Margot C Nash, MBBS FRACP MD
Consultant Paediatrician
Department of General Paediatrics
Royal Children's Hospital
Parkville, Victoria, Australia

Ms Jennifer Nayak
Specialist Speech and Language
  Therapist
Trent Regional Centre for Cleft Lip
  and Palate
Nottingham City Hospital
Nottingham, UK

Mr Ken K Nischal, FRCOphth
Consultant Ophthalmic Surgeon
Great Ormond Street Hospital for
  Children NHS Trust
London, UK

Dr Vas M Novelli, FRCP, FRACP, FRCPCH
Consultant and Lead Clinician in
  Paediatric Infectious Diseases
Clinical Infectious Diseases Unit
Great Ormond Street Hospital for
  Children NHS Trust
London, UK

Ms Valerie Pereira
Previously Part Time Visiting Assistant
  Professor
University of Hong Kong, Division of
  Speech and Hearing Sciences
London, UK

Dr Mark J Peters, MBChB MRCP FRCPCH PhD
Consultant Paediatric Intensivist
Great Ormond Street Hospital for
  Children NHS Trust
London, UK

Dr Andy J Petros, MBBS MSc FRCP FRCPCH FFARCSI MA
Consultant Paediatric Intensivist
Great Ormond Street Hospital for
  Children NHS Trust
London, UK

Dr Clarissa A Pilkington, MBBS BSc MRCP
Consultant Paediatric Rheumatologist
Great Ormond Street Hospital for
  Children NHS Trust
London, UK

Ms Katie Price
Specialist Speech and Language
  Therapist
Neurodisability
The Wolfson Centre
Great Ormond Street Children
  Hospital for Children NHS Trust
London, UK

Dr. Jon Pritchard, FRCPCH FRCPE
Consultant Paediatric Oncologist
Department of Oncology &
  Haematology
Royal Hospital for Sick Children
Edinburgh, UK

Dr Lesley Rees, MD FRCP FRCPCH
Consultant Paediatric Nephrologist
Great Ormond Street Hospital for
  Children NHS Trust
London, UK

Professor Sheena Reilly
Professor of Paediatric Speech
  Pathology
Royal Children's Hospital
Murdoch Children's Research Institute
La Trobe University
Melbourne, Australia

Professor Graham J Roberts, BDS PhD FDSRCS MDS MPhil ILTM
Consultant and Professor in Paediatric Dentistry
The Eastman Dental Hospital
University College Hospitals London and King's College London
London, UK

Dr Sushmita Roy, MBBS DCH MRCP MSc
Consultant Paediatrician
Calcutta Medical Research Institute and Institute of Child Health
Calcutta, India

Ms Martina Ryan
Specialist Speech & Language Therapist
Dysphagia Team – Team Leader
Speech & Language Therapy Department
Great Ormond Street Children Hospital for Children NHS Trust
London, UK

Dr Neil J Sebire, MBBS BClinSci MD DRCOG MRCPath
Consultant Paediatric Pathologist
Great Ormond Street Children Hospital for Children NHS Trust
London, UK

Dr Debbie Sell, PhD, Cert. MRCSLT, FRCSLT
Lead SLT, North Thames Regional Cleft Lip and Palate Service
Head of Speech and Language Therapy Department
Honorary Senior Lecturer – UCL Institute of Child Health and Great Ormond Street Children Hospital for Children NHS Trust
London, UK

Ms Caroleen Shipster
Specialist Speech & Language Therapist
Craniofacial Team – Team Leader
Speech & Language Therapy Department
Great Ormond Street Children Hospital for Children NHS Trust
London, UK

Dr Pete K Smith, BMedSci MBBS FRACP PhD
Associate Professor and Consultant Paediatric Allergist
Bond University, Gold Coast, Queensland, Australia

Professor Owen P Smith, MA MB BA FRCPCH FRCP FRCPI FRCPath
Consultant Paediatric Haematologist
Our Lady's Hospital for Sick Children, and St James's Hospital Dublin
Professor of Haematology, Trinity College Dublin, Ireland

Mr Brian C Sommerlad, FRCS
Consultant Plastic Surgeon
Great Ormond Street Children Hospital for Children NHS Trust
London, UK

Professor Lewis Spitz, MBChB PhD MD(Hon) FRCS FAAP(Hon) FRCPCH
Nuffield Professor of Paediatric Surgery
UCL Institute of Child Health
London, UK

Professor Stephan Strobel, MD PhD FRCP FRCPCH
Director of Clinical Education, Peninsula Postgraduate Health Institute
Professor of Paediatrics and Clinical Immunology and Consultant Paediatric Immunologist, Plymouth Hospitals NHS Trust
Plymouth, UK

Dr Richard S Trompeter, MB FRCP FRCPCH
Consultant Paediatric Nephrologist
Great Ormond Street Hospital for Children NHS Trust
London, UK

Dr William G van't Hoff, BSc MD FRCPCH
Consultant Paediatric Nephrologist
Great Ormond Street Hospital for Children NHS Trust
London, UK

Dr Colin E Wallis, MD FRCPCH
Respiratory Paediatrician
Great Ormond Street Hospital for Children NHS Trust
London, UK

Dr Bruce Whitehead, MD MPhil FRACP FRCP FRCPCH
Paediatric Respiratory & Sleep Specialist
Kaleidoscope John Hunter Children's Hospital
New Lambton, New South Wales, Australia

Dr Callum J Wilson, FRACP
Metabolic Consultant
Starship Children's Hospital
Auckland, New Zealand

The late Professor Robin M Winter, BSc FRCP PhD
Previously Professor of Clinical Genetics & Dysmorphology
UCL Institute of Child Health
London, UK

Dr Paul JD Winyard, MA MRCP PhD
Senior Lecturer in Paediatric Nephrology
Nephro-Urology Unit
UCL Institute of Child Health
London, UK

Dr Jackson YW Wong, MBBS DCH MRCP FRCPCH FHKAM FHKCPaed
Locum Consultant Respiratory Paediatrician
Department of Respiratory Medicine
Bristol Royal Hospital for Children
Bristol, UK

Professor Pat Woo, CBE BSc MBBS PhD FRCP FRCPH FMedSci
Professor of Paediatric Rheumatology
Great Ormond Street Hospital for Children NHS Trust
London, UK

Mr Victor J Woolf, MBBS FRCS
Consultant Orthopaedic Surgeon
North Middlesex University Hospital NHS Trust
London, UK

FOREWORD

Dr Charles West was the inspiration behind the first ever children's hospital in the United Kingdom, known as Great Ormond Street. The hospital opened its doors on 14 February 1852 with just 10 beds. The hospital's neighbour, who was a friend of Charles West, was none other than Charles Dickens, one of Britain's leading novelists. Charles Dickens was one of its first celebrity supporters and wrote a powerful article in his popular magazine 'Household Words' to publicise the hospital when it opened.

Great Ormond Street Hospital for Children is now one of the most famous children's hospitals in the world. The hospital receives referrals from a huge population, not only from London and the South East of England, but also from further afield in the United Kingdom and indeed, internationally. The staff of Great Ormond Street Hospital comprise experts in the whole range of child health, including all fields of paediatric medicine and surgery.

A major part of this accumulated experience is brought together in this wonderful compendium of paediatric practice and child health. It has been designed with the clinician in mind and is an effective and practical tool, useful to anyone caring for sick children. It will provide a valuable reference source for general practitioners, general paediatricians, community paediatricians and students of medicine of all ages.

Due to the hospital's excellent department of clinical photography and medical illustration, this book exceeds any other paediatric atlas in the comprehensive nature of its illustrations. The specialists of the hospital have immense teaching responsibilities and, over the years, they have utilised their resources to build up what I believe is an unrivalled collection of over 1100 illustrations and photographs. These show the presentation of both common and less common children's illnesses and their progress, as well as illustrating normal appearances. This latter point is important, because so often the task is to reassure oneself and the family concerned what is normal.

It is no easy task to bring together such a large number of authors and such a huge amount of material into an easily accessible and digestible form. I think the authors and editors have succeeded in this extremely difficult task that they set themselves, and that this book will be on and off a large number of bookshelves all over the world over the next few years.

I personally wish all the authors and editors success with what I believe is an excellent paediatric handbook. I look forward to using this and subsequent editions in the future.

Sir Cyril Chantler

Chairman
Great Ormond Street Hospital

PREFACE

This Colour Handbook comprises concise text and clinical photographs covering the full spectrum of childhood diseases. It is the culmination of many years of hard work and we hope the final product will be well accepted and used for many years to come.

The book encompasses every paediatric medical and surgical specialty. The number of authors (73) testifies to the scope and extent of the text. Most of the authors either trained at Great Ormond Street Hospital NHS Trust or are current or past consultants at the Trust. Others have been co-opted to provide expertise in their special area of interest. One of us, Stephen Marks, was brought into the editorial team at a relatively late stage. He has provided the additional impetus to drive the project forward to its completion.

Special thanks are due to Patrick Daly and latterly to Ayala Kingsley for coordinating the contributions, and to Michael Manson and his team for their patience and forbearance.

We hope the book will be used not only in medical libraries and personal collections but will be freely accessible on paediatric wards and in general practice, for use by medical and nursing staff. The book aims to inform all of us who care professionally for children, and to help explain to parents the details of their child's condition and the help which is available.

The Editors
London

Emergency Medicine

David Inwald
Andy Petros
Mark Peters

INTRODUCTION

A simple, structured approach to an acutely ill child has been the focus of the recent initiatives of Advanced Paediatric Life Support (APLS), Paediatric Advanced Life Support (PALS) and European Paediatric Life Support (EPLS) courses.

The advantages of this structured approach are clear: clinical problems are addressed in order of urgency and the chances of significant omissions are reduced. In all acutely ill children the **A** airway, **B** breathing and **C** circulation should be assessed (and supported if inadequate) before a more detailed assessment is undertaken.

This chapter will outline the emergency management of the most common conditions requiring treatment in paediatric practice. In contrast to the APLS/EPLS approach we include details of ongoing care. This does not mean to distract from the vital importance of the initial assessment and resuscitation. All readers involved in the care of acutely unwell children are encouraged to train in APLS/EPLS.

ANAPHYLAXIS

Anaphylaxis is a type I hypersensitivity reaction triggered by crosslinking of IgE on mast cells. It occurs when enough antigen enters the systemic circulation to activate circulating basophils and tissue mast cells. This results in the release of inflammatory mediators, particularly histamine, prostaglandins and leukotrienes. These mediators cause massive peripheral vasodilation (cardiorespiratory arrest, shock), increased vascular permeability (angiooedema, airway obstruction and urticaria), intense contraction of non-vascular smooth muscle (bronchoconstriction), abdominal pain, nausea, vomiting and tachycardia. Anaphylaxis may be due to drugs, insect stings (**1.1**), foods, plants, chemicals or latex.

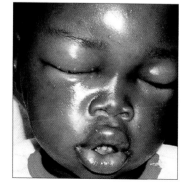

1.1 Severe anaphylaxis in a 11-month-old baby caused by bee stings with oedematous eyelids and lips, wheeze and shock.

Anaphylaxis may progress slowly or rapidly and may range from a mild cutaneous reaction to circulatory arrest.

RECOGNITION

Clinical assessment should include rapid physical examination, with attention to airway, breathing and circulation, measurement of peak expiratory flow rate (PEFR) in children able to perform the technique and pulse oximetry. Children should be examined for generalized oedema, angiooedema, erythematous rash and urticaria (**1.2**) and a history taken for substance exposure (with particular reference to drugs or foodstuffs).

IMMEDIATE MANAGEMENT

Mild anaphylaxis

Mild reactions such as urticaria should respond to treatment with antihistamines and steroids. Drug treatment should be followed by a period of observation to ensure a more serious response does not occur.

Severe anaphylaxis

Patients should be treated with high flow oxygen, artificial ventilation and cardiac massage if necessary. If stridor is present, airway angiooedema is likely and senior anaesthetic assistance should be summoned to secure the airway. Intramuscular adrenaline should be administered as soon as possible in anaphylactic shock (**Table 1.1**). The intravenous route should be reserved for extreme emergency when there is doubt as to the adequacy of the circulation. The dose for intravenous epinephrine is 10 micrograms/kg (0.1 mL/kg of the dilute 1 in 10,000 epinephrine injection) by slow intravenous injection. However, when intramuscular injection might succeed, time should not be wasted seeking intravenous access. Adrenaline doses may be repeated at 5-minute intervals if necessary. Hypotension in anaphylaxis is due to vasodilatation and capillary leak and resuscitation with colloid is necessary to restore circulation. Steroids and antihistamines should be given and if the patient's condition is not stable an adrenaline infusion should be commenced. Bronchospasm, if present, may resond to adrenaline and steroids. If mechanical ventilation is necessary, a slow rate and long expiratory time should be used to allow full expiration to occur. Refractory bronchospasm should be treated as severe asthma (see also 'Respiratory Medicine' chapter).

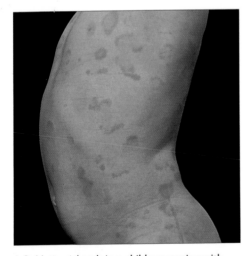

1.2 Urticarial rash in a child presenting with mild anaphylaxis caused by food allergy. If no other features are present this can be safely treated with antihistamines and allergen avoidance.

Table 1.1 Dose of intramuscular injection of adrenaline for anaphylactic shock

Under 6 months: epinephrine 50 micrograms (0.05 ml of adrenaline 1 in 1,000 (1 mg/ml)

6 months to 6 years: epinephrine 120 micrograms (0.12 ml of epinephrine 1 in 1,000 (1 mg/ml)

6–12 years: epinephrine 250 micrograms (0.25 ml of epinephrine 1 in 1,000 (1 mg/ml)

Adult and adolescent: epinephrine 500 micrograms (0.5 ml of epinephrine 1 in 1,000 (1 mg/ml)

FOLLOW UP

The causative allergen may be identified by taking a careful history. Further investigation may include skin prick testing (SPT). Radio-absorbent assays (RAST) for specific IgE is often performed but 50% of those with positive SPT/RAST will have no symptoms and 50% of those with confirmed allergy will have negative SPTs. The gold standard test for diagnosis of food allergy remains the food challenge. This should be carried out in a centre with adequate resuscitation facilities.

Any child who has had a serious reaction to peanuts should avoid all peanut products including oil. Peanuts are legumes and, although it is uncommon for patients to react to other legumes, cross-reactivity with tree nuts can occur. Peanut sensitive individuals should be introduced to these singly and with caution.

If there is evidence of a severe food or other allergy, the findings should be clearly documented and explained to the patient. Management primarily consists of avoidance. However, patients should also be instructed to carry a hand held summary and to wear a warning bracelet or necklace. Patients or parents of children at risk of anaphylactic reactions to foods, environmental allergens, chemicals, or plants should carry injectable adrenaline at all times and know how to use it in an emergency.

UPPER AIRWAY OBSTRUCTION

See also 'Respiratory Medicine' chapter.

Stridor is an inspiratory noise related to obstruction of the extrathoracic airway. Dynamic intrathoracic airway obstruction can also result in expiratory stridor in conditions such as broncho- or tracheomalacia. Obstruction of the extrathoracic airway is most commonly due to viral tracheitis (**1.3**) but can also occur in bacterial tracheitis (**1.4**),

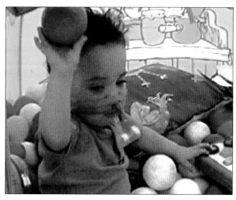

1.3 A two-year-old child with viral tracheitis intubated in the ICU. As the lungs are unaffected he does not require mechanical ventilation. A humidification device is attached to the end of the tube to prevent secretions drying in the airway.

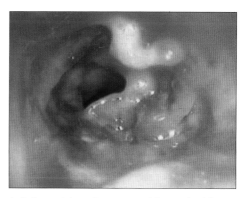

1.4 Bacterial tracheitis in an 18-month-old child who presented with a high pyrexia, shock and stridor.

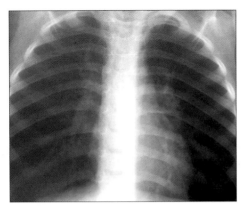
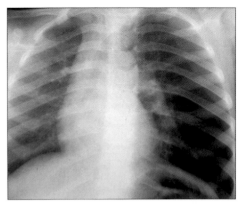

1.5 and **1.6** Inspiratory (left) and expiratory (right) chest radiographs in a four-year-old child with an inhaled peanut in the left main bronchus. Though foreign bodies usually cause occlusion of the entire airway lumen and distal collapse, in this case the peanut is causing a ball-valve effect and the left lung does not deflate on expiration.

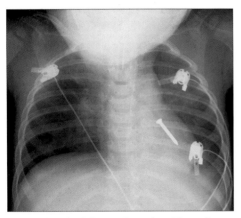

1.7 Nail in the left main bronchus. This will require removal with a rigid bronchoscope. Physiotherapy and flexible bronchoscopy are contraindicated, as both may cause the foreign body to slip further down the airway.

foreign body aspiration (**1.5–1.7**) and other conditions such as quinsy and epiglottitis. As these conditions have very different management, part of the assessment involves a process of differentiation between them.

IMMEDIATE ASSESSMENT AND MANAGEMENT
Initial assessment should include rapid physical examination of the airway, breathing and circulation, with particular attention to the work of breathing (ie, respiratory rate, recession, use of accessory muscles) and pulse oximetry.

Cyanosis, distress, exhaustion or oxygen saturations of <92% in air are all signs of severe obstruction and impending collapse. Children with these signs may require urgent intubation and ventilation and senior anaesthetic help should be summoned. Children with milder obstruction may require intravenous fluids in addition to more specific management (see below). The presence of a high fever in a toxic looking child should raise the possibility of bacterial tracheitis or epiglottitis. If the child is stable, a brief history should be taken with regard to recent coryzal illness (suggestive of viral tracheitis), foreign body aspiration and haemophilus influenza immunization.

INVESTIGATIONS
Radiological investigations are not routinely required. Lateral neck x-rays are rarely helpful and immediate management (including intubation if necessary) is more important. A lateral neck film and chest radiograph should only be performed when the child is stable. Laboratory investigations need only be performed if intravenous access is required.

FURTHER MANAGEMENT
Bacterial tracheitis and viral tracheitis
Children with mild or moderately severe viral tracheitis who do not require immediate intubation should be commenced on steroids, which have been shown to be of benefit in randomized controlled trials. However, children with bacterial tracheitis or severe viral tracheitis occasionally require intubation. A senior anaesthetist should be called as the child will almost certainly require inhalation anaesthesia. The use

of paralysing agents in this setting is not recommended as when muscle tone is lost the airway may completely obstruct. While waiting for help nebulized adrenaline can be helpful in reducing airway oedema, but this should only be given in a high dependency area as reactive hyperaemia with worsening obstruction can occur when the nebulizer is completed. Children with suspected bacterial tracheitis (**4**) may be septic and will require volume resuscitation prior to intubation. They should also have blood cultures sent and be commenced on antibiotics with good *Staphylococcus* and *Streptococcus* cover such as cefuroxime and flucloxacillin.

Foreign body

Aspiration of a foreign body (**1.5–1.7**) may result in an asymptomatic child or cardiorespiratory collapse. Clearly, partial or complete obstruction at the level of the larynx or trachea may require urgent resuscitation. Again, senior anaesthetic help should be summoned. It may be possible to remove the foreign body at laryngoscopy with a Magill's forceps. If not, urgent tracheostomy may be required as a temporizing measure. A foreign body further down the airway may cause partial or complete obstruction of one or more major bronchi. A chest radiograph may demonstrate areas of hyperinflation or collapse, depending on the degree of airway obstruction. If in any doubt, inspiratory and expiratory films and the radiographic appearance of the pulmonary vascular tree will help to determine which lung is abnormal. These children will need to be referred to a specialist centre where rigid bronchoscopy can be performed to remove the foreign body.

Other

Epiglottitis has become extremely rare since the introduction of Haemophilus influenza immunization. If it is suspected, however, senior anaesthetic, ENT and paediatric advice should be sought. The airway will require securing, by tracheostomy if necessary, and the child will need volume resuscitation and antibiotic therapy with cefotaxime, which has good *Haemophilus* spp. cover.

Quinsy (peritonsillar abscess) can often be seen on a lateral neck radiograph and will require incision and drainage, sometimes with a period of airway support while postoperative oedema settles.

Airway haemangiomas and tonsillar hypertrophy may require specific surgical management (**1.8–1.10**).

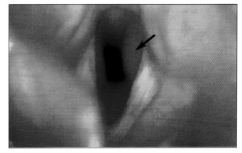

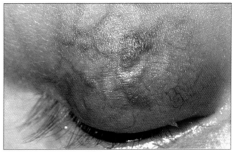

1.8 An airway haemangioma in a six-month-old child who presented with stridor. These lesions often present during viral lower respiratory tract infections when they are unmasked by additional airway swelling. The clue to the diagnosis may be the presence of haemangiomas elsewhere, **1.9**. Treatment is with local or systemic steroids. They usually regress at around two years of age, but some infants require a tracheostomy.

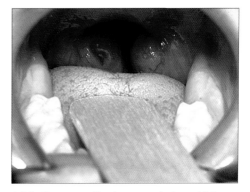

1.10 Gross tonsillar hypertrophy in a child with recurrent tonsillitis and obstructive sleep apnoea who presented with airway obstruction. The airway must be secured before the tonsils are removed at surgery.

ASTHMA

See also 'Respiratory Medicine' chapter.

Asthma is a chronic disease characterized by reversible airflow obstruction, particularly in the bronchi, with recurrent bouts of wheezing and breathlessness. However, all that wheezes is not asthma and important differential diagnoses of acute severe asthma include foreign body aspiration and bronchiolitis. Asthma has increased in prevalence over recent years and now affects 10–20% of children in the UK. Acute exacerbations of asthma represent 10–15% of all acute medical admissions in children. About 20 children and about 1600 adults die in the UK every year due to acute severe asthma. Common factors leading to acute exacerbations include viral respiratory infections, irritants, exercise, and allergens.

RECOGNITION

Clinical assessment should include rapid physical examination, with attention to airway, breathing and circulation, measurement of peak expiratory flow rate (PEFR) and pulse oximetry (see box below). Routine blood gas analysis is not recommended as arterial puncture is painful and may cause acute decompensation. Clinical assessment is more useful than blood gas analysis. Assessment of pulsus paradoxus is no longer recommended.

Recognizing asthma symptoms	
Severe	**Life-threatening**
Age 1–5	
• Tachycardia	• Cyanosis
• Flaring	• Silent chest
• Accessory muscles	• Fatigue
• Recession	• ↓ Conscious level
• Head retraction	
• Unable to feed	
Age >5	
• Tachycardia	• Cyanosis
• Accessory muscles	• Unable to speak
• Recession	• Silent chest
• PEFR <50% best	• Fatigue
	• ↓ Conscious level
	• PEFR <33% best

IMMEDIATE MANAGEMENT

Severe asthma without life-threatening features should be treated with high-flow oxygen, nebulized salbutamol and ipratropium bromide, and oral steroids. Salbutamol and ipratropium can safely be given continuously until improvement has occurred, when the dose frequency can be reduced. Oxygen should be given before, during and after administration of inhaled bronchodilators, to avoid hypoxaemia. The safest way to do this is via an oxygen driven nebulizer rather than a holding chamber.

If life-threatening features are present, senior help and an experienced anaesthetist should be summoned. In the meantime the airway should be maintained, oxygen should be administered by a rebreathing mask and intravenous access secured for administration of steroids and bronchodilators. Proven effective intravenous bronchodilators include bolus salbutamol, aminophylline, and magnesium sulphate. These should be given with cardiac monitoring, as salbutamol and aminophylline can cause arrhythmias.

INVESTIGATIONS

A chest radiograph should be obtained after initial stabilization in any child with features of severe or life threatening asthma, or with a first episode of wheeze, to exclude a foreign body, pneumothorax and mucus plugging (**1.11– 1.13**). Routine chest radiographs in all cases of acute asthma are not necessary.

INDICATIONS FOR VENTILATORY SUPPORT

- Patients who are tired.
- Those with a reduced conscious level.
- Those who continue to deteriorate despite maximal therapy.

Blood gas analysis is not a substitute for clinical assessment and the focus should remain on the clinical state of the patient.

Intubation

The patient should be pre-oxygenated and 10–20 mls/kg colloid given electively. Patients with acute severe asthma are often volume depleted and vasodilated. Ketamine (which has some bronchodilator activity) is a useful induction agent.

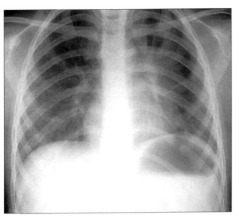

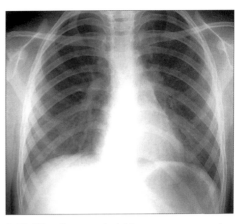

1.11 Plugging of the left lingular bronchus in acute severe asthma in an eight-year-old girl. The left heart border is indistinct but the left diaphragm is clearly seen.

1.12 The plug seen in 1.11 was expectorated after bronchodilators were given.

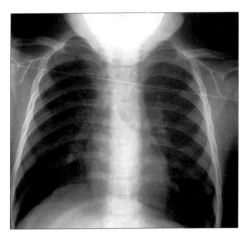

1.13 Acute severe asthma in a 13-year-old child. The lungs were grossly hyperinflated but there is no evidence of a pneumothorax. This child was ventilating at the top of his functional residual capacity and had little reserve.

Ventilation strategies

High airway resistance may lead to a very prolonged expiratory phase during artificial ventilation, and slow ventilation rates may be required (10–15 breaths per min). Blood gases should not be normalized and very high $PaCO_2$ values may be tolerated without harm ('permissive hypercapnia') provided the pH remains >7.2. Some PEEP is necessary to counteract intrinsic PEEP. Neuromuscular paralysis should be discontinued as soon as possible as the combination of steroids and paralysing agents is associated with an increased risk of critical illness neuropathy.

WHILE VENTILATED

Key in the management are generous humidification and physiotherapy to mobilize secretions and mucus plugs (**1.11, 1.12**). Drug treatment can include continued neuro-muscular paralysis, ketamine by continuous infusion (for both sedative and bronchodilator effect) and intravenous bronchodilators such as salbutamol and aminophylline. Some inhala-tional anaesthetic agents also have some bronchodilator activity. Heliox (a mixture of oxygen and helium with a lower density than air) has been used to ventilate patients with very high airway resistance. Weaning from mechanical ventilation can be difficult.

Table 1.2 Common errors in resuscitation and subsequent management of asthma

Common errors	Action
• Failure to give high-flow oxygen to children with severe or life threatening features.	Nebulize salbutamol and ipratropium with high-flow oxygen. Give high-flow oxygen before and after nebulizers. DO NOT use a holding chamber (spacer).
• Frequent blood gas analysis or examination for pulsus paradoxus.	Focus on clinical state of child. Pulse oximetry is a useful adjunct.
• Failure to recognize hypovolaemia.	Ensure adequate volume resuscitation prior to intubation.
• Intubation and ventilation not initiated until cardiorespiratory arrest.	Consider semi-elective intubation and ventilation in presence of: • Decreased conscious level • Exhaustion • Worsening respiratory failure.

BRONCHIOLITIS

See also 'Respiratory Medicine' chapter.

Bronchiolitis is a clinical syndrome of infancy characterized by respiratory distress with both crepitations and wheezes on auscultation. It is often preceded by a coryzal illness and usually has a viral aetiology: respiratory syncytial virus (RSV), influenza, parainfluenza and adenovirus are common. Secondary bacterial infection is rare. Small airway obstruction leading to hyperinflation is typical, although many severe cases also have localized or diffuse atelectasis (**1.14**).

RECOGNITION

Clinical assessment should include rapid physical examination, with attention to airway, breathing and circulation and pulse oximetry. In very sick infants, capillary or venous blood gases can help to guide treatment. However, clinical assessment is still more important than blood gas analysis.

IMMEDIATE MANAGEMENT

- Oxygen therapy. Humidified oxygen via headbox or nasal cannula should be given to maintain saturations >92%.
- Intravenous fluids. Colloid may be given to maintain intravascular volume then crystalloid at 67% maintenance if the child is unable to feed. Orogastric may be preferred in the acute phase as a nasal tube will increase airway resistance.
- Monitoring should include clinical assessment, pulse oximetry, apnoea monitoring and, in severe cases, blood gas analysis.
- Bronchodilators, including nebulized adrenaline, do not shorten the length of admission or alter outcome. However, in some studies, nebulized adrenaline improved both oxygenation and symptoms.
- Antibiotics are not routinely recommended.
- Ribavirin, is not of any clear benefit.

INVESTIGATIONS

If severely unwell, alternative diagnoses such as pneumonia and empyema should be considered. This group of infants will require a chest radiograph. Further investigations should include a nasopharyngeal aspirate for viral immunofluorescence. A sweat test to exclude cystic fibrosis and serum immunoglobulins to exclude hypogammaglobulinaemia should be considered in those infants with severe or persistent symptoms.

INDICATIONS FOR VENTILATORY SUPPORT

Assisted ventiation is required in a small proportion of infants, who often fall into one of the high risk groups (see box below).

Ventilatory support may be required in infants who are tired, who have a reduced conscious level or who continue to deteriorate with worsening respiratory failure with progressive hypoxaemia or hypercarbia. As with asthma, blood gas analysis is not a substitute for clinical assessment and the focus should remain on the clinical state of the patient.

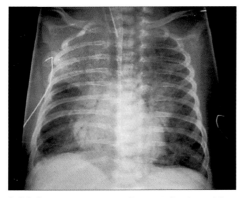

1.14 Respiratory syncitial virus infection with features of acute respiratory distress syndrome, showing generalized air space shadowing in addition to areas of collapse and hyperinflation.

Recognizing bronchiolitis symptoms

Severe	Life-threatening
• Tachycardia	• Cyanosis
• RR >50	• Getting tired
• Flaring	• ↓ Conscious level
• Accessory muscles	• Saturation <92%
• Recession	despite O_2
• Head retraction	therapy
• Unable to feed	• Rising pCO_2

Intubation

Ventilation is rarely required and is often accompanied by a transient worsening of gas exchange.

Ventilation strategies

CPAP via a nasal prong may be all that is required. If mechanical ventilation is required, a low tidal volume lung protective strategy should be adopted with tidal volumes of 4–7 mls/kg, PIP <35, rate of 10–20 bpm, I:E ratio of 1:2 and permissive hypercapnia, allowing the pH to go down to 7.2. Some PEEP is necessary to counteract intrinsic PEEP.

WHILE VENTILATED

There is no proven treatment for bronchiolitis other than good supportive care. Exogenous surfactant is sometimes used. Modified cardio-pulmonary bypass or extracorporeal membrane oxygenation (ECMO) has been used in very severely affected infants with excellent results (99% survival).

Infants at risk of severe disease

- Age less than 6 weeks
- Chronic lung disease of prematurity (**1.15**)
- Other pre-existing pulmonary conditons (e.g. cystic fibrosis) (**1.16**)
- Congenital heart disease
- Immunocompromised host

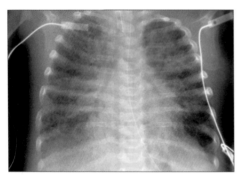

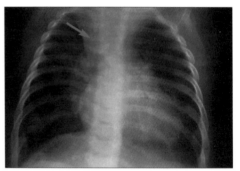

1.15 Respiratory syncitial virus infection in a one-year-old baby with chronic lung disease of prematurity. Areas of collapse and hyperinflation are seen on a background of cystic changes consistent with bronchopulmonary dysplasia.

1.16 Respiratory syncitial virus infection in an 11-month-old baby with failure to thrive, who was subsequently diagnosed to have cystic fibrosis. Gross hyperinflation with areas of streaky atelectasis and right upper lobe collapse are seen.

Table 1.3 Common errors in resuscitation and subsequent management of bronchiolitis

Common errors	Action
Frequent blood gas analysis	Focus on clinical state of child. Pulse oximetry is a useful adjunct.
Nasogastric feeding	Consider orogastric feeding or, if severely unwell, stop enteral feeds.
Failure to recognize hypovolaemia	Ensure adequate volume resuscitation prior to intubation.
Overhydration	Give crystalloid maintenance at 2/3 of daily requirement after adequate colloid resuscitation.
Intubation and ventilation not initiated until cardiorespiratory arrest	Consider intubation and ventilation in presence of: • Decreased conscious level • Exhaustion • Worsening respiratory failure.

CARDIAC EMERGENCIES

Cardiac emergencies in childhood are rare. Cyanosis, cardiogenic shock and arrhythmia are the common modes of presentation.

CYANOSIS

Cyanosis in a newborn infant should raise suspicion of a right to left shunt due to congenital heart disease but can also be due to persistent pulmonary hypertension of the newborn. In later life it is possible though now extremely rare for children with missed congenital left to right shunts to develop pulmonary hypertension and for the shunt to reverse, causing cyanosis. This situation is known as Eisenmenger's syndrome but is now almost unheard of. Primary pulmonary hypertension can, however, can present with cyanosis in later childhood (**1.17**).

Any newborn child with persistent cyanosis which cannot be explained by a respiratory cause should be presumed to have a cardiac lesion. Prostaglandin E2 should be commenced to maintain ductal patency and the infant referred to a paediatric cardiology centre for further management. Prostaglandin E2 may cause apnoea and transfer may require the airway to be secured with an endotracheal tube. Well, older children presenting with cyanosis will usually have an undiagnosed cardiac or pulmonary shunt and should be referred to a paediatric cardiologist for diagnosis and management.

CARDIOGENIC SHOCK

Cardiogenic shock can occur in the newborn period, most commonly when the duct closes in duct-dependent lesions with left heart obstruction, for example hypoplastic left heart syndrome, coarctation of the aorta or critical aortic stenosis. An aberrant left coronary artery can have the same presentation, usually a few weeks later (**1.18**). Cardiogenic shock may also

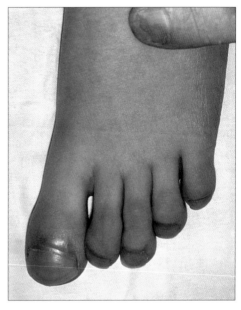

1.17 Cyanosis and clubbing in an eight-year-old with primary pulmonary hyptertension. The thumb shown for contrast is that of a healthy sibling.

1.18 12-lead electro-cardiograph of a six-week-old infant with anomalous origin of the left coronary artery from the pulmonary artery (ALCAPA). The infant presented with poor feeding, lethargy and tachypnoea. Q waves are present in lead I and aVL, ST segment elevation in aVL and ST segment depression in II, III, and aVF and the anterior chest leads consistent with a full thickness anterior infarct.

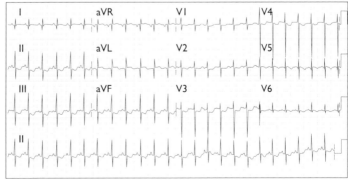

occur secondary to acquired disease at any time, the most common of which in childhood is viral myocarditis or dilated cardiomyopathy (**1.19**). However, coronary occlusion can occur in Kawasaki disease (see 'Infectious Diseases' and Rheumatology' chapters) and can have a similar presentation (**1.20, 1.21**).

Infants presenting with cardiogenic shock in the newborn period should be presumed to have a duct-dependent circulation until proven otherwise and prostaglandin E2 should be commenced. The differential diagnosis includes sepsis, and infants should be commenced on broad spectrum intravvenous antibiotics after blood cultures have been taken. An enlarged liver is often a clue to a cardiac diagnosis. These infants are often profoundly acidotic and may require airway support, mechanical ventilation, fluids, bicarbonate and inotropes to maintain cardiac output. Central venous access and measurement of central venous pressure is useful to optimize filling pressures. If there is any suspicion of a hypoplastic left heart or a univentricular circulation, high concentrations of inspired oxygen should be avoided as the pulmonary vascular bed can become hyper-perfused at the expense of systemic circulation. Older, previously well children presenting with cardiogenic shock will require similar management but without attention to the possibility of duct dependent circulation or univentricular heart.

ARRHYTHMIAS

The commonest arrhythmias in the newborn period are congenital complete heart block (often secondary to maternal SLE and trans-placental carriage of anti-Ro antibodies) or supraventricular tachycardia due to an aberrant conduction pathway such as in Wolff-Parkinson-White syndrome (**1.22**). In later life, supra-ventricular tachycardia is also the commonest arrhythmia (**1.23**). Ventricular arrhythmias are extremely rare in childhood and almost always due to a non-cardiac cause, for example poisoning, hyperkalaemia or acidosis.

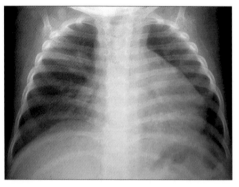

1.19 Cardiomegaly and congested pulmonary vessels in a one-year-old infant with dilated cardiomyopathy. The left lower lobe has collapsed due to extrinsic compression of the airway by the enlarged left atrium.

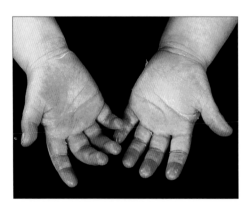

1.20 Desquamation of the hands in a four-year-old with Kawasaki disease.

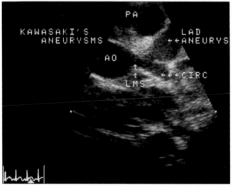

1.21 Echocardiograph showing left anterior descending coronary artery aneurysm in Kawasaki disease. Short axis view shown. Key: AO aorta; LMS left main stem; LAD left anterior descending; CIRC circumflex; PA pulmonary artery.
(Courtesy of Dr Robert Yates)

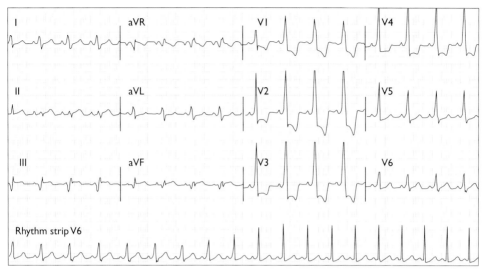

1.22 12-lead electrocardiograph showing characteristic features of Wolff-Parkinson-White syndrome with short PR interval, delta waves and ventricular repolarization abnormalities.

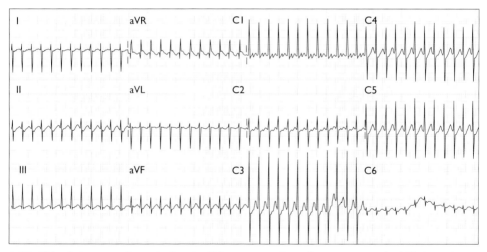

1.23 12-lead electrocardiograph showing AV re-entry tachycardia in a six-month-old baby with an accessory AV pathway. The ventricular rate is about 200–250, P waves are absent and the QRS complexes are narrow with normal morphology.

SEPTIC SHOCK AND MULTI-ORGAN FAILURE

Sepsis is 'the systemic response to infection'. This is defined by changes in temperature, heart rate, respiratory rate and white cell count. 'Septic shock' is inadequate organ perfusion in addition to the above changes. The characteristic pattern of worsening cardiovascular, respiratory and subsequently other organ system dysfunction is termed 'multiple organ failure'. While the most extreme cases of severe sepsis are seen with gram-negative infections (classically *Neisseria meningitidis*) (**1.24**) the pattern can be seen in response to many organisms including viruses and fungi.

INITIAL ASSESSMENT AND RESUSCITATION

The immediate care of a child with suspected septic shock must follow the principles of **A**, **B**, **C** (**A**irway, **B**reathing and **C**irculation) followed by specific therapy for the probable causative organism. Depressed conscious level (GCS ≤9), poor airway reflexes, tachypnoea and requirement for supplemental oxygen indicate impending need for assisted ventilation. Such signs will usually be accompanied by significant shock and hence induction presents a significant risk. This can be minimized by: aggressive volume replacement, pre-oxygenation, and intravenous atropine. An adrenaline bolus should be prepared and available. A range of ETT sizes should also be prepared (a good fit may be necessary to ensure adequate ventilation in the face of pulmonary oedema).

Optimal drugs for induction include fentanyl and/or ketamine. Myocardial depression agents such as thiopentone, midazolam or propofol are not good choices in children with septic shock. Rapid sequence induction may be necessary and should be performed by the most experienced staff available. Children with meningococcal disease should be orally intubated unless a coagulopathy has been excluded.

The heart rate, blood pressure and capillary refill time (normal <2 seconds) should be noted and secure intravenous access obtained. If the child is in shock peripheral (or central) venous access should not be attempted for more than 90 seconds. Initial resuscitation via an anterior tibial intraosseous needle is easy and effective. A prolonged capillary refill time should be immediately treated with 20 ml/kg of intravenous colloid (e.g. 4.5% human albumin solution, Haemocel, Gelofusin) which can be safely repeated while management is continuing.

INVESTIGATIONS

These should include full blood count, clotting screen (including fibrinogen and d-dimers or fibrin degradation products to look for evidence of disseminated intravascular coagulopathy), urea and electrolytes, calcium, magnesium, phosphate, liver function tests, blood and urine for culture and rapid antigen screening and/or PCR where available. **Lumbar puncture should not be performed in children with coagulopathy or with a reduced conscious level.**

FURTHER MANAGEMENT

Antibiotics

Appropriate antibiotic therapy should be commenced as soon as possible, ideally after taking blood and urine for culture. The only exception to this is in meningococcal disease, where the primary care provider may have already administered parenteral benzylpenicillin.

Circulatory support

Some children require vast amounts of fluid resuscitation: 100–200 ml/kg. Ideal subsequent management will involve the siting of central venous access to titrate fluids to maintain right heart filling pressures (usually 8–12 cmH$_2$0) to avoid pulmonary oedema. If pulmonary oedema is present it should be

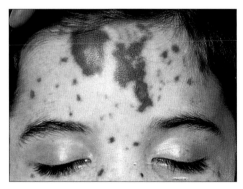

1.24 Rash of meningococcal disease with purpura and petechiae.

managed with ventilation and high-end expiratory pressure rather than diuretics. The use of FFP or packed cells as volume should be considered to correct coagulopathy and to maintain haematocrit. In the absence of CVP monitoring the effect of hepatic compression or leg elevation on BP and HR can give a rough guide to the consequences of further fluid administration.

In the presence of persistent hypotension despite adequate filling, inotropic support should be initiated. The choice of inotropic agent varies but a reasonable starting regimen would be dopamine, followed by adrenaline if there is no response (**1.25**).

Coagulopathy

Profound coagulopathies should be treated with FFP. Low fibrinogen concentrations suggesting DIC can be replaced with cryoprecipitate. Low platelet counts in the absence of clinical bleeding should not be supplemented. More aggressive FFP therapy with or without fibrinolytic and anticoagulant therapy may be considered in the presence of severe dermal thrombosis and impending necrosis.

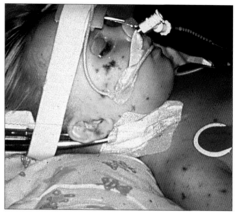

1.25 Some children with meningococcal disease develop severe cardiovascular failure. While most cases respond to inotropic support, this child has required support with an extracorporeal membrane oxygenator (ECMO). (Courtesy of Dr Allan Goldman)

Table 1.4 Common errors in resuscitation and subsequent management of septic shock/MODS

Common errors	Action
• Failure to establish intavenous access in a severely shocked child	Attempt peripheral IV access (for a maximum of 1.5 minutes. If unsuccessful, intra-osseous needle placement into anterior tibia allows high fluid infusion rates and drug administration.
• Inadequate fluid resuscitation	20 ml/kg colloid boluses initially, repeated as required; may need total of 100–200 ml/kg. (High requirement for colloid indicates severe disease. Consider ventilation and titration of fluid administration to central venous pressure).
• Intubation and ventilation not initiated until cardiorespiratory arrest	Consider semi-elective intubation and ventilation in presence of: • Decreased conscious level • Severe cardiovascular compromise (e.g. profound hypotension, high colloid requirement) • Significant respiratory dysfunction (e.g. increasing requirement for supplementary oxygen) • Presence of markers of severe disease (see below).
• False security after initial response to resuscitation	Disease severity indicators must be assessed. Likely severe disease if: • Low WCC • Low platelet count.

THE HEAD-INJURED CHILD

Head injury is the major cause of death in children after infancy. The majority of cases in this age group are the result of pedestrians being struck by cars (~50%) with falls and unrestrained passenger road traffic accident injuries responsible for most of the remainder. In infancy, most serious head injuries are non-accidental, resulting from shaking with or without an impact against a hard surface (see "Child Protection" chapter). Such mechanisms are relatively rare after 12 months of age. The majority of head injuries seen in emergency departments are minor. The probability of a serious injury is increased by a violent mechanism of injury (e.g. pedestrian versus car, fall from a height), reduced conscious level – either on history or still present on examination, any focal neurological signs and penetrating injury. A combination of these factors makes a serious injury very likely (**1.26–1.29**).

INITIAL ASSESSMENT AND RESUSCITATION

The initial assessment and management of the severely head-injured child follows the routine of **A** airway (and cervical spine), **B** breathing and **C** circulation. Direct airway trauma is rare but loss of the airway due to reduced conscious level and absent cough and gag reflexes is common. The child's conscious level must be assessed and any concern about the ability to protect the airway should be aggressively managed with elective intubation and ventilation to avoid hypoxaemia or hypercarbia. The airway reflexes should be assessed in all cases in which there is evidence of a reduced conscious level. All children with serious head injuries should be considered to have sustained a cervical spine injury, even in the presence of a normal lateral neck x-ray (because of the relatively high risk of ligamentous injury in childhood). Only when a child has regained full consciousness and has both a normal neurological clinical examination and no neck pain, in addition to a normal lateral neck x-ray, can cervical spine precautions be removed. If these criteria cannot be met, then the cervical spine should be immobilized and specialist neuro-radiological advice sought (**1.30**).

Fundoscopy (**1.31**) may reveal subhyaloid haemorrhages suggestive of a non-accidental injury. Specialist ophthalmology advice should be sought when the child is stable and appropriate clinical images taken.

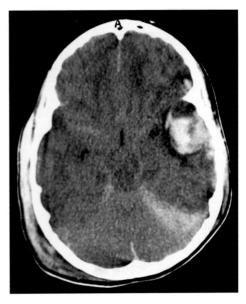

1.26 Traumatic brain injury with intracerebral haematoma in contused left temporal lobe with mass effect. Generalized cerebral oedema is also present. A small amount of blood is also seen on the surface of the tentorium cerebelli.

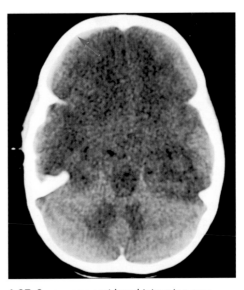

1.27 Severe non-accidental injury in a two-year-old child. There is a right subdural haematoma and severe cerebral oedema.

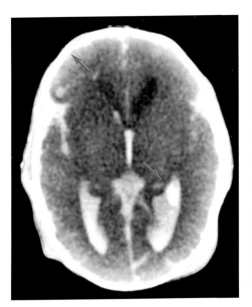

1.28 Traumatic brain injury with intraventricular and subarachnoid blood. Generalized cerebral oedema is also present.

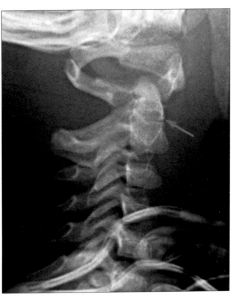

1.30 Multiple fractures of the atlas (CI) with dislocation of CI on C2 in a three-year-old child who was involved in a road traffic accident.

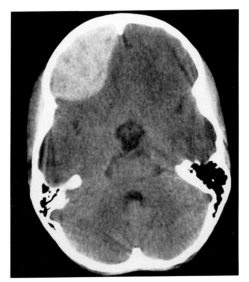

1.29 Acute extradural haematoma in the right frontal region with mild mass effect but no oedema.

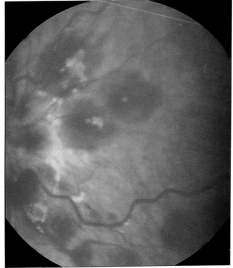

1.31 Multiple domed subhyaloid retinal haemorrhages in a case of non-accidental injury caused by shaking. The white spots in the centre of the haemorrhages are light reflexes. Fundoscopy should be performed in all infants presenting with significant head injuries.

Hypoventilation raises arterial carbon dioxide levels leading to cerebral vasodilatation and increased intra-cranial pressure (ICP). The aim of respiratory support in severe head injury is to avoid hypercarbia and maintain $PaCO_2$ at 4.5–5.3 Kp_a. Lower levels are detrimental and may contribute to cerebral ischaemia via excessive cerebral vasoconstriction. Hypotension must be avoided in order to maintain cerebral perfusion. Fluid resuscitation may be required, but in cases with severe cerebral oedema, inotrope or vasopressor treatment may be essential to maintain cerebral perfusion pressure (CPP). A child who has been ventilated with a severe head injury must receive both sedation and analgesia to assist in the control of raised ICP.

MANAGEMENT AFTER INITIAL STABILIZATION

Primary brain injury occurs on impact and is, as yet, untreatable. The care of the child with head injury is aimed at avoiding secondary brain injury. This can be summarized as providing a 'well-perfused and well-oxygenated brain.' Three principle mechanisms lead to the generation of secondary brain injuries: hypoxaemia, reduced cerebral perfusion and metabolic disturbances (e.g. hypoglycaemia, hyponatraemia). Raised ICP may occur due to a rapidly expanding intracranial haematoma or acute hydrocephalus resulting in a decrease in cerebral perfusion – a neurosurgical emergency. However, raised ICP is more commonly the result of diffuse cerebral oedema in children. In this scenario, the circulation must be supported to maintain cerebral blood flow.

There is little consensus on the on-going intensive care management of head-injured children. Treatments commonly employed include head up 30° tilt, midline head position, sedation, analgesia, intra-cranial pressure monitoring with circulation support (fluid and vasopressors) to maintaining cerebral perfusion pressure. Mannitol may be useful to decrease ICP prior to emergency neurosurgical intervention. The use of phenytoin as seizure prophylaxis reduces the incidence of early seizures. Hyperventilation can be harmful as it reduces cerebral perfusion and is no longer recommended. Hypertonic saline, barbiturates, hypothermia and steroids are not of any proven benefit.

THE CHILD WITH MULTIPLE INJURIES

Few paediatricians will be regularly involved with the resuscitation of children with multiple injures. Such cases must be approached in a structured way (**A, B, C**) in order to identify and treat life-threatening injuries. The care of a child with multiple injuries requires careful organization and can be best achieved in large centres with all the relevant specialities available onsite (e.g. anaesthesia/ICU, radiology, orthopaedics, neurology, general, cardiothoracic, maxillofacial and plastic surgery).

INITIAL ASSESSMENT AND RESUSCITATION

This is identical to that already described for the head-injured child. As before the patient should be considered to have a cervical spine injury until they are awake and able to demonstrate normal neurology in the absence of neck pain and with a normal lateral neck x-ray. Airway assessment must include an assessment of the airway reflexes and conscious level as well as the effects of any direct trauma or foreign body (**1.32**).

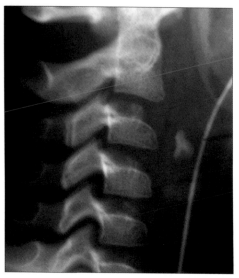

1.32 Inhaled tooth after facial trauma.

Chest wall contusion should be noted and the possibility of fractured ribs considered. Acute tension pneumo- or haemo-pneumothorax may require emergency aspiration and drainage (**1.33**). Haemorrhagic shock is the main threat to the circulation in multiple trauma. The priority is early secure intravenous or intra-osseous access (ideally away from the site of obvious injuries) and fluid resuscitation of 20 ml/kg repeated as necessary. Blood samples for blood count, coagulation screen, grouping and cross-matching should be taken as early as possible. Resuscitation must continue while sites of potential blood loss are assessed in the secondary survey.

MANAGEMENT AFTER INITIAL STABILIZATION

After immediately life-threatening ABC problems have been addressed, a careful examination to detail all injuries must be undertaken. This includes log-rolling to examine the back and thoraco-lumbar spine. It is at this stage that imaging (which must include a chest x-ray and lateral neck film) appropriate to the injures (e.g. CT head, ultrasound or CT abdomen) should be performed if stability can be obtained. The management of individual injuries must be planned with the relevant surgical teams.

Blood loss from fractures (especially to the pelvis or femora) is easily underestimated and often requires early fixation. Hepatic, renal or splenic injuries are all sites of potentially lethal haemorrhage though many such injuries can be managed without surgical intervention (**1.34, 1.35**). Injury to the aorta or mediastinum requires further imaging and discussion with a cardiothoracic surgeon.

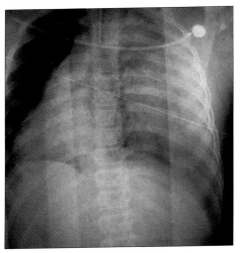

1.33 Right side haemothorax (and contusion of underlying lung). This required urgent drainage.

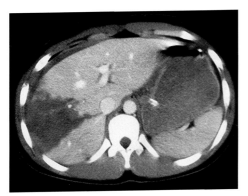

1.34 Large hepatic contusion after a fall down stairs. This was successfully treated with conservative management.

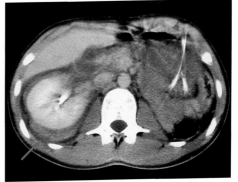

1.35 Right perinephric haematoma after a road traffic accident. Note this child has congenital absence of the left kidney. Conservative treatment only was required.

BURNS

The initial management of a child with severe burns can be summarized as 'forget about the burn'. The priorities remain **A**irway, **B**reathing and **C**irculation. If the mechanism of burn is unclear or there is co-existent trauma then cervical spine precautions must be observed. Analgesia must also be addressed urgently.

GENERAL APPROACH TO THE CHILD WITH BURNS

Reduced conscious level and airway obstruction from facial (**1.36**) or inhalational burn injury are the major causes of airway obstruction in burns. A child with facial or airway burns should be assessed for early intubation because of the high risk of swelling tissue.

Smoke inhalation or reduced chest wall movement from circumferential burns must be considered. High flow oxygen should be administered to cases in which smoke inhalation is possible (to limit the effects of carbon monoxide poisoning). Large fluid losses will occur though areas of burned skin in proportion to the area affected (**1.37, 1.38**). Complex formulae exist for calculating fluid replacement required but this should not confuse the initial management. Immediate circulation support should be as for shock from any cause with 20 ml/kg of colloid/crystalloid. If shock is present it should not be ascribed to fluid losses through the burn without considering the possibility of associated fractures, abdominal and thoracic injuries.

After the initial resuscitation, ongoing care including fluid management should be undertaken in combination with the specialized burns centre and/or paediatric intensive care unit.

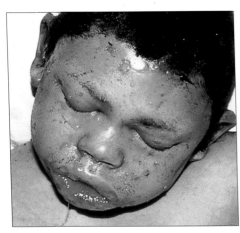

1.36 Facial oedema with eyelid and lip swelling caused by a flash burn. Swelling occurs up to 24 hours after the injury and the airway must be secured with an endotracheal tube.

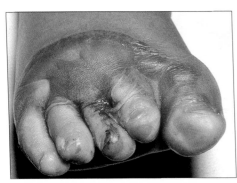

1.37 Full thickness electrical burn of the foot. An entry point is clearly visible between the second and third toes. Respiratory failure and cardiac dysrhythmias may require immediate treatment. Urgent exploration and debridement is usually required.

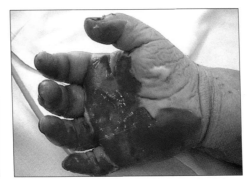

1.38 Partial thickness burn of the palm of the hand caused by grasping a hot object. This sort of injury, sustained during exploration of the environment, is likely to be accidental.

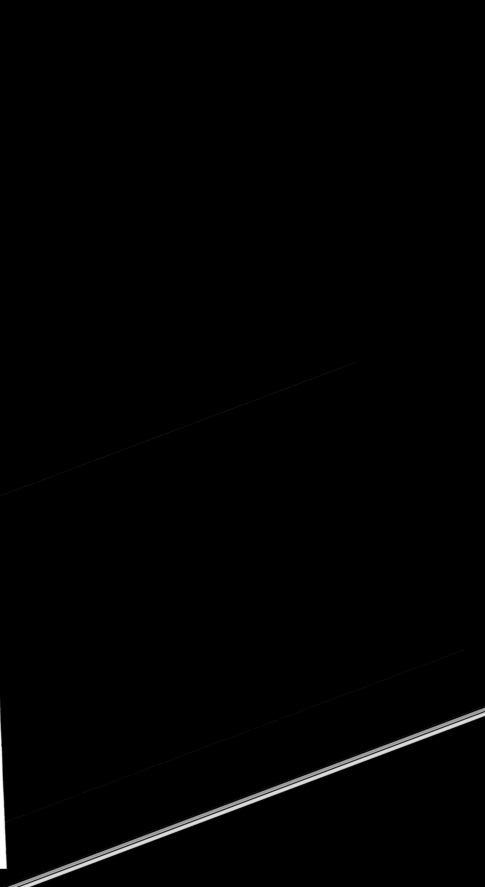

DIABETIC KETOACIDOSIS

See also 'Endocrinology' chapter.

Diabetic ketoacidosis (DKA) is the common presentation of insulin dependent diabetes mellitus (IDDM) in childhood. The primary cause is insufficient endogenous or therapeutic insulin to allow adequate cellular uptake of glucose and inhibition of ketogenesis. This decompensation is frequently precipitated by an infective illness. The main clinical picture is of dehydration resulting from hyperglycaemia-induced osmotic diuresis, and a profound metabolic acidosis (with an increased anion gap) from the accumulation of acidic ketone bodies. DKA requires intensive medical and nursing input, however the vast majority of cases can be effectively managed by following some very simple rules.

INITIAL ASSESSMENT AND RESUSCITATION

As with all acutely ill children the initial assessment of a child with DKA focuses on airway, breathing and circulation. Altered conscious level on presentation is an important poor prognostic factor and should trigger the early involvement of senior help. Reduced conscious level and airway obstruction are the principal risks to the airway. Cases of DKA will be tachypnoeic as they attempt to compensate for metabolic acidosis by reducing $PaCO_2$. A low pH (<7.0) or low $PaCO_2$ (<2.5 kPa) indicate severe disease with a high risk of cerebral oedema. In the rare cases that require artificial ventilation for exhaustion or shock, the initial target $PaCO_2$ must be similar to the value that the patient was achieving. This will prevent worsening of acidosis and cerebral oedema. The heart rate, blood pressure and peripheral perfusion must be regularly assessed. Shock should be treated promptly with 20 ml/kg of normal (0.9%) saline and the circulation reassessed. The possibility of a serious infection precipitating DKA must be considered.

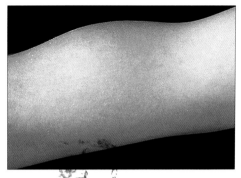

1.39 Fat hypertrophy in a 12-year-old with insulin-dependent diabetes, caused by injecting insulin repeatedly at the same site rather than rotating the sites. She presented with keto-acidosis caused by poor insulin absorption.

Any significant reduction in conscious level should prompt discussion with anaesthetic and/or paediatric intensive care unit staff. Cerebral oedema in DKA is unpredictable but is associated with a low $PaCO_2$ on presentation, rapid changes in osmolarity and the use of bicarbonate solution. Treatment of cerebral oedema is essentially supportive as with raised intra-cranial pressure after head-injury. Control of $PaCO_2$, support of the circulation and avoiding low plasma osmolarity are the main strategies. Invasive intra-cranial pressure monitoring should not be used in these cases.

INITIAL INVESTIGATIONS

These should include glucose, urea and electrolytes, bicarbonate, creatinine, plasma osmolality, liver and bone profile, FBC, PCV, arterial blood gas, urinalysis (for ketonuria and glycosuria) and partial septic screen (e.g. MSU, blood cultures). Hourly blood glucose levels should be performed. Urea and electrolytes with at least venous blood gas should be performed 2–4 hourly for the first 12 hours, and then 6-hourly for the next 12 hours. Sudden changes in glucose, osmolarity, pH and potassium levels can therefore be addressed promptly.

FURTHER MANAGEMENT

If **A**, **B**, **C** are satisfactory, the child should be assessed as follows:

Fluids

Although fluid resuscitation for shock should be undertaken promptly, there is no rush for rehydration, pH or electrolyte correction. Therefore rehydrate slowly over 48 hours with normal (0.9%) saline or 0.45% saline (if hypernatraemic). Check serum electrolytes and osmolarity two hours later and act accordingly. Place a urinary catheter, in the presence of oliguria or reduced conscious level, monitor urine output.

Insulin therapy

Once fluid replacement has commenced, the glucose level will start to reduce and a continuous infusion of rapid-acting soluble insulin (e.g. velosulin or actrapid) must be commenced. The initial dose is 0.1 units/kg/hour, but this may need adjustment to maintain a smooth trend towards nomoglycaemia. The dose of insulin should remain at 0.1 U/kg/h until resolution of ketoacidosis. To prevent a precipitous drop in plasma glucose, glucose should be added to the inravenous fluid when plasma glucose falls to about 14–17 mmol/l.

Potassium replacement

Potassium replacement therapy should be started immediately if the patient is hypokalaemic. If the patient is hyperkalaemic, potassium replacement therapy should be deferred until there is urine output. Otherwise, potssium should be started with insulin therapy and should continue while the patient is on intravenous fluids.

Bicarbonate replacement

Bicarbonate administration is not necessary or justified in DKA. It has been associated with an increased risk of cerebral oedema.

Nasogastric tube

A nasogastric tube should be sited in all cases with any reduction in conscious level or if there is a history of vomiting. Large volumes of gastric aspirate should be replaced with 0.45% saline plus 10 mmol/L potassium chloride.

STATUS EPILEPTICUS

Generalized convulsive (tonic–clonic) status epilepticus (CSE) is defined as a generalized convulsion lasting 30 minutes or longer, or repeated tonic–clonic convulsions occurring over a 30 minute period without recovery of consciousness between each convulsion. CSE in childhood is a life threatening condition with a serious risk of neurological sequelae. Although the outcome from an episode of CSE is mainly determined by its cause, duration is also important. In addition, the longer the duration of the episode, the more difficult it is to terminate.

From 0.4–0.8% of children will experience an episode of CSE before the age of 15 years, and 12% of children's first seizures are CSE. CSE in children has a mortality of approximately 4%. Neurological sequelae of CSE, such as epilepsy, motor deficits, learning difficulties, and behaviour problems, occur in 6% of children over 3 years but in 29% of children under 1 year.

The consensus guideline shown here was developed by the British Paediatric Neurology Association and is primarily designed for a child presenting in the Accident and Emergency Department with an acute tonic–clonic convulsion.

RECOGNITION

Initial assessment and resuscitation should address, as always, the airway, breathing and circulation (A, B, C). High-flow oxygen should be given and the blood glucose level measured by stick testing. A brief history and clinical examination should be undertaken to confirm genuine seizure activity.

Although the definition of CSE implies that the seizure should last 30 minutes, treatment should start within 10 minutes of continuous generalized tonic–clonic seizure activity. The times of drug administration in the guideline are from the time of arrival in A&E. It has been assumed that the convulsion will have been continuing for at least five minutes prior to arrival.

IMMEDIATE MANAGEMENT

If intravenous access is available, lorazepam 0.1 mg/kg should be given. Lorazepam is equally or more effective than diazepam and causes less respiratory depression. Lorazepam also has a longer duration of anti-seizure effect (12–24 hours) than diazepam (15–30 minutes). In children, when immediate intravenous cannulation has failed, rectal diazepam 0.5 mg/kg should be given. If after 10 minutes the convulsion has not stopped or another convulsion has begun, a second dose of lorazepam (0.1 mg/kg) should be given, assuming intravenous access is established.

If, following the first dose of rectal diazepam, no intravenous or intra-osseous access is established and the child is still convulsing, rectal paraldehyde 0.4 ml/kg mixed with an equal volume of olive oil should be given. Arachis oil should be avoided because of the risk of peanut allergy. Intramuscular paraldehyde should be avoided because the injection is painful and there are risks of sciatic nerve damage and sterile abscesses.

If seizure activity continues for a further 10 minutes and in the unlikely event that intravenous access is still not possible, an intraosseous needle should be inserted. Continuing convulsive activity indicates a longer acting intravenous anticonvulsant is required. Phenytoin is recommended as it causes less respiratory depression than phenobarbitone. Heart rate, ECG, and blood pressure monitoring during infusion are recommended as intravenous phenytoin can cause arrhythmias. In children already receiving phenytoin as a maintenance oral anticonvulsant, intravenous phenobarbitone should be given.

INVESTIGATIONS

Once seizure activity has ceased, a full examination including examination of the central nervous system and fundoscopy should be performed. Focal seizures or residual focal neurology suggest a structural cause for the seizures and neuroimaging may be required. Fundoscopy may reveal retinal haemorrhages suggestive of non-accidental injury (see "Child Protection" chapter). Children with no previous history of a seizure disorder who remain encephalopathic should be presumed to have an infective aetiology until proven otherwise, particularly if a fever is present, and given acyclovir, cefotaxime and erythromycin.

When intravenous or intraosseous access is obtained, blood should be sent for a full blood count, urea and electrolytes, anticonvulsant calcium and magnesium levels and blood glucose. Monitoring should include ECG, blood pressure, pulse oximetry, core temperature, blood glucose and sometimes blood gases. Appropriate specimens should also be sent for bacterial, viral and mycoplasma culture, serology and PCR. Lumbar puncture should be avoided until it is clear that intracranial pressure is not raised. Further investigation when the child is stable may include neuro-imaging and neurophysiological investigation (**1.40–1.42**).

INDICATIONS FOR VENTILATORY SUPPORT

If, 20 minutes after intravenous phenytoin or phenobarbitone has commenced, the child remains in CSE, then rapid sequence induction of anaesthesia should be performed using thiopentone. If neuromuscular paralysis is used this should be short acting so as not to mask the clinical signs of the convulsion. At this stage, children under three years of age with a prior history of chronic, active epilepsy who present with an episode of established CSE should be treated with intravenous pyridoxine in case the seizures are pyridoxine-dependent or pyridoxine-responsive (**1.43–1.45**).

The child will need to be nursed on a paediatric intensive care unit (PICU) and advice on ongoing management should be sought from a paediatric neurologist.

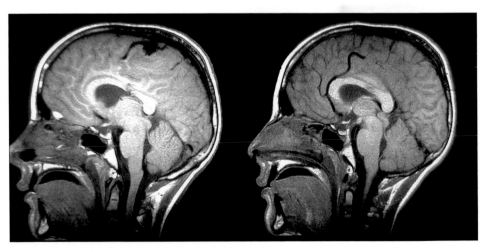

1.40 Tl-weighted magnetic resonance image in sagittal section of a five-year-old who presented with intractable seizures. The diagnosis was an arteriovenous malformation (the tortuous black lesion seen arising anterior to the corpus callosum).

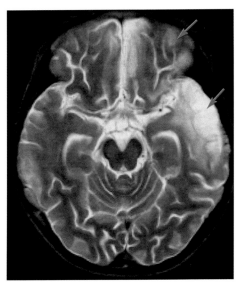

1.41 T2-weighted magnetic resonance image in transverse section of a two-year-old with intractable seizures due to herpes simplex encephalitis. Increased signal, representing oedema, is seen in the left prefrontal and temporal lobes.

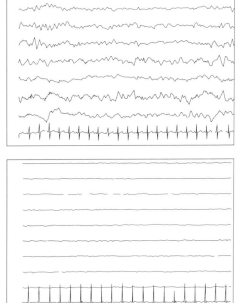

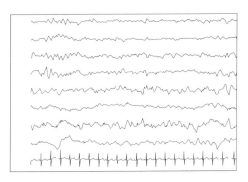

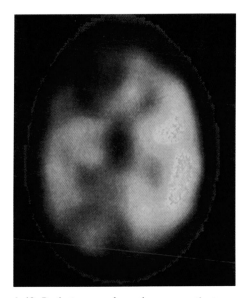

1.42 Perfusion scan from the same patient showing increased uptake in the same area.

1.43–1.45 EEGs of a five-month-old child with a history of neonatal seizures responding to phenobarbitone presented with increasingly severe and prolonged seizures with tonic–clonic and myoclonic elements.

Top: During status epilepticus, high amplitude (note the change in calibration) repetitive sharp waves are seen continuously.

Middle: Following an injection of pyridoxine the EEG activity disappears, returning after 8 to 9 hours.

Bottom: An interictal EEG shows age appropriate activity. The child had pyridoxine-dependent seizures and was maintained fit-free on regular pyridoxine after the diagnosis was made. (Courtesy of Dr Stuart Boyd)

POISONING

Suspected poisoning in children results in 40,000 visits to Accident and Emergency departments in England and Wales every year and 15–20 deaths. Poisoning may occur accidentally in a young child or toddler, intentionally in teenagers or deliberately in some cases of child abuse and Munchausen syndrome by proxy (see *Child Protection* chapter).

RECOGNITION AND ASSESSMENT

Primary assessment should be directed to airway patency, adequacy of breathing and circulation and neurological status. Acidotic breathing is seen in salicylate or ethylene glycol poisoning. QRS prolongation and ventricular tachycardia are seen in tricyclic antidepressant poisoning. A depressed conscious level suggests poisoning with opiates, sedatives, antihistamines or hypoglycaemic agents. Small pupils suggest opiate poisoning but large pupils suggest amphetamines, atropine or tricyclic poisoning. Convulsions are associated with many drugs, particularly tricyclic antidepressants.

IMMEDIATE MANAGEMENT

Airway patency should be maintained, with intubation if necessary (**1.46**). Children with cardiorespiratory failure or a decreased conscious

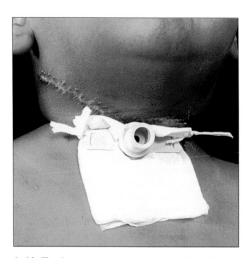

1.46 Tracheostomy in a two-year-old child after ingestion of caustic soda. Caustic soda causes severe burns and scarring to the oropharynx, oesphagus and stomach, which, in this case, has required surgical debridement and eventually resulted in airway obstruction necessitating a tracheostomy.

level should receive high-flow oxygen through a face mask with reservoir if the airway is patent. Shock should be treated with fluid boluses rather than inotropes as inotropes can cause arrythmias in combination with some toxins. Cardiac dysrhythmias caused by poisons need specific treatment, which should be discussed with a Poisons Centre. Hypoglycaemia should be treated with intravenous 10% dextrose and convulsions treated with diazepam or lorazepam. Naloxone should be given if the pupils are very constricted or there is a history of opiate poisoning.

INVESTIGATIONS

When intravenous access is obtained, blood should be sent for a full blood count, urea and electrolytes, paracetomol and salicylate levels, toxicology, and blood glucose. Urine specimens should be collected and sent to the laboratory. Monitoring should include ECG, blood pressure, pulse oximetry, core temperature, blood glucose and sometimes blood gases.

FURTHER MANAGEMENT
Gut decontamination

Activated charcoal can be given as a single dose (50 g for children over 12 years, 1 g/kg body-weight for a child up to 12 years) up to one hour after ingestion of toxin. Beyond this time adsorption is reduced. Charcoal should not be given if the airway cannot be protected because of the risk of aspiration pneumonia. Gastric lavage should only to be used within 60 minutes of overdose and only with drugs not adsorbed to charcoal. Syrup of ipecacuanha is now rarely used as an emetic as there is no evidence that it decreases morbidity or mortality. Whole gut irrigation with polyethylene glycol should be considered when patients have ingested potentially lethal substances, such as iron or lithium, which are not adsorbed to activated charcoal, or sustained release or enteric coated preparations.

Paracetamol poisoning

N-acetyl cysteine should be given as soon as possible after a large overdose of paracetamol or if levels are toxic 4 hours after ingestion. The management of patients presenting 15 hours or more after ingestion or patients taking staggered overdoses of more than 150 mg/kg/day or 12g for a child over 12 is controversial. Advice should be taken from a poisons unit and a liver transplant unit.

OTHER

Management for other poisons should be guided by advice from a poisons centre (**1.47**, **1.48**) and includes chelating agents and antidotes.

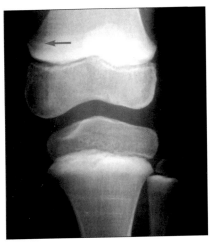

1.47 Lead poisoning causing a dense metaphyseal line at the growing ends of long bones. Chelation can be effected with dimercaprol, edetate calcium disodium and 2,3 dimercaptosuccinic acid. Management should be undertaken in conjunction with the local poisons unit.

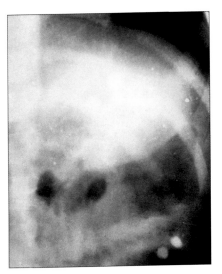

1.48 Multiple dense opacities seen in stomach and left flank in a two-year-old boy who had ingested his mother's iron tablets. He was treated with desferrioxamine and made a full recovery.

SEDATION IN PICU

Sedative drugs relieve anxiety, whereas hypnotic agents produce sleep. Commonly used sedatives include benzodiazepines, phenothiazines, chlormethiazole and buterophenones (**Table 1.5**).

Oral sedation is a frequently employed route in paediatrics and agents such as chloral hydrate and trimeprazine are used. Intravenous sedation involves the use of incremental doses of primarily benzodiazapines to reduce the child's level of consciousness and allow relatively minor yet stimulating procedures to be performed (**Table 1.6**).

It must be remembered that sedatives are not analgesics and this can result in restlessness and agitation when using sedation alone. Children are unable to localize the pain or discomfort they are experiencing. Hence the judicious combination of sedative and analgesia can produce ideal conditions for minor procedures and results in calm, cooperative children.

Table 1.5 Drugs commonly used for sedation in children

- Benzodiazepines
- Phenothiazines
- Buterophenones
- Antihistamines
- Chloral Hydrate
- Ketamine
- Barbiturates
- Opioids

Table 1.6 Levels of consciousness when using sedation

Conscious sedation
Medically induced state of CNS depression in which communication is maintained so that the child can respond to verbal command.

Deep sedation
Medically induced state of CNS depression in which the child is essentially unconscious and so does not respond to verbal command.

General anaesthesia
Medically controlled state of CNS depression in which the child is unconscious and in which the protective reflexes and the ability to independently maintain a patent airway is lost.

However, the combined use of sedation and analgesia for noxious procedures is potentially hazardous as it may result in the loss of protective laryngeal airway reflexes and should only be employed by doctors trained in resuscitation. Full resuscitation equipment must be available and those providing deep sedation should ideally by trained in advanced paediatric life support (APLS).

The use of intravenous sedation can also be hazardous in children as the margin between sedation and anaesthesia is very narrow. Therefore, standards of monitoring should be the same for deep sedation as they are for anaesthesia. These should include continuous monitoring of heart rate and peripheral oxygen saturation. The use of sedation so deep as to cause loss of protective airway reflexes should be avoided by all but anaesthetists.

BENZODIAZEPINES

The most commonly used drugs for sedation are benzodiazepines. They are anxiolytic, anticonvulsant and sedative. Their main site of actions are in the limbic and reticular activating system. They act by facilitating gamma amino butyric acid (GABA) the main inhibitory neurotransmitter in the central nervous system. GABA normally opens chloride channels, hyperpolarize neurones and decrease their excitability. Benzodiazepines facilitate GABA by increasing the frequency of the chloride channel opening.

Because of their lipid solubility benzodiazepines have a large volume of distribution and are metabolized in the liver. Renal excretion is not an important route of elimination. For some benzodiazepines the production of active metabolites and enterohepatic recirculation prolongs their duration of action. The active metabolite of diazepam is methyldiazepam which results in a half-life of up to 90 hours (**Table 1.7**).

MIDAZOLAM

This agent is probably the most commonly used benzodiazepine in the last 15 years and is still the drug of choice in combination with morphine to provide sedation and analgesia on the PICU. It has a half-life of 2–4 hrs. Respiratory depression can occur if given in excess or too rapidly. Withdrawal symptoms can occur after modest duration of use. Its advantage is that it has a number of routes of administration which has given it an important role in the acute treatment of seizure disorders.

BENZODIAZEPINE ANTAGONISTS

Flumazenil is a specific benzodiazepine antagonist. It has a short half-life and can cause seizures, cardiac arrhythmias as well as acute withdrawal symptoms. It is given intravenously and because of its short half-life the actions of the benzodiazepine can recur.

CHLORMETHIAZOLE

Related to vitamin B1, this drug also acts by affecting GABA transmission. It is given intravenously in a 0.8% solution in 5% dextrose. It is 50% bound to plasma proteins and has a half-life of 3–5 hours. If given slowly it can produce sedation. However, it can also produce respiratory depression.

PHENOTHIAZINES

Phenothiazines have potent central anticholinergic sedative effects as well as properties. Trimeprazine 2–4 mg/kg (Vallergan) is a commonly used sedative in children, particularly as a pre-medication. They produce sedation in 30–40 minutes.

BUTEROPHENONES

Potent sedatives which act on various neurotransmitters including dopamine and norepinephrine and have similar effects to phenothiezines (but are not commonly used in children).

Table 1.7 Half-lives for commonly-used benzodiazapines

Drug	Half-life (hours)	Active metabolites
Diazepam	20–90	Yes
Lorazepam	10–20	No
Midazolam	2–4	No
Temazepam	2–4	No

BARBITURATES

One of the oldest classes of agents used for sedation with its respiratory depressant function, being dose-dependent. Thiopentone and pheno-barbitone are probably the most commonly used, with half-lives of about 6–12 hours.

CHLORAL HYDRATE

This agent only has sedative properties and is dependent upon enteral absorption. It is metabolized in the liver to trichlorethanol which is the active agent. It is then further metabolized to trichloracetate and trichlorethanol glucuronide which depend upon renal excretion. The half-life in neonates is 8–66 hours.

KETAMINE

This agent produces dissociate anaesthesia. It has profound analgesic and sedative properties. It also has bronchodilator properties and is the agent of choice to provide sedation in children with status asthmaticus. It produces excess salivation and can have unpleasant psychological side effects which can be attenuated with simultaneous administration of benzodiazapines.

PROPOFOL

Whilst being the mainstay of sedation in adult intensive care, there have been an increasing number of reports of deaths using continuous infusion of propofol in children. In the UK, the Committee on Safety of Medicine has advised against the use of propofol in children under 16 years of age as continuous infusion. It should therefore not be used as a sedative agent on the PICU.

Table 1.8 Guidelines for route of administration, bolus and infusion doses of commonly used sedative agents in children

Drug	Route	Dosage
Diazepam	IV	Bolus: 0.2–0.4 mg/kg Infusion: NOT RECOMMENDED
Midazolam	IV	Bolus: 0.1–0.2 mg/kg Infusion: 1–4 mcg/kg/min
Morphine	IV	Bolus: 0.1–0.2 mg/kg Infusion: 20–40 mcg/kg/hour
Chloral hydrate	Oral	30–50 mg/kg, 6–8 hourly
Trimeprazine	Oral	2–4 mg/kg, 6–8 hourly
Triclofos	Oral	30–50 mg/kg, 6–8 hourly
Chlormethiazole	IV	Bolus: 1–2 ml/kg Infusion: 0.5–1.0 ml/kg/minute
Ketamine	IV	Bolus: 1–2 mg/kg Infusion: 0–20 mcg/kg/minute
Lorazepam	IV	Infusion: 10–100 mcg/kg/hour
Fentanyl	IV	Infusion: 2–4 mcg/kg/hour

PAIN MANAGEMENT

OPIOIDS

Useful for the treatment of pain mediated by C fibres, dull, visceral pain (**Table 1.9**). Opioids are all drugs, synthetic or naturally occurring which bind to opioid receptors. The μ and κ opioid receptors are associated with analgesia. However centrally mediated respiratory depression is also μ and κ associated. Morphine is a μ agonist.

MORPHINE

Morphine is one of the most frequently used opioids in PICU to provide sedation, analgesia. and anxiolysis. It is frequently the only agent used in neonates but is combined with midazolam infusions in infants and children. Its elimination half-life is about 9 hours in the preterm, about 7 hours in the neonate but only about 5 hours in the older infant. The active metabolite morphine-6-glucuronide further prolongs its activity.

FENTANYL

Fentanyl is 100 times more potent than morphine and is cardiovascularly stable over a wide range of doses. There is a large variability in requirements to achieve similar levels of sedation.

REMIFENTANIL

This is a very short acting potent opioid ideal for stimulating procedures such as physiotherapy or chest drain removal. Also useful as a short acting sedative agent and may replace propofol in PICU. Ideal for neurosedation as it can be stopped and allow the child to awake to get a window of consciousness.

METHADONE

The potency of methadone is about the same as that of morphine but it has a much longer duration of action, with a half-life of 12–24hrs. The dose is 0.1–0.2 mg/kg 6–12 hourly, orally and can be used to wean from morphine dependency.

CLONIDINE

A centrally acting alpha-2 agonist has sedative and anxiolytic properties. It also has a significant role in reducing symptoms of withdrawal. Dose 3–5 μg/kg.

ANTI-INFLAMMATORY DRUGS

Prostaglandins do not produce pain, they sensitize peripheral nerve endings to agents such as histamine and bradykinins. Most non-steroidal anti-inflammatory drugs (NSAIDs) (**Table 1.10**) work by inhibiting cyclo-oxygenases which produce prostaglandins.

When stable non-steroidals per rectum may be very useful. Care should be taken in renal clotting and platelet disorders.

PARACETAMOL

This is not an anti-inflammatory but has centrally acting analgesic and antipyretic properties. It is metabolized in the liver and renally excreted. Rectal pararcetamol can be useful in providing analgesia. Higher doses are required when used rectally, 40 mg/kg initially, then 30 mg/kg 6-hourly. The oral dose is 15 mg/kg.

Table 1.9 Potency and half-life of commonly used opioids

Drug	Potency	Half-life (hours)
Morphine	1	2–3
Pethedine	0.1	2–3
Methadone	1	12–24
Alfentanil	20	0.2–0.3
Fentanyl	100	0.3–0.5
Remifentanil	100	0.1
Sufentanil	1000	0.2–0.4

Table 1.10 Anti-inflammatory drugs

Drug	Dose	Interval
Diclofenac	1mg/kg	8–12 hourly
Ibuprofen	2.5–10 mg/kg	6–8 hourly
Ketorolac	0.2 mg/kg	4–6 hourly

METHODS OF OXYGEN DELIVERY

OXYGEN MASK
- A simple oxygen masks deliver 35–60% oxygen at flow rates of 6–10 L/min.
- Partial rebreathing masks consist of a simple face mask with a reservoir bag and deliver 50–60% oxygen at flow rates of 10–12 L/min.
- Non-rebreathing masks have a facemask, a device to prevent entrainment of room air during inspiration and a valve between bag and mask to prevent flow into the bag. An inspired concentration of 95% can be achieved with flow rates of 10–12 L/min.

OXYGEN HOOD
Oxygen hoods are clear plastic containers that cover the child's head. On some occasions hoods are better tolerated then nasal cannula in infants. They allow easy access to the baby. They also permit control of inspired oxygen concentration and gas temperature. They need flow rates of 10–15 L/min. They can achieve an oxygen concentration of 80–90%, but are not ideal for children above one year of age.

OXYGEN TENT
This is a larger device that covers the upper half of the child. It achieves about 50% oxygen concentration and allows more movement within the tent.

NASAL CANNULA
This is a simple low-flow delivery device ideal for infants and children who need just a little extra oxygen. The catheter has two small prongs which insert into the anterior nares. Oxygen is then delivered directly into the nasopharynx. The oxygen provided is not humidified and at flow rates >4 L/min the gas irritates the nasopharynx by drying it out (**Table 1.11**).

NASAL PRONG
This consists of a short endotracheal tube about 6–8 cm long and measured from nares to anterior tragus on the ear. The catheter is placed in one nostril and advanced to the pharynx behind the uvula. Although it provides oxygen directly above the laryngeal inlet, some argue that it is no better than nasal cannula.

OROPHARYNGEAL AIRWAYS
This is a curved piece of plastic through which an air channel passes. There are eight sizes – 000, 00, 0, 1, 1A, 2, 3, and 4.

Table 1.11 Fresh gas flow requirement for weight

Weight (kg)	Flow rate (litres per minute)
<10	2
10–50	4
>50	6

SUCTION DEVICES
Suction force for infants and children – 80–120 mmHg. Maximum from wall-mounted suction provides a negative pressure of 300 mmHg and flows of 30 L/min.

REFERENCES

Mackway-Jones K, Molyneux E, Phillips B, Wieteska S (eds). *Advanced Paediatric Life Support* (3rd edn). London: BMJ Books, 2001.

Appleton R, Choonara I, Martland T, *et al* (Status Epilepticus Working Party). The treatment of convulsive status epilepticus in children. *Arch Dis Child* 2000; **83:** 415-419.

British guideline on the management of asthma. *Thorax* 2003; **58 (Supp I)**.

Carcillo JA, Fields AI (American College of Critical Care Medicine Task Force Committee Members). Clinical practice parameters for hemodynamic support of pediatric and neonatal patients in septic shock. *Crit Care Med* 2002; **30:** 1365-78.

Dunger DB, Sperling MA, Acerini CL, *et al.* European Society for Paediatric Endocrinology; Lawson Wilkins Pediatric Endocrine Society ESPE/LWPES consensus statement on diabetic ketoacidosis in children and adolescents. *Arch Dis Child* 2004; **89:** 188-194.

Guidelines for the acute medical management of severe traumatic brain injury in infants, children, and adolescents. *Ped Crit Care Med* 2003; **4:** Supp.

Hartling L, Wiebe N, Russell K, Patel H, Klassen TP. Epinephrine for bronchiolitis (Cochrane Review). In: *The Cochrane Library*, Issue 1. Chichester: Wiley, 2004.

Jones AL, Volans G. Management of self poisoning. *BMJ* 1999; **319:** 1414-1417.

Randolph AG, Wang EEL. Ribavirin for respiratory syncytial virus infection of the lower respiratory tract (Cochrane Review). In: *The Cochrane Library*, Issue 1. Chichester: Wiley, 2004.

Russell K, Wiebe N, Saenz A, et al. Glucocorticoids for croup (Cochrane Review). In: *The Cochrane Library*, Issue 1. Chichester: Wiley, 2004.

Child Protection
Paul Hargreaves

FORMS OF CHILD ABUSE

Child abuse takes many forms, which may occur through physical acts, or through neglect and inappropriate care. A physically abused child is defined as any child who receives physical injury (or injuries) as a result of acts (or omissions) on the part of his/her parents or guardians. Within this definition, hitting a child does not constitute physical abuse unless it results in injury, e.g. bruise or fracture.

Child abuse has existed since the dawn of time, and in all cultures maltreatment of children is seen as unacceptable. Which acts constitute child abuse is an area of heated debate with conflict between different cultures and their beliefs, and the human rights of the child. Following a series of inquiries into notable child deaths in the UK, the Children Act came into being in 1989, which has helped to greatly strengthen Child Protection procedures. These are mentioned later.

Child abuse is often classified into four main areas: physical abuse, emotional abuse, sexual abuse and neglect (from 'Working Together', 1999).

Suspected child abuse in any form requires reporting to Social Services and will need to be fully investigated with the co-operation of all appropriate agencies.

PHYSICAL ABUSE

This may involve hitting, shaking, burning, scalding, suffocating, drowning, or otherwise causing physical harm to the child. Physical harm may also be caused when a parent or carer feigns the symptoms of, or deliberately causes ill health to a child. This is termed factitious illness of Munchausen syndrome by proxy.

EMOTIONAL ABUSE

This is persistent ill treatment such as to cause severe and persistent adverse effects on the child's emotional and behavioural development. This form of abuse often accompanies the others.

SEXUAL ABUSE

This involves forcing or enticing a child to take part in sexual activities. The activities may include physical contact or non-contact activities.

NEGLECT

Neglect is the persistent failure to meet a child's basic physical and/or psychological needs, likely to result in the serious impairment of the child's health or development.

INCIDENCE

The incidence of child abuse is difficult to quantify. Changes in figures over time reflect changes in awareness, recognition and reporting, as well as changes in the epidemiology of abuse.

UK DATA

As can be seen in the diagram below (2.1), in 1999 the Department of Health estimated that out of 11 million children nationally, 4 million 'vulnerable' children live in families with less than half the average household income, and a significant number are 'in need'. 'Looked after' children and children on the child protection register represent a small percentage of those families who may need additional support. There are many thousands of families who would benefit from additional support, but currently the children who are 'looked after' and on the child protection register receive the most input.

Table 2.1, taken from DfES data, shows the numbers of children on the child protection register has been declining over the past few years. The majority of registrations are under the category of neglect and sexual abuse is very rarely used as a category for registration. This may be because in sexual abuse cases often Social Services may decide to institute care proceedings earlier and children may be removed earlier.

US DATA

Recent data for 2002 has shown that the incidence of child abuse is 12.3 per 1,000 children. Figures for 2004 show an estimated 1,400 children die as a result of abuse per year, which approximates to 4 per day. Of these children, 74% were aged less than 3, and 41% under the age of 1 year. In the USA, neglect remains the most common form of abuse, with 60% of cases being due to this; physical abuse comprises 19%, sexual abuse 10% and emotional abuse 6%. In addition, another 19% of children experienced such 'other' types of maltreatment as 'abandonment,' 'threats of harm to the child,' and 'congenital drug addiction.' Many children may be registered under several categories. Child abuse is reported to Social Services Departments every 10 seconds, i.e. 3 million children per year, and around 60% of these referrals are investigated.

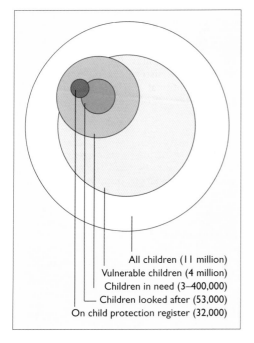

All children (11 million)
Vulnerable children (4 million)
Children in need (3–400,000)
Children looked after (53,000)
On child protection register (32,000)

2.1 Representation of extent of children 'in need' in England at any one time (from 'Framework for the Assessment of Children in Need and their Families', Department of Health 2002.

Table 2.1 Children and young people on child protection registers at 31st March (DIES)

Category of abuse	1999	2000	2001	2002	2003
Neglect	13,900	14,000	12,900	10,100	10,600
Physical abuse	9,100	8,700	7,300	4,200	4,300
Sexual abuse	6,600	5,600	4,500	2,800	2,700
Emotional abuse	5,400	5,500	4,800	4,500	5,000
Categories not recommended by 'Working Together'	460	310	440	–	–
No category available (transfer pending conferencing)	170	110	80	–	–
Mixed / not recommended by 'Working Together'	–	–	–	4,100	4,000
Total of all abuse categories	35,630	34,220	30,020	25,700	26,600

PHYSICAL ABUSE

Physical abuse can take many forms and involve various implements. Children may be slapped, assaulted with straps, canes, ropes, slippers and various other implements. From the pattern and distribution of the marks inflicted, it is often possible to differentiate accidental from non-accidental injuries.

BITE MARKS

Bite marks inflicted by humans are crescent-shaped with the teeth imprints being similar in size, shape and prominence (2.2). Human bites are less likely to result in puncturing of the skin, unless very aggressive. The size of the bite mark tends to be larger in adults, with the intercanine distance being over 3.0 cm, where-as children inflict smaller bites. Saliva from the bite mark may be collected by swabs, and may be used to identify the blood group of the perpetrator, and DNA analysis may be possible. Photography (including ultraviolet light) may be useful to compare the mark with dental mould of suspected perpetrators (with the help of a forensic odontologist).

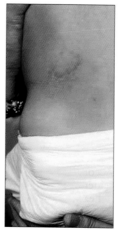

2.2 Bite marks on the back of an eight-month-old girl.

BRUISES

Bruises are present in the vast majority of physically abused children. However, a physically abused child may not have visible bruises on any given day of examination. In a bruise, blood is lost from the intravascular space into the skin and surrounding tissues. Significant trauma is usually required, except in the rare situation of children with bleeding problems. Because of the serious implications associated with non-accidental injury, it is important to consider excluding rare bleeding disorders (e.g. idiopathic thrombocytopenic purpura – ITP, haemophilia, platelet dys-function) with a family history, FBC and detailed clotting studies. Also important to consider in the differential diagnoses are Mongolian blue spots in babies and infants, sepsis (including meningococcal infection), disseminated intravascular coagulation (DIC), and various skin diseases such as Ehlers-Danlos syndrome and erythema nodosum.

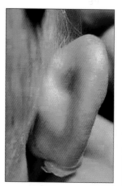

2.3 Bruising to pinna suggestive of excessive pinching.

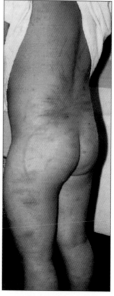

2.4 Multiple bruises of various colours and shapes suggestive of physical abuse.

Ageing of bruises

The time taken for a bruise to develop depends on the force used and the depth of the injury; deeper bruises take longer to appear. Numer-ous studies have been undertaken to assess ageing of bruises but no consensus has been met. Many bruises do not undergo the typical

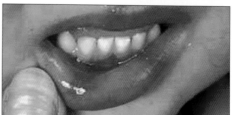

2.5 Torn frenulum.

development from purple to yellow over a period of time. All one can say with some degree of certainty is that yellow bruises are over 18 hours old but other colours are not useful for ageing purposes. Multiple bruises of different size and colour may indicate multiple episodes of trauma and are highly suggestive of physical abuse.

Distribution of bruises
If bruises are identified, the mechanism of alleged injury and the age of the child should be taken into account. According to a recent paper, in babies most accidental bruises were found on the face and head, with smaller numbers being found on the shins. Older children are more mobile and tend to have bruises over the forehead and shins, but also accidental bruises are found in the upper limbs caused by falls.

Characteristic patterns of bruises over the head and neck may help to identify slap marks, or the use of implements. Bruising to the pinna of the external ear (**2.3**) suggests a punch or significant pinching and the use of force. Non-accidental bruises are often found on the buttocks, lower back and inner thigh (the latter may be associated with sexual abuse) (**2.4**). Injuries to the upper lip associated with a torn frenulum (**2.5**) are also highly suggestive of abuse, but may also occur accidentally after a fall onto the mouth.

Finger marks associated with a slap may leave characteristic parallel bruises with areas of no bruising in between. Slap marks are commonly found on the sides of the face and over the buttocks. Strangulation marks over the neck may be associated with finger marks or the use of ligatures. Fine petechiae may be found in the head and neck area suggesting venous congestion, which occurs in attempted strangulation or suffocation.

BURNS AND SCALDS
Burns and scalds are the cause of 10% of all accidental deaths in children with over 30,000 attendances in Accident and Emergency departments per year. The majority of children affected are aged less than 4 years and boys outnumber girls by 3:2. Most of the injuries occur in the home when the toddler seeks out new things to play with. Kitchen appliances (such as pans, kettles), and electrical appliances (such as irons, electric fires and curling tongs) are a common source of danger.

Depth and distribution of burns
With scalds from tap water, the higher the temperature the shorter the contact time required to cause significant burns. At a water temperature of 65°C, a one-second contact may cause a partial thickness burn, and 10 seconds may lead to a full thickness burn.

When assessing the distribution of the burn, one should take into account the history and the developmental stage of the child. Accidental burns due to a pan or kettle of hot water being pulled onto a child tend to result in burns to the head, neck, shoulders and upper trunk. There may be splash marks on the body. Deliberate immersion burns may have a glove and stocking distribution to hands and/or feet, and tend to have little splash marks (indicating restraint). If the child is immersed in the bath, there may be areas of skin spared, e.g. soles of the feet or between the buttock creases ('hole in the doughnut' effect).

Burns caused by grabbing at hot objects tend to involve the fingertips and the palm of the hand (**2.6**).

Burns to the dorsum of the hand are more worrying and indicate abuse. Deliberate burns may show the imprint of whatever is used very clearly, e.g. iron burns.

Cigarette burns
These may be single or multiple, and may be found anywhere on the skin, especially on the limbs. Accidental burns of this nature occur after a brief contact and have an elliptical shape with a tail. Abusive cigarette burns are different, being completely circular and with a visible crater suggestive of longer contact. It is important to differentiate these marks from those associated with impetigo and chicken pox scars.

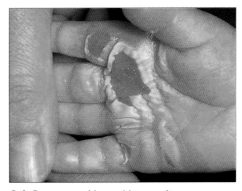

2.6 Burn caused by grabbing curling tongs.

FRACTURES

Incidence

Fractures of the long bones occur in approximately 5% of physically abused children. (See also 'Orthopaedics and Fractures' chapter.)

Presentation

Fractures may present with pain, swelling and bruising, but loss of function may be the only indicator in younger children. A major fracture may present with symptoms or signs, the effects of which cannot be ignored by the regular carers. Whenever physical abuse is suspected social services should be informed and it is imperative that a skeletal survey should be performed. This is because many of the fractures caused by abuse are clinically silent in that they are not associated with overlying swelling or bruising.

Imaging

The skeletal survey should be performed in normal working hours after explaining the reasons for it to the carers. Two health professionals should remain with the baby throughout the examination and they should initial each film. The skeletal survey should include:

- Skull: AP and Lateral
- Spine: Lateral
- Chest: AP
- Upper and lower limbs: AP
- Pelvis: AP
- Both hands: PA
- Both feet: DP

Additional views may be necessary such as oblique views of the chest to identify rib fractures: coned views of the metaphyseal regions when these are not clearly seen on the limb views, lateral long bone views when a fracture has been identified to evaluate displacement, and a Townes view when an occipital fracture is suspected. Delayed images after a few days or weeks may help in dating fractures. Early new bone formation (soft callus) at the site of a fracture is first seen 7 days after the injury (**2.7**) and then gradually increases in size and consolidates (hard callus) (**2.8**) before remodelling takes place.

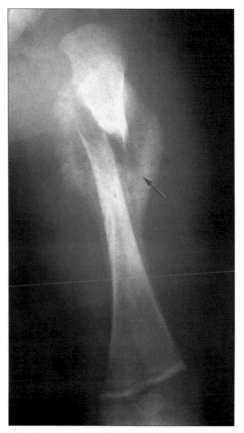

2.7 Soft callus formation after a femoral shaft fracture.

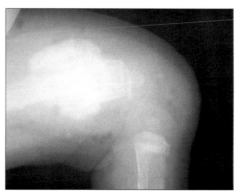

2.8 Hard callus formation.

When the fracture is relatively undisplaced remodelling has occurred by about 12 weeks. If fractures are identified then other children under the age of two years with the same carers should have a skeletal survey performed. A radioisotope bone scan is not a routine investigation and should not replace the skeletal survey, but as an adjunct it may identify unrecognized injuries (spine and ribs).

Diaphyseal fractures

The commonest presenting fracture is of a diaphyseal long bone fracture, most commonly affecting the humerus (**2.9**). The fracture may be spiral, caused by an applied twisting force below the site of the fracture, or transverse (oblique), caused either by a direct blow at the site of the fracture or by an applied levering force with the pivot or fulcrum at the site of the fracture. Diaphyseal fractures are not specific for non-accidental injury but there would need to be an appropriate accidental explanation of a significant incident to account for such a fracture. The specificity would increase if an additional injury is present, there is an inappropriate history, or if there has been delay in presentation. Diaphyseal fractures are usually associated with overlying soft tissue swelling which may extend up and down the injured limb. The baby experiences pain on movement of the injured limb, is reluctant to use it and the limb appears floppy.

Metaphyseal fractures

These occur at the ends of the long bones, commonly around the knees and consist of a thin rim of bone detached from the adjacent metaphysis. Depending on their angulation relative to the x-ray beam they may have a 'bucket-handle' (**2.10**) appearance or appear as 'corner' fractures. They are considered to be highly specific for non-accidental injury as they are caused by applied gripping, twisting and pulling forces applied to the ends of the bones. Rarely they are caused by shaking. They are difficult to date as they may heal without callus formation, gradually consolidating to the adjacent metaphysis (**2.11**). They are rarely associated with overlying soft tissue swelling or bruising and therefore are not apparent on clinical examination. Metaphyseal fractures result in tenderness on direct palpation of the injured area for a few days.

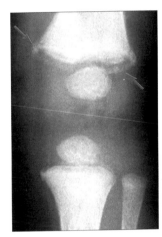

2.10 Metaphyseal fracture of the distal humerus.

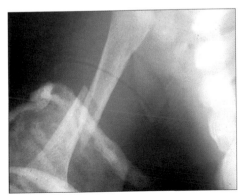

2.9 Fracture of humeral shaft.

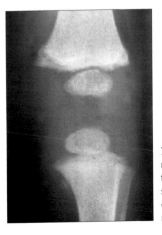

2.11 Healing metaphyseal fractures showing exuberant metaphysis.

Rib fractures

These are caused by severe compressive forces to the chest and may occur at any point along the ribs although posterior fractures are thought to be more specific for non-accidental injury (**2.12**).

They are not usually associated with superficial changes but cause ongoing pain when the baby is picked up, for a period of a few days. They may not be identified until healing periosteal new bone is seen around seven days after they have occurred. Occasionally underlying lung contusion or haemothorax may occur. The squeezing force causing rib fractures may be associated with a shaking action resulting in subdural haemorrhages.

Periosteal reactions

These may occur along the shafts of long bones from gripping and twisting shearing forces around the limbs. If due to trauma they usually extend down to the metaphyses, and may be asymmetric or layered (**2.13**). They need to be differentiated from normal physiological periosteal reactions, which are seen in about 40% of babies under the age of four months, are usually symmetrical and affect only the mid-diaphyses.

Unusual fractures

In infants these are considered to be highly specific for non-accidental injury. They include fractures of the acromial processes (**2.14**), short tubular bones of the hands and feet, pubic rami, vertebrae and long bone epiphyseal separation fractures. As they are unusual, it may be difficult to be certain of their precise mechanisms of causation.

Skull fractures

These may occur as a result of accidental or non-accidental injury and presentation may be as a result of the identification of an overlying soft, boggy swelling. Patterns of skull fractures more commonly associated with non-accidental injury include fractures affecting more than one bone, multiple fractures, those crossing sutures, or are fissured or branching, or affect the occipital bone, or are depressed (**2.15**).

The commonest skull fracture is that of a single, linear, hairline parietal fracture which may be seen either as a result of accidental or non-accidental injury. Accidental skull fractures need an appropriate history of a significant incident, usually of a fall from several feet onto a firm or hard surface, to account for them. Fractures resulting from accidental domestic falls rarely result in intracranial injuries. Skull fractures do not heal by developing callus and cannot be dated from the radiographic appearances. If soft

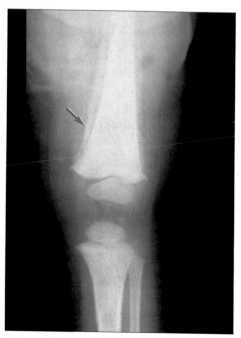

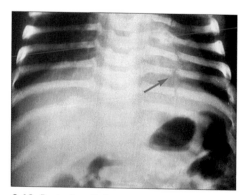

2.12 Posterior rib fractures.

2.13 Exuberant periosteal reactions of the femur.

tissue swelling is present overlying the fracture it is likely to have occurred within the previous seven days.

Any fracture occurring in a non-ambulant infant, without an appropriate incident to account for it should be regarded as being the result of non-accidental injury. It should be remembered however that sometimes an accident has occurred which the carer is unable to admit and the whole family and social circumstances should be evaluated. Medically it is important to exclude any skeletal disorder, which may predispose to fractures, such as osteogenesis imperfecta, a metabolic bone disease or underlying neurological disorder. When more than one fracture is present, or there is evidence of other forms of abuse, and when they have occurred on more than one occasion without appropriate explanations then the diagnosis of non-accidental injury becomes more certain.

SHAKEN BABY SYNDROME

This was first recognized over 30 years ago but it is being increasingly recognized. The typical scenario is of a baby less than 6 months of age who has been subjected to violent shaking and possible thrown onto a surface. Children of this age have a relatively large head and weak neck muscles compared to older children and therefore are prone to significant harm from shaking. The shaking leads to intracerebral and subdural haemorrhages within the skull, and also to bleeding in the retinae.

There may or may not be visible bruises on the head or limbs, but there is often extensive intracranial damage. The baby may present with severe shock (often resembling septic shock or metabolic conditions) associated with fits. Blood tests may reveal a significant metabolic acidosis with anaemia. CT or MRI scans of the brain shows subdural haematomas (which may be of different ages), and ophthalmological examination reveals extensive retinal haemorrhages. X-rays of the limbs may show metaphyseal fractures as a result of the limbs flailing during the abusive episode.

Recent Canadian data have shown that in babies subject to this form of abuse, 1 in 5 die, 3 in 5 have some neurological injury and only 1 in 5 survive intact.

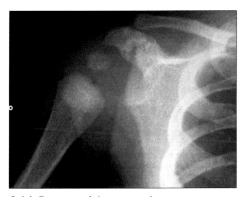

2.14 Fracture of the acromial process.

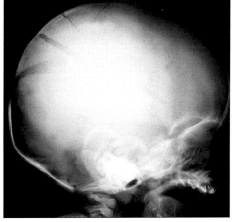

2.15 Branched skull fracture emanating from the occipital bone.

FABRICATED OR INDUCED ILLNESS

The fabrication of illness in a child by a carer is rarely recognized and it has an estimated incidence of 1–2 per 100,000 children in the UK. The child may have had extensive, unnecessary medical investigations carried out in order to establish the underlying causes for signs and symptoms reported by a carer. The child may also have treatments prescribed or operations that are unnecessary.

The abusive carer is often the mother, and they may have a medical background. They often have inappropriate behaviour on the wards, and they may have a previous history of chronic physical or mental ill health. Munchausen syndrome by proxy may manifest in several ways:

- Deliberately inducing symptoms by administering medication, or other substances – e.g. adding blood to urine specimens, adding salt to feeds, altering thermometer readings
- Interfering with medical treatments – e.g. by overdosing, not giving prescribed medicines, or manipulating with intravenous lines
- Obtaining multiple specialist opinions for conditions which do not warrant them
- Exaggeration of symptoms, causing doctors to carry out numerous and often invasive investigations.

Reports have shown that up to 10% of such children may die, and 50% may experience long-term morbidity as a consequence of such abuse.

There have been many controversies in this difficult area with regard to how these children are identified. The relevant authorities should be alerted and a strategy discussion should be held. Consideration should be given to covert video surveillance, but this should only be done after discussion with senior hospital and medical staff, and the Police should be responsible for the surveillance. Covert video surveillance should be used only if there is no other ways of proving this form of abuse. It is important for the Police to monitor the situation locally so that the carers can be arrested quickly if abuse is seen.

NEGLECT

INCIDENCE

It is difficult to assess how many children are neglected in the UK. As mentioned earlier, neglect is increasingly being used as a category to register children on the Child Protection Register, but we are only seeing the tip of the proverbial iceberg here.

In the USA, data has suggested that out of every 1,000 children, 8 experience physical neglect, 4.5 experience educational neglect, and 3 experience emotional neglect. These are probably gross underestimates.

PREDISPOSING FACTORS

Neglect, both physical and emotional, is usually associated with other forms of abuse. There are many social factors that predispose to neglectful parenting. Some of the factors are listed below:

- Lower social class (IV and V)
- Lone parent or large family
- Low income and poor housing
- Poor physical and/or mental health in the carers or children themselves
- Substance abuse
- School failure
- Families from ethnic minorities
- Families who move frequently and are unable to access services properly.

These families often have increased rates of:
- Low birth weight
- Perinatal and infant mortality and morbidity
- Accidents
- Poor dental health
- Infectious disease.

Neglected children may present to doctors in various ways. Suspicions should be roused when children present with the following:
- Recurrent accidents (e.g. falls, scalds, road traffic accidents)
- Inadequate growth (non-organic failure to thrive)
- Failure of immunisation
- Failure of attendance at clinics for check-ups
- Poor development.
- Unkempt and dirty appearance

CLINICAL FEATURES

Examination of these children should specifically look for evidence of poor clothing, dirty hair and skin, poor dentition and recurrent skin infections (including nappy rash in babies). There may be evidence of poor growth when reviewing the centile charts, and general muscle bulk may be reduced, in particular subscapular skin thickness.

Detailed developmental assessment will often reveal delay in several areas, and this may be particularly evident in social communication (including speech), and fine motor skill areas. These children may have associated behavioural problems and may either be extremely passive and difficult to engage, or they may be over-active and difficult in structured environments such as nursery or school. Various labels such as 'autistic spectrum disorder' or 'attention deficit hyperactivity disorder (ADHD)' may be used erroneously. Psychological input, together with family support is extremely valuable in such difficult cases.

ASSESSMENT AND TREATMENT

Multidisciplinary assessment is useful in identifying specific medical and developmental needs. Involvement of social services is necessary to carry out a thorough assessment and provide a programme of support for the family. If the parenting skills do not improve with such a programme, then serious consideration should be made to accommodate the child elsewhere. Problems within the family that may be intractable and not amenable to change may include parental mental ill health, serious interpersonal difficulties, and limited resources.

SEXUAL ABUSE

INCIDENCE

Although sexual abuse accounts for a minority of Child Protection Registrations in the UK, it is often unrecognized and therefore frequently missed. It has been estimated that up to 100,000 children per year have a potentially harmful sexual experience in the UK. A recent NSPCC survey of 18–24 year olds found that 1% alleged they had been sexually abused by a parent or carer and a further 3% had been sexually abused by another relative.

Sexually abused children may not manifest any signs or symptoms, and will often not disclose any information. These children are more likely to grow up into adults who have significant adjustment problems and other forms of mental ill health. This transgenerational phenomenon is not specific to this form of abuse. Very worryingly, they may go on to become parents who abuse their own children in a similar fashion to the way they were abused themselves as children. It is therefore very important to identify these children to break this cycle of abuse.

SYMPTOMS AND SIGNS

These may be present or absent and may take the form of various behaviours or signs.
Physical indicators:
• Rectal or vaginal bleeding
• Dysuria, frequency and enuresis
• Constipation and encopresis
• Vulvovaginitis and recurrent PV discharge
• Sexually transmitted disease (STD)
• Recurrent headaches, abdominal pains and anorexia.
Behavioural indicators:
• Sexually explicit play or language inappropriate to developmental age
• Self-mutilation and other forms of deliberate self-harm (e.g. overdoses)
• Sleep disturbance.

DIAGNOSTIC PROCESS

Most children who have been sexually abused are abused by someone known to them, who may live within the same household. They may have been abused over a long period of time, may have been sworn to secrecy and thus other family members may be unaware of it.

The concerns about possible sexual abuse may come from various sources (e.g. parents, neighbours, teachers, social worker). If the perpetrator is believed to live within the child's household, the child may be at significant risk of further abuse. In this very difficult situation, it may be necessary to inform social services and convene a strategy discussion. Further investigations may proceed if there are sufficient concerns.

If the abuse is very recent, it is important to carry out a thorough examination as soon as possible, to collect valuable forensic evidence. The child should be interviewed at a separate occasion to this examination; this may occur before or afterwards.

INTERVIEW PROCESS

Children are often interviewed in a specially designed child-friendly suite that may have facilities to record on videotape for future court proceedings. Staff experienced in this situation should carry out this interview. It is vital that children are not questioned by the health professionals who may have initial contact with the child. They should have a thorough understanding of child development and behaviour. Open non-directive questions should be asked before leading to more focussed questions. The use of anatomically correct dolls may be very useful in acting out previous experiences.

EXAMINATION

Examination of such children should be carried out by an experienced senior doctor (usually a consultant who has undergone necessary training). This is carried out in the presence of an adult responsible for the child and who is chosen by the child.

The examination of the anogenital area follows on from examination of other systems and a detailed history covering general health, hygiene, bowel and urinary habits, and discharges. The examination of the genital area is usually in the frog-legged position, and the anal region in the left lateral position. There should be adequate lighting, and a colposcope may be used to take pictures. It is vital that the child is fully aware and happy with what is happening. They should be aware that swabs might need to be taken. These swabs should be handled and labelled by the doctor and treated as chain of evidence specimens.

It is worth noting that examination of the anogenital area in children who have been sexually abused may be completely normal. If there has been recent trauma or penetration there may be abnormal findings and specimens should be analysed for semen, saliva, hair and other substances.

It is important to look at the all the anatomical structures and to describe any findings accurately (**2.16**). There is much variation in normal anatomy, and this is dependent on the age of the child. The size of the hymenal orifice is very small in babies and normally increases 1mm per year thereafter. Larger orifices suggest penetration.

The descriptions of markings around the hymen are likened to that of a clock face. Tears of the posterior fourchette (between 3 and 9 o'clock) are highly suggestive of abuse (**2.17**), as are transactions of the hymen.

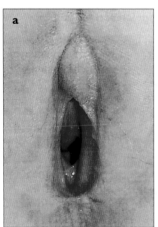
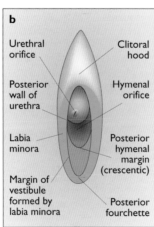

Urethral orifice

Clitoral hood

Posterior wall of urethra

Hymenal orifice

Labia minora

Posterior hymenal margin (crescentic)

Margin of vestibule formed by labia minora

Posterior fourchette

2.16 Anatomy of genitalia in a normal five-year-old girl.

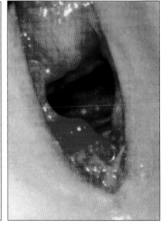

2.17 Laceration of the hymen and posterior fourchette following a rape one week previously.

Other abnormalities may include erythema, bruising, scarring, increased vascularity and oedema. Examination of the anal margin may also reveal abnormalities suggestive of trauma. Reflex anal dilatation (RAD) occurs when the anus dilates to reveal the rectum after separating the buttocks for up to 30 seconds. This sign has been commonly found in non-abused children with constipation, and other children who may have poor anal tone. RAD on its own should *not* be used as indicator of sexual abuse.

At the conclusion, it is essential to depict the examination findings on a line drawing. Photographs may be used later in court proceedings.

MANAGEMENT OF CHILD ABUSE

Internationally, any suspicion of child abuse should be alerted to the relevant authority, (in the UK this is the Social Services Department) and they have a duty to investigate. Suspicions may come from parents, relatives, neighbours, school and health professionals.

Health professionals should be aware that, in the course of their jobs, if any concerns of a child protection issue arise, then they have a duty to inform the relevant authorities. This overrides any such duty of keeping medical information confidential.

Health professionals who have expertise in Child Protection may examine children for signs of abuse. It is important that consent for this is given by someone with Parental Responsibility (PR). The natural mother always has PR and if a couple is married, both parents have PR. In unmarried couples, the father can acquire PR through an agreement with the mother, by subsequently marrying the mother, or by being mentioned on the Birth Certificate of the child.

In the UK, the Children Act 1989 was the first comprehensive piece of legislation that simplified and integrated the law regarding children. The main principles were:
* The child's welfare is paramount
* The upbringing of children is primarily the responsibility of parents
* Parents continue to have parental responsibility, even if their children are no longer living with them
* Any help offered to the child should be in partnership with the family, meet the child's individual and cultural needs, and be open to review.

The Act includes a number of court orders that are still used today.

EMERGENCY ORDERS
Emergency Protection Order (EPO)
The child may be removed to, or kept in a place of safety for up to 8 days, and this can be extended by a further 7 days. Parents may challenge this order after 72 hours. Social Workers and NSPCC officers can apply for this Order.

Power of Police Protection
This is an order allowing a child to be taken into a place of safety for up to 72 hours. Any police officer can instigate this.

NON-EMERGENCY ORDERS
Child Assessment Order
This order is for up to 7 days and is used if parents are uncooperative and there is need to assess whether there is significant harm.

Interim Care and Interim Supervision Order
If the court decides that the child is at significant risk within the home and further investigations may be required, it may grant this order. This order may last for 8 weeks but subsequent orders may last no longer than 4 weeks.

Care and Supervision Orders
These may last several years and allow the child to be accommodated by the local authority, ideally by relative, foster parents or in residential care. In this case, the local authority shares parental responsibility (PR) with the parents. Arrangements should be made for parental access.

FURTHER PROCEDURES
Under 1989 Children Act, children can be identified who are at risk of 'significant harm'. Usually, if this is the case, a child protection conference is convened to which all the agencies involved and parents are invited. If there is sufficient concern, the child's name may be placed on the Child Protection Register under any of the four categories mentioned at the beginning of the chapter.

The child usually remains with the family, and support is offered (e.g. health visitor input, day care support). A key worker is appointed to oversee all support. The child may however be accommodated elsewhere. Once a child is registered, the conference should be re-convened at 3 months and then at 6-monthly intervals to decide if registration is to continue.

The assessment framework

In 1995 and 1999, the 'Working Together' documents were published. They drew from studies carried out since 1989 and highlighted the need for reform of child protection procedures.

In 2000, the 'Framework for the assessment of children in need and their families' document was produced to aid Social Services in their assessment of families in response to Child Protection concerns. The Assessment Framework looks at three domains, i.e. the child's health and development, the parenting capacity of the parents, and family and environmental factors (**2.18**). Current Social Services guidelines stipulate that this assessment has to be completed within 35 days of initial referral.

In 2003, the Department of Health issued the pamphlet 'What to do if you're worried a child is being abused'. In contrast to previous documents, this is a very short and user-friendly publication which gives professionals advice about how to report concerns and what their responsibilities are with regard to Child Protection. This document also gives useful advice when and how to share information that professionals may have about families.

In 2005, it is expected that the Children's Bill will be passed by Parliament. This Bill will introduce many measures to try and improve the welfare of children generally and hopefully identify children 'in need' earlier, before they become children 'in need of protection'.

REFERENCES

Working Together to Safeguard Children: a Guide to Inter-agency Working to Safeguard and Promote the Welfare of Children. Department of Health, 1999.

Framework for the Assessment of Children in Need and their Families. Department of Health, 2000.

Statistics of education: referrals, assessments and children and young people on child protection registers: year ending 31 March 2003. Department for Education and Skills, 2004.

National Clearinghouse on Child Abuse and Neglect Information
http://nccanch.acf.hhs.gov/pubs/factsheets/fatality.cfm
http://www.acf.hhs.gov/programs/cb/publications/cm02/index.htm

King WJ, MacKay M, Sirnick A, and The Canadian Shaken Baby Study Group. Shaken baby syndrome in Canada: clinical characteristics and outcomes of hospital cases. *Canadian Medical Association Journal* 2003; **168** (2).

Child Maltreatment in the United Kingdom. NSPCC, 2000

Physical signs of sexual abuse in children 2nd edition. Royal College of Physicians of London, 1997.

Children Act 1989. HMSO.

What to do if you're worried a child is being abused. Department of Health, 2003.

Framework for the assessment of children in need and their families. Department of Health, 2000.

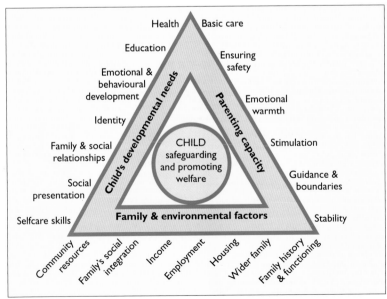

2.18 The assessment framework.

Infectious Diseases

Vas Novelli
Huda Al-Ansari

BACTERIA

DIPHTHERIA
Incidence
The disease is endemic in most of the developing world. Infection is acquired via droplet inhalation or via direct contact with infected skin lesions. Epidemics have been caused by contaminated milk. Cases in most developed countries are usually imported. There has been a recent resurgence of diphtheria in Eastern Europe.

Aetiology/pathogenesis
Corynebacterium diphtheriae is a gram positive, nonmotile, pleomorphic bacillus. Three colony types are recognized (mitis, gravis and intermedius). Following transmission of *C diphtheriae* to a susceptible contact, the bacilli tend to remain localized at mucosal surfaces of the nose and upper respiratory tract. They initiate an inflammatory response with local tissue necrosis and eventually the formation of an adherent greyish 'pseudo-membrane' which may cause respiratory obstruction. Exotoxin production by *C diphtheria* depends on the presence of a lysogenic B-phage which carries the gene encoding for the toxin. Myocarditis and neuritis are the result of systemic absorption of the toxin and end-organ damage.

Clinical presentation
The initial clinical presentation depends on the anatomic location of the infection and diphtheric membrane (nasal, tonsillo-pharyngeal, laryngeal, conjunctival, skin and genital). Nasal diphtheria (**3.1**) is mainly seen in infants who usually present with a foul smelling, profuse, mucopurulent nasal discharge leading to excoriation of the nose and lips. Tonsillopharyngeal diphtheria is a more severe form of the disease.

Initially there is anorexia, malaise, low grade fever and pharyngitis, followed in 1–2 days by the appearance of a white-grey adherent membrane covering the tonsils, uvula, pharynx and larynx. Cervical adenitis is sometimes noted with tissue oedema (bull neck) (**3.2**). Laryngeal diphtheria may present as a croup-like illness. Complications of diphtheria include respiratory obstruction, myocarditis (second week of illness), thrombocytopenia, and neuritis (vocal cord palsy, Guillain-Barré syndrome) which occurs after several weeks.

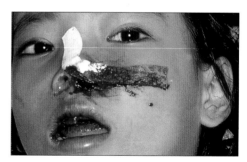

3.1 Nasal diphtheria.

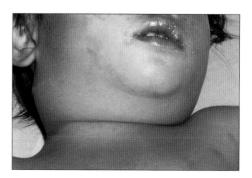

3.2 Diphtheria. Bull neck.

Diagnosis

Definitive diagnosis depends on isolation of the organism. Cultures should be obtained from the nose and throat (from beneath the membrane). Strains should then be tested for toxigenicity.

Treatment

Equine diphtheria antitoxin should be given as soon as possible. The dose prescribed depends on the site and size of the diphtheric membrane, degree of toxicity and duration of the illness (severe disease – 80,000 U). Penicillin or erythromycin is given for 14 days to eradicate the organism. General supportive measures are also important (bed rest, hydration, serial ECG, suction of secretions).

Prognosis

Present mortality is less than 5%. The more extensive the diphtheric membrane, the more severe the disease. Delayed treatment is also associated with an increased mortality.

Prevention

Prevention is carried out by active immunization. Booster doses of toxoid should be given every 10 years. Patients recovering from the disease should be vaccinated.

TETANUS

Incidence

The disease occurs world-wide but is more frequent in developing countries and in hot climates. In developed countries, Tetanus is usually seen in older individuals (> 60 years), following waning of immunity. A high incidence of neonatal tetanus occurs in those countries with low immunization rates and no vaccination programmes of pregnant women.

Aetiology/pathogenesis

Clostridium tetani is a gram-positive, motile rod which under certain environmental conditions forms spores that remain in soil for years. In the presence of tissue injury and low oxygen tension, contaminating spores change into vegetative forms. They multiply and produce a specific toxin (tetanospasmin) which affects the motor nerve endings, spinal cord, brain and sympathetic nervous system. This results in the onset of spasms and sympathetic dysfunction.

Clinical presentation

Tetanus is seen in two forms, generalized or local. The most common presentation is the generalized form, which is manifested as trismus (tonic spasms of the masseter muscles/ risus sardonicus) (**3.3**) in over 50% of the cases. Other manifestations may include irritability, difficulty in swallowing and rigidity of abdominal muscles. Slight external stimuli may precipitate a sudden burst of painful tonic contractions of all groups of muscles leading to the characteristic opisthotonus posture.

Local tetanus is a generally mild disease, characterized by painful rigidity of groups of muscles near the site of entry of *Clostridium tetani*. It may be an antecedent of generalized tetanus. Cephalic tetanus is a form of local tetanus that occurs following injuries to the face, scalp, neck, or eye. It may also follow otitis media and tonsillectomy. Cranial nerve palsies (III, IV, VII, IX, X, XII) are commonly seen. Neonatal tetanus (**3.4**) is a major cause of mortality in developing countries. The disease is related to unhygienic practices carried out on the umbilical cord at birth, as well as the use of unclean instruments to cut the umbilical cord.

Diagnosis

There is no specific laboratory test, although any wound should be cultured. The diagnosis depends on maintaining a high index of suspicion in those patients with a history of injury and signs of muscle spasm.

Treatment

Human tetanus immune globulin (TIG) 3000–6000 units is given as soon as possible to neutralize the effect of the toxin. Penicillin G is administered intravenously for 10 days to eradicate the toxin producing organisms. All wounds should be debrided, including the umbilical stump in neonatal tetanus. Supportive care includes the use of diazepam to contol spasms and endotracheal intubation, ventilation and, if necessary, tracheostomy to stabilize the airways. Tetanus toxoid should be given later.

Prognosis

Case fatality is highest in neonates and elderly (40–90%). In those areas of the developing world where some intensive care facilities may be available, mortality may be considerably less. A poor outcome is associated with a short incubation period (2–10 days), short period elapsing between the onset of tetanus and the first spasm, cephalic tetanus and neonatal tetanus.

Prevention

Following the administration of a primary vaccination course, booster doses should be given every 10 years. Vaccinating unimmunized pregnant women with two doses of toxoid is highly protective against tetanus neonatorum. Tetanus prone wounds (i.e. contaminated with dirt, faeces, etc.) should be cleaned or debrided. Toxoid or toxoid/ TIG should be administered.

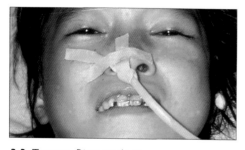

3.3 Tetanus. Risus sardonicus.

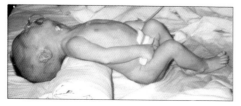

3.4 Neonatal tetanus.

MENINGOCOCCAL INFECTIONS

Incidence

In England and Wales, in 2001, there were 2,053 cases of invasive meningococcal infections, with peak incidence occurring in children younger than two years. Disease rates were 3–4 per 100,000 population per year, with around a 5% mortality. 40% of cases were meningitis alone, while the remainder were meningococcaemia ± meningitis. The disease tends to be sporadic with very occasional small outbreaks. In sub-Saharan Africa, there are regular epidemic outbreaks of disease (serogroup A), which tend to abate with the coming of the rainy season.

Aetiology/pathogenesis

Neisseria meningitidis is a Gram-negative diplococcus. Nine serotypes of meningococci are recognized by their different capsular polysaccharide antigen. Most epidemics in developing countries are caused by group A or C. In the UK, group B strains are responsible for the majority of cases, while group C constitutes a decreasing number, due to the introduction of the meningococcal C conjugate vaccine.

Asymptomatic carriage of meningococci in the upper respiratory tract may occur in 5–15% of the population. Transmission of meningococci occurs from person to person via respiratory droplet spread. In some individuals, meningococci are able to invade the circulation with resultant release of bacterial products, including endotoxin, thereby initiating an inflammatory process. The end result is vascular endothelial damage which results in capillary leak syndrome (responsible for severe hypovolemia), and intravascular thrombosis with consequent vascular occlusion leading to extensive organ damage.

Clinical presentation

These may present as either meningococcaemia and/or meningitis. Meningococcaemia is usually manifested by an abrupt onset of fever, malaise and a characteristic petechial rash (**3.5**) which may initially be maculopapular. In its most devastating form, DIC (**3.6**), shock and coma lead to a rapidly fatal outcome, despite appropriate therapy. The presentation of meningococcal meningitis is much the same as other forms of meningitis with fever, headache, vomiting and neck stiffness. Complications of invasive meningococcal disease include arthritis, pericarditis, endophthalmitis and pneumonia.

Diagnosis

Blood and/or CSF cultures are usually positive. Culture of petechial scrapings may be helpful, as may a Gram-stain of the scraping and/or buffy coat. Latex agglutination tests to detect antigen in CSF, serum and urine may be useful for rapid diagnosis or in cases of partially treated disease. However sensitivity is a problem with the use of these reagents (50% sensitivity). PCR techniques are increasingly being used for epidemiological diagnosis.

Treatment

Early recognition, initiation of antibiotic therapy (intramuscular or intravenous benzyl-penicillin 1200 mg for children >10years of age, 600 mg for those aged from 1–9 years, and 300 mg for those younger than 1year) and prompt referral to hospital is essential for a good outcome. Inpatient treatment consists of benzylpenicillin, high dose intravenous, for 7 days. Cefotaxime or ceftriaxone should be the initial empirical therapy until confirmation of the aetiology of the invasive disease. Hypo-volaemia evident by cold peripheries, poor capillary refill, tachycardia and oliguria should be corrected promptly with boluses of intra-venous fluid (colloids or crystalloids). Patients should be admitted to the paediatric intensive care unit, and elective ventilation may be required for severely ill patients. Correction of DIC and maintenance of the circulation are priorities.

Prognosis

Mortality has fallen in recent years (5%), but is higher in patients with shock.

Prevention

All household contacts (apart from pregnant women) should receive rifampicin 10 mg/kg twice daily for two days. Day-care contacts and healthcare personnel in close contact with an index case should also be considered for rifampin prophylaxis. Other antibiotics used for chemoprophylaxis include ceftriaxone and ciprofloxacin.

The specific serogroup vaccine has also been administered to control outbreaks of serogroup A and C strains (i.e. Group A + C vaccine, and the Group A,C,Y,W-135 combined vaccine). Travellers to epidemic areas in Africa/Asia should be vaccinated with one of the combined meningococcal vaccines prior to departure. As of November 1999, a meningococcal group C conjugate vaccine has been introduced into the immunization schedule in the UK with spectacular success. Effective serogroup B vaccines are still in the development stage.

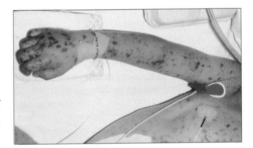

3.5 Meningococcal infections. Petechial rash.

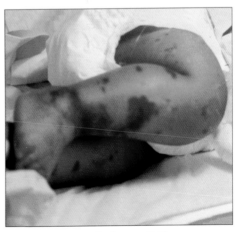

3.6 Meningococcal infection. DIC.

TUBERCULOSIS

Incidence
There has been a dramatic resurgence of tuberculosis (TB) worldwide. In developed countries, this increase is strongly associated with poverty, homelessness, urban overcrowding, the AIDS pandemic, the breakdown in TB control programmes and the increase in the number of immigrants from areas of high endemicity. In the UK there are currently 6,000 cases being notified annually, with around 500 paediatric cases per year.

Aetiology/pathogenesis
M tuberculosis, an acid-fast bacillus, is the major cause of human tuberculosis. Transmission occurs via inhalation of droplet particles, usually from an adult with 'open' pulmonary tuberculosis (cavitary tuberculosis). The inhaled organisms multiply in alveolar macrophages and spread via lymphatics to regional lymph nodes. The primary complex (Ghon) consists of local disease at the portal of entry and the involved regional lymph nodes.

While this is developing, some tubercle bacilli spread via the bloodstream to establish metastatic infection in the lungs, reticulo-endothelial system and various other organs. After 6–8 weeks, cell-mediated immunity develops (skin test conversion), and is usually followed by progressive healing of infected foci. In a small proportion of patients, symptomatic disease will develop at the time of primary infection. In general, complications in children occur commonly within the first year after initial infection.

Clinical presentation
Most children infected with *Mycobacterium tuberculosis* are asymptomatic. Clinical manifestations of tuberculous disease may occur 1–6 months after infection. Patients may present with radiographic abnormalities consistent with hilar or mediastinal lymphadenopathy, cervical adenitis, pulmonary involvement (atelectasis, consolidation, pleural effusion) (**3.7**, **3.8**), miliary disease (**3.9**) or meningitis. Later manifestations may include bone and joint involvement, renal and cutaneous disease. The classic symptoms of tuberculosis of fever, night sweats, and loss of weight are rare in young children. Extrapulmonary disease occurs in around 25% of patients.

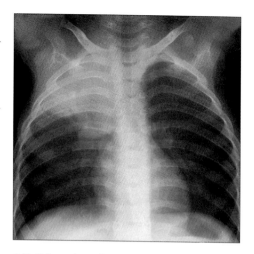

3.7 Tuberculosis. Pulmonary involvement.

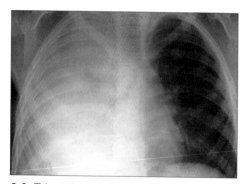

3.8 Tuberculosis. Right pleural effusion.

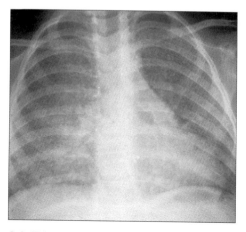

3.9 Tuberculosis. Miliary disease.

Diagnosis

Definitive diagnosis is made via the identification and isolation of *M tuberculosis* from early morning gastric aspirates or from other normally sterile body fluids (CSF, pleural fluid, urine, sputum). Recovery of organisms may take up to 10 weeks by conventional methods (using the BACTEC radiometric system, this can be reduced to 2 weeks). Newer more rapid methods of diagnosis, including PCR and the use of DNA probes, are currently being evaluated in children. A positive skin test (Mantoux reaction >10 mm induration) is suggestive of either infection (in an asymptomatic individual) or disease, in a symptomatic patient.

Treatment

It is important to differentiate between infection and disease. Asymptomatic tuberculin positive cases with normal chest x-rays (infection) are treated with isoniazid (INH) 10 mg/kg for 6–9 months (chemoprophylaxis). Pulmonary disease, including TB adenitis, requires short-course chemotherapy which consists of a 2-month course of INH (10 mg/kg), rifampicin (15 mg/kg) and pyrazinamide (30 mg/kg), followed by INH and rifampicin for a further 4 months. Miliary TB and TB meningitis are treated for a total of 12 months, often with streptomycin added for the first 2-month period (streptomycin, INH, pyrazinamide, rifampicin), followed by 10 months of INH and rifampicin. If resistant tuberculosis is suspected, patients should be treated with at least four drugs (ethambutol or streptomycin as additional drugs).

Prognosis

Although overall some 10% of patients infected with *M tuberculosis* will develop disease, this is more likely to occur in young infants. 45% of infected infants younger than 1 year will develop disease, 25% of those aged 1–5 years, and 15% of those aged 11–15 years. Mortality rates in children are around 0.6%.

Prevention

In some trials, vaccination with BCG has been thought to reduce the risk of childhood infection and disseminated disease (miliary and TB meningitis) by up to 60%. Screening the contacts of TB-infected patients is an essential public health measure. A baseline chest x-ray and skin test are performed, and in patients with a high risk of developing disease (e.g. an immunocompromised host or young infants) preventive therapy with INH is started. Chest x-rays and skin tests are repeated after 3 months and, if there is no evidence of infection, INH is stopped.

TUBERCULOUS MENINGITIS (TBM)

Incidence

Tuberculous meningitis constitutes 2–3 % of total TB cases. It is characteristically a disease of infants and children. The disease usually develops within 3–6 months of the primary infection. There is often a history of recent contact with an adult who has active tuberculosis.

Aetiology/pathogenesis

The organism is *M tuberculosis*, an acid-fast bacillus. CNS infection occurs following haematogenous spread from a primary focus in the lungs. Metastatic caseous lesions develop in cerebral tissue or in the meninges. These subsequently 'discharge' tubercle bacilli into the subarachnoid space resulting in meningitis and characterized by the formation of a thick gelatinous exudate at the base of the brain. In severe cases this invariably leads to obstructive hydrocephalus, generalized thrombophlebitis and infarction. Meningitis may also occur as part of a disseminated miliary tuberculosis and is found in 50% of such cases.

Clinical presentation

Presentation is usually sub-acute over a number of weeks with weight loss, anorexia, pallor, night sweats and low-grade fever the non-specific early symptoms. These are subsequently followed by the appearance of CNS manifestations: headache, vomiting, neck stiffness, seizures and deterioration of conscious level. Focal neurological signs may be present and usually involve cranial nerves, III, IV and VII, as well as the appearance of pyramidal tract signs. The MRC has proposed a classification of disease on presentation which is related to prognosis:

- Stage I: Conscious, non-specific symptoms.
- Stage II: Some depression of conscious state.
- Stage III: Coma, focal neurological signs.

Diagnosis

CSF changes include a pleocytosis with predominant lymphocytosis, low CSF sugar and high protein. CSF culture for acid-fast bacilli (AFB) is positive in 50% of cases. Commercial PCR tests to demonstrate specific DNA sequences of *M tuberculosis* are currently being evaluated. CT scans of the brain invariably show hydrocephalus (**3.10**), basilar enhancement or tuberculoma formation (**3.11**). The chest x-ray may show abnormalities in half of the cases, while the Mantoux test may only be positive in 30% of cases.

Treatment

INH 10 mg/kg/day and rifampicin 10–15 mg/kg/day are given for a total of one year. Pyrazinamide 30 mg/kg/day and streptomycin 20–30 mg/kg/day are also given for the first two months. There is some evidence that steroids are beneficial and these should be administered for the first 4–6 weeks. Early surgical intervention, in the form of placement of a ventriculo-peritoneal (V-P) shunt or external ventricular drain, may be required for management of hydrocephalus and severe disease.

Prognosis

The outcome is better when treatment is initiated early in the disease. Before the advent of anti-TB therapy, TBM was uniformly fatal. Morbidity and mortality are worst for Stage III patients, among whom there is approximately 50% mortality with 60–70% having neurological sequelae. Stage II patients have a cure rate of around 85%, with some 50% of survivors having some sequelae. For Stage I patients, cure rates are high, with relatively little in the way of sequelae.

Prevention

BCG vaccination is helpful in reducing the risk of this serious complication of tuberculosis.

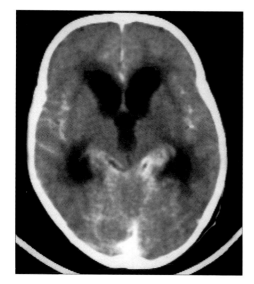

3.10 Tuberculous meningitis. CT scan showing hydrocephalus.

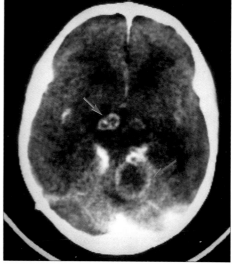

3.11 Tuberculous meningitis. CT scan showing tuberculoma formation.

NON-TUBERCULOUS MYCOBACTERIAL INFECTIONS (NTM)

Incidence

There is marked variation of disease incidence in different geographical regions. In developed countries, non-tuberculous mycobacterial infections are becoming more common, especially with the advent of AIDS. In the developing world, chronic adenitis is most often due to *Mycobacterium tuberculosis.*

Aetiology/pathogenesis

Non-tuberculous mycobacteria are acid-fast bacilli, the most common species in children being *M avium-intracellulare, M marinum* and *M scrofulaceum.* The organisms are ubiquitous and are found in soil, food and water. Transmission is by aspiration (lymphadenitis and pulmonary diseases) and inoculation (cutaneous and soft tissue diseases) of organisms. The disease causes a granulomatous reaction and subsequent symptoms at the portal of entry or in regional lymph nodes.

Clinical presentation

The most common presentation is the development of chronic localized lymphadenopathy, usually unilateral, and in the form of a neck lump. Affected nodes tend to be in the anterior cervical chain and submandibular area (less commonly there is involvement of the pre-auricular, post-auricular and sub-mental lymph nodes). The affected nodes are usually firm, painless and may be fixed to underlying tissues. They often develop an overlying, superficial, dark reddish or purplish hue (**3.12**). The natural history is for fluctuance to develop with eventual chronic discharging sinus formation and scarring. Occasional low grade fever may be present but no other constitutional symptoms are usually seen. Some children may present with either bony involvement, cutaneous disease or lung disease. Disseminated disease, characterized by multiple organ (lung, liver, and spleen) and bony involvement, persistent fever and failure to thrive, may be seen in immuno-compromised patients (**3.13**), including patients infected with HIV.

Diagnosis

Isolation and identification of non-tuberculous acid-fast bacilli from specimens taken from sterile sites such as blood, CSF, bone marrow or lymph node aspirate is required for a definitive diagnosis. A positive Mantoux test of less than 10 mm of induration is suggestive of NTM in a child with a negative CXR and negative family history of tuberculosis. Skin testing using atypical mycobacterial antigens may also be helpful in the diagnosis (antigens are not standardized, and are not available in some countries). Cases with disseminated disease should be evaluated for immuno-deficiency.

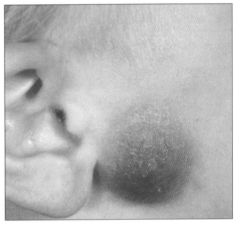

3.12 Non-tuberculous mycobacterial infection (NTM). Lymphadenopathy.

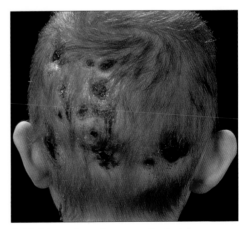

3.13 Non-tuberculous mycobacterial infection affecting skull.

Treatment

Complete surgical excision of involved lymph nodes is the definitive treatment. If this is not possible, then a period of antituberculous chemotherapy may be necessary (6–9 months). Pending results of sensitivity testing, a 2–3 drug regimen should be prescribed from the following antituberculous agents:

- Clarithromycin 15 mg/kg/day.
- Rifabutin 5 mg/kg/day.
- Ciprofloxacin 15–20 mg/kg/day.
- Clofazimine 1–2 mg/kg/day.
- Ethambutol 15 mg/kg/day.

Management of cutaneous disease and disease at other sites may also require both chemotherapy and surgical debridement. Triple or quadruple antituberculous therapy is generally indicated for disseminated disease in immunocompromised patients.

Prevention

Human to human transmission does not occur, hence no isolation precautions are necessary. Patients with AIDS and low CD4 counts may benefit from long term Clarithromycin chemoprophylaxis. All patients with severe immunodeficiency may also benefit from the use of sterilized/boiled water, as water-borne transmission of organisms may occur.

Prognosis

Most infections involving lymph nodes, even if untreated, eventually resolve, although with disfiguring scarring. Disseminated disease in immunocompromised patients may be fatal if not treated with combination chemotherapeutic agents.

STAPHYLOCOCCAL TOXIC SHOCK SYNDROME (TSS)

Incidence

Although initially described in the USA in children, most cases of toxic shock syndrome (TSS) occur in young menstruating women using tampons. Some 40 cases of TSS occur each year in the UK, although only half are definitely confirmed. 60% of cases are associated with menstruation, and there are around 2–4 deaths annually. Non-menstrual cases have been associated with cutaneous or subcutaneous lesions, surgical wound infections, and other focal staphylococcal infection.

Aetiology/pathogenesis

The most common aetiologic agent is TSST-1 producing strains of *S aureus*. Often the *S aureus* is merely a colonizer of a body site and does not cause a focal infection. The toxin produced has superantigen properties and is able to cause widespread activation of the immune system with consequent endothelial damage. This results in multi-system organ damage secondary to capillary leak syndrome, loss of intravascular volume and tone, and interstitial oedema.

Clinical presentation

An acute febrile illness characterized by the onset of a diffuse macular rash, mucositis (**3.14**), myalgia, gastrointestinal symptoms, hypotension, and often multi-organ system dysfunction including renal failure. A flaky desquamation of the trunk (**3.15**) begins after 7 days, followed by involvement of the palms and soles.

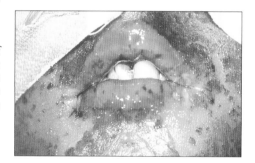

3.14 Staphylococcal toxic shock syndrome. Mucositis.

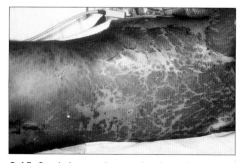

3.15 Staphylococcal toxic shock syndrome. Flaky desquamation of the trunk.

Diagnosis

Diagnosis is based on established clinical criteria. Typically, fever, rash, myalgia, headache, diarrhoea and vomiting, along with hypotension, occur on day 1. These signs and symptoms are followed on day 2–3 by mucositis and mental confusion, and later by skin desquamation. Laboratory abnormalities usually include anaemia, clotting derangements, thrombo-cytopaenia, elevated CPK, and in some patients evidence of liver and/or kidney damage. Isolates of *Staphylococcus aureus* (from superficial and potential infected sites) should be examined for their ability to produce toxic shock syndrome toxin-1 (TSST-1).

Treatment

This consists of management of the multisystem organ failure, antibiotic therapy with an anti-staphylococcal agent, and eradicating the source of toxin production (removal of any foreign body and/or irrigation of wound). Due to the severe capillary leak, fluid replacement in excess of 200–300 ml/kg may be required to restore intravascular volume. There is a role for intravenous immunoglobulin and this agent should be considered as an adjunct in any severely ill patient, or one who remains unresponsive to the usual therapy. The addition of Clindamycin may also be useful, as it may have an effect on decreasing toxin production. Steroids are of uncertain value.

Prognosis

TSS can be a serious and even fatal disorder. With treatment, the mortality is in the order of 3%. Death is usually due to myocardial or pulmonary failure.

Prevention

To lower the risk of menstrual TSS, the use of high-absorbency tampons should be avoided. Localized staphylococcal infections should be treated.

PYOGENIC LIVER ABSCESS

Incidence

Although rare in childhood, pyogenic liver abscess tends to occur in younger children and in those with underlying disease (e.g. immunodeficiency, biliary atresia, chronic inflammatory bowel disease and haemoglobinopathies). In one autopsy series, the incidence was 38 per 1,000 in children under 15 years of age. Retrospective hospital series suggest lower incidences of 3 per 100,000.

Aetiology/pathogenesis

In around 50% of cases, the aetiology is polymicrobial with gram positive cocci (*Staphylococcus aureus*, streptococci, 33% of isolates), enteric gram negative bacilli (33%), and anaerobes as the predominant agents.

Most cases in children follow systemic haematogenous spread (80%), and usually occur in those with abnormalities of host-defence. About 10–15 % occur following portal vein inflammation and bacteraemia, secondary to appendicitis/peritonitis or chronic inflammatory bowel disease. A small number either follow extension of infection from contiguous structures (e.g. from biliary tract as in ascending cholangitis), or are cryptogenic in origin.

Clinical presentation

Often presents with non-specific manifestations such as fever, nausea, vomiting, anorexia, malaise and abdominal pain. A pyrexia of unknown origin (PUO) with abdominal pain should alert the practitioner to the possibility of a liver abscess, especially in an immuno-compromised patient (e.g. chronic granulomatous disease). Hepatomegaly is present in more than half the patients although jaundice is uncommon.

Diagnosis

Ultrasound and CT scanning are used initially as non-invasive diagnostic techniques. On CT scan, liver abscesses appear as areas of low attenuation (**3.16**), and should differentiate from hydatid cysts. Amoebic liver abscesses are an important differential diagnosis (although they tend to be a single, solitary abscess) and need to be excluded by obtaining serum antibody titres to *Entamoeba histolytica*.

A microbiological diagnosis is made, following

culture of fluid/pus obtained from either needle aspiration (for multiple abscesses) (3.17), or percutaneous drainage in the case of a single solitary abscess. Blood cultures may be positive in some cases. Other laboratory features include an elevated white cell count, anaemia, and a raised ESR; abnormal LFTs are unusual.

Treatment
For the single solitary liver abscess, percutaneous needle aspiration and drainage (pigtail catheter placed into the abscess cavity under CT scan guidance), and antibiotic therapy for 6 weeks is the treatment of choice. Multiple liver abscesses are more difficult to treat as drainage is not possible; diagnostic aspiration, however, is often performed and prolonged antibiotic therapy (intravenously for 2–4 weeks) for 3–4 months is necessary, as well as the treatment of any underlying disease. Initial antibiotic combinations used for liver abscesses include:
- Piptazobactam/amikacin.
- Penicillin/gentamicin/metronidazole.
- Clindamycin/gentamicin.

Prognosis
Mortality from undrained and untreated lesions tends to be high (up to 100%). However, since the introduction of percutaneous aspiration and drainage techniques, mortality in some adult series has fallen appreciably (around 20%). Complications that may occur include peritoneal spillage, haemorrhage and spread to other organs (e.g. empyema).

VIRUSES

HIV INFECTION AND AIDS
Aetiology/pathogenesis
HIV infection is due to a human cytopathic RNA retrovirus (usually HIV-1, less commonly HIV-2), which is trophic for CD4 T-lymphocytes. Transmission is via one of three routes:
- Perinatal infection.
- Transfusion of infected blood products.
- Sexual transmission.

The virus is able to integrate its genome into the host's genome (mainly in CD4 cells) through the action of reverse transcriptase enzyme. There follows a long incubation period (around 10 years in adults) prior to the development of symptoms. It is now known that viral expression and replication are occurring continuously during this period; hence there is also a large turnover of CD4 cells to compensate. The eventual consequences of infection are a gradual CD4 T-cell depletion and a mainly cell-mediated immuno-deficiency. With the occurrence of a major opportunistic infection or cancer (AIDS-defining illness), the diagnosis is then one of AIDS.

Incidence
The World Health Organization estimates that in 2003, 35 million people world-wide were infected with HIV (2–3 million children), the majority being in sub-Saharan Africa. In the UK, as of 2004, more than 1,200 children were known to have been infected with HIV.

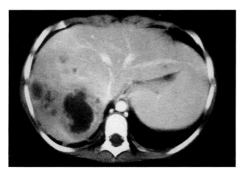

3.16 Pyogenic liver abscess. Appearance on CT scanning.

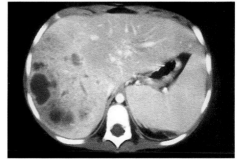

3.17 Appearance of CT scan of patient in 3.16 after contrast enhancement, showing multiple liver abscesses.

In the Inner London area, it has been estimated that 1 in 250 pregnant women is HIV-infected. The perinatal transmission rate varies from 2% to 15% in the UK, depending on whether interventions to prevent vertically-acquired HIV infection are taken up by mothers during pregnancy and the perinatal period.

Clinical presentation
The majority of children are asymptomatic for the first few years of life. Generalized lymph-adenopathy, hepatosplenomegaly, failure to thrive, parotitis (**3.18**) and lymphocytic interstitial pneumonitis are often seen in combination when children become sympto-matic. Around 25% of children, however, present in the first year with an AIDS-defining illness (PCP, recurrent bacterial infections, HIV encephalopathy, CMV retinitis, etc.).

Diagnosis
A positive HIV antibody test (ELISA) is diagnostic of HIV infection in children over 18 months. Confirmatory results are often also carried out to make the diagnosis secure (e.g. Western Blot). In younger infants, because placentally-transmitted antibody may persist for up to 18 months, the diagnosis is dependent on the demonstration of virus (viral culture, p24 antigen) or viral DNA (HIV PCR). By using these tests most children can be diagnosed by the age of 3–6 months. Other laboratory findings may show low CD4 cells (both absolute percentage and total number), lymphopenia, hypergammaglobulinaemia and thrombocytopenia.

Aids-defining illness
Pneumocystis carinii pneumonia (PCP)
This is the most common AIDS-defining illness occurring in up to 30% of children with an AIDS diagnosis. Presentation is usually in the first year of life, often with cough, dyspnoea and tachypnoea. The chest x-ray shows an interstitial pattern of pneumonitis (**3.19**); diagnosis is via broncho-alveolar lavage (BAL) with demonstration of typical protozoal cysts. Treatment is supportive (infants often require ventilation), along with the administration of high dose co-trimoxazole and steroids.

Lymphocytic interstitial pneumonitis (LIP)
This presents as a slowly progressive pulmonary disorder, often with associated cough and obstructive airway symptoms. Generalized lymphadenopathy and parotitis are often common accompaniments with the presence of digital clubbing indicating severe disease. The chest x-ray shows a reticulonodular infiltrate bilaterally (**3.20**). Definitive diagnosis is via a lung biopsy, however in practice a presumptive clinical diagnosis is usually made, after other causes have been excluded (especially miliary TB). LIP may be asymptomatic; the more severe forms are considered AIDS-defining. The aetiology is not known, although EBV may play a part in the pathogenesis. Treatment is symptomatic and may include broncho-dilators, oxygen therapy, steroids and anti-retrovirals. A common complication is superadded viral or bacterial pneumonia.

Recurrent bacterial infections
Children with HIV infection are prone to the development of recurrent bacterial infections, including bacteraemia and meningitis, due to the encapsulated organisms (pneumococcus, *Haemophilus influenzae* type b). The most common infections tend to involve the respiratory tract: pneumonia (**3.21**), sinusitis, otitis media. Despite the hypergamma-globulinaemia, there is B-cell dysfunction and in some patients IgG2 sub-class deficiency. Broad spectrum antibiotics (third-generation cephalosporins) are given intravenously for serious disease. PCP prophylaxis with daily co-trimoxazole tends to provide some protection against recurrent bacterial infections.

Failure to thrive

This is highly prevalent in developing countries where in the adult HIV population, the malnutrition associated with AIDS, is known as 'slim disease'. Due to the progressive immunodeficiency in HIV infection, gastro-intestinal pathogens (e.g. cryptosporidium, campylobacter, salmonella) often initiate the damage to the gut epithelium leading to chronic diarrhoea and malnutrition. HIV infection itself is probably responsible for a malabsorptive syndrome (**3.22**). Treatment consists of specific therapy for any enteric pathogens isolated and dietary manipulation to decrease the malabsorption and increase calorific intake through the use of an elemental formula. In some cases, continuous overnight nasogastric feeding regimens may be required to provide the necessary calories.

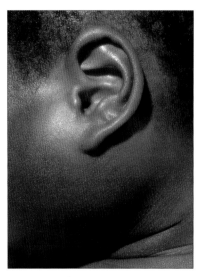

3.18 HIV infection. Parotitis.

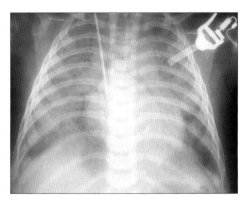

3.19 HIV infection. PCP pneumonitis.

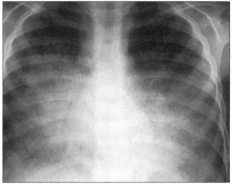

3.20 HIV infection. Reticulonodular infiltrate suggestive of LIP.

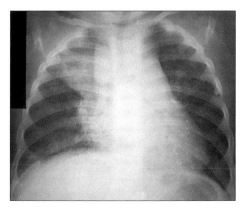

3.21 HIV infection. Bacterial pneumonia.

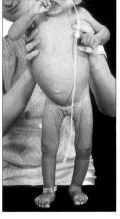

3.22 HIV infection. Malabsorptive syndrome.

HIV encephalopathy

A common early sign is the development of spastic diplegia. There may also be failure to achieve developmental milestones, and in the latter part of the disease, developmental regression and seizures may occur.

Opportunistic infections of the CNS, common in adults, need to be excluded. CT scan findings may show cerebral atrophy (**3.23**) or basal ganglia enhancement/calcification. Treatment with highly active antiretroviral therapy (HAART) may lead to some improvement, with reversal of the cognitive and neurological deficits. Without any treatment, the prognosis is bleak (median survival is 11 months).

CMV retinitis

CMV retinitis occurs in around 1–2% of HIV-infected children. It is the most common paediatric ocular infection. White granular lesions with irregular borders and centred around blood vessels (haemorrhagic lesions may be present) are seen on fundoscopy (**3.24**). It occurs as a result of systemic infection with CMV which may be otherwise asymptomatic. Young children do not usually complain of visual loss, but tend to present with bilateral ocular involvement, unless adequate screening regimens are in place which will detect early disease. Some centres screen all patient with low CD4 counts (i.e. CD4 + <100), and/or who are viraemic with CMV.

Treatment is with ganciclovir (or foscarnet, if no response). Patients, who have a degree of immune reconstitution as a result of combination antiretroviral therapycan stop long-term suppressive therapy with ganciclovir.

Kaposi's sarcoma

This is a rare AIDS-defining illness in children. It usually presents as a lymphadenopathic variant with massive enlargement of groups of lymph nodes (**3.25**). Progressive visceral involvement may occur as well as skin infiltration (**3.26**). Recurrent blood-stained pleural effusions, indicating pulmonary/pleural Kaposi's sarcoma, is one manifestation of visceral disease (**3.27**). The disease is now thought to be associated with a new herpes virus (HHV-8). Treatment in children has consisted of administration of various chemotherapeutic agents :

- Vincristine, bleomycin and doxorubicin.
- Liposomal daunorubicin.
- Interferon-alpha.

These agents are mainly used for control of disease rather cure. The prognosis is generally poor in those patients with advanced immunodeficiency who have no access to HAART.

Prognosis

As far as the natural history of HIV/AIDS is concerned, two patterns are seen in children with perinatally-acquired disease. In around 20–25% of patients, severe immunodeficiency develops in the first year of life with resultant severe opportunistic infections and/or encephalopathy developing. The prognosis in this group of patients is poor, with the majority dying by the age of 2 years. The other 75–80% of infected children have a slower, progressive disease, as is seen in adults. This is also the case in those HIV-infected children who acquired disease via blood products.

Combination antiretroviral therapies have led to a decrease in mortality and hospitalisation rates in infected children. It is also likely that the natural history of the disease will also change in young infants as a result of the increased use of combination antiretroviral therapy, as well as the use of PCP prophylaxis in the first year of life.

Prevention

Apart from educating teenagers with regard to the dangers of unprotected sexual intercourse, the main emphasis in preventative strategies has been to try and decrease perinatal transmission rates, through the administration of AZT (or other HIV therapies) to mothers during the latter part of pregnancy and the intrapartum period, and to the neonate for the first 6 weeks of life. This has been shown to decrease transmission rates by 66%.

Elective Caesarian section has also been shown to exert a protective effect. When these two approaches are combined, with the avoidance of breast-feeding, HIV perinatal

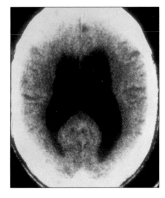

3.23 HIV infection. CT scan showing cerebral atrophy.

transmission rates can be decreased to 1–2%. All of this is obviously dependent on an effective antenatal screening programme being in place.

Treatment

Combination antiretroviral therapy (HAART) is indicated for patients with an AIDS diagnosis, severe symptomatic disease, and in patients with a progressively falling CD4 cell count (CD4 20% of total lymphocytes and/or absolute CD4 counts of less than 250–300), and rising HIV viral loads (>50,000 copies per ml).

It is usual to start with two nucleoside reverse transcriptase inhibitors (NRTI), such as zidovudine (360 mg/mg/m² /day in 2 doses) and lamivudine, (8 mg/kg/day in 2 divided doses), as well as a protease inhibitor (PI), such as nelfinavir (90–150 mg/kg/day in 2 divided doses) or an NNRTI such as Nevirapine. This combination would need to be changed if, or when, there was evidence of therapy failure. Prophylaxis with daily co-trimoxazole (30 mg /kg/day) is important in the prevention of PCP and recurrent bacterial infections.

All immunizations are indicated in this group of patients, except perhaps BCG, and oral polio vaccine (inactivated polio vaccine is preferred). BCG may be considered for asymptomatic children in those countries with high incidence of tuberculosis. Pneumovax, Hib vaccines and meningococcal C conjugate vaccine should also be given.

It is essential that infected children and their families receive comprehensive care that addresses both the medical and psychosocial aspects of this disease. This is best done in a 'family clinic', where both parents and children can be assessed/treated by a multidisciplinary team which would include an adult physician, a paediatrician, psychologist, social worker, HIV counsellor, physiotherapist and dietician.

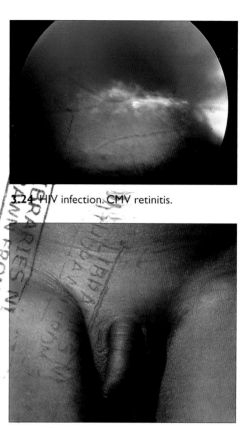

3.24 HIV infection. CMV retinitis.

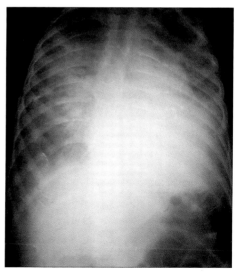

3.25 HIV infection. Kaposi's sarcoma: femoral lymphadenopathy.

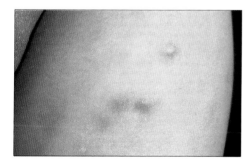

3.26 HIV infection. Kaposi's sarcoma: skin infiltration.

3.27 HIV infection. Kaposi's sarcoma: pulmonary involvement.

INFECTIOUS MONONUCLEOSIS

Clinical presentation

Typical manifestations of the disease include fever, exudative pharyngitis (**3.28**), lymphadenopathy, hepatosplenomegaly, and atypical lymphocytosis. Complications include upper-airway obstruction, thrombocytopaenia, jaundice, and CNS problems (aseptic meningitis, encephalitis, Guillain-Barré syndrome). Infection in the immunocompromised patient may lead to fatal lymphoproliferative disease (e.g. X-linked lymphoproliferative disease). Burkitt B-cell lymphoma and nasopharyngeal carcinoma are associated with EBV infection in Africa and Asia respectively.

Incidence

Although infection usually occurs early in life, an acute primary EBV infection is usually sub-clinical and is not synonymous with infectious mononucleosis, unless typical clinical findings are present. The incidence of infectious mono-nucleosis (IM) is highest in the adolescent age group (15–24 years). The virus is excreted in the saliva and spread by direct contact (kissing disease). It is also spread by blood transfusion.

Diagnosis

Laboratory diagnosis generally rests on serology: non-specific tests such as mono-spot or the Paul-Bunnell test (heterophile antibody tests), and the more specific tests of identifying antibody against the various viral components of EBV (VCA, EA [D & R], EBNA). Acute infection is characterized by the presence of IgM against VCA (viral capsid antigen). Isolation of virus from oropharyngeal secretions and detection of virus via PCR is possible but does not necessarily indicate acute infection. Non-specific laboratory changes include an absolute lymphocytosis (>10% atypical lymphocytes) often with neutropaenia, rarely a haemolytic anemia with pancytopenia, and frequently raised liver enzymes.

Aetiology/pathogenesis

Epstein-Barr virus is a herpes virus which has special affinity for B-lymphocytes. Initial infection takes place in pharyngeal epithelial cells followed by spread to B-lymphocytes. In acute stages of IM, the number of infected circulating B-cells may be high as 5–20%. Proliferation of EB virus is regulated by natural killer cells and T-cytotoxic suppressor cells. Atypical lymphocytes represent T-lymphocytes responding to infected B cells.

Treatment

IM is a self-limited disease, hence treatment is supportive. Steroids have been shown to be beneficial in the upper-airway obstruction due tonsillar hypertrophy and adenopathy. Acyclovir has activity against EBV, but clinical trials do not show any clear benefit. Nevertheless, children with EBV induced lymphoproliferative disease are usually initially treated with acyclovir (or ganciclovir), as well having their immuno-suppressive therapy decreased. Specific monoclonal antibodies (anti-CD20) such as Rituximab have have been shown to be beneficial in some groups of patients.

Prognosis

Most cases of IM resolve over a period of 2–3 weeks. Death from IM is rare. It is usually the result of overwhelming infection in the immunocompromised host or as a result of complications of the disease.

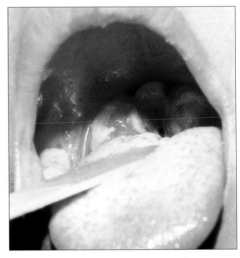

3.28 Infectious mononucleosis. Exudative pharyngitis.

NEONATAL HERPES SIMPLEX VIRUS (HSV) INFECTIONS

Incidence
HSV infection of the neonate can be acquired during the intrauterine, intrapartum or post-natal period. More than 85% of cases occur following intrapartum transmission. In the UK, the incidence of neonatal HSV infection is much less than in the USA.

Aetiology/pathogenesis
The majority of neonatal HSV infections are due to HSV-2 (70%). Following direct exposure to the virus at delivery, the newborn will develop localized disease on the skin, eye or mouth. In some patients, infection will progress to involve the brain, perhaps by intraneuronal transmission of viral particles, or disseminated disease may occur following the development of viraemia. A higher incidence of neonatal herpes has been documented in babies born to mothers with primary (33%) as compared to recurrent genital herpes infection (3%).

Clinical presentation
The hallmark of infection is a vesicular eruption (clusters of vesicles on an erythematous base) on the skin (**3.29**). Presentation is usually within the first 2–4 weeks of life, and most neonatal infections with HSV can usually be divided into one of the following categories:
- Disease localized to the skin, eyes or mouth (40%).
- Localized central nervous system disease (usually encephalitis) (35%).
- Disseminated disease with multiple organ involvement, including lung and liver (25%).

Unfortunately the diagnosis can sometimes be difficult, as skin lesions may not be seen in some patients with disseminated or CNS disease. Disseminated infection may also present with a picture of severe liver dysfunction, mimicking a metabolic disorder, or primarily a sepsis syndrome.

Diagnosis
Herpes simplex virus can be easily cultured from infected tissues. Acute and convalescent sera show rise in antibodies to HSV. Intrathecal synthesis of Herpes antibodies can also be detected in HSV enecephalitis, as can HSV DNA in the CSF by the polymerase chain reaction.

Treatment
Aciclovir, 60 mg/kg/day in three divided doses, intravenously for 14 days (21days for encephalitis or disseminated disease) is recommended. Disease may relapse after discontinuation of therapy. Long term oral suppressive therapy for 6–12 months is controversial, but should be considered. Babies with ocular involvement (keratoconjunctivitis) should also receive a topical antiviral drug (3% vidarabine).

Prognosis
If the diagnosis can be made early when the disease is localized (i.e. skin, eye and/or mouth), antiviral therapy leads to zero mortality and normal development in >90% of infants. Involvement of the brain and disseminated disease leads to mortality rates of 14–50%, with as many as 50% of surviving patients having some form of neurological sequelae.

Prevention
Women with active genital lesions at the time of delivery should be delivered by Caesarian section. Infants born vaginally to mothers with active genital lesions should be observed closely and have HSV cultures taken at 24–48 hours (eyes, mouth, skin, rectum, CSF). If cultures are positive or should the infant develop symptoms, antiviral therapy should be started. Some authorities recommend starting empiric therapy with aciclovir, at birth, pending results of cultures.

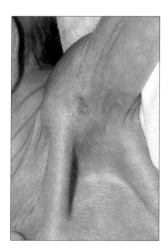

3.29 Neonatal herpes simplex virus (HSV) infection. Vesicular eruption.

VARICELLA (CHICKEN POX)

Incidence
Chicken pox is a highly contagious disease with an estimated 90% of susceptible household contacts developing the disease after exposure. Varicella tends to occur seasonally (late winter, early spring) and in epidemics. In the UK, virtually the whole of the annual birth cohort (600,000) will develop the infection.

Aetiology/pathogenesis
The varicella zoster virus is a herpes virus and primary infection with this agent results in varicella. The incubation period is usually 14 days (ranging between 10–21 days). Transmission occurs from person to person by direct contact or via airborne spread from respiratory secretions. Virus replication occurs in regional cervical lymph nodes following infection of conjunctivae and/or mucosa of the nasopharynx. A primary viraemia ensues in 4–6 days, with viral replication occurring in the liver, spleen and other organs. A secondary viraemia occurs at 10 days, with spread of virus to the skin and subsequent appearance of rash.

Clinical presentation
Varicella is generally a benign illness characterized by the appearance of a maculo–papular vesicular rash, fever, malaise and anorexia. The rash, which may be pruritic, usually crusts over in 5 days and occurs in a centripetal distribution with a characteristic feature of lesions at all stages (macules, papules, vesicles, crusts) being present together (**3.30**).

The most common complication is secondary bacterial infection. Other complications include pneumonitis (**3.31**), hepatitis, encephalitis and orchitis (**3.32**). In the immunocompromised patient, varicella can be life-threatening. There is a progressive eruption of numerous, umbilicated and haemorrhagic vesicles, associated with a high grade fever (**3.33**). Pneumonitis is a common manifestation of disseminated disease in this population.

Diagnosis
Varicella zoster virus can be isolated from vesicular fluid early in the illness. Specific diagnosis can also be accomplished by the staining of vesicle scrapings with fluorescein-tagged VZV specific monoclonal antibodies. Electron microscopy of vesicular fluid will identify a 'herpes virus', while a Tzanck smear will demonstrate multinucleated giant cells with intracellular inclusions. The most reliable serologic tests to detect specific VZV IgM and IgG are the fluorescent antibody to membrane antigen test (FAMA) and the ELISA assay. PCR tests are also being increasingly used.

Treatment
Oral aciclovir is not recommended routinely for treatment of uncomplicated chicken pox in otherwise healthy children. It may be considered for the older child (>12 years), or for those patients taking short courses of steroids (or inhaled steroids). Infection in the immunocompromised host should be treated with intravenous aciclovir $1.5g/m^2/day$ in 3 divided doses for 7–10 days. Children with varicella should not receive salicylates because of the risk of Reye's syndrome.

Prognosis
Five percent of normal children will develop complications, the most common being secondary bacterial infection. In untreated immunocompromised children, one-third of patients will develop disseminated disease, with a mortality of 7%. Varicella is responsible for 20–30 deaths per year in the UK.

Prevention
Strict isolation of cases in negative-pressure rooms is necessary if patients are admitted to hospital. Infectivity occurs from 24–48 hours before, until 5 days after the appearance of the rash. Varicella zoster immunoglobulin should be given to susceptible individuals, in contact with chickenpox, if they are at risk of developing severe varicella. A live-attenuated varicella vaccine is available (and licensed for normal children) in the USA. It is available in the UK on a named-patient basis.

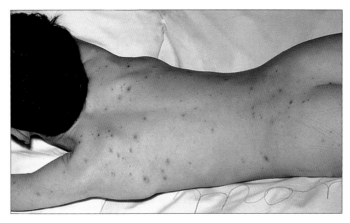

3.30 Varicella (chicken pox). Characteristic lesions.

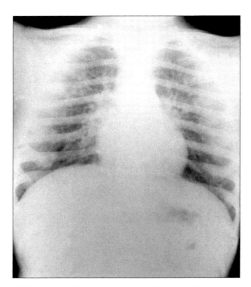

3.31 Varicella (chicken pox). Pneumonitis.

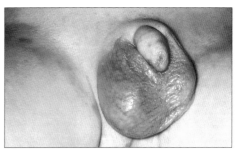

3.32 Varicella (chicken pox). Orchitis.

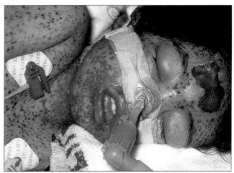

3.33 Varicella (chicken pox). Immuno-compromised patient.

HERPES ZOSTER (SHINGLES)
Incidence
Herpes zoster infection is less common in children than in adults. It is a more common event in the immunosuppressed patient, especially post bone-marrow transplantation (BMT). There is an association between the early development of chickenpox and the appearance of zoster in later childhood.

Aetiology/pathogenesis
Shingles occur as a result of reactivation of latent VZV in the dorsal root ganglia after primary infection with chicken pox. When cell mediated immunity to VZV declines (e.g. onset of immunodeficiency, old age), the virus starts replicating in the ganglia and is transported along the axon to the sensory nerve endings in the skin. Thereafter it replicates locally to produce the characteristic vesicular lesions.

Clinical presentation
The eruptive phase of herpes zoster infection in children starts with the appearance of grouped red papules, which are dermatomal in distribution. These rapidly progress to vesicles, pustules and scab formation in around 5–10 days. The lesions are usually unilateral and may be accompanied by fever and malaise. Pain and tenderness is often felt along the dermatomal distribution, a few days before the onset of the rash. The most commonly affected dermatomes tend to be the thoraco–lumbar (**3.34**) and the trigeminal, especially the ophthalmic division (**3.35**). Immunosuppressed children may have lesions that are outside the involved dermatomes; prolonged eruption of vesicles may occur as well as disseminated visceral disease.

Diagnosis
The characteristic lesions and their distribution usually make the clinical diagnosis. Viral culture of vesicular fluid and specific serological tests to detect rises in VZV IgG may be helpful. Vesicular scrapings to detect multinucleated giant-cells and electron microscopy to detect herpes viruses are less specific tests. PCR tests to detect viral DNA are helpful.

Treatment
Immunocompromised children with zoster should receive intravenous aciclovir $1.5g/m^2/$ day in 3 divided doses for 7–10 days. Healthy children with uncomplicated zoster do not require systemic antiviral therapy.

Prognosis
30% of patients develop zoster in the first year after BMT, with close to 50% having disseminated disease.

Prevention
There is some evidence to suggest that live varicella vaccine may be protective in some groups of immunosuppressed children (haematological malignancies in remission, or on maintenance chemotherapy) against the development of subsequent zoster, compared to a control group who were infected with wild-type virus.

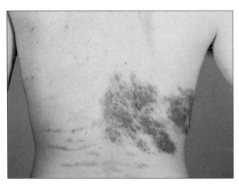

3.34 Herpes zoster (shingles). Thoraco–lumbar infection.

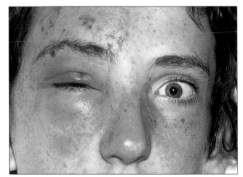

3.35 Herpes zoster (shingles). Ophthalmic infection.

MEASLES
Clinical Presentation
Measles begins with a prodromal period of 3–5 days which is characterized by a fever, cough, runny nose and conjunctivitis. Koplik's spots (grayish-white dots) (**3.36**) appear on the buccal mucosa opposite the upper and lower premolar teeth some 24–48 hours before the onset of rash. These are a pathognomonic exanthem of measles and may persist up to 2–3 days after the rash has appeared. The characteristic rash usually appears around the fourth day, as the fever peaks. It is an erythematous, blanching maculopapular eruption (**3.37**) that starts at the hairline and spreads down, eventually involving the hands and feet. The rash tends to become confluent and after 2–3 days starts to fade, with clearing over 2–3 days. A brawny desquamation of the skin often follows.

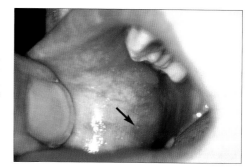

3.36 Koplik's spots present on the buccal mucosa.

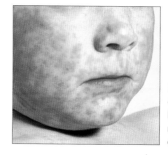

3.37 Measles exanthem – a blanching, maculopapular eruption

Incidence
Prior to immunization programmes being instituted, measles was common in childhood, with epidemics occurring every 2–3 years. In the UK, following the introduction of MMR in 1988, the incidence decreased from around 150,000 cases per year to less than 10,000 cases in 1993. Measles is till responsible for around 1–2 million deaths per year, mainly in developing countries.

Diagnosis
Clinical diagnosis is based on the presence of a characteristic rash, fever, conjunctivitis, rhinitis, and cough. Salivary tests for detecting the presence of anti-measles IgM antibodies are available for confirming the diagnosis. Serologic tests (ELISA) are also used to detect IgG and IgM antibodies. A nasopharyngeal aspirate can also be used to confirm the diagnosis by performing immunofluorescence testing for the presence of measles antigen. Viral isolation is rarely performed.

Aetiology/Pathogenesis:
Measles is caused by the measles virus, which is an RNA virus of the genus Morbillivirus, of the *Paramyxoviridae* family. It is transmitted by droplet infection, with the virus replicating intially in the respiratory tract. During the prodromal period, and for a short time after the rash appears, it is found in nasopharyngeal secretions, blood and urine. Patients are infectious from 4 days before the rash appears, until 4 days after its appearance.

Complications
Complications of measles include otitis media, pneumonia, laryngotracheitis, and encephalitis. These may occur as a result of the primary viral illness or due to secondary bacterial invasion. SSPE (subacute sclerosing panencephalitis) is a rare and late complication of measles infection, occurring many years after primary infection. It is characterized by the onset of gradual intellectual deterioration, incoordination and seizures.

Management
Prevention through routine immunization with MMR (2 doses – 15months, 4 years) is the priority. Treatment of disease remains symptomatic. Patients require appropriate isolation, hydration, and administration of antibiotics for any secondary bacterial infections (pneumonia, otitis media). Respiratory support may be required for severe croup, whilst steroids have proven of some use for measles encephalitis. Vitamin A should be given to children who are malnourished, Vitamin A deficient or immunodeficient. Antiviral therapy (Ribavirin, Interferon-alpha) for giant-cell pneumonia in the immunodeficient host is not established.

PROTOZOA / FUNGI / TROPICAL DISEASES / MISCELLANEOUS

CONGENITAL TOXOPLASMOSIS (CT)

Incidence

The incidence of maternal toxoplasmosis in the UK is thought to be around 1:500 pregnancies. The transmission rate to the fetus is thought be about 40%, with a higher risk of congenital infection being associated with the latter stages of pregnancy. Most infants with congenital toxoplasmosis (CT) are asymptomatic at birth (90%). The BPSU estimates that about 14 infants per year may be born in the UK with severe symptomatic CT.

Aetiology/pathogenesis

Toxoplasma gondii is an intracellular coccidian parasite with a world-wide distribution. Members of the cat family are the definitive hosts. Humans acquire the disease by consumption of poorly cooked meat or ingestion of oocysts from soil or contaminated food. When the disease is acquired in pregnancy, transplacental transmission of the parasite may occur with potentially serious sequelae for the fetus and newborn. The severity of CT is related to the period of gestation when maternal disease was acquired: infection in early pregnancy results in the more severe form of congenital disease.

Clinical presentation

The clinical manifestations include the 'classic triad' of hydrocephalus, intracranial calcification (**3.38**), and choroidoretinitis. Other non-specific features which may be seen include jaundice, hepatosplenomegaly, thrombocytopenia, maculopapular rash, dysmaturity, lymphadenopathy, microphthalmia and seizures.

Diagnosis

A diagnosis of CT can be made by detection of specific toxoplasma IgM or IgA (ELISA/ISAGA), the persistence of specific IgG antibodies beyond 12 months (passively transmitted antibodies usually disappear by this time in an uninfected child), or the isolation of the parasite by mouse inoculation.

Toxoplasma PCR is available in some centres to detect the presence of parasite DNA in blood, CSF or amniotic fluid. Other investigations that may be helpful include computerized tomography of the head, and CSF examination (pleocytosis and high protein).

Treatment

All infants with CT should be treated irrespective of clinical findings. Therapy should be for a total of 12 months and should include the combination of pyrimethamine (2 mg/kg/day for the first 2 days, followed by 1 mg/kg/day – maximum of 25 mg/day), sulfadiazine (100 mg/kg/day, q6h), and folinic acid (5 mg three times weekly) for the first 6 weeks. This is followed by thrice-weekly pyrimethamine and folinic acid, and daily sulfadiazine for the rest of the treatment course. Steroids are given for choroidoretinitis when there is macular involvement.

Prognosis

Most congenital infections are asymptomatic at birth (90–95%). There is significant mortality among those neonates who are severely symptomatic at birth; most who survive have neurological sequelae. Up to 80% of congenitally infected neonates who are asymptomatic at birth may present later in life with visual impairment, learning disabilities, or mental retardation.

Prevention

Pregnant women should avoid contact with cats and cat litter, and gardening should not be undertaken. Hands should be washed after handling raw meat and vegetables; all meat should be thoroughly cooked before eating.

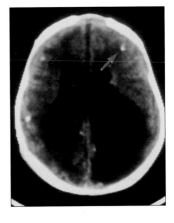

3.38
Congenital toxo-plasmosis. Intracranial calcification.

CRYPTOSPORIDIOSIS

Incidence
Disease prevalence is higher in underdeveloped countries (8.5% compared with 2.1% in industrialized communities). The highest incidence is in young children aged 6–24 months. Symptoms appear after an incubation period of 2–14 days. The main source of transmission is person-to-person, although animal to human (farm livestock) and waterborne outbreaks have occurred.

Aetiology/pathogenesis
Cryptosporidium parvum is an intracellular coccidian protozoan parasite which invades the epithelial lining of the intestinal and respiratory tracts. Following ingestion of oocysts, excystation occurs with the release of sporozoites which attach to intestinal epithelial cells, forming parasitiphorous vacuoles (**3.39**). An asexual intestinal cycle leads to reinfection of enterocytes and a sexual intestinal phase produces oocysts that are excreted in the stools.

Clinical presentation
Infection in immunocompetent individuals results in a self-limited diarrhoeal illness (average of 10 days), associated with low-grade fever, anorexia, abdominal pain and weight loss. The infection in immunocompromised patients, especially those with defective cellular immunity, is characterized by chronic profuse watery diarrhoea, malabsorption, extreme weight loss and, in some cases, a fatal outcome. Disseminated disease (pulmonary, biliary tract) may also be seen in this population.

Diagnosis
Definitive diagnosis is made by microscopic identification of oocysts in stool specimens stained with a modified acid-fast technique, or by identification of the organism in jejunal tissue obtained at biopsy. At least three separate stool specimens should be examined before considering the test to be negative.

Treatment
To date there is no fully effective therapeutic agent against cryptosporidium. Paramomycin, azithromycin, nitazoxanide and hyperimmune bovine colostrum have all been used with limited success. Supportive therapy, along with adequate fluid replacement (with or without parenteral nutrition) is important.

In HIV patients, anti-diarrhoeal agents are also often used as symptomatic treatment.

Prevention
Immunocompromised patients should boil their drinking water and avoid contact with potential sources of infection (such as farm animals and pets). People with diarrhoea should not use public swimming pools.

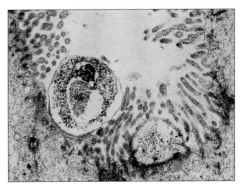

3.39 Cryptosporidiosis. Appearance of parasitiphorous vacuoles at biopsy.

CYSTICERCOSIS (NEUROCYSTICERCOSIS)

Incidence

The disease is endemic in rural areas of Latin America, South East Asia and Africa. Autopsy studies in some areas show that up to 3.5% of the population have cysticercosis.

Aetiology/pathogenesis

The disease is caused by infection with the larval stage (cysticerci) of the pork tapeworm, *Taenia solium*, (**3.40**). It is acquired by ingesting eggs of the pork tapeworm which are shed in the faeces of human carriers of tapeworm (these acquire the adult tapeworm through eating inadequately cooked pork). Autoinfection is also a recognizable route of infection. Between 24 and 72 hours after the eggs are ingested, larvae hatch and penetrate the small intestinal wall and then migrate via the circulation, to sites throughout the body. Symptoms appear when a granulomatous reaction eventually ensues around dead or dying cysts.

Clinical presentation

Symptoms depend on the location, size and number of cysticerci. Any tissue can be affected, the most common being brain, subcutaneous tissue, muscle and eye. Painless lumps under the skin are characteristic of subcutaneous cysticerci. Involvement of the central nervous system (neurocysticercosis) presents mainly as epilepsy in more than half of affected patients, some 4–8 years after infection. Other neurological symptoms that may be seen include transient hemiplegia, obstructive hydrocephalus and meningitis.

Diagnosis

Neurocysticercosis is diagnosed by a CT scan of the head (**3.41**) or MRI (**3.42**). These show multiple enhancing and non-enhancing cysts which later may become calcified. The enzyme-linked immunotransfer blot detects antibody to *Taenia solium* and is the best serologic test available.

Treatment

Cysticidal therapy is beneficial in those children with multiple cysts, viable cysts,or symptomatic disease. Praziquantel (50 mg/kg/day in 3 divided doses for 2 weeks) is the treatment of choice. Dexamethasone is usually also given in the first week of treatment to reduce the inflammatory reaction induced by the dead larvae. Albendazole (15 mg/kg/day in 2 divided doses for 4 weeks) should be tried if praziquantel is not effective.

Prognosis

Between 80% and 90% of patients respond to medical therapy with complete disappearance or regression in cyst volume. Around 60% of patients remain seizure-free after cysticidal therapy. Patients who have a single ring-enhancing lesion often have spontaneous resolution of the lesion.

Prevention

Eating raw or undercooked pork should be avoided. Stool examination of the patient and close family contacts should be carried out. Those harbouring the adult tapeworm should be treated.

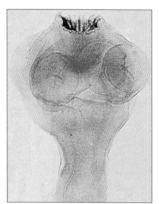

3.40 Cysticercosis. *Taenia solium.*

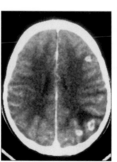

3.41 Cysticercosis. Appearance of head (CT scan).

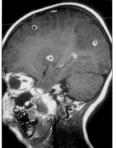

3.42 Cysticercosis. Appearance of head (MRI).

INVASIVE ASPERGILLOSIS

Incidence

Aspergillus species are ubiquitous saprophytic moulds present in the environment. The incidence of disease varies between 4–8% in various groups of immunocompromised patients (BMT, SCID, CGD). They are second only to *Candida* species in the frequency of opportunistic mycoses. Outbreaks of disease have been reported on transplant units in close proximity to building sites.

Aetiology/pathogenesis

Infection with the organism is usually initiated by inhalation of air-borne spores. In the immunocompromised host, *Aspergillus* tends to invade blood vessels resulting in infarction, necrosis and haematogeneously disseminated disease. *A fumigatus* is the usual cause of invasive disease, although *A flavus* is also important.

Clinical presentation

Occurs almost exclusively in immunocompromised patients, especially those with prolonged and profound neutropenia. The most common clinical presentation is pulmonary aspergillosis. These patients present with persisting fever not responding to antibiotics, abnormal chest x-ray (often with new infiltrates appearing) (**3.43**), cough, haemoptysis and pleuritic chest pain. Other clinical syndromes include: cutaneous disease (**3.44**), spinal osteomyelitis, cerebral abscess (**3.45**), and renal involvement.

Diagnosis

Definitive diagnosis requires histopathological evidence of *Aspergillus* hyphae in tissue as well as isolation of an *Aspergillus* species in culture.

Treatment

Amphotericin B in high doses is the treatment of choice, with or without the addition of flucytosine for at least 6 weeks. Other antifungals that have been used include liposomal amphotericin B (ambisome) or itraconazole. Ambisome should be considered for patients who are intolerant to standard amphotericin B, or in those who are not responding (doses from 3-7.5 mg/kg have been used). In some units, ambisome has replaced standard Amphoterecin B as the main antifungal agent. Voricanozole, which is undergoing trials at present, is a new parenteral azole that is effective against *Aspergillus* species. Surgical resection of localized lesions may be required in some patients.

Prevention

Some evidence supports the use of oral itraconazole as fungal prophylaxis in high risk patients. Nursing patients in air-filtered areas (HEPA) also decreases exposure of patients to high *Aspergillus* counts.

Prognosis

Mortality rates are around 70%, with the highest rate being observed in subgroups of children undergoing BMT for SCID or haematological malignancies. Earlier diagnosis and therapy as well as the future development of effective prophylactic regimens will lead to lower mortality rates.

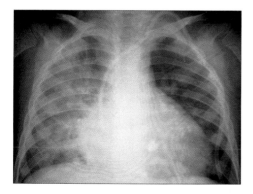

3.43 Invasive aspergillosis. Chest x-ray.

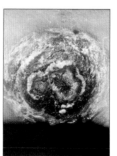

3.44 Invasive aspergillosis. Skin lesion.

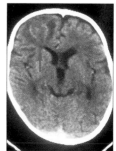

3.45 Invasive aspergillosis. Cerebral abscess.

MALARIA

Incidence

Each year, world-wide, there are 200 million cases, with around 1 million deaths (mainly African infants). In the UK, 2,000 cases of imported malaria are seen each year. Most cases (60%) are due to *P falciparum* acquired in Africa with between 5 and 10 deaths reported each year.

Aetiology/pathogenesis

Malaria is caused by invasion of erythrocytes by one of the species of intracellular protozoa of the genus *Plasmodium*. Those species infecting humans are: *P falciparum* (**3.46**), *P vivax*, *P malariae* and *P ovale*. Transmission of the parasite is usually through the bite of an infected female *Anopheles* mosquito.

The severe complications seen in *P falciparum* malaria are the result of the high parasitaemia, followed by sequestration of parasitized red blood cells in deep vascular beds (including the cerebral vasculature). Vascular occlusion subsequently occurs with resultant tissue anoxia and the development of clinical symptoms, including a diffuse encephalopathy in cerebral malaria.

Clinical presentation

Symptoms tend to be paroxysmal with high fever, chills, sweating and headaches in a cyclical pattern. Jaundice and anaemia as a result of haemolysis, as well as hepatosplenomegaly may be found on physical examination. *Plasmodium falciparum* tends to cause the most severe disease, ranging from cerebral malaria (**3.47**), renal failure, shock, pulmonary oedema, hypoglycaemia and haemoglobinuria ('blackwater fever').

Diagnosis

A thick smear, stained by Giesma, identifies the presence of malarial parasites in the peripheral blood and a thin smear identifies the type of malarial species causing disease.

Treatment

All children with malaria due to *P falciparum* require admission to hospital. Treatment with parenteral quinine is recommended in severe or complicated cases. A loading dose of intravenous (IV) quinine 15mg/kg of salt, given over 2 hours in 20 ml normal saline, is followed by a maintenance dose of IV quinine 20 mg/kg/day in two divided doses until oral therapy can be started (quinine 30 mg/kg (salt)/day, in three divided doses). Therapy is for 7 days; one dose of fansidar is usually also given at the end of treatment (<1 yr – ¼ tablet; 1–3 years – ½ tablet; 4–8 years – 1 tablet; 9–14 years – 2 tablets). For other strains of malaria, chloroquine is the drug of choice (25 mg/kg of base, over 48 hours).

Prognosis

In endemic areas, infants, young children, and non-immune visitors are at highest risk of infection. In cerebral malaria, which occurs in about 1% of patients infected with *P falciparum*, there is a mortality rate of 10–30%, with focal neurological damage in 10%.

Prevention

The following general measures should be adopted to prevent mosquito bites: use of bed nets impregnated with Permethrin, wearing of appropriate clothing (i.e. long sleeves, trousers), and the use of insect repellants. Prophylactic anti-malarials should be taken 1–2 weeks before departure to an endemic area and continued for 4 weeks after returning.

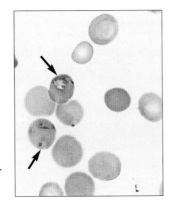

3.46 Malaria. *Plasmodium falciparum.*

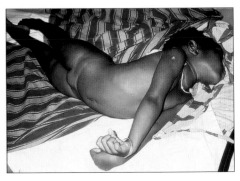

3.47 Cerebral malaria.

SCHISTOSOMIASIS (URINARY)

Incidence

The disease is endemic in Africa and Southwest Asia. The presence of the specific snail host and the inappropriate disposal of human excreta in the environment are essential in maintaining endemicity of the disease. World-wide, 200 million are infected with the five major species of schistosomes.

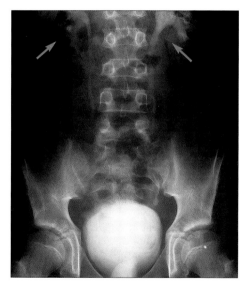

3.48 Schistosomiasis (urinary). Hydronephrosis.

Aetiology/pathogenesis

Schistosoma haematobium is a blood fluke (trematode) that inhabits the venous plexuses of the urinary bladder. Large numbers of eggs are laid by the female every day. Eggs retained in the tissues cause a tissue reaction with the formation of multiple granulomas and eventual fibrotic lesions, leading to obstructive uropathy. The expelled eggs hatch in fresh water and the liberated miracidiae invade the snail intermediate host. Cercariae are eventually released which penetrate the skin of a human swimmer, and then migrate to the lung and liver and finally to the venous plexus of the bladder.

Clinical presentation

The early manifestations in children infected with *S haematobium* are frequency, dysuria and terminal hematuria. Symptoms of obstructive uropathy (straining, dribbling, incomplete emptying of the bladder and constant urge to urinate) occur in advanced infection. End-stage disease results in hydronephrosis (**3.48**) and uraemia. CNS involvement is occasionally seen.

Diagnosis

Microscopic examination of centrifuged urine, collected between 12 and 2 pm, demonstrates the characteristic *S haematobium* eggs with the lateral spine (**3.49**). Egg viability should be determined by hatch test. Biopsy of the bladder mucosa may be necessary if urine tests are negative. IVP and cystoscopy indicate the extent of the disease. Serologic tests (ELISA, RIA) to detect schistosomal antibodies are available.

Treatment

Praziquantel: 2 oral doses of 20 mg/kg in 1 day. Some authorities recommend this to be repeated after 2 weeks.

Prognosis

Egg/worm burden has been shown to be related to severity of disease. Urinary tract lesions are reversible if treatment is initiated early in the course of the illness. In advanced disease, despite parasitologic cure, surgical intervention may be required. An association between chronic schistosomiasis and bladder cancer has been noted.

Prevention

Health education, along with treatment of infected hosts and proper disposal of human excreta are the mainstays of prevention. Travellers should avoid freshwater streams and lakes.

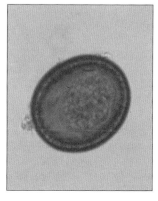

3.49 Schistosomiasis (urinary). Characteristic *S. haemotobium* egg, with lateral spine.

KAWASAKI DISEASE

See also 'Emergency Medicine' (page 26) and 'Rheumatology' chapters.

Incidence

The disease is most prevalent in Japan, where epidemics occur every three years. In the UK there are around 100 cases reported each year with an estimated incidence of 15 per million children, which is probably an underestimate of the true incidence of the disease. About 80% of affected patients are under 4 years of age. There is little evidence for person-to-person transmission, although siblings and some contacts of index cases have been affected.

Aetiology/pathogenesis

Clinical features suggest an infectious aetiology, however a microbial agent has not been conclusively implicated. Current evidence suggests the disease is the result of superantigen activity (i.e. a toxin with superantigen properties is able to cause widespread activation of the immune system with massive cytokine release and consequent initiation of generalized inflammatory changes and vasculitis). The pathological lesion in Kawasaki disease is thus a vasculitis affecting small to medium-sized musculo-elastic arteries throughout the body but with a predilection for the coronary vessels. Medial disruption and formation of coronary artery aneurysms (CAA) may occur.

Clinical presentation

Kawasaki disease is an acute febrile illness of unknown aetiology, affecting predominantly infants and young children. It is a leading cause of acquired heart disease in children. It is characterized by a prolonged remittent fever, mucositis (**3.50**), conjunctivitis, polymorphous skin rash (**3.51**), cervical adenopathy and oedema of the hands and feet with subsequent desquamation (**3.52**). Cardiac involvement with coronary arteritis and aneurysm formation (**3.53**) may occur, with fatal consequences.

Diagnosis

The diagnosis is based on the presence of five of six principal clinical criteria (mentioned above), without other explanation for the illness. Laboratory investigations are non-specific: normochromic normocytic anaemia, leukocytosis, thrombocytosis (in the second week), raised ESR and CRP, along with hypoalbuminaemia may be present.

Treatment

A single high dose of intravenous immunoglobulin (2 g/kg) given over 10–12 hours, within the first 10 days of the illness, along with the initiation of high dose aspirin therapy (100 mg/kg/day in 4 divided doses) is the mainstay of treatment. Once the fever has defervesced (or on the 14th day) the aspirin is changed to 3–5 mg/kg once daily as antiplatelet therapy and continued for 2–3 months. Some patients may require additional doses of immunoglobulin if symptoms persist.

Echocardiograms are obtained at diagnosis, 1 week into the illness and at 4–6 weeks after the start of the illness. If CAA are detected, dipyridamole may be added to the aspirin therapy and continued indefinitely.

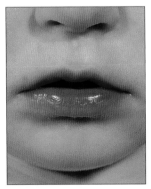

3.50 Kawasaki disease. Mucositis.

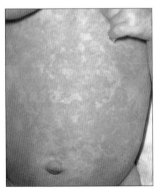

3.51 Kawasaki disease. Polymorphous skin rash.

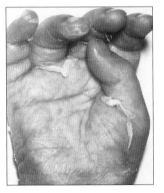

3.52 Kawasaki disease. Desquamation of the hand.

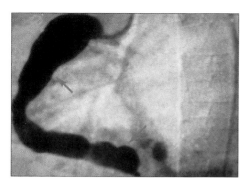

3.53 Kawasaki disease. Multiple right coronary artery aneurysms on angiogram.

Prognosis

In patients not receiving high-dose immuno-globulin within the first 10 days of the illness, the incidence of CAA is 15–30%. In treated patients the incidence is less than 5%. Regression of CAA may occur in around 50% of patients over a 1–2 year period. Sudden death from coronary thrombosis and myocardial infarction occurs in approximately 1–2% of untreated patients.

REFERENCES

Diphtheria
Feigin RD, Stechenburg BW, Aguilar LK. (1998) Diphtheria. In: Feigin RD, Cherry JD (eds). *Textbook of Pediatric Infectious Diseases* (4th edn). Philadelphia: Saunders, 1998: 1169–1175.

Meningococcal infections
Pollard AJ, Faust SN, Levin M. Meningitis and meningococcal septicaemia. *J Roy Coll Phys* 1998; **32**: 319–328.

Tetanus
Brook I. (2003) Clostridium tetani (Tetanus). In Long S, Pickering L, Probeer C (eds). *Principles and Practice of Pediatric Infectious Diseases* (2nd edition). Churchill Livingstone, 2003: 981–984.

Tuberculosis
Shingadia D, Novelli V. Diagnosis and treatment of tuberculosis in children. *Lancet Infect Dis* 2003; **3**: 624–632.

Tuberculous meningitis
Farinha N, Razali B, Holzel H, Morgan G, Novelli VM. Tuberculosis of the central nervous system in children: a 20 year survey. *J Infect* 2000; **41**: 1–8.

Non-tuberculous mycobacterial infections
Starke JR. Nontuberculous mycobacterial infection in children. *Advan Ped Infect Dis* 1994; 7: 121–159.

Staphylococcal toxic shock syndrome
Lowy FD. Staphylococcal aureus infections. *N Engl J Med* 1998; **339**: 520–532.

Pyogenic liver abscess
Kaplan S. Pyogenic Liver Abscess. In: Feigin RD, Cherry JD (eds). *Textbook of Pediatric Infectious Diseases* (4th edn). Philadelphia: Saunders, 1998: 655–658.

HIV infection and AIDS
Gibb D, Butler K, Klein N et al. *Guidelines for Management of Children with HIV Infection* (3rd edn). Horsham, West Sussex: AVERT, 1998.
Katz BZ. Epstein-Barr Virus (Mononucleosis and Lymphoproliferative Disorders). In: Long S, Pickering L, Prober C (eds.). *Principles and Practice of Pediatric Infectious Diseases*. New York: Churchill Livingstone, 2003: 1059–1068.

Neonatal herpes simplex virus (HSV) infections
Whitley RJ. Herpes Simplex Infections. In: Glaser R, Jones JE (eds). *Herpes Virus Infections*. New York: Marcel Decker, 1994: 1–58.

Varicella (chicken-pox)
Al-Ansari H, Novelli V. Acyclovir in the treatment of chicken-pox. *Matern Child Health* 1995; **20**: 248–253.

Herpes zoster (shingles)
Grose C. Varicella Zoster Virus Infection: Chickenpox, Shingles and Varicella Vaccine. In: Glaser R, Jones JE (eds). *Herpes Virus Infections*. New York: Marcel Decker, 1994: 117–185.

Measles
Maldonado Y. (2004) Measles. In Behrman RE, Kliegman RM, Jenson HB (eds): *Nelson Textbook of Pediatrics*. 17th edition. Philadelphia, WB Saunders Co. 2004: 1026–1032.

Congenital toxoplasmosis
American Academy of Pediatrics. Toxoplasma Gondii Infections. In: Pickering LK. (ed). *2000 Red Book: Report of the Committee on Infectious Diseases* (26th edn). Elk Grove Village, Ill: American Academy of Pediatrics, 2003: 631–635.

Cryptosporidiosis
American Academy of Pediatrics. Cryptosporidiosis. In: Pickering LK. (ed). *2000 Red Book: Report of the Committee on Infectious Diseases* (26th edn). Elk Grove Village, Ill: American Academy of Pediatrics, 2003: 255–257.

Cysticercosis (neurocysticercosis)
St Geme JW, Maldonado YA, Enzmann D et al. Consensus: diagnosis and management of neurocysticercosis in children. *Ped Infect Dis J* 1993: **12**: 455.

Invasive aspergillosis
Walmsley S, Devi S, King S et al. Invasive Aspergillus infections in a pediatric hospital: a ten year review. *Ped Infect Dis J* 1993; **12**: 673–682.

Malaria
Crawley J. Malaria : new challenges, new treatments. *Curr Paed* 1999, **9**: 34–41.

Schistosomiasis (urinary)
Maguire JH. Trematodes (Schistosomes) and Other Flukes. In: Mandell GL, Bennett JE, Dolin R (eds). *Principles and Practice of Infectious Diseases* (6th edn). New York: Churchill Livingstone, 2005: 3276–3285.

Kawasaki disease
Brogan PA, Bose A, Burgner D, Shingadia D, Tulloh R et al. Kawasaki disease: an evidence based approach to diagnosis, treatment, and proposals for future research. *Arch Dis Child*. 2002; **86**: 286–290.

Respiratory Medicine

Robert Dinwiddie
Colin Wallis

CYSTIC FIBROSIS

INCIDENCE
The incidence is approximately 1 in 2,500 in Caucasians with a wide variation, although usually lesser frequency, in other ethnic groups. Carriers are normal healthy individuals with a population frequency of 1 in 20 to 1 in 25.

AETIOLOGY / PATHOGENESIS
Cystic fibrosis (CF) is an autosomal recessive disease caused by a gene defect on the long arm of chromosome 7. The most common mutation in Caucasians is delta F508, accounting for some 70% of the gene types seen in Northern Europeans. Over 1,000 other mutations have been described, a number of which are specific to other ethnic groups. A combination of any two similar or different CF genes will cause the disease.

Clinically, different genotypes do not usually produce disease of significantly varying severity.

The gene defect codes for an abnormal protein called the cystic fibrosis transmembrane regulating protein (CFTR). This principally controls chloride and the associated sodium transport across cell membranes which, when abnormal, results in unusually viscid and sticky secretions especially in the lung and the pancreas. It may also have a role in the immune defence of the respiratory epithelium thus promoting bacterial infection. There is also an absence of the vas deferens in males in intrauterine life which leads to infertility in almost all cases. Diabetes is also an increasingly common complication with age. The liver is also affected over time leading to hepatic cirrhosis. Gene therapy for the respiratory complications is under investigation but is not a treatment option at the present time.

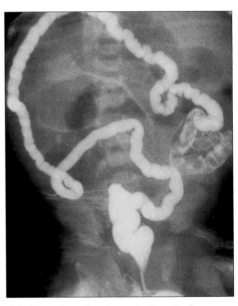

4.1 Meconium ileus in cystic fibrosis. Contrast study showing micro-colon.

CLINICAL PRESENTATION
The most common presentation is with recurrent chest infection, failure to thrive and steatorrhoea. Other modes of presentation include neonatal bowel obstruction due to meconium ileus in about 10–15% of cases (**4.1**), hypoproteinaemia, anaemia and oedema, nasal polyposis, hepatic cirrhosis and, rarely, infertility in young adulthood. Other cases may be detected by neonatal screening where this is practised or by a family history of siblings with the illness.

DIAGNOSIS

Diagnosis is by identification of the genotypes, which is possible in over 90% of cases.

Elevated levels of sodium and chloride in sweat remain major diagnostic criteria in those with typical clinical features in whom two genes cannot be specifically identified. Most children develop respiratory symptoms early in life. These are highly variable in severity but arise from recurrent infections, initially viral but subsequently due to infection with bacteria especially *Staphylococcus aureus, Haemophilus influenzae* and *Pseudomonas aeruginosa.*

TREATMENT

Prophylactic flucloxacillin commences from diagnosis to delay the onset of chronic Staphylococcal infection as long as possible. As age increases there may be persistent symptoms of cough, chronic sputum production and wheeze related to the development of long term airway damage and bronchiectasis (**4.2**). The major pathogen which increases in prevalence with age is *Pseudomonas aeruginosa.* When initial infection occurs it should be treated with oral ciprofloxacin and inhaled colomycin. Prophylactic inhaled colomycin or tobramycin may be needed long-term. Intensive two-week courses of intravenous antibiotics are often necessary to control *Pseudomonas*-related lung infection.

Burkholderia cepacia is another important organism, usually multi-resistant, which can cause severe and even fatal lung disease in a small but important number of cases. Cross-infection between patients is best prevented by separation and avoidance of intimate physical contact. Treatment of the chest requires physiotherapy by a number of techniques in almost all cases on a daily basis

Bronchodilators and inhaled steroids are useful for those with significant wheeze or asthma. Mucolytic agents such as nebulized acetylcysteine can be helpful in selected cases. Hypertonic saline may have similar effects. DNase is also of significant benefit in children with CF who have reduced lung function and significant cough and sputum production. Heart/lung transplantation is an option for those with end stage lung disease. However the supply of donors is very limited, with survival rates in the order of 70% at one year and 60% at five years post transplant. Pancreatic insufficiency is seen in over 90% of cases and requires supplementation with pancreatic enzymes. Given in sufficient amounts a normal or energy-rich diet is well tolerated. The exact dose of enzymes has to be limited to the individual on a day to day basis. There is a small risk of fibrosing colonopathy if too much enzyme is given and current recommendations suggest that the daily lipase intake is kept below 10–15,000 units per kilogram body-weight per day.

Other important bowel related problems include distal intestinal obstruction syndrome (DIOS) which requires treatment with lactulose, oral acetylcysteine, gastrografin or 'kleen prep' depending on its severity. Intestinal obstruction can occur due to this problem or secondary to adhesions from previous surgery or stricture formation. CF related diabetes is seen in 1–2% of children and as many as 15% of adults. Urinalysis for glycosuria should always be carried out when the patient has shown weight loss for no other obvious reason. Liver dysfunction leading to hepatic cirrhosis is another problem seen in 10–15% of children, especially in adolescence. This can lead to splenomegaly, portal hypertension, oesophageal varices and haematemesis. The use of ursodeoxycholic acid may be helpful in slowing the progress of hepatic disease over time. Liver transplantation is useful in those with end-stage disease.

PROGNOSIS

Long-term survival in cystic fibrosis is increasing steadily with a current median life expectancy of 31 years in the best centres. A life expectancy of 40 years can be predicted for a newborn with CF today.

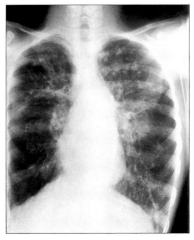

4.2 Chest x-ray of a child with advanced cystic fibrosis lung disease. There is severe over-inflation, generalized bronchial-wall thickening and bilateral bronchiectasis.

ASTHMA AND RECURRENT WHEEZE

INCIDENCE
Current estimates suggest that 20–30% of children will wheeze during the first three years of life.

AETIOLOGY / PATHOGENESIS
The major precipitant is viral lower respiratory tract infection (see also 'Emergency Medicine' chapter). Approximately 60% of these children who are non-atopic will outgrow this tendency and will not have significantly more wheeze than those who did not wheeze during early life. Maternal smoking in pregnancy, which can affect lung growth *in utero* and reduce small airway diameter at birth, may be an important predisposing factor to recurrent wheeze in these children. Those who go on to have typical asthma in later childhood are much more likely to be atopic with a positive family history of asthma, hay fever, food allergy, allergic conjunctivitis or eczema (**4.3**).

DIFFERENTIAL DIAGNOSIS
Differential diagnosis in childhood is important. It has been said that 'all that wheezes is not asthma and all that's asthma does not wheeze'. Other conditions to consider include post-bronchiolitis wheeze, recurrent aspiration with or without gastro-oesophageal reflux, cystic fibrosis, cilia dyskinesia, immune deficiency, foreign body aspiration, vascular ring, vocal cord dysfunction, tracheobroncho-malacia, cysts or glands pressing on the airway, congenital lobar emphysema, cardiac failure and drug reactions (for example, to propranolol).

DIAGNOSIS
Individual case investigation will vary greatly in complexity depending on the clinical certainty of diagnosis. Where there is doubt, full investigation to exclude other conditions is warranted. Alternatively, if there is a clear family history and an individual background of atopy with typical clinical features then the diagnosis of asthma can be made on clinical grounds alone. The most important conditions to exclude when there is doubt are cystic fibrosis, recurrent aspiration with or without reflux and immune deficiency.

TREATMENT
This needs to be tailored to the individual in relation to the frequency and severity of attacks. There are now well established guidelines for the best approach to management. Initially this will involve the use of inhaled bronchodilators (such as the beta-2-agonists salbutamol or terbutaline). Ipratropium bromide is also useful, especially in infants. If treatment is required more than three times weekly then prophylaxis with an inhaled steroid (such as beclo-methasone, budesonide or fluticasone) is indicated. The dosage schedule recommended is clearly set out in the guidelines. If control is not achieved then other agents (such as inhaled salmeterol, eformoterol or occasionally oral theophylline) may be useful. The use of oral steroids on a daily basis is largely confined to acute exacerbations but is required, preferably on an alternate day basis, in a small number of severe cases. The leukotriene antagonists are a useful adjunct to treatment in those where asthma control with inhaled steroids and other agents is unsuccessful.

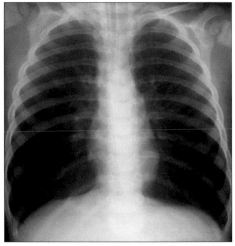

4.3 Severe over-inflation in asthma.

BRONCHIOLITIS

See also 'Emergency Medicine' chapter.

INCIDENCE

This mainly affects children between 3 months and 2 years of age and occurs seasonally between late autumn and early spring. Respiratory syncytial virus (RSV) is also a major cause of pneumonia in children of this age group.

AETIOLOGY / PATHOGENESIS

It is an acute infection in which the main effects are seen at the bronchiolar level in the lung. It is caused principally by viruses, especially RSV which accounts for around 70% of cases. Influenza, parainfluenza and adenovirus can also cause this illness.

There is widespread inflammation, oedema and hypersecretion in the lower airways. This leads to significant small airway obstruction causing hyperinflation, air trapping and wheezing. These changes are exacerbated in those who have underlying lung disease such as bronchopulmonary dysplasia or cystic fibrosis.

DIAGNOSIS

Auscultation of the chest reveals high pitched wheezing throughout both lung fields and also widespread crackles. Chest x-ray typically shows hyperinflation bilaterally (**4.4**) with patchy areas of collapse or consolidation. Other complications include presentation with apnoea or occasionally convulsions. Diagnosis can be made by rapid antigen screen for respiratory viruses, especially RSV.

TREATMENT

This is principally supportive and will include the use of oxygen as necessary to maintain saturation levels above 92%. Adequate hydration is important but should not be excessive. This should be provided by a fine nasogastric tube or intravenously in those who have significant respiratory distress. The use of bronchodilators is controversial but ipratropium bromide or salbutamol can be tried in children over the age of 6 months. Response can be monitored by changes in oxygen saturation. The use of nasal continuous positive airway pressure (CPAP) can be helpful in those who have significant respiratory failure before they reach a stage requiring ventilation.

Ribavirin, a specific anti-viral agent against RSV should only be used in those with severe disease associated with underlying problems such as cystic fibrosis, immune deficiency, bronchopulmonary dysplasia or major cardiac disease. The use of antibiotics, oral or inhaled steroids has not been of proven benefit in this condition. Those who fail to respond to treatment should be investigated further for immune deficiency especially acquired immune deficiency syndrome (AIDS) and cystic fibrosis. A significant number of children have recurrent wheezy episodes after this illness. Continuing airway abnormalities may be detected on lung function tests over several years. Clinically, however, these children usually make a satisfactory recovery and the recurrent wheeziness decreases with age. In a very small number of cases where other viruses, particularly adenovirus, are implicated, there may be permanent lung damage with major hyperinflation and chronic wheezing over many years. This, however, is unusual. The use of RSV monoclonal antibody (palivizumab) is under investigation and may be a helpful prophylaxis in susceptible infants.

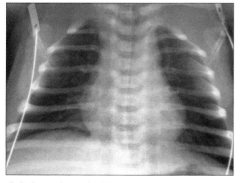

4.4 Acute bronchiolitis in a one month old infant showing hyperinflation and peribronchial thickening.

PNEUMONIA

INCIDENCE
Pneumonia can cause severe morbidity and mortality at any age but especially in infants and young children. Severity is likely to be increased where there is overcrowding, poor housing, parental smoking, malnutrition or underlying disease such as immune deficiency, chronic lung disease of prematurity, cystic fibrosis, a congenital anomaly of the lung, immotile cilia syndrome or a neurological problem leading to recurrent aspiration.

AETIOLOGY / PATHOGENESIS
During early life viruses are the most common pathogens, especially respiratory syncytial virus (RSV), influenza and parainfluenza. Others such as adenovirus and cytomegalovirus are potentially more damaging in the longer term. Modern diagnostic techniques such as immuno-fluorescence have facilitated rapid identification of these organisms in affected infants. During the neonatal period less common agents such as *Ureaplasma urealyticum* and *Chlamydia trachomatis* are found.

Bacterial pathogens such as *Streptococcus pneumoniae* become increasingly prevalent in community-acquired pneumonia as age increases. Pertussis remains a major cause of morbidity and death where immunization rates are low (**4.5**). Children in hospital are more likely to acquire organisms such as *Staphylococcus aureus, Haemophilus influenzae, Eschericia coli, Klebsiella pneumonia* or *Pseudomonas aeruginosa*. Fungal infections with *Candida* or *Aspergillus species* are particularly seen in the immunocompromized. *Pneumocystis carinii* is another major pathogen in this group. Anaerobic bacteria are probably important in children with recurrent aspiration but are difficult to identify. *Mycoplasma pneumoniae* is more prevalent in the older child and adolescent. Tuberculosis is an important pathogen world-wide and atypical mycobacteria are increasingly seen in the immunocompromised.

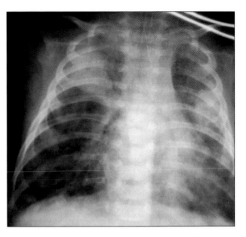

4.5 Widespread patchy consolidation due to Bordetella pertussis infection. Note segmental consolidation in right upper lobe.

CLINICAL PRESENTATION
Typical presenting features include fever, tachypnoea, cough with or without sputum production, increasing respiratory difficulty including use of accessory muscles of breathing, inspiratory indrawing and expiratory grunting. As the illness progresses central cyanosis appears. Physical examination reveals decreased air entry to affected areas, dullness to percussion, bronchial breathing, and conducted secretory noises with coarse or fine crackles over the affected areas. It is also possible to have significant pulmonary consolidation with no obvious externally elicitable physical signs. Wheeze may or may not be present depending on the underlying pathology and whether or not the patient has a history of asthma.

DIAGNOSIS

These should include chest x-ray (**4.6**) full blood count, C-reactive protein, sputum culture, rapid antigen screen, immunofluorescence for respiratory pathogens and viral antibody levels. Other investigations such as Mantoux test, antibodies to less common organisms such as *Chlamydia*, and bronchoscopic or non-bronchoscopic alveolar lavage should be undertaken when appropriate.

TREATMENT

This depends on the presumed underlying pathogen and whether or not there is considered to be secondary bacterial infection. Viral infection requires supportive therapy such as oxygen and attention to fluid intake and feeding. Antibiotics are not indicated and bronchodilators and inhaled steroids are widely used but not of proven value. Infants and young children who are severely unwell are usually covered with broad spectrum antibiotics including an aminoglycoside such as gentamicin or tobramycin in combination with a penicillin or third generation cephalosporin. Antifungal agents such as amphotericin or 5-flucytosine are used when clinically indicated. *Pneumocystis carinii* pneumonia is treated with co-trimoxazole (trimethoprim-sulphamethoxazole) in conjunction with corticosteroids.

PROGNOSIS

The outcome for the immunocompetent child is usually complete recovery. Some children go on to develop acute complications such as pleural empyema (see page 95). This is usually associated with a return to complete normality in the majority of cases. Long term complications such as bronchiectasis are more likely to occur where there is an underlying abnormality including recurrent aspiration, immune deficiency, malnutrition or cystic fibrosis.

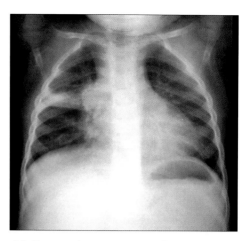

4.6 Segmental pneumonia in right upper lobe. Note loss of the right heart border, indicating right middle lobe consolidation.

CHRONIC ASPIRATION

AETIOLOGY

Aspiration into the lower respiratory tract is a major problem at any age. Acute aspiration with a foreign body is covered on page 100. Chronic aspiration principally of liquid or semi-solid foodstuffs is a major cause of respiratory pathology in children. It is often associated with gastro-oesophageal reflux and is exacerbated by underlying conditions which result in swallowing incoordination. Principal presenting features include recurrent episodes of wheezing and lower respiratory tract infection with over-inflation of the lungs seen on x-ray. When major aspiration occurs the episodes may be life threatening.

The condition is exacerbated by oesophageal anomalies such as tracheo-oesophageal fistula or hiatus hernia. These conditions may be associated with impaired oesophageal motility. In children with underlying neurological abnormalities which cause incoordination of sucking or swallowing, the risk of aspiration is greatly increased. Rarely there may be a more direct connection between the oesophagus and the airway such as occurs in cleft larynx or in isolated tracheo-oesophageal fistula. A number of children who recurrently aspirate have no cough reflex so that inhaled material is not expelled from the lungs as it should be under these conditions.

DIAGNOSIS

This should include a contrast swallow to evaluate oesophageal motility and to rule out underlying anatomical defects such as hiatus hernia, pyloric narrowing resulting in hold up to gastric emptying or malrotation of the upper small bowel. A video fluoroscopy examines the swallowing reflex in specific detail especially with different consistencies of food including liquids, semi-solids and solids (**4.7**, previous page). This will demonstrate spill-over or recurrent aspiration into the trachea and also the efficiency of the cough reflex in the face of such stimulation. A tracheo-oesophageal fistula requires specific investigation with an oesophagram carried out by an experienced radiologist. Gastroesophageal reflux also requires investigation with a pH study or a radio isotope milk scan if the pH study is difficult to perform or is not readily available.

TREATMENT

This depends on the nature of the underlying lesion and varies from feeding of specific consistencies of food to complete abstinence of oral feeding in those with the worst problems. Gastroesophageal reflux can be treated with thickening of the feeds and prokinetic agents such as Domperidone and H2 antagonists or proton pump inhibitors. Physically propping up the infant to no greater than 30 degrees may help to control reflux.

If medical measures fail then a Nissen's fundoplication with or without gastrostomy is the treatment of choice.

PROGNOSIS

Many children with swallowing difficulties who are otherwise neurologically normal outgrow these problems with time although those with major difficulties or those who have an associated underlying neurological abnormality may require long term gastrostomy feeds.

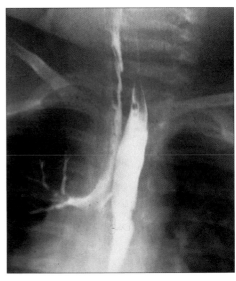

4.7 Contrast swallow showing acute aspiration into the tracheobronchial tree.

PNEUMOTHORAX

AETIOLOGY

Pneumothorax occurs when there is presence of air in the pleural space outside the lung (**4.8**). This can occur either due to rupture of the lung surface itself or by external puncture of the thoracic wall. Pneumothorax occurs for a variety of reasons which are shown in **Table 4.1**. Spontaneous pneumothorax is not uncommon in adolescent males even in the absence of other underlying lung pathology. In other cases there may be intrinsic pulmonary anomalies such as congenital cysts or connective tissues disorders, (e.g. Ehlers-Danlos syndrome). Some cases are familial. External trauma to the chest including direct injury can allow puncture of the pleural surface to occur with air escape.

CLINICAL PRESENTATION

This includes the sudden onset of chest pain in association with breathlessness and cyanosis. Physical examination may reveal mediastinal shift and hyper-resonance to percussion on the affected side. If the air is under tension this is a dangerous situation and there will be tracheal shift to the opposite side. The condition may be associated with air leak elsewhere such as surgical emphysema onto the chest wall, abdomen, into the neck or down the arm.

DIAGNOSIS

Chest x-ray will show the pneumothorax and any associated air leaking elsewhere such as into the mediastinum or subcutaneous tissue.

TREATMENT

This consists of direct evacuation of air from the pleural cavity by chest tube drainage. In those with minor symptoms spontaneous recovery can occur and is assisted by the administration of oxygen which increases its content in the pneumothorax space and therefore hastens absorption. Otherwise a large chest tube should be inserted into the appropriate area under local or general anaesthesia and placed on direct suction. The drain should be placed under a water seal so that air does not leak back into the pleural cavity. If the chest drain shows continuous bubbling this is an indication that there is a bronchopleural fistula and that other interventions such as surgical correction or pleurodesis may be required. Nowadays, thoracoscopic intervention can be particularly helpful in this situation.

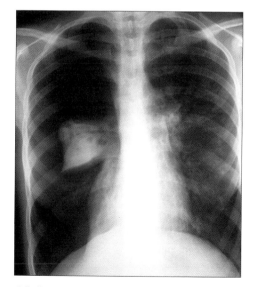

4.8 Pneumothorax in a patient with cystic fibrosis.

Table 4.1 Causes of pneumothorax

• **Spontaneous**	Idiopathic Familial e.g. Ehlers-Danlos syndrome
• **Trauma**	Penetrating or blunt chest injury
• **Foreign body**	
• **Asthma**	
• **Cystic Fibrosis**	
• **Iatrogenic**	Intubation Ventilation Venous cannulation Bronchoscopic biopsy
• **Pneumonia**	Bacterial Viral
• **Rare diseases**	Histiocytosis Lobar emphysema Marfan syndrome
• **Toxic inhalation**	Cocaine or marijuana smoking

EMPYEMA

AETIOLOGY / PATHOGENESIS

Empyema is due to the accumulation of purulent material in the pleural cavity. It is a relatively uncommon but serious complication of pneumonia in childhood. If not treated aggressively there may be prolonged and unnecessary morbidity. The condition occurs secondary to a wide variety of infecting organisms but is particularly associated with *Staphylococcus aureus, Streptococcus pneumoniae, Haemophilus influenzae* and *Mycoplasma pneumoniae*.

CLINICAL PRESENTATION

Patients tend to present in the pre-school age group. The most common symptoms are cough and fever associated with chest pain and difficulty in breathing. Cyanosis occurs in approximately 20% of patients. Some children present with abdominal pain and this should be remembered as an important differential diagnosis for this condition. Chest x-ray usually shows pulmonary consolidation and a marked pleural effusion. This will be confirmed on ultrasound and if necessary by CT scan (**4.9**).

DIAGNOSIS

These should include a chest x-ray, full blood count, blood culture, serology for appropriate organisms and rapid antigen screening and chest ultrasound.

TREATMENT

After chest ultrasound a diagnostic tap is performed and the aspirated fluid is sent for microscopy and culture. Intravenous antibiotics are then commenced against the most common organisms. This is followed by the insertion of a chest tube, usually under general anaesthesia and instillation of urokinase.

The clinical status is monitored by white blood cell count and C-reactive protein levels which should fall as response to treatment occurs. The chest drains are usually required for a median time of around 8 days. If treatment fails a thoracoscopic or open decortication may be required. Oral antibiotics may be continued after intravenous therapy has finished if there is continuing evidence of inflammation.

PROGNOSIS

The vast majority of immunocompetent patients recover completely after such an illness and chest x-ray can be anticipated to be normal within 6 months.

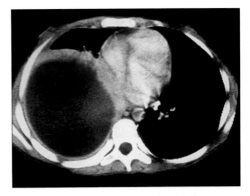

4.9 CT scan showing large right-sided empyema.

BRONCHIECTASIS

AETIOLOGY / PATHOGENESIS

Bronchiectasis is caused by dilatation of the major bronchi usually secondary to chronic infection in which there is ongoing bronchorrhoea with persistent cough and sputum production. It may result from a number of causes in childhood particularly secondary to pneumonia and chronic or recurrent lower respiratory tract infection. This can be precipitated, for example, by foreign body inhalation especially if removal is delayed or by particular organisms such as *adenovirus* which causes bronchiolitis or *staphylococci* which can occur as a complication of cystic fibrosis.

Bronchiectasis also occurs in the presence of recurrent aspiration of foreign material into the lower respiratory tract. This is especially likely to occur in those who have swallowing incoordination or where there is major gastroesophageal reflux when gastric contents can also spill over into the lower respiratory tract.

Congenital anomalies within the lung tissue such as cystic adenomatoid malformation or pulmonary sequestration or other underlying conditions such as primary cilia dyskinesia can also lead to the development of this problem.

DIAGNOSIS

This should include chest x-ray and CT scan (**4.10**) of the chest which can show localized abnormalities and is also used for sequential follow up over the long term. Ventilation perfusion lung scan can show regional abnormalities and may also be useful in long term follow up. Bronchoscopy will identify specific areas of affected lung and is useful for the clearance of secretions and the exclusion of

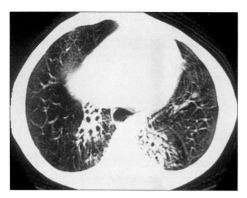

4.10 CT scan showing bilateral bronchiectasis.

other problems such as foreign body, severe tracheobronchomalacia and mucus plugging. Bronchoalveolar lavage may identify important infective organisms.

Investigations should rule out underlying causes such as cystic fibrosis (by sweat test or genotype), recurrent aspiration (by pH study and video swallow), immune deficiency (with examination of T-cell function and immuno-globulins) and family history (to exclude rare recessive disorders such as Familial Dysauto-nomia). In those with chronic immune defi-ciency prolonged parenteral immunoglobulin therapy and prophylactic antibiotics may be particularly helpful in preventing progress of the lung damage over time.

TREATMENT
This consists of daily physiotherapy, physical exercise and appropriate antibiotics to treat acute infection and to prevent further recur-rence over the longer term. Some recovery can take place if aggressive treatment is started early in the illness. If a limited area of lung is perma-nently damaged then surgical removal may be appropriate. This, however, is difficult if there is bilateral lung disease, which is often the case when there is another major underlying abnormality such as cystic fibrosis. In developed countries this condition is less frequent than it was in the past due to improved general health and nutrition, and active immunization in particular against *Haemophilus influenza* type B, measles, pertussis and diphtheria. Pneumococcal vaccine is recommended for those with persistent changes and annual influenza vaccine is useful for all those with long-term symptoms.

PIERRE ROBIN ANOMALAD

INCIDENCE
The incidence of Pierre Robin anomalad is probably about 1:30,000 live births. The micrognathia is usually obvious at birth and results in significant airway obstruction. This varies greatly in severity causing minimal problems in some and major airway obstruction in others. These infants often have significant feeding problems.

AETIOLOGY / PATHOGENESIS
There is a combination of upper airway anom-alies including micrognathia, glossoptosis and cleft palate. It is usually sporadic but must be differentiated from other conditions such as Stickler syndrome (see 'Genetics' chapter) where there is an associated myopia and hypotonia and which has an autosomal dominant inheritance.

TREATMENT
In the mildest cases prone positioning may be sufficient to overcome airway obstruction. However, in those with significant problems, the best approach is the use of a nasopharyngeal tube. This is inserted through the nose to lie just above the epiglottis but over the back of the tongue, so relieving the airway obstruction. Positioning of the airway is critical and should be confirmed by a lateral neck x-ray (**4.11**). Many infants will need supplemental nasogastric feeding for satisfactory calorie intake and normal growth. In most cases the airway can be removed by 6 months of age.

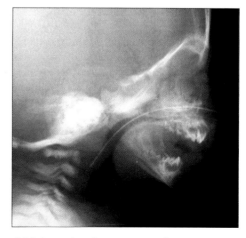

4.11 Lateral neck x-ray in an infant with Pierre Robin anomalad (nasopharyngeal tube *in situ*.).

CHARGE ASSOCIATION

The CHARGE association is a very rare disorder characterized by a number of features. These include

- **C** olobomata of the iris.
- **H** eart disease.
- **A** tresia of the choanae.
- **R** etarded growth and development of the central nervous system.
- **G** enital hypoplasia.
- **E** ar anomalies.

The condition is also associated with a number of other problems particularly cleft lip and palate.

AETIOLOGY / PATHOGENESIS

The condition is sporadic but a proportion of cases have an anomaly on chromosome 22 close to the deletion seen in Di George syndrome (see 'Immunology' chapter). Many children have feeding difficulties resulting from weakness of the pharyngeal muscles which results in recurrent aspiration (**4.12**). This leads to chronic lung disease which may be fatal. The specific cardiac defects which are seen include tetralogy of Fallot, patent arterial duct, double outlet right ventricle with an atrioventricular canal, ventricular or atrial septal defect and right sided aortic arch.

PROGNOSIS

The long-term outcome is extremely variable dependent on the success of treatment and clinical support of their supervising clinicians in addition to a major physical and emotional input from the parents.

TRACHEOBRONCHOMALACIA

AETIOLOGY

Tracheomalacia is due to softening of the tracheal wall either intrinsic or extrinsic. It is frequently found in extremely pre-term infants but may also occur secondary to extrinsic compression or with other lesions such as tracheo-oesophageal fistula in association with oesophageal atresia or a vascular ring.

CLINICAL PRESENTATION

These lesions result in dynamic airway changes during breathing which can cause acute respiratory distress especially during expiration when the airway may collapse completely. This can result in major apnoeic episodes which can be life threatening. Additionally there is retention of tracheobronchial secretions especially during recurrent infections and this leads to prolonged respiratory illness and also wheezing because of distal small airway obstruction.

TREATMENT

This consists of correction of the underlying anomaly such as a tracheo-oesophageal fistula or division of a vascular ring but if the condition is intrinsic then more detailed investigation with a bronchogram may be necessary to delineate the extent and severity of the problem and the pressures which are required to overcome the tracheobronchial narrowing (**4.13**). In selected cases surgery may be indicated, including resection, tracheal splinting with a stent, or an aortopexy. A number of these patients respond to long term CPAP or biPAP treatment but this may require many weeks or months in hospital before gradual recovery occurs.

PROGNOSIS

The long-term outcome for those who survive this initial period is good because of the natural growth and increased stability of the tracheo-bronchial tree with age. However, there is a very significant morbidity and mortality in the early years of life.

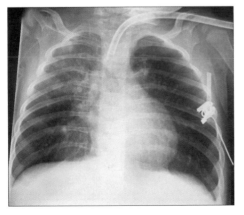

4.12 CHARGE association: Chest x-ray showing patchy consolidation due to aspiration in the right middle and lower lobes.

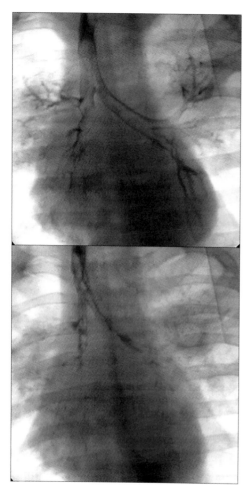

4.13 Bronchogram showing bilateral bronchomalacia with collapse on expiration (bottom panel).

DIAPHRAGMATIC HERNIA

INCIDENCE / AETIOLOGY
Congenital diaphragmatic hernia occurs when part of the abdominal contents migrate into the chest through a congenital defect in the diaphragm. The incidence is between 1:2,000 and 1:5,000 live births. There is a high incidence of associated congenital anomalies in these children occurring in 30–50% of cases. The incidence is much more common on the left side compared with the right. The most common lesion is through a postero-lateral herniation via the foramen of Bochdalek. If the lesion occurs in early gestation there is an accompanying hypoplasia of the lung on the affected side.

DIAGNOSIS
Chest x-ray typically shows bowel in the chest, with lung compression unilaterally or bilaterally. After birth, as the bowel distends with air, the lungs are compressed and this contributes to major respiratory distress. The condition can be confused with cystic adenomatoid malformation of the lung, although, in this condition, a chest x-ray will usually show the gastric bubble below the diaphragm. The position of the abdominal contents can be confirmed by the use of contrast medium (**4.14**).

TREATMENT
Treatment is supportive initially, until surgical correction can be undertaken.

PROGNOSIS
An associated pulmonary hypoplasia on the affected side can lead to significant long-term lung pathology even in those who recover from the initial illness. The condition still carries a high mortality in those who are diagnosed *in utero*.

4.14 Contrast study showing right-sided diaphragmatic hernia, with the stomach in the right hemithorax.

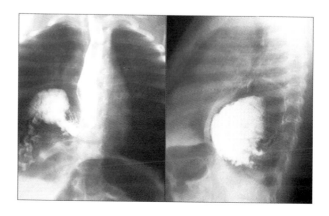

FOREIGN BODY

See also 'Emergency Medicine' chapter.

The inhalation of a foreign body into the airways most commonly occurs in the toddler age group. There may be a history of coughing or gagging whilst eating or playing with small toys. Occasionally a foreign body will completely obstruct the larynx or trachea and be a cause of sudden death. More commonly, however, the foreign body passes through the larynx and trachea and lodges in one of the main bronchi.

CLINICAL SIGNS

The common symptoms and signs are stridor or audible wheeze, sternal retraction, cough and hoarseness. Sudden onset of wheeze, especially unilateral, is highly suspicious of an inhaled foreign body. The most common site for impaction is the right main stem bronchus followed by the left main stem bronchus (**4.15**) and the trachea.

INVESTIGATIONS

X-rays of the neck and anterior-posterior chest need to be closely inspected for a radio-opaque object. Chest x-rays should be taken in inspiration and expiration; the classical feature on the expiratory film is overinflation of the lung on the affected side, secondary to airway obstruction. A foreign body can have two pathophysiological effects: it can cause a complete blockage and collapse, or can result in an incomplete blockage and ball-valve effect. A foreign body is not always static. This can lead to changing signs both clinically and radiologically.

When the plain film is normal and there is a strong clinical suspicion of foreign body aspiration, then rigid bronchoscopy (**4.16**) is required. Removal of foreign bodies, in particular laryngeal foreign bodies, can be difficult and an experienced endoscopist and anaesthetist will need to undertake the procedure. Failure to detect a foreign body can lead to long term chronic changes and bronchiectasis in the distal lung tissue.

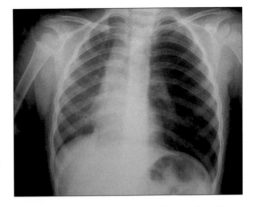

4.15 Peanut in left main bronchus with ball-valve effect and overinflation of left lung.

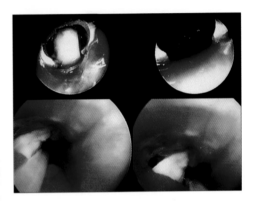

4.16 Rigid bronchoscopy images of peanut.

MILIARY PATTERN ON CHEST IMAGING

The presence of fine, discrete nodules less than 5 mm in size and extending uniformly throughout the lung fields on plain chest radiograph (**4.17**) or CT scan (**4.18**) is a distinctive and not uncommon finding in paediatric practice. The underlying aetiology incorporates a wide differential diagnosis (important considerations are listed in the table).

In countries in which tuberculosis is prevalent this pattern of densities is commonly encountered and receives the descriptive term 'miliary tuberculosis'.

In endemic areas, disseminated histoplasmosis may display this radiographic pattern. This appearance is encountered in children who test positive for human immunodeficiency virus and have lymphoid interstitial pneumonitis.

Haematogenous or lymphangitic spread of malignant neoplasms such as leukaemia, lymphoma, rhabdomycosarcoma, neuroblastoma and carcinoma of the thyroid all need consideration.

Miliary pattern on chest radiograph: causes of diffuse, fine (1–4 mm), sharply-defined nodules

Category	Specific disease
Infectious diseases	Tuberculosis
Fungal	Disseminated histoplasmosis, coccidioidomycosis, blastomycosis aspergillosis, and cryptococcosis
Bacterial	Nocardiosis
Viral	Varicella zoster
Metastases	Thyroid carcinoma, melanoma, and lymphangitic carcinomatosis
Granulomatous diseases	Eosinophilic granulomata and sarcoidosis
Inhalational disorders	Berylliosis, silicosis, pneumoconiosis, siderosis, and extrinsic allergic alveolitis
Inherited disorders	Niemann-Pick disease, Gaucher disease, and pulmonary alveolar microlithiasis
Other disorders	Hemosiderosis

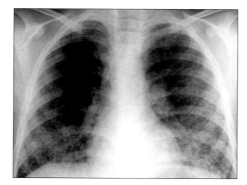

4.17 Chest x-ray demonstrating diffuse bilateral miliary changes representing metastases from thyroid carcinoma.

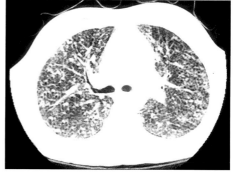

4.18 CT scan of the chest demonstrating the miliary changes in the patient described in 4.17.

PRIMARY CILIARY DYSKINESIA

Primary ciliary dyskinesia or immotile cilia syndrome represents a group of conditions whose essential feature is either an absent or severely reduced ciliary motility. There is considerable phenotypic variation. In children with classical symptoms of bronchiectasis and situs inversus (**4.19**) together with recurrent sinusitis the term Kartagener syndrome is often applied. There are a number of cases that show autosomal recessive inheritance. Male infertility is also a feature. The phenotypic variation is highlighted by the fact that only 50% of cases show situs inversus.

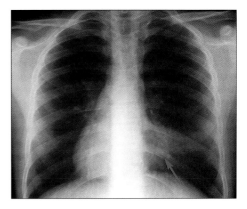

4.19 Situs inversus with left-sided infection.

CLINICAL PRESENTATION

The condition is present from birth and can produce symptoms in the neonatal period. Usually, however, chest symptoms with cough, nasal obstruction and recurrent chest infections appear early in infancy. If treatment is not introduced at this stage, lung infection and bronchiectatic changes progress during childhood.

DIAGNOSIS

Cilia can be obtained by a special brushing technique. Motility is assessed using a light microscope and an electron microscope reveals the variety of structural defects which must be present in at least 50% of the cilia examined. The abnormalities include defective dynein arms, defective or missing radial spokes and microtubular abnormalities (**4.20, 4.21**). More recently, it has been documented that low levels of exhaled nitric oxide are also characteristic of this syndrome and NO levels could be become a useful screening tool.

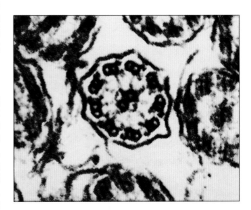

4.20 Electromagnetic image of normal ciliary structure.

MANAGEMENT

Bacterial infection requires control and airways need to be kept clear of secretions. Physiotherapy is a mainstay of treatment and antibiotics are used frequently according to the microbial sensitivities obtained from sputa specimens. Particular attention may need to be paid to the treatment of conductive hearing loss and sinusitis may require surgical intervention. Adult males require appropriate testing and counselling for infertility.

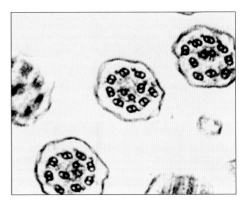

4.21 Electromagnetic image of abnormal cilia with radial spoke defect.

MYCOPLASMA PNEUMONIAE

Mycoplasma pneumoniae is a common cause of pneumonia. It is characterized by an upper respiratory tract infection, dry cough and breathlessness, with highly variable diffuse x-ray changes to which the term 'atypical pneumonia' is often attached.

Members of the mycoplasma genus have no cell wall and represent some of the smallest free-living organisms. They are unaffected by antibiotics such as the betalactams. They act as an extra-cellular organism attaching to ciliated epithelial cells by a specialised terminal organelle, resulting in ciliary damage and airway inflammation.

CLINICAL PRESENTATION

Spread of this organism is by droplet inhalation with an incubation period of 14–21 days. Infected children may present with a wide range of symptoms from asymptomatic or mild pneumonia to acute respiratory failure and death. Children of school age are mostly affected, and infection typically occurs in three- or four-yearly cycles (**4.22**).

Initial presentation includes fever, headaches, malaise and nocturnal sweating. Cough usually begins 3–5 days after the onset and is a common finding. Crackles and wheezing can be heard but respiratory signs may be surprisingly unimpressive when compared to the severity of the symptoms, especially if there is pleuritic chest pain. Some patients continue to wheeze for months after recovery and there is an association with the subsequent development of asthma. There are a number of extra-pulmonary manifestations such as pericarditis, arthritis and haemolytic anaemia, which may be secondary immunological phenomena.

DIAGNOSIS

The chest x-ray typically shows patchy shadowing although lobar consolidation and hilar adenopathy are also found (**4.23**). The white cell count is usually normal although the ESR may be raised. There can be considerable difficulty in culturing the organism from the throat or nasopharynx but successful growth usually clinches the diagnosis. Cold agglutinins may be positive in anywhere between 72% and 92% of patients but are also common in viral infections. Complement fixation tests require a four fold increase in titre over a 2–3 week period. ELISA tests for *M pneumoniae* serology allow for detection of IgM and IgG antibodies and PCR testing is currently under development.

MANAGEMENT

The current treatment of choice is a macrolide antibiotic given for 10–14 days.

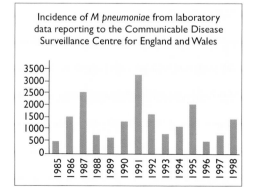

Incidence of *M pneumoniae* from laboratory data reporting to the Communicable Disease Surveillance Centre for England and Wales

4.22 *Mycoplasma pneumoniae.* Annual detected incidence in England and Wales.

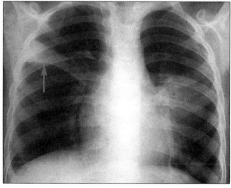

4.23 *Mycoplasma pneumoniae* affecting the right upper lobe and lingula.

ASPHYXIATING THORACIC DYSTROPHY

Asphyxiating thoracic dystrophy (also known as Jeune syndrome) is a heterogeneous multisystem disorder. The main characteristic is an abnormally small narrow thorax with rib abnormalities and pulmonary hypoplasia (**4.24**). Severely affected children die from respiratory insufficiency in infancy but there is a wide phenotypic spectrum and some children may survive into adulthood.

A variety of associated skeletal manifestations have been described including hypoplastic iliac wings, flattening of the acetabular roof (**4.25**), shortening of the long bones, abnormalities of the epiphyses and small hands with fusion between the epiphyses and the metaphyses of the middle and distal phalanges.

Renal, pancreatic and hepatic involvement are not uncommon and additional findings include retinal degeneration and hydrocephalus. There has also been a recent report of an association with Hirschsprung's disease (**4.26**).

AETIOLOGY / PATHOGENESIS
It is inherited as an autosomal recessive disorder.

TREATMENT
In children with significant restrictive lung disease and underlying pulmonary hypoplasia the condition is not usually compatible with life. In milder cases, however, attempts have been made to increase the thoracic cage dimensions by various rib and sternal distraction techniques. The outcome from these procedures is very variable and not universally successful.

In children with milder variants, long term follow up is recommended, especially in relation to their respiratory, ocular, renal and hepatic functions.

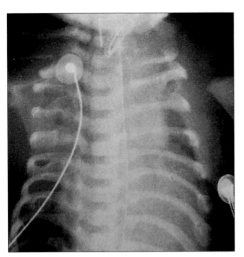

4.24 Asphyxiating thoracic dystrophy.

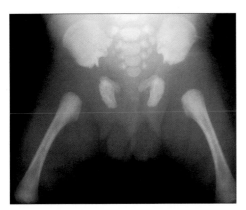

4.25 Classic bony changes in the pelvis in Jeune syndrome, including feathering of the acetabular roofs, hypoplastic iliac wings and characteristic spurs.

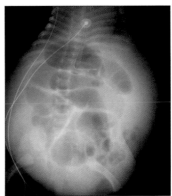

4.26 Jeune asphyxiating dystrophy with Hirschsprung's disease.

PULMONARY AGENESIS AND APLASIA

In pulmonary agenesis, there is no development of the lung beyond the carina. Bilateral pulmonary agenesis results when this occurs at the single respiratory bud stage and is incompatible with life. In unilateral pulmonary aplasia, it is common to find either a rudimentary bronchus that ends blindly or enters a very underdeveloped and non-functioning lung (**4.27**). The unaffected lung or lobes can function normally apart from the compensatory overinflation to fill the empty hemithorax. The underlying pathogenesis for the two defects is likely to be similar.

CLINICAL PRESENTATION

Children may present with lung agenesis or aplasia as an isolated finding. Frequently, however, there are other associated anomalies (often on the ipsilateral side) such as renal aplasia, ear or limb defects. Curiously, congenital abnormalities are more associated with right sided agenesis.

DIAGNOSIS

Chest x-rays following a clinical impression of decreased breath sounds or mediastinal displacement. A CT scan is usually warranted to identify the underlying anatomy more accurately and can be useful in revealing lung remnants not readily visible on the plain film.

PROGNOSIS

Many children suffer no ill-effects and can lead healthy lives. Pulmonary hypertension is very rare.

Some children can be troubled with chest infections, air flow problems and wheezing or respiratory distress on effort. Treatment remains supportive. Occasionally surgery is offered in children where the remnant bronchial pouch in aplasia is thought to be acting as a reservoir for infection.

CONGENITAL LOBAR EMPHYSEMA (CLE)

Over-distension of a lobe or lobule following partial bronchial obstruction and a ball-valve effect can result in emphysematous-like changes to the lobe. Purists will point out that the term emphysema in this situation is incorrect and alveolar over-distension with normal paren-chymal architecture is more accurate. In spite of attempts to change nomenclature, the term continues. In congenital lobar emphysema, a bronchial obstruction is only clearly identified in less than a quarter of the cases and in many lesions, no cause is found.

CLINICAL PRESENTATION

Usually the abnormality is confined to a lobe and the left upper lobe is the most common. Most present in the neonatal period, with respiratory distress due to compression by the over-distended lobe.

DIAGNOSIS

Diagnosis is usually evident on plain x-ray (**4.28**) although CT scans demonstrate the

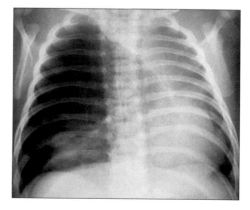

4.27 Chest x-ray showing opacity of the left hemithorax; a penetrated view of the large airways revealed the presence of a carina with left-sided aplasia.

4.28 Congenital lobar emphysema. Plain film showing CLE of right upper lobe.

changes well and may image the offending bronchial lesion (**4.29**). A ventilation perfusion (VQ) scan (**4.30**) will confirm the matched perfusion/ventilation defect that is represented by the emphysematous lobe.

MANAGEMENT

Severe respiratory distress requires urgent surgical intervention. Selective intubation of the unaffected lung can significantly improve the cardiorespiratory status during preparation for surgery. For milder cases, a period of observation can prove very useful. Unless there is significant air-trapping with a space-occupying effect (which can develop slowly over the first weeks to months of life and therefore present 'late').

PROGNOSIS

CLE can be an asymptomatic finding and produce no long-term effects or vulnerabilities. As such it represents one of only a few congenital abnormalities of the developing lung that can be satisfactorily managed conservatively.

BRONCHOGENIC CYST

Abnormal budding of the bronchial tree can occur either in early gestation, producing a mediastinal or central cyst or later during lung development, producing peripheral lesions. The cysts are thin-walled, with ciliated columnar lining that may contain cartilage, smooth muscle, glands or even gastroesophageal mucosa. They can be fluid or air-filled (**4.31**).

CLINICAL PRESENTATION

Functionally most bronchogenic cysts are asymptomatic at birth, although the central lesions may compress the airway and impact on ventilation. Peripheral lesions may have a space-occupying effect that may not be present immediately after birth.

INVESTIGATION

The plain chest x-ray may be sufficient to diagnose the cyst, although a CT scan is often useful to delineate the structure in the mediastinal forms (**4.32**). A ventilation perfusion scan will demonstrate the functional effects and

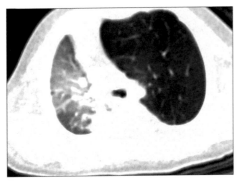

4.29 Congenital lobar emphysema. CT image of CLE of left upper lobe.

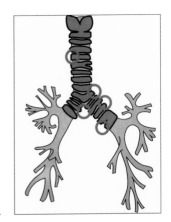

4.31 Common sites for bronchogenic cysts (circles).

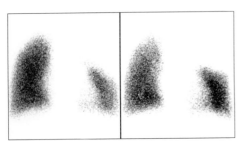

4.30 Congenital lobar emphysema. VQ scan showing matched defects in left upper lobe.

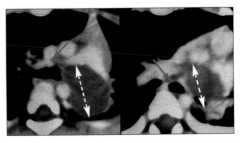

4.32 CT images showing a bronchogenic cyst (white arrow) closely related to the right main bronchus (red arrow).

is a useful investigation following removal of the lesion to document post-surgical recovery of the affected lung.

MANAGEMENT

Surgical resection of these lesions is recommended even if asymptomatic due to the high incidence of infection. Reports suggest that 75–95% of these cysts become infected although the number of asymptomatic lesions in the general population is unknown.

CONGENITAL CYSTIC ADENOMATOID MALFORMATION (CCAM)

Congenital cystic adenomatoid malformations are a result of an antenatal abnormality of lung development. Adenomatous overgrowth of tissue is lined by proliferating bronchial or cuboidal epithelium with intervening normal portions of lung. There are three histological types:
- Type 1 with multiple large thin walled cysts.
- Type 2 with multiple even spaced cysts.
- Type 3, which is a bulky firm mass with small regular spaced cysts (**4.33**).

CLINICAL PRESENTATION AND MANAGEMENT

The lesion is frequently detected antenatally and if very large and associated with other congenital abnormalities may affect the long-term future of the pregnancy. Postnatally a CCAM can present in different ways:
- A large mass may present as a space occupying lesion. Clinically there is evidence of respiratory distress with mediastinal shift and a plain chest x-ray reveals a large cystic lesion (**4.34**) with the anatomy further defined on CT imaging. (**4.35**) Surgical removal is indicated and outcome depends on the degree of hypoplasia of the remaining lobes following the intra-uterine compression. With improved surgical outcome there are now reports of good long term results even with large lesions.
- A common presenting feature is infection. A child who has a severe pneumonia (especially repeated involvement of the same area) or fails to achieve radiological clearance of the infection needs detailed imaging to exclude a congenital cystic lesion. Current accepted management is surgical removal of the lesion once the child has been treated for infection.

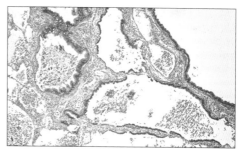

4.33 Histopathology of congenital cystic adenomatoid malformation.

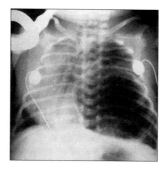

4.34 Congenital cystic adenomatoid malformation on the left, with mediastinal shift.

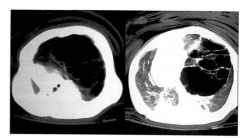

4.35 CT findings of a large left-sided CCAM.

- A CCAM can be an incidental finding or asymptomatic lesion. Antenatal scanning may document a CCAM that is either completely asymptomatic at birth or very small such that it is not clearly seen on plain chest x-ray. Although some practitioners advocate removal of the lesion thereby preventing any risk of infection or malignant change the natural history of an asymptomatic CCAM is not well described.
- A CCAM may also form part of a lobar pulmonary sequestration with abnormal systemic feeding vessels.

SCIMITAR SYNDROME

Scimitar syndrome applies to a dysmorphic condition of the right lung classically represented by hypoplasia of the right lung with a corresponding mediastinal shift where the entire right lung drains into the right atrium or inferior vena cava and systemic collaterals are present. There are many variations on both arterial supply and venous drainage but the syndrome pertains particularly to abnormalities of the whole lung.

CLINICAL PRESENTATION

Children can present with recurrent respiratory tract infection or the abnormality may be an incidental finding on plain chest films (**4.36**). X-rays show right-sided pulmonary hypoplasia and often, but not always, demonstrate the scimitar sign of a shadow produced by the draining vein. A case of left-sided scimitar syndrome has been reported but almost always it occurs as a dysplastic right lung.

DIAGNOSIS

Pulmonary function is rarely compromised. The lesion may present as an incidental finding.

TREATMENT

Occasionally excess blood flow to the lung can result in shunting with breathlessness or exercise limitation. In this situation it is possible to embolise the abnormal artery. Surgical correction of other vascular anomalies may also be indicated. If the area has become infected and there is significant lung damage then removal of the affected area is recommended as it may become bronchiectatic.

DESQUAMATIVE INTERSTITIAL PNEUMONITIS/ FIBROSING ALVEOLITIS

INCIDENCE

Some cases are familial in type and overall the recurrence risk within a family is of the order of 10%.

CLINICAL PRESENTATION

This is a rare condition in paediatric practice. It can present at any age, although it is most common in infancy. It is manifested by the gradual onset of tachypnoea, a dry cough and increasing respiratory distress on exercise or feeding. As the disease progresses, hypoxia increases and the child becomes cyanosed. In some cases, especially in older children, the first diagnostic feature is finger clubbing.

It is important to note that in many of these cases oxygen saturation at rest is normal, but falls as soon as any exercise is taken.

DIAGNOSIS

Examination of the chest may be normal, with no added sounds or may demonstrate widespread crackles in all lung fields, especially on deep inspiration. The differential diagnosis is wide and in approximately 40% of cases an underlying diagnosis is found (e.g. sarcoidosis, alveolar proteinosis, rheumatoid lung disease or pulmonary haemosiderosis). It is important to perform a lung biopsy whenever possible to confirm the diagnosis and to evaluate underlying disease severity which is important for the determination of prognosis.

In idiopathic cases, a wide spectrum of histological changes are seen. These vary from desquamation of alveolar macrophages into the alveoli to widespread interstitial fibrosis.

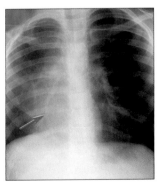

4.36
Scimitar syndrome. Chest x-ray shows hypoplasia of the right lung and a visible scimitar vein along the right heart border.

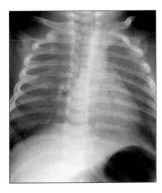

4.37
Chest x-ray demonstrating bilateral ground-glass appearance in fibrosing alveolitis.

The outcome is extremely variable, and except in the most severe cases, it is not directly related to the severity of histological change, unlike the picture seen in adults.

Chest x-ray will typically show widespread interstitial shadowing in both lung fields (**4.37**); some cases have a honeycomb appearance and in advanced cases multiple cystic lesions may also be seen. These findings should be confirmed on CT scan which is particularly useful for assessing regional severity of lung disease and acts as a baseline for disease progression in the future. Investigation should also be undertaken to exclude other underlying pathological conditions which may be the primary cause of the lung disease as described above. Recurrent aspiration should also be ruled out as should major immune deficiency.

TREATMENT

This depends on the severity of the disease, its activity and the rate of progression. Some children may require only additional oxygen for a limited period of time. More commonly, specific anti-inflammatory treatment with oral prednisolone or monthly pulsed intravenous methylprednisolone is needed, with or without an anti-fibrotic agent such as hydroxychloroquine. In less severe cases hydroxychloroquine on its own may be sufficient. Other immunosuppressive agents are occasionally used in patients who fail to respond to standard treatment and lung transplantation is an option for those with end stage lung disease.

PROGNOSIS

Mortality is about 15% and is highest in infancy

REFERENCES

Cystic fibrosis
Keresmar CM. The Respiratory System. In: Kliegman B (ed). *Nelson Essentials of Pediatrics.* Philadelphia: Saunders, 1998: 459–496.
Dinwiddie R (ed). *Diagnosis and Management of Paediatric Respiratory Disease.* Edinburgh : Churchill Livingstone, 1997: 197–245.
Valerius NH, Koch C, Hoiby N. Prevention of chronic Pseudomonas infection in cystic fibrosis by early treatment. *Lancet* 1991; **338**: 725–726.
Hodson ME, Shah PL. DNase trials in cystic fibrosis. *Eur Respir J* 1995; **8**: 1786–1791.
Whitehead BF, Rees PG, Sorenson K *et al*. Results of heart-lung transplantation in children with cystic fibrosis. *Eur J Cardiothorac Surg* 1995; **9**: 1–6.
British guideline on the management of asthma. *Thorax* 2003; vol 58 (S1).

Asthma and recurrent wheeze
Martinez FD, Wright AL, Taussig LM *et al.* Asthma and wheezing in the first six years of life. *N Eng J Med* 1995; **332**: 133–138.
Stein RT, Holberg CJ, Morgan WJ *et al.* Peak flow variability, methacholine responsiveness and atopy as markers for detecting different wheezing phenotypes in childhood. *Thorax* 1997; **52**: 946–952.
Dinwiddie R (ed). *Diagnosis and Management of Paediatric Respiratory Disease.* Edinburgh: Churchill Livingstone 1997: 167–196.
Warner JO, Naspitz CK. Third International Pediatric Consensus Statement on the Management of Childhood Asthma. International Pediatric Asthma Consensus Group. *Pediatr Pulmonol* 1998; **25(1)**: 1–17.

Bronchiolitis
Soong W-J, Hwang B, Tang R-B. Continuous positive airway pressure by nasal prongs in bronchiolitis. *Ped Pulmonol* 1993; **16**: 163–166.

Pneumonia
Kercsmar CM. The Respiratory System. In: Kliegman B (ed). *Nelson Essentials of Pediatrics* (3rd edn). Philadelphia: Saunders, 1998: 459–496.
Dinwiddie R (ed). *Diagnosis and Management of Paediatric Respiratory Disease.* Edinburgh: Churchill Livingstone 1997: 103–134.

Pneumothorax
Panitch HB, Papastamelos C, Schidlow DV. Abnormalities of the pleural space. In: Taussig LM, Landau LI (eds). *Paediatric Respiratory Medicine.* St Louis: Mosby, 1999: 1178–1196.

Empyema
Chan PWK, Crawford O, Wallis C, Dinwiddie R. Treatment of pleural empyema. *J Paed Child Health* 2000; **36**: 375–377.

Pierre Robin anomalad
Dinwiddie R (ed). *Diagnosis and Management of Paediatric Respiratory Disease.* Edinburgh: Churchill Livingstone 1997: 81–102.

CHARGE association
Sporik R, Dinwiddie R, Wallis C. Lung involvement in the multi-system syndrome CHARGE association. *Eur Respir J* 1997; **10**: 1354–1355.

Diaphragmatic hernia
Beresford MW, Shore MJ. Outcome of congenital diaphragmatic hernia. *Paed Pulmonol* 2000; **30**: 249–256.
Davis CF, Sabharwal AJ. Management of congenital diaphragmatic hernia. *Arch Dis Child* (Fetal and Neonatal edition) 1998; **79**: 1–3.

Desquamative interstitial pneumonitis/fibrosing alveolitis
Fan LL, Langston C. Interstitial Lung Disease. In: Chernick V, Boat T, Kendig L (eds). *Disorders of the Respiratory Tract in Children.* Philadelphia: Saunders, 1998: 607–616.
Barbato A, Panizzolo C. Chronic interstitial lung disease in children. *Paed Respir Rev* 2000; **1**: 172–178.
Dinwiddie R, Sharief N, Crawford O. Idiopathic interstitial pneumonitis in children: a national survey in the United Kingdom and Ireland. *Ped Pulmonol* 2002; **34**: 23–29.

Cardiology
Magdi H El Habbal

VENTRICULAR SEPTAL DEFECT (VSD)

INCIDENCE
Ventricular septal defect (VSD) is the commonest congenital heart disease (**5.1**). It occurs in any part of the ventricular septum, most commonly in the perimembranous region.

AETIOLOGY / PATHOGENESIS
The cause of the majority of ventricular septal defects is unknown. Inlet type of defects may occur in association with Down syndrome.

CLINICAL PRESENTATION
Clinical features are generally related to the size of the defect. Site is also important as defects in the membranous region may involve the aortic valve. Symptoms vary from asymptomatic (small defect), recurrent chest infection (moderate size defect) to heart failure and failure to thrive (large defect). The apex of the heart is that of left ventricular type (localized and shifted inferolaterally from the normal position). Right ventricular impulse (diffuse parasternal pulsation) is palpable in complicated defects (very large or pulmonary hypertension). There may be a thrill with a small VSD. The first heart sound is invariably normal in isolated defects. The second heart sound is normal with a small VSD and single in a large defect (loud P2).

A ventricular septal defect is recognized by the presence of a systolic murmur (indicating left to right shunt). However, the murmur may not be usually heard until the 8th week after birth (when pulmonary pressure starts to drop). Therefore, the presence of a pansystolic murmur indicates that the pulmonary resistance is lower than the systemic resistance thus allowing left to right shunting. The murmur may vary from short early systolic (in muscular defect) but may be absent (in very large defects). The louder the murmur, the smaller the defect. A mid diastolic rumbling murmur may be heard at the apex in a large defect (with the bell of the stethoscope and the patient on his/her left side), secondary to increased flow across the mitral valve.

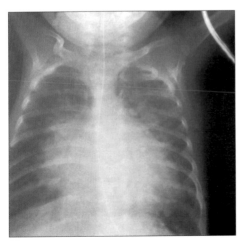

5.1 A chest x-ray of a child with an isolated large ventricular septal defect. Note the presence of pulmonary plethora, pulmonary oedema, large heart and dilated left atrium.

DIAGNOSIS

Electrocardiogram (ECG). In small defects the ECG is normal. The changes in the ECG reflect the haemodynamic burden of the shunt and may help in identifying the site of the defect. The presence of left axis deviation raises the suspicion of an inlet defect (more common in children with Down syndrome). The degree of left ventricular hypertrophy has significant correlation with the magnitude of shunting, whereas the right ventricular hypertrophy pattern has a reliable correlation to the elevation of the pulmonary pressure. Biventricular hypertrophy is expected in large defects and in moderate defects that are left for a number of years.

Chest x-ray. The x-ray is mainly to confirm the severity of shunting. The presence of pulmonary plethora is a reliable sign of a significant left to right shunt. In the absence of an atrial septal defect, the left atrium becomes dilated. This is recognized by a wide angle of the tracheal bifurcation and double shadow with a double right border of the heart.

Echocardiography. This will delineate site and size of the defect. With the help of Doppler the left to right shunting can be reliably measured (**5.2**). The pulmonary pressure can also be estimated.

TREATMENT

Treatment of large defects is by surgical closure. Some lesions in the muscular septum may be amenable to device closure. Long term antibiotic prophylaxis to prevent endocarditis is mandatory. Following complete closure, no treatment is required. The presence of residual defects requires long-term prophylaxis.

PROGNOSIS

The majority of VSD may close spontaneously within the first year of life (almost 90%). Large defects should be repaired in infancy because of the likelihood of developing pulmonary vascular disease. If there are no convincing signs of the defect getting smaller (patient is becoming asymptomatic, murmur is getting louder or fading away, pulmonary second sound is normal) confirm with echocardiographic examinations and consider closure. A VSD with a significant shunt may result in the development of pulmonary vascular disease that causes cyanosis (pulmonary hypertension) and reduce life expectancy.

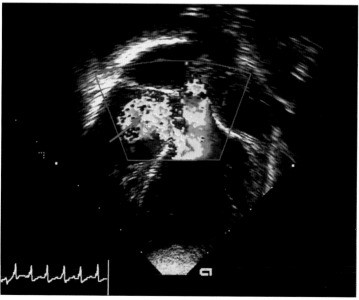

5.2 An echocardiographic view with colour-flow Doppler showing muscular ventricular septal defect with left to right shunt.

ATRIAL SEPTAL DEFECT (ASD)

INCIDENCE

ASD is a common congenital heart disease. It may occur in any part of the atrial septum (primum defect, secondum, sinus venosus, fossa ovalis, coronary sinus). It is not unusual that it remains undiagnosed and recognized only after the occurrence of a systemic embolism.

Aetiology/pathogenesis

Unknown and most cases are isolated. ASD can occur as a clinical association of many syndromes including Down, Holt-Oram, and Klinefelter syndromes.

Clinical presentation

This depends on the size of the defect (amount of shunting), with small defects being asymptomatic. Moderate and large defects usually manifest in late teen and early twenties with easy fatigue and/or recurrent chest infection. However, large defects may present with symptoms at a young age (occasionally in infancy). The arterial pulse is of small volume. There is diffuse left parasternal pulsation (right ventricular volume overload), a mid-systolic ejection murmur in the pulmonary area and wide split and fixed second heart sound.

DIAGNOSIS

Electrocardiogram. In moderate and large defects, the QRS axis may be normal or deviated to the right with right ventricular enlargement (**5.3**). In a primum defect, the axis is deviated to the left with long PR interval (> 0.11 sec) and rSR pattern in the right chest leads (incomplete right bundle branch block) (**2.2**). Right bundle branch block reflects delayed conduction into a dilated right ventricle.

Chest x-ray. The presence of pulmonary plethora, enlarged heart (in a large defect) and dilated main pulmonary artery is almost diagnostic (**5.4**).

Echocardiogram and Doppler. This confirms the diagnosis and determines the type of defect. Transoesophageal echocardiography is most valuable in identifying small defects.

Treatment

This must begin before the onset of symptoms of congestive cardiac failure. Traditionally surgical closure in pre-school children or increasingly acceptable device closure via cardiac catheterization if the lesion is small or moderate.

Prognosis

Most children will be recognized at an early stage and the defect is closed. The natural history is that of spontaneous closure in only 40% by 10 years of age. Congestive heart failure develops more commonly after the age of 40, whereas pulmonary vascular disease is rarer (5–10%). It is recognized that atrial arrhythmias may occur in adult patients with ASD whether it was closed or not.

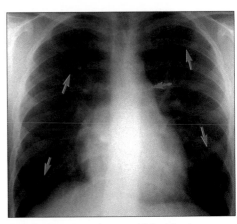

5.3. A 12-lead electrocardiogram from a child with ostium secondum ASD. The QRS axis is shifted to the right, PR interval is normal (< 0.11 sec) and rSR pattern in V1.

5.4 A chest x-ray from a child with a large secondum ASD. Note the increase in pulmonary vascularity, dilation of the pulmonary artery and small aortic knuckle.

COARCTATION OF THE AORTA

INCIDENCE
This is a not uncommon congenital heart disease occurring more often in boys than girls.

AETIOLOGY
Any condition leading to reduced flow through the aortic isthmus may predispose to coarctation formation, for example ventricular septal defect. In addition, remnants of ductal tissue may exist within the wall of the aorta and coarctation may develop when this tissue contracts during ductal closure. Coarctation may be associated with Turner syndrome.

CLINICAL PRESENTATION
Patients may present with severe heart failure (usually newborn), hypertension or a cardiac murmur. The diagnostic clinical sign is weak or absent femoral artery pulsation in the presence of good right brachial artery pulsation. Blood pressure is usually elevated with pressure difference between the right arm and right leg. In a newborn, the right ventricle is enlarged, whereas in an older child the left ventricle is enlarged. A mid systolic ejection murmur is usually heard at the mid left sternal edge and radiates to the back between the scapulae.

DIAGNOSIS
Electrocardiogram. ECG shows right ventricular enlargement in a newborn and left ventricular enlargement in older child.
Chest x-ray. This shows an enlarged heart; rib notching (rare in children) may occur in adults who develop collateral, prominent aortic arch with a prominent descending aorta giving it the shape of an inverted figure 3.
Echocardiogram and Doppler. This confirms the diagnosis. The abdominal aorta is usually less pulsatile. Doppler signals at the site of the narrowing may show the flow extending to diastole.

TREATMENT
Surgical treatment is the gold standard. Balloon angioplasty (**5.5**) and stent implantation are contemplated in primary lesions and are usually applied in recurrent coarctation (restenosis after surgery). In a newborn, maintain patency of the ductus while awaiting for surgery by using a prostaglandin E infusion. Patients are followed up for life. Antibiotic prophylaxis for endocarditis is recommended.

PROGNOSIS
If left untreated, it causes death from severe heart failure or cerebrovascular complications (from associated aneurysms of the circle of Willis or from hypertension). Recurrence rates are variable. There is no pattern of increased recurrence with reconstruction techniques.

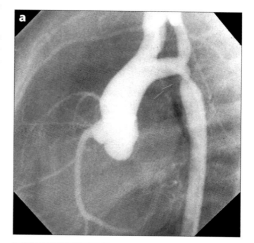

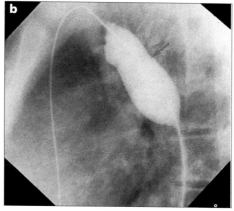

5.5 An angiographic still frame of a patient with coarctation of the aorta before (**a**) and during (**b**) balloon angioplasty.

PATENT ARTERIAL DUCT (PAD)

INCIDENCE
This is the second most common congenital heart disease. In a term infant, the ductus arteriosus closes spontaneously within 72 hours. Patency of the ductus beyond 6 weeks is abnormal.

AETIOLOGY / PATHOGENESIS
The most common association is prematurity.

CLINICAL PRESENTATION
The size of the defect determines the clinical findings. In moderate and large defects, the arterial pulse is of large volume (bounding pulses). There is left ventricular pulsation with the apex shifted out of the mid-clavicular line and down from the 4th intercostal space. There is classically (but unusually) continuous (machinery) murmur heard at the upper left sternal edge midway below the clavicle. However, there may be an early systolic murmur heard only at the upper left sternal edge. The patient may present with symptoms of heart failure (large PAD), recurrent chest infection (moderate PAD) or be asymptomatic (only a murmur in small defect). In premature infants, the increasing oxygen requirements usually alert the neonatologist to the presence of a PAD. A silent duct refers to a large PAD, which is not associated with a murmur; but the other physical findings are present.

DIAGNOSIS
Electrocardiogram. ECG may be normal (in small duct) or show evidence of left atrial and ventricular enlargement when there is a large shunt.
Chest x-ray. In small PAD, the chest x-ray is normal. There may be increased pulmonary vascularity in moderate size and large PAD. The heart is enlarged in large defects. The angle between the pulmonary trunk and aortic arch (knuckle) is obliterated by the PAD, with enlargement of the left atrium.
Echocardiography. This shows the presence of the PAD and dilated left atrium and ventricle in large shunts (**5.6**).

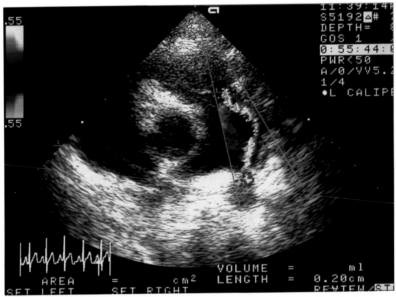

5.6 An echocardiographic left parasternal short axis view with colour flow Doppler, characteristic of PAD.

TREATMENT (5.7)

In premature infants the treatment is with diuretics and fluid restriction. Intravenous indomethacin (1–3 doses) may close the PAD. Failure of this treatment may warrant surgical closure of the PAD. In older children, an occlusion device (by using cardiac catheterization) may achieve total closure of the ductus. Surgical (or thoracoscopic) closure is still an option in some patients (very large duct or on patient request). There are suggestions that asymptomatic or clinically undetectable PAD (only identifiable on echo-Doppler studies by accident) should be left alone. Antibiotic prophylaxis is usually recommended for patients with PAD.

PROGNOSIS

PAD does not usually close spontaneously. If left untreated it may cause complications (such as endo-arteritis), significant shunt may cause pulmonary vascular disease, reversal of the shunt (Eisenmenger complex), aneurysm formation and rupture and calcification. The general recommendation is therefore to close a significant PAD when it is found.

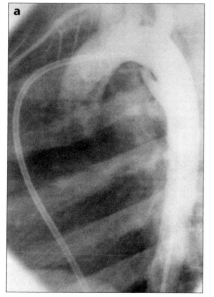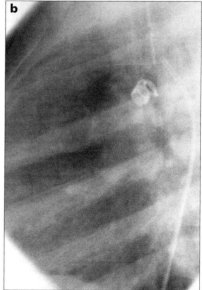

5.7 Angiographic view of PAD before (**a**) and after (**b**) transcatheter coil implantation.

TETRALOGY OF FALLOT (ToF)

INCIDENCE

This is the most common cyanotic congenital heart disease. Its components are; subvalvular pulmonary stenosis, large perimembranous ventricular septal defect, right ventricular hypertrophy and overriding aorta (in severe form, >50% of overriding makes the diagnosis of double outlet right ventricle). Pulmonary stenosis and ventricular septal defect will produce the same physiology as Tetralogy of Fallot (ToF).

AETIOLOGY / PATHOGENESIS

Chromosome 22q11 microdeletions have been associated with 12% of children with ToF with pulmonary stenosis, and 33% of ToF with pulmonary atresia. There is a greater tendency to inheritance by maternal microdeletion.

CLINICAL PRESENTATION

Patient may pass unrecognized until cyanosis occurs. Long standing hypoxia causes clubbing of fingers (**5.8**) and toes. Cyanotic episodes and/or attacks of increased cyanosis with shortness of breath and tachycardia are characteristic of the disease (cyanotic spells). Many children with this condition squat instinctively to increase their stroke volume to temporarily reverse the cyanotic spell. Many children do this before they even experience shortness of breath. The praecordium is quiet to palpation. There may be a palpable second heart sound (aorta close to the chest wall). On auscultation, the first heart sound is normal and the second heart sound is single and loud. There is usually a mid-systolic ejection murmur at the third and fourth intercostal space near the left sternal border. The louder the murmur the milder the subpulmonary stenosis. In cyanotic spells the murmur may disappear.

DIAGNOSIS

Electrocardiogram. This shows right axis deviation and right ventricular hypertrophy with the transition lead at V3-4 (**5.9, 5.10**).

Chest x-ray. This shows pulmonary oligaemia in significant stenosis. The chest x-ray in mild stenosis is similar to that in ventricular septal defect. The shape of the heart is characteristic (round apex which is tilted upwards, increased pulmonary artery bay which makes the heart looks 'boot shaped') The aortic arch is on the right sided in 30 % of cases (**5.11**).

Echocardiogram. It confirms the diagnosis and determines the severity of subpulmonary stenosis and size of pulmonary arteries.

Catheterization and angiography. This is no longer needed for diagnosis or assessment of simple Fallot. Magnetic resonance imaging can provide detailed anatomy of the pulmonary arteries.

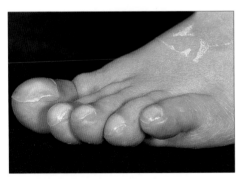

5.8 A third-degree clubbing of the toes.

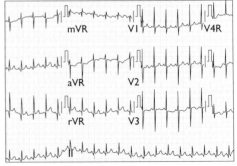

5.9 Electrocardiogram before surgical repair of ToF. Note the presence of right ventricular hypertrophy before the repair.

TREATMENT

All cases of ToF must be repaired unless there is a contraindication. Palliative surgery is in the form of a systemic to pulmonary artery shunt (e.g. a modified Blalock-Taussig shunt). In cyanotic spells, position the child in a squatting position. Avoid any factors that distress the child. Intravenous propranolol is usually needed to help relieve the episode. If these measures fail then surgical intervention is indicated. Prophylactic propranolol may be used in some patients while awaiting surgery.

PROGNOSIS

Untreated patients with ToF have a short life span. They develop severe cyanosis, polycythaemia and die from cerebrovascular and/or cardiac events. They may develop collateral circulation and reach adult life. Sudden death may occur later in life from ventricular arrhythmia and therefore regular follow up is needed. Patients may require further heart surgery to insert a pulmonary valve, which is usually rendered incompetent at the time of the initial repair, where progressive right ventricular dilation is identified.

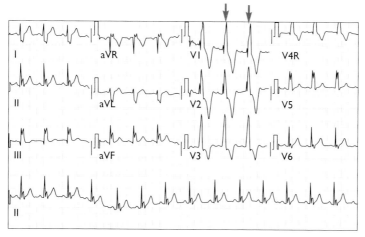

5.10 Electrocardiogram of the patient in 5.9 after surgical repair of ToF. Note complete right bundle branch block after repair.

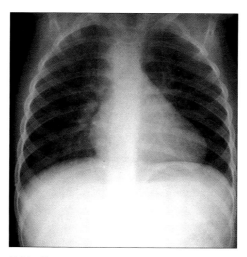

5.11 Chest x-ray of a child with ToF. Note the presence of right aortic arch.

PULMONARY STENOSIS

INCIDENCE

Isolated pulmonary stenosis is a common form of congenital heart disease. Stenosis may be valvular, subvalvular or supravalvular.

AETIOLOGY / PATHOGENESIS

It may occur in association with congenital rubella, Alagille (peripheral pulmonary stenosis), Williams or Noonan syndromes (see 'Gastroenterology' and 'Genetics' chapters). Subvalvular lesions are associated with ventricular septal defect and are a component of tetralogy of Fallot.

CLINICAL PRESENTATION

The physical findings are similar to those of atrial septal defect. However, the second sound may be widely split and the pulmonary component may be quiet or absent. There is usually an ejection click (valvular stenosis) heard maximally at the pulmonary area. There is a mid-systolic ejection murmur. In valvular stenosis, the loudness of the murmur correlates positively with the severity of stenosis. However, this is not the case in subvalvular or supravalvular stenosis where the murmur is louder towards the axillae or the back in peripheral pulmonary stenosis, and at the 3rd left intercostal space in subvalvular stenosis. Severe lesions may cause cyanosis because of right to left shunting at the atrial level. Low cardiac output may present as easy fatigue and poor exercise tolerance.

DIAGNOSIS

Electrocardiogram. This shows right ventricular enlargement of various degrees. The changes in the right praecordial leads are a reliable indicator to the severity of right ventricular hypertrophy and pulmonary stenosis.
Chest x-ray. This may show normal pulmonary vascularity, dilated pulmonary artery (post-stenotic dilatation) and a round upward-tilted apex. The x-ray is similar to that of ASD but with normal pulmonary vascularity. Severe pulmonary stenosis is associated with pulmonary oligaemia on Chest x-ray.
Echocardiogram and Doppler. The gradient between the right ventricle and pulmonary artery may be calculated to determine the severity of the stenosis. Echocardiography (**5.12**) can also measure the size of the pulmonary annulus for intervention.

TREATMENT

Mild lesions are usually left untreated, but moderate and severe stenoses are relieved by balloon angioplasty. In the newborn, surgery is rarely required. Prophylaxis for bacterial endocarditis is not usually required.

PROGNOSIS

An untreated mild lesion may regress with time but moderate and severe lesions usually progress and can be fatal if untreated. Balloon angioplasty, if performed adequately, often does not need to be repeated.

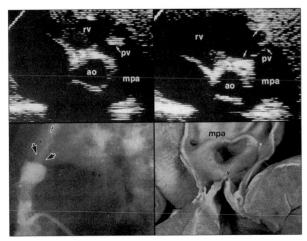

5.12 Echocardiograms showing pulmonary valve stenosis during diastole and systole (top), Angiographic view of pulmonary valve stenosis (lower left) and corresponding heart specimen (lower right).

ao = aorta
rv = right ventricle
pv = pulmonary valve
mpa = mean pulmonary artery

AORTIC STENOSIS

INCIDENCE
The stenosis can be valvular, sub-valvular or supra-valvular.

AETIOLOGY / PATHOGENESIS
This is mainly unknown. Aortic valvular stenosis may be secondary to bicuspid or unicuspid aortic valve, acquired due to rheumatic fever or other systemic diseases such as glycogen storage disease. Supra-valvular stenosis is associated with William syndrome. Subvalvular lesion is also known as fixed subaortic stenosis

CLINICAL PRESENTATION
Patients may complain of chest pain and syncope. Although these symptoms are associated with severe lesions they may also occur in less severe cases. In moderate and severe aortic stenosis, the arterial pulse is weak with slow upstroke (pulsus parvus et tardus). Pulse pressure is low unless associated with aortic regurgitation. There is left ventricular pulsation, which is sustained. There may be a systolic thrill palpable at the aortic area (valvular), third left intercostal space (sub-valvular) or first right intercostal space (supra-valvular). The murmur is located at the same sites but may radiate as well as the thrill to the neck. The presence of an ejection click indicates stenosis of the aortic valve. The second heart sound shows weak aortic component which, in severe cases, may be heard after the pulmonary second sound (reversed splitting).

DIAGNOSIS
Electrocardiogram. This may show left ventricular hypertrophy. There may be ST depression and T wave inversion in severe cases, indicating left ventricular subendocardial ischaemia.

Chest x-ray. This is usually normal in mild lesions. It may show left ventricular enlargement and dilated ascending aorta in valvular stenosis (post-stenotic dilatation).

Echocardiogram and Doppler. This confirms the diagnosis and locates the site of stenosis (**5.13**). Measurement of the aortic root is needed to aid treatment decision (size of angioplasty balloon and/or type of surgery).

TREATMENT
Valvular stenosis is usually treated by balloon angioplasty. Surgery is considered for small children, failed balloon dilatation, sub-valvular and supra-valvular stenosis. In the presence of a small aortic root, replacement or augmentation of the root may be carried out (Kono procedure) Exercise levels may need restriction. All patients will require prophylactic antibiotic for endocarditis.

PROGNOSIS
Patients with mild lesions and those that are adequately treated have a normal life expectancy (if left ventricular hypertrophy and ischaemia is totally reversed to normal). Severe lesions cause severe heart failure and patients may die suddenly. Subvalvular stenosis is a progressive disease and may be associated with aortic regurgitation. Incomplete resection of sub-valvular stenosis may recur. All patients are at risk of endocarditis. Critical aortic stenosis is a duct-dependent lesion.

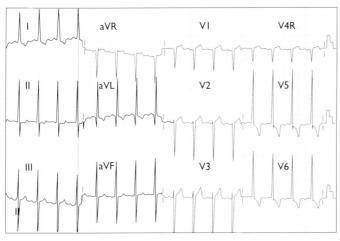

5.13 A long axis view (echocardiogram) from a patient with discrete subaortic stenosis.

CARDIOMYOPATHY

INCIDENCE
This may be dilated, hypertrophic or restrictive cardiomyopathy.

AETIOLOGY / PATHOGENESIS
The hypertrophic form has a genetic predisposition and is familial. It may be associated with lentiginosis. The dilated form may follow any severe heart disease as well as several systemic diseases and can be idiopathic or familial. It may cause dilated cardiomyopathy.

CLINICAL PRESENTATION
Dilated and restrictive cardiomyopathy usually presents with symptoms of heart failure (shortness of breath, fatigue, poor feeding, failure to thrive). Hypertrophic cardiomyopathy may present with sudden death, chest pain, syncope, recurrent tachycardia (ventricular) or heart failure. There may be symptoms of the systemic disease. The jugular venous pulse is prominent in restrictive cardiomyopathy with rapid Y descent. In severe cases, systemic hypotension is noted. The liver may be enlarged (in heart failure)and the respiratory rate increased. Peripheral oedema may be noted in the periorbital area and the dorsum of hands and feet. Ankle oedema occurs in ambulant children.

There are usually third and fourth heart sounds with tachycardia, producing a galloping rhythm. There may be a pansystolic murmur of mitral regurgitation (at the apex and radiating to the axilla) or tricuspid regurgitation (at the lower left sternal edge). In hypertrophic cardiomyopathy there may be a palpable third heart sound at the apex. There may also be a mid systolic ejection murmur at the 3rd left intercostal space. In restrictive cardiomyopathy, the praecordial impulses are reduced.

DIAGNOSIS
Electrocardiogram. This usually shows evidence of biventricular enlargement in dilated cardiomyopathy. Hypertrophic cardiomyopathy usually shows an enlarged left ventricle with ST segment and T wave changes. The P wave may be long and bifid. In restrictive cardiomyopathy, there is usually ST segment depression and/or T wave inversion with evidence of dilated left and right atria (tall P wave which is also biphasic).

Chest x-ray. The heart is enlarged and there may be pulmonary venous congestion. In hypertrophic cardiomyopathy, the heart size may appear normal but the left atrium may be dilated. There may be pulmonary oedema. In restrictive cardiomyopathy the cardio-thoracic ratio is not increased.

Echocardiography. This determines the type of cardiomyopathy and ventricular size and function. In restrictive cardiomyopathy the ventricles are not enlarged but the atria are dilated.

Cardiac catheterization is carried out prior to transplantation to assess the extent of pulmonary vascular disease. A myocardial biopsy will determine the cause of dilated cardiomyopathy.

TREATMENT
This is the same as for heart failure (diuretics, vasodilators and ACE inhibitors). Anticoagulation may be needed if there is evidence of embolism or intracavitary thrombosis. Beta-blockers are used in adults and there is some support for their use in children with heart failure. Beta-blockers are routinely used for hypertrophic cardiomyopathy and anti-arrhythmic agents may be necessary. In the presence of localized obstruction, surgical myectomy or myotomy may be performed. Repair or replacement of the mitral valve may be needed. Transplantation may be needed if ventricular function is poor and there is no sign of improvement.

PROGNOSIS
This depends on the aetiology. It is poor for hypertrophic cardiomyopathy, most metabolic causes (check availability of enzyme replacement) and idiopathic dilated cardiomyopathy. The outcome is often good after myocarditis. Transplantation is an option but sudden death may occur.

SUPRAVENTRICULAR TACHYCARDIA (SVT)

INCIDENCE

This is the commonest type of arrhythmia in children. It can be re-entrant, ectopic, or junctional type. Atrial flutter can be considered as supraventricular type of tachycardia.

AETIOLOGY / PATHOGENESIS

This is most commonly due to abnormal automaticity or a re-entrant circuit. Predisposing factors include electrolyte imbalances, atrial dilation, thyrotoxicosis, or myocarditis,

CLINICAL PRESENTATION

Patients may present with heart failure, dizzy episodes or palpitations. The hallmark of diagnosis is the finding of a rapid heart rate , exceeding 180 beats per minute in the newborn, or 160 beats per minute in children with a characteristic ECG. The heart rate during SVT may exceed 300 beats per minute in infancy.

DIAGNOSIS

Electrocardiogram. This is used for diagnosis and differentiates from atrial flutter (saw tooth appearance of flutter waves) and ventricular tachycardia (wide QRS complex with irregular R-R intervals) (**5.14**). Twenty-four hour ambulatory monitoring may be needed to disclose the type and frequency of arrhythmias.
Chest x-ray. This shows a normal heart, but occasionally the heart is enlarged from chronic paroxysmal tachycardia.

Echocardiogram and Doppler. This excludes any structural heart disease. Fetal echocardiography allows recognition of fetal tachycardia.

TREATMENT

Treat any precipitating factor. Atrial flutter is treated by synchronized direct cardioversion. Other forms of supraventricular tachycardia may be managed with Valsava manoeuvre, iced water 'diving', or chemically cardioverted with rapid acting intravenous adenosine. Anti-arrhythmic agents such as amiodarone or flecainide may be necessary for refractory or recurrent arrhythmias. Long-term treatment may be necessary. Transcatheter ablation is considered in resistant cases, particularly older children and adults.

PROGNOSIS

Young infants may present *in extremis*, however older children and adults are rarely haemodynamically compromised during episodes unless very longstanding. Anti-arrhythmic treatments are also associated with side effects, including other forms of arrhythmia. Junctional ectopic tachycardia after cardiac surgery is a serious problem. The natural history is to resolve over time, but haemodynamic compromise may be life threatening. Treatment involves cooling, atrial pacing and reduction of catecholaminergic support. Congenital junctional ectopic tachycardia carries a poor prognosis. Chronic recurrent atrial flutter may cause cardiomegaly and heart failure that is reversible with treatment.

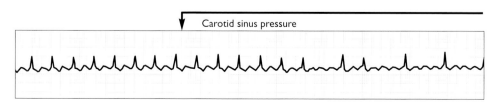

Carotid sinus pressure

5.14 An electrocardiogram of a child with atrial flutter. Note the saw-tooth appearance of the flutter waves.

PERICARDITIS AND PERICARDIAL EFFUSION

INCIDENCE
Pericarditis is inflammation of the pericardium. It may be acute or chronic and can be constrictive. Pericardial effusion is accumulation of fluid (transudate, exudate, purulent, haemopericardium) between the parietal and epicardial layers of the pericardium.

AETIOLOGY / PATHOGENESIS
It may be viral, bacterial (e.g. tuberculosis, *Staphylococcus aureus*), trauma (heart surgery), myocarditis (pancarditis such as rheumatic fever), a tumour invading the heart, systemic inflammatory disease or idiopathic.

CLINICAL PRESENTATION
The patient may present with chest pain which is characteristically reduced on leaning forward. Shortness of breath may occur with rapidly accumulating effusion (tamponade). Systemic manifestation of the underlying disease may be present. A jugular venous pulse is prominent in a large effusion. A rapid Y descent is usually noted in constrictive lesions and tamponade. The arterial pulse may be normal or may fluctuate during inspiration (reduced volume during inspiration, pulsus paradoxus). This can be confirmed by blood pressure measurement (systolic blood pressure reduced during inspiration by more than 10 mmHg). The praecordium is quiet to palpation. The heart sounds are usually muffled with pericardial effusion. A friction rub is heard in acute pericarditis.

A pericardial knock (metallic sound) may be heard during systole in constrictive pericarditits.

DIAGNOSIS
Electrocardiogram. ECG shows inverted T waves in most chest leads, with upward concavity of the ST segment. In large effusions, the QRS amplitude may be reduced in all chest leads.

Chest x-ray. The heart may be normal in acute pericarditis, constrictive form and small effusions. The heart is markedly enlarged in large effusions (**5.15**), often with pulmonary oedema.

Echocardiogram. This delineates the severity of the effusion and whether the right atrium or ventricle are being compressed (tamponade), and may reveal the thickness of the pericardium. Further investigations are required to disclose the aetiology.

TREATMENT
Treatment is for underlying disease and pain relief. Large and purulent effusions should be aspirated and/or drained. Steroids may be considered in selected cases to reduce the likelihood of constriction. Pericardiectomy is carried out to relieve cardiac constriction.

PROGNOSIS
Most cases resolve completely but may recur. Bacterial pericarditis may cause constriction. Pericardial constriction is usually difficult to relieve. Prognosis is usually poor in constrictive and post radiotherapy pericarditis, transplantation may be recommended.

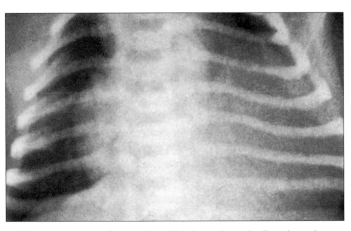

5.15 A chest x-ray of a one-day-old baby with markedly enlarged heart from massive pericardial effusion.

HEART BLOCK

INCIDENCE
Heart block indicates a failure of atrial activation to be transmitted to the ventricle, so the atria and ventricles are activated independently. It may be congenital or acquired and is rare.

AETIOLOGY / PATHOGENESIS
The cause is usually unknown. It may be acquired secondary to maternal systemic lupus erythematosus, heart surgery, drugs, myocarditis or an intracardiac tumour.

CLINICAL PRESENTATION
The patient may be asymptomatic and diagnosis is made during routine examination (slow heart rate) or on antenatal scan (fetal bradycardia). The patient may present with dizzy episodes or syncope with a heart rate that is slow for their age. There may be left ventricular pulsation due to enlargement of the left ventricle (large stroke volume). Pulse pressure is wide. In older children cannon a waves in jugular venous pulse may be noted.

DIAGNOSIS
Electrocardiogram. The typical picture of complete heart block shows no relation between P waves and QRS complex (**5.16**). In congenital form, the QRS complex is usually narrow (<0.12 sec). Heart rate in infants and young children may reach 100/minute due to fast nodal rhythm. Wide QRS complex suggests idio-ventricular rhythm (it may be wide due to heart surgery).

Chest x-ray. The heart may be normal in size, but it is usually enlarged.

Echocardiogram. This can demonstrate ventricular function and fetal echocardiography allows diagnosis of heart block antenatally.

TREATMENT
Asymptomatic children are treated conservatively. Symptomatic children, those with wide complex heart block, frequent ventricular ectopic beats and heart rate less than 55 beats per minute in an infant should receive pacemaker implantation. If the heart rate is very slow, intravenous isoprenaline can be given to increase the rate while awaiting pacemaker implantation.

PROGNOSIS
The natural history is progressive development of symptoms and if untreated can suddenly be fatal. The overall prognosis, even with a pacemaker, is guarded. A mother who has had a child with congenital heart block is at 8% risk of a second child with the same disease.

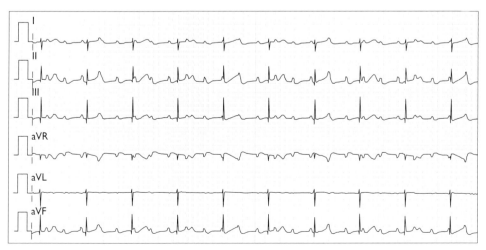

5.16 A 12-lead electrocardiogram from a newborn with congenital complete heart block. Note that there is no relationship between P waves and QRS complexes, which are narrow.

ANOMALOUS PULMONARY VENOUS DRAINAGE

INCIDENCE
A rare condition, pertaining to abnormal connection of the pulmonary veins to sites other than the left atrium (such as the superior vena cava, **5.17**). It may be total or partial, with some veins draining normally.

AETIOLOGY
The aetiology is unknown.

CLINICAL PRESENTATION
The patient is blue (or dusky). The clinical picture depends on whether the venous pathway is obstructed or not. If it is obstructed, the patient presents as a newborn with severe heart failure and pulmonary oedema requiring ventilation. Unobstructed veins may present later with heart failure and a hyperactive right ventricle. Partial anomalous venous connection may appear – for example, atrial septal defect, with the second heart sound widely split with an accentuated pulmonary component. The difference from ASD is that the splitting of the second heart sound is not fixed. There is usually an ejection systolic murmur at the pulmonary area.

DIAGNOSIS
Electrocardiogram. This shows right ventricular hypertrophy and right axis deviation.
Chest x-ray. This shows an enlarged heart and pulmonary plethora. In supra-diaphragmatic total anomalous venous connection it may show a figure of 8 (or snowman appearance). Partial anomalous venous connection may look similar to the x-ray of atrial septal defect. A sequestration of part of the right lung, associated with anomalous pulmonary venous drainage to the inferior caval or hepatic vein and abnormal arterial supply from the aorta or its branches, is often described as the Scimitar syndrome. The vertical common pulmonary vein causes a characteristic sword-like feature on chest x-ray. There is usually hypoplasia of the right lung.
Echocardiogram and Doppler. This confirms the diagnosis and identifies the anatomy of total or partial abnormalities and whether it connects to the systemic vein above or below the diaphragm. The right ventricle and atrium are dilated. There is always an atrial septal defect in patients with total anomalous connection. Absence of an ASD is incompatible with life.
Cardiac catheterization. This may be required to disclose details of the anatomy (**5.17**) in complex cases and to perform atrial septostomy if the atrial septal defect is small (can be performed under echo control).

TREATMENT
This is surgical. It is important to keep the patient haemodynamically stable until surgery is performed. Isolated anomalous small pulmonary veins (a shunt of less than 1.5:1) may be left untreated.

PROGNOSIS
Total anomalous venous drainage if left untreated is fatal. The outcome of surgical repair is influenced by the complexity of the anatomy and general condition of the child. Partial anomalous venous connection is similar to that of atrial septal defect. Surgical repair may result in complications, particularly damage to the sinus node, and residual pulmonary vein stenosis.

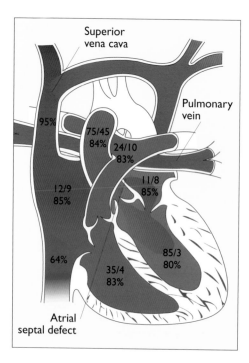

5.17 Cardiac catheterization findings (blood pressure and oxygen saturation) in an infant with total anomalous pulmonary venous drainage. Note the high O_2 saturation in the superior vena cava.

ENDOCARDITIS

INCIDENCE
This is an acute, subacute or chronic infection of the endocardium including valves.

AETIOLOGY / PATHOGENESIS
The commonest organism is *Streptococcus viridans.* but any organism can infect the heart. An underlying predisposing structural abnormality is usually found, although rarely it may occur in a normal heart. It is rare with atrial septal defect and pulmonary stenosis.

CLINICAL PRESENTATION
In the acute form, the patient presents with a high temperature and is seriously unwell. In the subacute form the patient tires easily, often with a low-grade temperature and sweating. The symptoms may be so vague that such patients may present with a fever of unknown origin. A history of a procedure and heart disease suggests the diagnosis. There may be clubbing of the fingers and toes and the spleen may be enlarged. Sub-conjunctival haemorrhage, Oslers nodes, subcutaneous nodules and splinter haemorrhage may be found. The previous heart murmur may change or a new murmur may appear. Systemic septic emboli may occur.

DIAGNOSIS
Blood culture. Blood cultures must be taken first, prior to treatment.
Electrocardiogram. This may be normal. If there is atrio-ventricular valve dysfunction, this may be reflected in abnormal P waves from atrial enlargement.
Chest x-ray. This may show evidence of pulmonary embolism.

Echocardiogram. This may show the site of the endocardial vegetation and disclose the underlying heart disease (**5.18**). A negative echocardiogram does not rule out bacterial endocarditis. Blood culture is the most important diagnostic test (3 consecutive blood cultures for both aerobic and anaerobic organisms). In negative blood cultures, endocarditis antibody titres of the suspected organism may help in the diagnosis.

Treatment
In the acute form, treatment with broad-spectrum antibiotics that cover both gram positive and negative organisms may be started while waiting for the culture sensitivity results. Changes are made based on the clinical condition and the results of the sensitivity tests. In the sub-acute form, treatment can be started after the results have been obtained (usually from 24–48 hours). Treatment should be continued for 6 weeks.

Prognosis
Acute endocarditis is fatal if not treated. Inadequate treatment (choice of drug or dosage) may cause resistant organism and can be fatal. The prognosis depends on the severity of infection, complications (e.g. residual valve lesion or papillary muscle rupture) and the invading organism. The risk of re-infection is increased.

Prevention
It is important to prevent this type of infection by using appropriate antibiotics prior surgical or dental treatment.

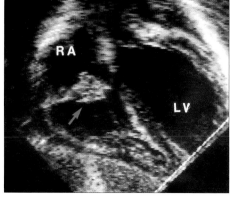

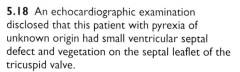

5.18 An echocardiographic examination disclosed that this patient with pyrexia of unknown origin had small ventricular septal defect and vegetation on the septal leaflet of the tricuspid valve.

TRICUSPID ATRESIA

INCIDENCE
This may be due to the absence of the inflow part of the right ventricle or an imperforate valve. Thus, the outlet for the right atrium is the interatrial septum (or patent foramen ovale). The right ventricle is small. The blood flows to the pulmonary artery via a ventricular septal defect, which if small causes sub-valvular stenosis, or via the patent ductus arteriosus.

AETIOLOGY
The aetiology is unknown.

CLINICAL PRESENTATION
The child is usually blue at birth. The spectrum may range from heart failure due to increased pulmonary flow via a large ventricular septal defect to severe cyanosis due to severe sub-pulmonary stenosis. A small restrictive atrial communication causes systemic venous congestion. The right ventricular pulsations are reduced or absent. There is a left ventricular apex, which may be shifted. The first heart sound is single (difficult to recognize). The second heart sound may be single (large VSD) or split with a delayed pulmonary component (severe sub-pulmonary stenosis). There may be a mid-systolic ejection murmur (sub-pulmonary stenosis) at the 3rd left intercostal space.

DIAGNOSIS
Electrocardiogram. Characteristically, it shows left axis deviation and reduced right ventricular forces in the right chest leads (**5.19**).

Chest x-ray. The heart tends to have a straight right border. The pulmonary vascularity may be normal, reduced or increased according to the size of the ventricular septal defect.
Echocardiography. This delineates the anatomy and confirms the diagnosis.
Cardiac catheterization. This may be indicated to assess the size of the pulmonary arteries and pulmonary resistance. Particularly important prior to decision-making on the type of surgical repair.

TREATMENT
This is surgical and depends on the child's condition and age. Palliation may be in the form of systemic to pulmonary arterial shunt (Blalock-Taussig-type shunt) or systemic venous to pulmonary artery connection (Glenn-type procedure). The total repair is to establish a Fontan-type circulation by connecting the systemic venous return to the pulmonary artery (or total caval anastomosis to the pulmonary arteries). The criteria for this type of repair are good left ventricular function, low pulmonary vascular resistance, good size pulmonary arteries and normal function mitral valve.

PROGNOSIS
The outcome of the Fontan procedure is guarded because of the long-term complications, including treatment resistant arrhythmias, ventricular failure, pulmonary oedema, systemic venous obstruction and pulmonary vein compression.

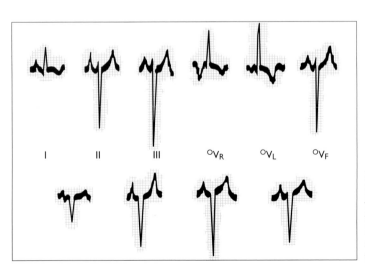

5.19
Electrocardiogram from a child with tricuspid atresia. Note left axis deviation and absence of right ventricular forces.

TRANSPOSITION OF GREAT ARTERIES

INCIDENCE
This is an uncommon congenital malformation. The aorta arises from the right ventricle and the pulmonary artery from the left ventricle. Thus, the aorta is anterior and to the right of the pulmonary artery (although it may vary). See **5.22** (next page).

AETIOLOGY
This is unknown.

CLINICAL PRESENTATION
Although appearing normal at birth, the child may become unwell, blue (central cyanosis), and breathless. This may occur because the patent arterial duct may be patent and of good size during the hospital stay and mislead the neonatologist. The diagnosis is made when the child presents with the above symptoms. There may be a murmur (usually from associated lesions such as ventricular septal defect, or associated sub-pulmonary stenosis). The praecordium may be more active than normal, although this often is not observed in the newborn. The right ventricular impulse is very easy to feel. In neonates with cyanosis, the hyperoxia test is positive. This differentiates between cyanotic congenital heart disease and respiratory disease.

DIAGNOSIS
Electrocardiogram. In the first few days of life a normal neonatal pattern is observed. Later right ventricular enlargement may be seen.

Chest x-ray. This typically shows the appearance of an egg on its side (**5.20**), because the aorta and pulmonary artery shadows are overlapping, producing a narrow pedicle. The pulmonary vascularity is normal. If there is a large patent arterial duct or ventricular septal defect, it may be increased.

Echocardiogram. This confirms the diagnosis and shows the anatomy of the coronary arteries and assesses the size of the atrial septal defect (**5.21**).

Cardiac catheterization. This may be required to delineate the anatomy of the coronary arteries and any associated lesions.

TREATMENT
Initially infants most often require balloon atrial septostomy. The arterial switch operation is the recommended surgery for newborns before 6 weeks of age. Beyond that age limit the left ventricle may have involuted, being faced with the low afterload of the pulmonary vascular bed. Retraining may therefore be necessary by pulmonary artery banding, to increase left ventricular mass and contractility pending a delayed arterial switch operation.

PROGNOSIS
Transposition of the great arteries is a fatal disease if left untreated. The mid term outcome of an uncomplicated switch operation is good. However, later complications were observed particularly supra-valvular pulmonary and/or aortic stenosis. Damage to the myocardium due to coronary complications affects life expectancy.

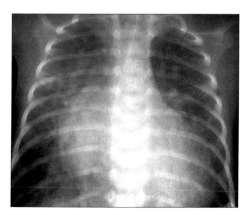

5.20 X-ray showing large heart with 'egg on side' appearance.

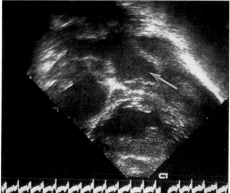

5.21 A long-axis view (echocardiogram) showing the pulmonary artery arising from left ventricle, identified on the second day of life.

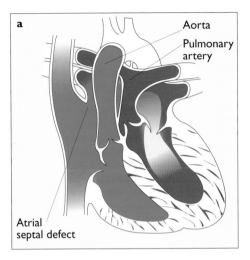

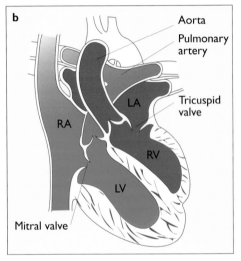

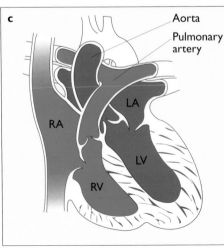

CORRECTED TRANSPOSITION OF GREAT ARTERIES

INCIDENCE
This is a rare, complicated, congenital anomaly. In this condition, the arrangement of the heart chambers is as follows:
- The right ventricle is on the left side receiving blood from the left atrium.
- The left ventricle is on the right side receiving blood from the right atrium .
- The aorta arises from the right ventricle and is located anterior and to the left of the pulmonary artery.
- The pulmonary artery arises from the left ventricle and is located posterior and to the right of the aorta.

Thus, the blood flow (oxygenated and non-oxygenated) is normal (**5.22**).

AETIOLOGY
This is unknown.

CLINICAL PRESENTATION
In isolation this disease may pass unknown for many years. The presentation is usually because of associated lesions, most commonly ventricular septal defect. Patients are at more risk of complete heart block, either congenitally or following surgical closure repair of intracardiac defect.

DIAGNOSIS
Electrocardiogram. Characteristically it shows deep Q wave in Vl-2 which is absent from V5-6 (because left ventricle is anterior). It may show complete heart block.

Chest x-ray. The left border of the heart may appear like a straight line (ascending aorta is on the left side). The heart may be enlarged if there is an associated lesion. Pulmonary vascularity is normal unless there is associated defect.

Echocardiogram. This is a diagnostic test which delineates the anatomy. In many cases this is not recognized until an echocardiogram is carried out for other purposes.

Cardiac catheterization. This is (rarely) carried out to confirm the diagnosis in doubtful cases, and more usually to clarify other associated lesions.

5.22 A diagram of transposition of great arteries (**a**) and congenitally corrected transposition of great arteries (**b**), compared with a normal heart (**c**).

TREATMENT
Uncomplicated cases are usually not diagnosed. However, some centres are carrying out double switch procedures (atrial switch and arterial switch) to keep the left ventricle in the systemic circulation. This has a very high mortality rate because of the process of left ventricular training by pulmonary artery banding associated with injury of the left ventricle itself. A pacemaker is required for cases of heart block.

PROGNOSIS
The life expectancy of uncomplicated cases is shorter than normal because the right ventricle is the systemic ventricle. There may be a role of measuring ischaemia to the RV based on isotope/perfusion studies. The anatomical substrate for right ventricular ischaemia is established. Complications are those of heart block, systemic atrioventricular valve regurgitation and heart failure. The prognosis is worsened by the presence of associated lesions.

VASCULAR RING

INCIDENCE
This is an anomaly caused by blood vessels that circle the trachea and causes its compression. The most common cause is a left-sided aortic arch with an aberrant right subclavian artery and right arterial duct or ductal ligament causing compression. A right sided aortic arch and aberrant left subclavian artery with left arterial duct or ductal ligament may also cause similar airways compression, although this is rare. A true double aortic arch ((5.23) is rare, but when present will cause a vascular ring. The only 'ring' to give an anterior oesophageal indention is a pulmonary artery sling.

AETIOLOGY
This is unknown.

CLINICAL PRESENTATION
The child usually presents with stridor and/or dysphagia. There may be associated congenital heart disease.

DIAGNOSIS
Chest x-ray. This may show right aortic arch.
Barium swallow. The most useful diagnostic investigation is barium swallow, which most commonly shows posterior indentation of the oesophagus.
Electrocardiogram. Non-specific changes may be seen.
Echocardiogram. It discloses the anatomy of the vascular ring.
Cardiac catheterization. This is to confirm the diagnosis and may be needed prior to surgical treatment.

TREATMENT
This is surgical division of the vascular ring. In double aortic arch, aortopexy may be necessary using a sling to reduced the pressure on the trachea.

PROGNOSIS
This is good if the ring is divided. The outcome depends on associated lesions.

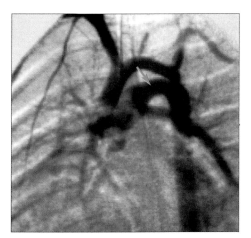

5.23 Angiogram showing double aortic arch and patent ductus arteriosus.

REFERENCES

Ventricular septal defect (VSD)
Hoffman JI. Congenital heart disease: incidence and inheritance. *Ped Clin N Am* 1990; **37**: 25–43.
Karr SS. New Doppler techniques for the evaluation of regurgitant and shunt volumes. *Curr Opin Cardiol* 1998; **13**: 56–58.
Hollman A. Ventricular septal defect. *B Heart J* 1967; **29**(6): 813–815.

Atrial septal defect (ASD)
Staffen RN, Davidson WR. Echocardiographic assessment of atrial septal defects. *Echocardiography* 1993; **10**: 545–552.
O'Laughlin MP. Catheter closure of secundum atrial septal defects. *Tex Heart Inst J* 1997; **24**: 287–292.
Espino-Vela J, Alvarado-Toro A. Natural history of atrial septal defect. *Cardiovasc Clin* 1971; **2**: 103–125.

Patent ductus arteriosus (PDA)
Srivastava D, Olson EN. A genetic blueprint for cardiac development. *Nature* 2000; **407**: 221–226.
Driscoll DJ. Left-to-right shunt lesions. *Ped Clin N Am* 1999; **46**: 64–68.

Coarctation of the aorta
McCrindle BW. Coarctation of the aorta. *Curr Opin Cardiol* 1999; **14**: 448–452.
Johnson MC, Canter CE, Strauss AW, Spray TL. Repair Of coarctation of the aorta in infancy – comparison of surgical and balloon angioplasty. *Am Heart J* 1993; **125**: 464–468.

Tetralogy of Fallot
Lu JH, Chung MY, Hwang B, Chien HP. Prevalence and parental origin in Tetralogy of Fallot associated with chromosome 22q11 microdeletion. *Pediatrics* 1999; **104**: 87–90.
Pacifico AD, Kirklin JK, Colvin EV, McConnell ME, Kirklin JW. Tetralogy of Fallot: late results and reoperations. *Semin Thorac Cardiovasc Surg* 1990; **2**: 108–116.

Pulmonary stenosis
Snellen HA, Hartman H, Buis-Liem TN, Kole EH, Rohmer J. Pulmonic stenosis. *Circulation* 1968; **38**: 93–101.
Rao PS. Balloon pulmonary valvuloplasty: a review. *Clin Cardiol* 1989; **12**: 55–74.

Aortic stenosis
Glancy DL, Epstein SE. Differential diagnosis of type and severity of obstruction to left ventricular outflow. *Prog Cardiovasc Dis* 1971; **14**: 153–191.
El Habbal MH, Suliman R. The aortic root in subaortic stenosis. *Am Heart J* 1989; **117**: 1127–1133.

Cardiomyopathy
McKenna WJ. The natural history of hypertrophic cardiomyopathy. *Cardiovasc Clin* 1988; **19**: 135–148.
Kopecky SL, Gersh BJ. Dilated cardiomyopathy and myocarditis: natural history, etiology, clinical manifestations, and management. *Curr Prob Cardiol* 1987; **12**: 569–647.
Bruns LA, Chrisant MK, Lamour *et al.* Carvedilol as therapy in pediatric heart failure: an initial multicenter experience. *J Pediatr* 2001; **138**: 505–511.

Supraventricular tachycardia
Case CL, Gillette PC. Automatic atrial and junctional tachycardias in the pediatric patient – strategies for diagnosis and management. *Pacing Clin Electrophysiol* 1993; **16**: 1323–1335.
Etheridge SP, Judd VE. Supraventricular tachycardia in infancy: evaluation, management, and follow-up. *Arch Ped Adolesc Med* 1999; **153**: 267–270.

Pericarditis and pericardial effusion
Hancock EW. Pericarditis and other pericardial diseases. *Curr Opin Cardiol* 1991; **6**: 428–434.

Heart block
Pordon CM, Moodie DS. Adults with congenital complete heart-block – 25-year follow-up. *Clevel Clin Med* 1992; **59**: 587–590.
Michaelsson M, Riesenfeld T, Jonzon A. Natural history of congenital complete atrioventricular block. *Pacing Clin Electrophysiol* 1997; **20**: 2098–2101.

Anomalous pulmonary venous drainage
Hammon JW. Total anomalous pulmonary connection – then and now. *Ann Thorac Surg* 1993; **55**: 1030–1032.

Endocarditis
Martin TM, Neches WH, Wald ER. Infective endocarditis: 35 years of experience at a children's hospital. *Clin Infect Dis* 1997; **24**: 669–675.

Tricuspid atresia
Franklin RCG, Spiegelhalter DJ, Sullivan ID *et al.* Tricuspid-atresia presenting in infancy – survival and suitability for the Fontan operation. *Circulation* 1993; **87**: 427–439.

Transposition of great arteries
Van Praagh R, Jung WK. The arterial switch operation in transposition of the great arteries: anatomic indications and contraindications. *Thorac Cardiovasc Surg* 1991; **39**: 138–150.

Corrected transposition of the great arteries
Connelly MS, Liu PP, Williams WG *et al.* Congenitally corrected transposition of the great arteries in the adult – functional status and complications. *J Am Coll Cardiol* 1996; **27**: 1238–1243.

Vascular ring
Lowe GM, Donaldson JS, Backer CL. Vascular rings – 10-year review of imaging *Radiographics* 1991; **11**: 637–646.

Dermatology
Alan Irvine
Debra Lomas
David Atherton
John Harper

VIRAL WARTS

INCIDENCE / GENETICS
Viral warts are one of the commonest infections in man and one of the commonest dermatological conditions presenting to primary care physicians.

CLINICAL PRESENTATION
Cutaneous viral warts present as discrete, raised lesions on any body surface. The appearance is often dependent on the body site affected. The commonest site is the hands (**6.1**); warts on the nose are often filiform or pedunculated (**6.2**).

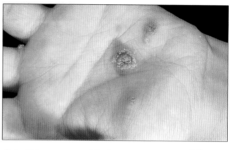

6.1 Palmar warts. Viral warts are one of the commonest infections.

AETIOLOGY / PATHOGENESIS
Viral warts are caused by infection with the double-stranded DNA human papilloma virus. At least 82 different types of papilloma virus have been characterized and almost certainly many more remain unidentified. Some viruses have oncogenic potential (see anogenital warts).

Inherited susceptibility to HPV infection may be relevant in the general population, but the best evidence for genetic determination is the rare condition epidermodysplasia verruciformis, an autosomal recessive disease characterized by increased susceptibility to the oncogenic HPV5. Recently this condition has recently been attributed to two genes, *EVER1* and *EVER2*, located on chromosome 17q25.

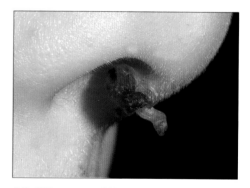

6.2 Filiform warts. Warts on the nose are often filiform in character.

DIAGNOSIS
The diagnosis is usually clinically obvious.

TREATMENT

There are no easy, painless treatments available for removing viral warts. A decision to treat must be made with the knowledge that warts are usually self-limiting and most treatments will require several applications. The simplest treatments, which are often successful, are based around salicylic acid, and are available as over-the-counter preparations. Recalcitrant warts may be treated with liquid nitrogen cryo-therapy, which is effective but does have the drawback of pain on application and, rarely, scarring after treatment. These side-effects, along with the need for repeated applications, limits the use of liquid nitrogen in paediatric dermatology.

PROGNOSIS

In otherwise fit and well individuals, viral warts will usually resolve with time. In immuno-suppressed patients, warts may become more extensive with time.

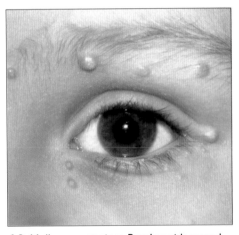

6.3 Mollusca contagiosa. Papules with central umbilication are characteristic of mollusca contagiosa. It is caused by a pox virus and the papules always resolve spontaneously. They can be widespread in children with atopic eczema and in immunocompromised individuals.

MOLLUSCUM CONTAGIOSUM

See also 'Ophthalmology' chapter.

INCIDENCE / GENETICS

The disease is common throughout the world. It is, however, rare under the age of one year, perhaps due to maternally transmitted immunity and the long incubation period. In hotter countries, where children are lightly dressed and in close contact, the peak incidence is between two and three years. In cooler clim-ates, infection tends to occur later.

It is likely that the great majority of children are infected at some time, but most infections probably go unnoticed because there is only a single lesion. The impression that mollusca are commoner in patients with atopic eczema is false; these children tend to have larger num-bers of lesions and therefore more often seek medical advice. Unusually widespread lesions may be seen in the immunocompromised, reflecting the role of cell-mediated immunity in the control and elimination of the infection.

AETIOLOGY / PATHOGENESIS

The molluscum contagiosum virus is a pox virus. Infection follows inoculation by infected persons, probably most often via the fingernails.

CLINICAL PRESENTATION

The incubation period of this pox virus is estimated at 14 days to 6 months. The indivi-dual lesion is a shiny, pearly-white, hemispherical papule which becomes umbilicated as it matures. It enlarges slowly and may reach a diameter of 5–10 mm in 6–12 weeks, though individual lesions may become considerably larger (**6.3**). After several months, inflammation occurs spontaneously as part of the immune response, resulting in eczematous changes, pruritus, suppuration, crusting and eventual destruction of the lesion. Patients may have just one or two lesions, or many hundreds.

The distribution of the lesions largely reflects the initial site of viral entry and the pattern of subsequent self-inoculation. For example, children with atopic eczema commonly have large numbers of lesions because of scratching. In otherwise healthy subjects, facial lesions are frequent, particularly on the eyelids, but they may, in practice, occur on any part of the body surface. Mollusca contagiosa are also commonly seen on the genital and perineal skin, and abuse should not be regarded as likely unless there are other suspicious features. Molluscum conta-giosum lesions may Köebnerise.

DIAGNOSIS
The diagnosis is usually clinically obvious. Direct microscopic examination of a curetted lesion crushed on a slide will reveal large hyaline bodies (molluscum bodies) in the central core of the lesion; this manoeuvre is however only very rarely necessary.

TREATMENT
It is usually best to leave mollusca to resolve spontaneously rather than using freezing, diathermy or curettage.

PROGNOSIS
Spontaneous resolution will generally occur within six to 24 months, but can take longer. Scarred pits may remain, but these improve with time.

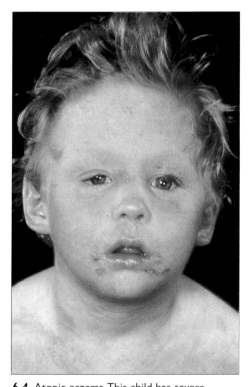

6.4 Atopic eczema. This child has severe erythrodermic eczema, which commenced at three months of age. Itching is a troublesome symptom. This disease waxes and wanes with acute exacerbations after being precipitated by secondary skin infections.

ATOPIC DERMATITIS (ATOPIC ECZEMA)

INCIDENCE / GENETICS
The terms dermatitis and eczema are used synonymously. Approximately 10% of children under five years have atopic dermatitis. In 80%, the onset is within the first year of life.

AETIOLOGY / PATHOGENESIS
There is a recognized genetic background, with some 70% of children having a positive family history of atopy (eczema, asthma or hayfever). The pathogenesis of atopic dermatitis represents a complex inter-relationship between genetic, immunological and pharmacological factors. Children with atopic dermatitis usually have an eosinophilia, a raised IgE and often produce multiple positive prick tests to a variety of common allergens.

A variety of factors can provoke or aggravate atopic dermatitis on a day-to-day basis, but these vary from one child to another and also relate to age and environmental exposure. They include food allergies (especially in infancy), viral infections and allergy to house dust mites and animal dander.

CLINICAL PRESENTATION
Atopic dermatitis often starts on the face in infancy, although any area can be affected (**6.4**). There is a predilection for the flexures, especially the antecubital and popliteal fossae (**6.5**). Sometimes the extensor aspects are affected. The predominant symptom of atopic dermatitis is itching, and the baby is fretful because of this. Rubbing and scratching the skin aggravates the dermatitis.

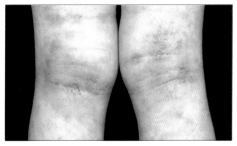

6.5 Atopic eczema. Extreme lichenification of long-standing eczema can be seen in this girl's popliteal fossae.

The disease typically waxes and wanes, and an acute exacerbation is frequently related to skin infection. These children are susceptible to infection because of scratching and fissuring of the skin. In older children, the affected skin becomes thickened, with accentuation of the normal skin creases, and is referred to as lichenification. The atopic child has characteristic facies, with darkened skin folds below the eyes, due to persistent rubbing. They usually have a dry flaky skin, and this dryness tends to exacerbate the itching. Many show deterioration during the winter months, when cold and low humidity increases the dryness of the skin; others are worse during the summer months, as a result of heat and increased sweating.

DIAGNOSIS
No investigation is essential. An immune work-up, including immunoglobulins (IgA, G, M and E), IgG subsets and specific IgE (RAST tests) to a battery of common allergens (cow's milk, soya, house dust mite, grass, dogs, cats) can be helpful in some cases.

TREATMENT
First-line treatment
- Avoidance of recognized aggravating factors
- Emollients
- Appropriate topical steroid
- Antihistamine

Second-line treatment
- Wet dressings with a weak topical steroid and/or moisturising agent
- Admission to hospital for intensive nursing care
- Topical immunomodulators such as tacrolimus ointment

Third-line treatment
(Used in specialist centres, for rare cases of severe refractory eczema.)
- Oral steroids
- Cyclosporin
- Azathioprine
- Phototherapy

General measures should include supportive care for the family, ideally with the help of a nurse specialist to liaise between the hospital, the general practitioner and the family. If food allergy is a problem, the involvement of a dietitian is useful. It is important that children with atopic dermatitis are kept cool and wear loose cotton clothes. It is important that they avoid contact with irritants such as synthetic or woollen fabrics, biological detergents and cigarette smoke.

PROGNOSIS
The prognosis is good, with a tendency towards spontaneous improvement through childhood. Over 90% of patients will not have a problem in adult life.

SCABIES

INCIDENCE / GENETICS
This infestation is common and found worldwide.

AETIOLOGY / PATHOGENESIS
Scabies is caused by the mite *Sarcoptes scabiei*.

CLINICAL PRESENTATION
Infestation with the *Sarcoptes* mite causes this highly contagious disorder. The infection is transmitted by close physical contact, although the incubation period can be as long as two months. The fertilized female mite burrows into the outer layers of the skin, where she lays her eggs. The characteristic burrow is seen as a fine, tortuous grey line (**6.6**). Typically, burrows are found in interdigital spaces, flexor aspects of the wrists and genitalia.

Babies may become infested on the palms and soles and, occasionally, on the face if suckling from infested nipples. In infants, lesions are commonly found on the soles and around the axillae.

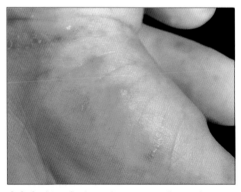

6.6 Scabies. Scabetic burrows and pustules are seen on the wrist and palm of this child's hand. Both soles were also affected. Topical pyrethroids such as permethrin are the treatment of choice.

There is intense itching with a widespread excoriated papular eruption, caused by a hypersensitivity reaction to the mite or its excreta. This may become eczematized and secondarily infected. Topical steroids may mask the cutaneous signs. The pruritus is worse when the patient is warm in bed.

DIAGNOSIS
Often the diagnosis is obvious. If confirmation of the diagnosis is needed then the female mite can be extracted from the blind end of the burrow with a needle and examined under the microscope.

TREATMENT
Treatment involves treating all members of the household and close contacts simultaneously. Written instructions should be given to the family. The treatments of choice for children are: malathion or permethrin.

PROGNOSIS
The outcome is excellent, if the treatment is carried out and is effective.

HAEMANGIOMA

INCIDENCE
Haemangiomas are very common, affecting about 1 in 20 babies with a higher incidence in premature infants and females.

AETIOLOGY / PATHOGENESIS
Haemangiomas arise from immature angio-blastic tissue developing as a protuberant vascular nodule.

CLINICAL PRESENTATION
Capillary haemangiomas or 'strawberry marks' are usually not obvious at birth and develop during the first few weeks of life. They grow, reaching a maximum size usually by six months (**6.7**). They then remain static for a variable period followed by spontaneous involution over three to five years. Deeper haemangiomas (cavernous type) appear as a soft lump in the skin with a bluish discolouration.

Often haemangiomas have a combination of both superficial and deep vascular components. Complications of haemangiomas relate to size and site. They can become ulcerated and infected, especially those around the mouth and genitalia. Haemangiomas around the eye may obstruct vision, requiring urgent intervention. Very rarely, extensive haemangiomas may present with bruising and bleeding, as a result of associated thrombocytopenia due to platelet trapping. This is known as the Kasabach-Merritt syndrome.

6.7 Haemangioma. This child is four months old and has a group of bluish-red tumours on the right side of the face, which started to develop shortly after her birth. Haemangiomas at this site carry a risk of interference with vision, either by direct obstruction of the visual axis or by causing pressure amblyopia if they affect the eyelids. These particular lesions show the greyish superficial opacification that indicates early resolution and there has been no increase in volume for several weeks. Highly satisfactory resolution can therefore be anticipated and there is no indication for intervention.

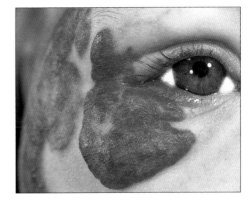

DIAGNOSIS

Investigation is usually not required. Larger complicated haemangiomas may require imaging, as well as a full blood count including platelets and a clotting screen.

TREATMENT

Reassurance is usually all that is required. Indications for active treatment are those lesions which, by virtue of their size and site, compromise vital structures, such as the airway or the eyes. In this situation the treatment of choice is a course of oral prednisolone (2–3 mg/kg per day initially). Other options for treatment include alpha interferon and embolization. Laser treatment is sometimes useful for ulcerated haemangiomas. Surgical excision is occasionally indicated.

PROGNOSIS

This is excellent as most haemangiomas will disappear completely. Sometimes the larger lesions leave behind some stretched redundant skin which can be surgically removed if necessary.

OROFACIAL HERPES SIMPLEX

INCIDENCE

HSV is one of the commonest infections of man throughout the world. Herpetic gingivostomatitis is the commonest clinical presentation of primary infection by herpes simplex virus type I (HSV I). Most cases occur between one and five years of age.

AETIOLOGY / PATHOGENESIS

There are two main antigenic types of HSV:
- Type I is classically associated with facial lesions.
- Type II is associated with genital lesions.

There is, however, considerable overlap. Both types persist in sensory nerve ganglia after primary infection, and may cause recurrent disease by travelling peripherally along the nerve fibre and replicating in the skin or mucosa. Viral particles are shed while the lesion is active, and this continues to a lesser degree in the weeks following an outbreak. Spread is by direct contact with or without droplets from infected secretions. Regardless of previous infection, the virus can be inoculated to any body site to cause a new infection.

CLINICAL PRESENTATION

Primary infections in children are usually minimal and often subclinical. After an incubation period of four to five days there may be fever and malaise, the gums may bleed easily and look red and swollen, and drinking and eating may be very painful (**6.8**). Vesicles presenting as white plaques may be seen inside the mouth. These plaques are followed by ulceration with a yellowish pseudomembrane. Regional lymph nodes may be enlarged and tender. The fever subsides after three to five days and recovery is usually complete within two weeks.

Recurrences tend to be around the mouth. The buccal mucosa is not usually involved in recurrent episodes, which are generally less severe than primary infections; vesicles tend to be smaller and more closely grouped and are often preceded by an itching or burning sensation. Healing occurs within ten days without scarring. Disseminated infection rarely occurs in healthy patients. If HSV involves the eye, an ophthalmological opinion should be sought.

DIAGNOSIS

Diagnosis of infection by culture of the virus from vesicle fluid usually requires one to five days. A quicker diagnosis may be made using immunofluorescence to detect viral antigen from scrapings of the lesion. If electron microscopy is readily available, rapid diagnosis may be made by electron microscopic identification of viral particles within the cell nucleus.

TREATMENT

Mild, uncomplicated eruptions require no treatment. Systemic administration of aciclovir is the treatment of choice for severe infection, but viral latency and recurrence rates after therapy are unaffected. Treatment should be started as soon as possible, and given for at least five days. Frequent recurrences can be suppressed by long-term treatment. Topical aciclovir is valuable in treating *Herpes labialis*, but is less effective than oral administration.

PROGNOSIS

Approximately 40% of patients with oral herpes simplex experience recurrence of the disease. Recurrence is commonly triggered by intercurrent infections and sun exposure.

PYOGENIC GRANULOMA

INCIDENCE / GENETICS

This common lesion affects both sexes and is most often seen in children and young adults. There may be a preceding history of a penetrating injury at the site; this stimulus is thought to be modified by genetic and/or hormonal factors, and to initiate vascular proliferation.

AETIOLOGY / PATHOGENESIS

Small blood vessels proliferate and erupt through a breach in the epidermis to produce a globular tumour composed of proliferating capillaries in a loose stroma.

CLINICAL PRESENTATION

The patient presents with a rapidly developing vascular nodule. The lesion is often more or less spherical, bright red and 5–10 mm in diameter. It cannot be fully blanched and does not pulsate. Older lesions may erode and crust and bleed easily. The commonest sites are hands (especially fingers), feet and face, especially around the lips (**6.9**). The initial evolution is rapid and, after a few weeks, growth ceases. Patients present complaining of the appearance, or recurrent bleeding; occasionally the lesion may be painful.

6.8 Herpes simplex. This child developed gradually progressive ulcerations on the face, from which herpes simplex virus could be cultured. This type of slowly progressive herpes simplex is characteristic of immunodeficiency.

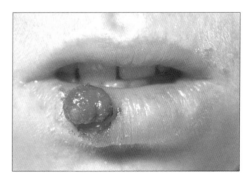

6.9 Pyogenic granuloma. The lip is a typical site for this reactive, benign, vascular proliferation. Profuse bleeding may be a problem.

DIAGNOSIS

In most cases the history and clinical appearance leave little doubt about the diagnosis. If the lesion seems at all atypical it would be important to consider the possibility of an amelanotic malignant melanoma, which is the most important differential diagnosis. In such a case, biopsy will provide reassurance.

TREATMENT

Protuberant lesions are easy to treat by curettage and cauterization, or diathermy coagulation of the base.

PROGNOSIS

Spontaneous disappearance may occur. A considerable proportion recur after treatment.

KELOID

INCIDENCE /GENETICS

Keloid is an overgrowth of dense fibrous tissue, which develops in the skin as a result of trauma, though in some cases the trauma may be trivial. The incidence of keloids increases throughout childhood to reach a maximum between puberty and the age of 30. Females are more often affected than males. There is a familial tendency to keloid formation; both autosomal dominant and recessive inheritance have been reported. Development of keloids is higher in the Afro-Caribbean population.

AETIOLOGY / PATHOGENESIS

Keloid formation may follow burns, the introduction of foreign materials into the skin (e.g., sutures or hairs), uncomplicated surgical incisions, or laser therapy.

CLINICAL PRESENTATION

The lesion becomes raised and thickened to form a well-defined, firm, pink or red plaque or nodule (**6.10**). Growth usually stops after a few months, sometimes resulting in lesions of bizarre configuration. The earlobes, chin, neck and upper chest are sites at which keloids are particularly likely to occur.

DIAGNOSIS

History and clinical appearance are usually sufficient for a diagnosis to be made without biopsy.

TREATMENT

Treatment may be difficult and non-essential surgery should be avoided in predilection sites in individuals who are individually or racially predisposed. Keloid scars usually recur following simple surgical excision, but a combination of excision with intralesional steroids, radiation or local compression may result in an improved aesthetic result. Early lesions may be successfully treated with intralesional steroids or by potent topical steroids applied under occlusion.

PROGNOSIS

Keloid scars will, in time, undergo considerable but not complete spontaneous resolution.

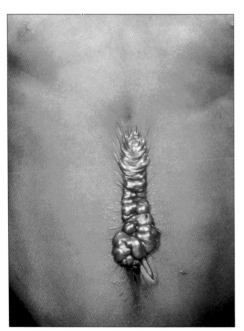

6.10 Keloid. This eight-year-old boy developed multiple nodules at the site of an abdominal surgical incision.

PITYRIASIS VERSICOLOR

INCIDENCE

Pityriasis versicolor is commoner in hot countries, and in the tropics 40% of some populations are affected, compared with 1% in cold climates. It is more often seen in teenagers than in younger children. Both sexes are equally affected. A positive family history among blood relations is found more often than chance would suggest, but whether this is due to a genetically determined host-susceptibility factor or a greater opportunity for fungal colonization is not determined. Conjugal cases rarely occur.

AETIOLOGY / PATHOGENESIS

When normal resident yeast flora increase in number, they may cause scaling and a pigmentary disturbance. The spherical yeast, *Pityrosporum orbiculare* is more likely to do this than the oval yeast *Pityrosporum ovale*. Malassezia furfur is the term used for the mycelial shift which is seen in pityriasis versicolor. It may be that affected patients have a poor cellular immune response to the specific fungal antigen, but there is no confirmed explanation for susceptibility. Application of oils to the skin may well promote pityriasis versicolor, as the organism is lipophilic. The oilier skin of the teenager probably explains the increased incidence in this age group.

CLINICAL PRESENTATION

The eruption typically presents as multiple oval, scaly, discoloured or hypopigmented macules, mainly on the upper trunk (**6.11**). It may spread to involve the upper arms, neck and abdomen and is often more extensive in tropical climates. Mild irritation is sometimes noticed. The term versicolor is particularly appropriate since in white skin the affected areas are usually darker and in dark skin the affected areas are commonly paler.

DIAGNOSIS

Examination under Wood's light reveals a typical yellow–green fluorescence. Direct microscopic examination of the scale reveals spherical thick-walled yeasts and coarse mycelium ('spaghetti and meatballs' appearance).

TREATMENT

2.5% selenium sulphide shampoo in a detergent base may be applied to the affected areas and washed off after a few minutes, or left to dry. This should be repeated daily for seven days. This treatment is cheap but may be an irritant to face and genitalia and may stain clothes and bedding. Ketoconazole shampoo or miconazole cream are less irritant and do not stain, but are more expensive. Oral ketoconazole or itraconazole are reserved for recalcitrant cases and may require just a one-week course.

PROGNOSIS

This mild, benign, chronic infection commonly relapses. Patients should be warned that reversal to normal pigmentation may take several months as otherwise they will report treatment failure.

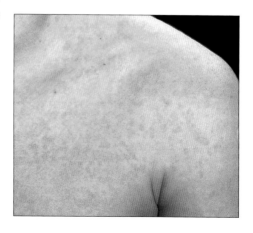

6.11 Pityriasis versicolor. This teenager exhibits the classical features of pityriasis versicolor, a superficial fungal infection caused by the yeast *Pityrosporum orbiculare*. There are discrete hyperpigmented and slightly scaly macules on the trunk and proximal parts of the arms. This patient was asymptomatic and responded well to treatment with a topical imidazole.

PITYRIASIS ROSACEA

INCIDENCE
Most cases occur between the ages of ten and 35. Pityriasis rosea is relatively common throughout the world and is more common in temperate regions during the winter months.

AETIOLOGY / PATHOGENESIS
The cause is unknown but it is most likely that a viral agent is implicated, possibly human herpes virus 7 (HHV7). Occasional family or household outbreaks occur.

CLINICAL PRESENTATION
In most cases the clinical pattern is remarkably predictable. Prodromal symptoms are usually absent and the first manifestation of the disease is usually the appearance of the 'herald patch' which is large and conspicuous. The herald patch is often mistaken for tinea corporis. Usually, between five and 15 days later a general eruption appears in crops at two- to three-day intervals for up to ten days. The eruption is classically of discrete oval macules, dull pink in colour, with fine dry scales and central clearing.

In children, the initial lesions may be papular or urticarial, particularly in more tropical climates. The long axes of the lesions characteristically lie parallel to the ribs in a 'Christmas tree' pattern. The rash, which is occasionally pruritic, is usually distributed on the trunk (6.12) and proximal limbs. The lesions may last from two weeks to two months. Pigmentary changes are usually short-lived.

DIAGNOSIS
The clinically distinctive nature of the condition usual makes biopsy unnecessary.

TREATMENT
The common asymptomatic and self-limiting cases require no treatment. If itch is troublesome or the appearance distressing, moderate strength topical steroids or ultraviolet light (UVB) may be helpful.

PROGNOSIS
This is an acute self-limiting disease. Relapse of a fading eruption is rare. Second attacks occur in 2% of cases.

VITILIGO

INCIDENCE
Approximately 1% of the population has vitiligo, although in some areas of the world, especially Asia, the incidence is purported to be higher.

AETIOLOGY / PATHOGENESIS
The cause is unknown. It has a genetic background, often associated with autoimmunity within the family. A biochemical defect in pigment metabolism has recently been suggested.

CLINICAL PRESENTATION
Vitiligo presents as ivory – white depigmented areas of skin appearing at any age, with approximately 50% starting in childhood (6.13). The most common site for an initial lesion in children is a leaf-shaped patch around one eye, although any area on the body can be affected.

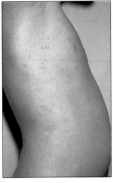
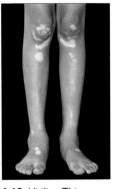
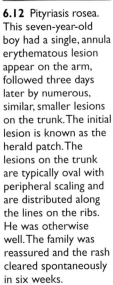

6.12 Pityriasis rosea. This seven-year-old boy had a single, annula erythematous lesion appear on the arm, followed three days later by numerous, similar, smaller lesions on the trunk. The initial lesion is known as the herald patch. The lesions on the trunk are typically oval with peripheral scaling and are distributed along the lines on the ribs. He was otherwise well. The family was reassured and the rash cleared spontaneously in six weeks.

6.13 Vitiligo. This young girl presented with depigmented patches in a symmetrical distribution. These gradually increased in size and further lesions appeared on her face and trunk. She also suffered from juvenile-onset diabetes mellitus. Spontaneous perifollicular repigmentation can occur in a proportion of cases. Prognosis for complete repigmentation is poor.

It usually spreads and is often strikingly symmetrical. Some lesions can repigment spontaneously but often the condition is progressive. A less common presentation is depigmentation localized to one area, called segmental vitiligo.

DIAGNOSIS
Investigations are not necessary. An autoantibody screen may be helpful, particularly if there is a family history of thyroid disease.

TREATMENT
There is no specific treatment for vitiligo at present. A short course of potent topical steroids may help early on to limit the extent of depigmentation. Phototherapy is often quoted as a treatment option for vitiligo, but the results are more often than not disappointing.

PROGNOSIS
The long-term prognosis for complete repigmentation is poor.

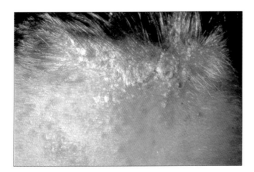

6.14 Psoriasis. Thick white scales along the hair margin and scalp in a child with chronic plaque psoriasis.

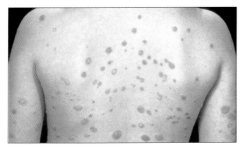

6.15 Guttate psoriasis. This is seen as an acute eruption of small erythematous scaly lesions mainly on the trunk. In this 12-year-old girl, it followed a streptococcal sore throat.

PSORIASIS

INCIDENCE / GENETICS
Approximately 1% of the population has psoriasis. There is a genetic predisposition to the development of psoriasis, with a polygenic inheritance pattern.

AETIOLOGY / PATHOGENESIS
This is a hyperproliferative disorder of keratinization, the cause of which is unknown. There is a genetic background.

CLINICAL PRESENTATION
Psoriasis is a chronic, relapsing, inflammatory skin disorder, characterized by red plaques covered with silvery scales (**6.14**). It is primarily a disease of young adults, but it can develop for the first time at any age although rarely before the age of three years. Typically, it relapses or remits spontaneously with variable disease-free intervals. In childhood, the onset may be related to streptococcal tonsillitis, otitis media or vaccination, although often there is no obvious precipitating cause. Psychological factors are sometimes implicated, but are difficult to assess. In adolescents and young adults, guttate psoriasis (an acute shower of small lesions – **6.15**) is common following a streptococcal infection. Rarely, psoriasis may present with an erythroderma or generalized pustular eruption.

DIAGNOSIS
Usually the diagnosis is obvious clinically, but if there is doubt a skin biopsy is confirmatory. For those patients with an acute onset, it is important to seek a source of infection and investigations should include a throat swab and an anti streptolysin (ASO) titre.

TREATMENT
Treatment includes oral antibiotics (penicillin or erythromycin) if there is an infection (usually caused by beta haemolytic streptococcus). Topical therapy includes mild/moderate strength steroids, tar and salicylic acid, vitamin D analogues and dithranol preparations. Ultraviolet light therapy can be helpful. For children with severe psoriasis unresponsive to conventional treatment, other options include methotrexate; ciclosporin and photochemotherapy (PUVA).

PROGNOSIS
The long-term prognosis is variable.

PORT WINE STAIN

INCIDENCE
Approximately 3 in 1,000 live births per year.

AETIOLOGY / PATHOLOGY
Port wine stains represent a vascular mal-formation involving mature capillaries.

CLINICAL PRESENTATION
This presents at birth as a flat, red area of skin, often unilateral and on the face (**6.16** and **6.17**). It persists and tends to become more purple with age. Port wine stains around the eye can be associated with glaucoma (see 'Ophthalmology' chapter). Those that are on the forehead and scalp have an increased incidence of meningeal blood vessel abnorm-alities and involvement of the cerebral cortex. This is known as the Sturge-Weber syndrome and can present with epilepsy, learning difficulties and, rarely, hemiplegia.

DIAGNOSIS
Ophthalmological assessment is essential for all port wine stains around the eye. If Sturge-Weber syndrome is being considered, imaging by MRI with gadolinium enhancement is the investigation of choice.

TREATMENT
The treatment of choice is laser therapy using a pulsed dye laser. The results are better in younger children and ideally treatment should be started within the first year. Normally four to six treatment sessions are necessary at three- to six-monthly intervals. The laser destroys the dilated blood vessels by selective photo-thermolysis.

PROGNOSIS
Laser treatment can improve the appearance considerably and hopefully reduce the psycho-logical problems associated with disfigurement.

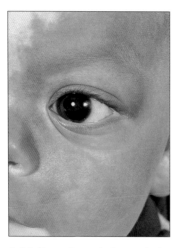

6.16 Port wine stain in a typical distribution. Port wine stains are typically flat and red and well demarcated. This little boy also had associated congenital glaucoma, which is a common complication of port wine stains around the eye.

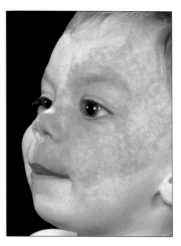

6.17 Port wine stain. After one treatment session with a pulsed dye laser, the treated spots demonstrate good clearance. Further treatments with the laser will be necessary to eliminate this reticulated appearance.

URTICARIA PIGMENTOSA

INCIDENCE
This condition appears to be an abnormality of development, without any genetic basis.

AETIOLOGY / PATHOGENESIS
Urticaria pigmentosa is a due to local proliferation or accumulation of mast cells. The cause is unknown. It belongs to a group of conditions collectively termed mastocytosis. In children, there are three varieties of mastocytosis: multiple (urticaria pigmentosa), solitary and diffuse (i.e. in which the skin is diffusely infiltrated with a dense band of mast cells). The diffuse variety is rare and generally presents with blistering during the neonatal period.

CLINICAL PRESENTATION
The onset is generally in the first few months of life. The commonest eruption consists of monomorphic, erythematous, pigmented, maculopapular or nodular lesions, with a widespread bilateral distribution, mainly on the scalp and trunk (**6.18**). Lesions may vary from a few millimetres to several centimetres across. Some lesions may appear urticated, and the diagnosis can be confirmed by demonstrating that gentle rubbing of a lesion causes local redness and whealing (Darier's sign). The lesions may be accompanied by dermographism.

The principal symptom is intense itching which is aggravated by rubbing or scratching. Some children may experience generalized flushing, which can be very variable.

Non-cutaneous lesions are almost always present. Occasionally these may be the source of the vaso-active substances that lead to flushing, and they may very rarely cause other problems such as diarrhoea or intussusception.

DIAGNOSIS
The diagnosis can almost always be made reliably on clinical grounds. Biopsy may occasionally be justified. There is no purpose in seeking out evidence of systemic involvement. It can be assumed that this will be present to a degree, and its presence is usually of little relevance to management.

TREATMENT
Patients with this condition should be advised to avoid certain well-recognized drugs that may degranulate mast cells, which include aspirin, opiates and certain drugs used in anaesthesia (e.g. scopolamine).

Pruritus may respond partially to antihistamines; non-sedative antihistamines such as cetirizine are preferred.

In severe cases, psoralen photochemotherapy (PUVA) may be helpful, but such treatment is rarely necessary.

PROGNOSIS
Urticaria pigmentosa carries a good prognosis with eventual spontaneous resolution in all cases, however severe. With time, the lesions become less itchy, less easily urticated but increasingly pigmented. The pigmentation may last into adolescence.

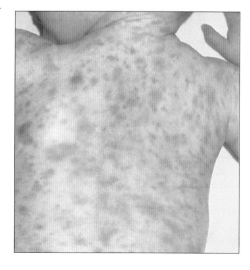

6.18 Urticaria pigmentosa. This baby presented with numerous erythematous lesions, mainly on the trunk, which when rubbed produced localized wheal and flare reactions and on one occasion a central blister. These lesions are foci of mast cells. With time these lesions become less active and acquire a brownish red colour. In the majority spontaneous resolution takes place by puberty.

ECZEMA HERPETICUM

INCIDENCE
Atopic eczema is by far the commonest predisposing condition for widespread or localized cutaneous infection with herpes simplex virus (HSV). Eczema herpeticum may present at any age.

AETIOLOGY / PATHOGENESIS
Most cases of eczema herpeticum arise from primary infection with HSV. Eczema herpeticum probably reflects the ease with which the virus can spread locally in eczematous skin.

CLINICAL PRESENTATION
After an incubation period of about ten days, vesicles, which rapidly become pustular, appear in crops; these may be very extensive in severe infections (**6.19**). New crops may appear for seven days. Fever, regional lymphadenopathy and severe constitutional symptoms may accompany the eruption. Permanent scarring is rare. Although eczema herpeticum tends to be more extensive in patients with severe eczema, it is also frequently seen in a more localized form in mild or quiescent cases.

DIAGNOSIS
See orofacial herpes simplex (page 136).

TREATMENT
Severe cases should receive prompt intravenous aciclovir to prevent progression, which may rarely be fatal. Less ill patients respond well to oral aciclovir. If aciclovir is being withheld, more cautious use of topical steroid therapy may be advisable until the viral lesions have healed. Whether heavy steroid use predisposes to herpetic infection or simply reflects the severity of the eczema is not known.

Awareness of the possibility of eczema herpeticum should be encouraged in patients with atopic eczema and their parents. Close contact with relatives and friends who have herpes labialis should be avoided.

PROGNOSIS
Recurrences of eczema herpeticum are commonly milder than the initial episode, but are sometimes of comparable severity.

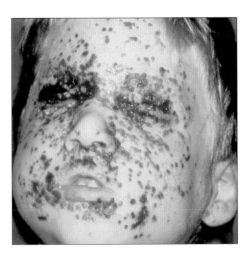

6.19 Eczema herpeticum. This disseminated vesicular eruption occurred in a child with preexisting eczema, following close contact with a relative who had active herpes labialis. She was seriously ill but responded to intravenous aciclovir. Occasional deaths still occur when there is delay in recognizing this frequent complication of atopic eczema.

ERYTHEMA MULTIFORME

INCIDENCE
Recurrent erythema multiforme is associated with HLA-B62, -B35 and DR53 types.

AETIOLOGY / PATHOGENESIS
Erythema multiforme may be precipitated by a variety of provocative factors. In children, the commonest associations are with a preceding herpes simplex virus, mycoplasma or group-A streptococcal infection. The interval between the infection and the onset of lesions is usually about three weeks. Drug sensitivities, especially to sulphonamides, antibiotics, anticonvulsants and non-steroidal antiinflammatory drugs are sometimes responsible for the erythema multiforme major. However, more often than not, it is impossible to identify a provoking factor, and drugs given for symptomatic relief during the prodrome are often inappropriately blamed.

Histologically, erythema multiforme is characterized by a variable degree of epithelial necrosis, associated with superficial dermal inflammation and oedema.

CLINICAL PRESENTATION
From a clinical point of view it is convenient to divide erythema multiforme into two broad categories, though there is good deal of overlap between these. They are:
- **Erythema multiforme minor** – cutaneous, mucosal, mucocutaneous.
- **Erythema multiforme major** (also known as Stevens-Johnson syndrome or toxic epidermal necrolysis).

The great majority of cases of erythema multiforme are of the minor type (**6.20**). This can present at any age, but appears to be rare in the first year of life. Lesions are dull red, flat or slightly raised and may remain small or increase in size within 48 hours, up to a diameter of about 3 cm. Typical cases usually show some target (or iris) lesions (**6.21**), which classically have three distinct zones:
- A central purpuric or bullous lesion.
- A surrounding pale oedematous ring.
- An outer ring of erythema with a well-defined edge.

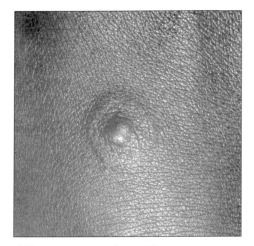

6.20 Erythema multiforme. This is a characteristic iris lesion with a central blister, seen on the dorsum of the hand (which is a common site). This patient was a black teenage boy who had a preceding history of herpes labialis, which is a common cause of erythema multiforme in children.

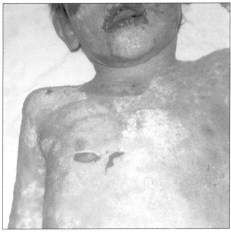

6.21 Stevens-Johnson syndrome (also known as toxic epidermal necrolysis). The more serious form of erythema multiforme is demonstrated in this young boy. He had extensive mucosal erosions and widespread cutaneous involvement; erythema multiforme of this severity has an appreciable mortality. Ocular and female genital tract scarring are the most important causes of long-term morbidity.

Lesions appear in crops for a few days and fade within two weeks. There may be few or many lesions and, classically, the distribution is predominantly acral (i.e. affecting the hands, which may be selectively involved, feet and wrists). The face is less commonly affected. The extensor surfaces of the elbows and knees are other predilection sites. Koebnerization may result in bizarre distributions. There may be a prodromal systemic illness, particularly in the more severe case, and there may be a previous history of an infectious illness or exposure to drugs.

In the mucosal form, the condition is limited to the mucosae of the oropharynx, the oesophagus, the anal canal, the eye, the urogenital tract and the nose. These may or may not be affected simultaneously. The oral mucous membrane characteristically shows extensive mucosal separation, with haemorrhagic crusting on the mouth and lips. Conjunctivitis is common and may be severe and purulent. Corneal ulceration is a frequent complication, and anterior uveitis or panophthalmitis may also occur. Genital lesions are frequent, and tend to be particularly severe in girls. Urethral involvement causes dysuria and may precipitate retention of urine.

Erythema multiforme major is a term given to the most severe attacks of erythema multiforme, usually of mucocutaneous type, but in clinical practice it can be difficult to draw the line between erythema multiforme minor and major. The cutaneous eruption is characteristically bullous and then erosive. Mucosal involvement is profound and distressing. The patient is almost invariably unable to speak, eat or drink.

DIAGNOSIS
Skin biopsy is rarely indicated. A search for causative infection is justifiable, but often fruitless.

TREATMENT
In mild cases, symptomatic treatment is all that is usually required. In cases of erythema multiforme major, first-class dermatological nursing is of paramount importance and an intensive care unit may be required. The value of systemic corticosteroids is still hotly debated, but it is increasingly felt that the three days of pulsed methylprednisolone (20–30 mg/kg/day up to 1 g/day, infused over 1–3 hours each day) is valuable, and can abort recurrent attacks if given early enough. Aciclovir may be given when there is good reason to believe that herpes simplex virus is responsible, the same is true for amoxycillin or ampicillin when group-A streptococcus is suspected.

Aciclovir may be helpful when used prophylactically for recurrent erythema multiforme, even when the herpes simplex virus has not been isolated.

Ocular involvement in erythema multiforme requires early ophthalmological referral.

PROGNOSIS
The condition generally resolves spontaneously with complete healing. Longer term sequelae may follow erythema multiforme major, particularly in the eye and the genital tract. Blindness can result. In the past, erythema multiforme major was associated with significant mortality from secondary sepsis.

All forms of erythema multiforme are prone to recur; repeated attacks associated with herpes simplex virus are particularly characteristic.

ANOGENITAL WARTS

INCIDENCE
Anogenital warts are relatively uncommon in children.

AETIOLOGY / PATHOGENESIS
Anogenital warts are caused by human papilloma virus, types 6 and 11 being common. In children, they cause alarm because they may reflect sexual abuse. Transmission of HPV to children may occur by two main routes:

- Intra-partum (i.e. the child is infected from the mother's genital tract at delivery; the virus may then remain latent for over three years).
- In the post-natal period, when transmission from adults with genital warts may occur non-sexually (e.g. by sharing a bath with an infected person) or sexually.

The long and variable incubation period, the possibility of latent or subclinical infection in the source, and the problems in eliciting an accurate account of sexual contact can make it difficult to decide which applies in the individual case.

CLINICAL PRESENTATION
Anogenital warts are often asymptomatic, but may cause discomfort, discharge or bleeding. Typically, lesions are soft, pink and elongated. They may be filiform or pedunculated; a few are flat. They are often multiple, especially on moist surfaces (**6.22**).

DIAGNOSIS
Typing of the causative human papilloma virus (HPV) may be useful in investigating cases in which sexual abuse is suspected. Identifying the same HPV type present in a suspected abuser does not provide proof of sexual abuse; however, a different HPV type would be strong evidence against the possibility.

TREATMENT
Viral warts can be expected to resolve spontaneously and without trace in the great majority of cases. Therefore, unless they are causing substantial discomfort, they should probably not be treated. Treatments that can be considered include topical podophyllin, cryotherapy and excision.

PROGNOSIS
The duration of anogenital warts varies from a few weeks to several years. The main long-term concern is the risk of cervical dysplasia and neoplasia in females, but the risk when infection occurs in early childhood has never been quantified. It is clearly important, for this reason, to identify active infections in the mother so that she can be treated and followed up appropriately.

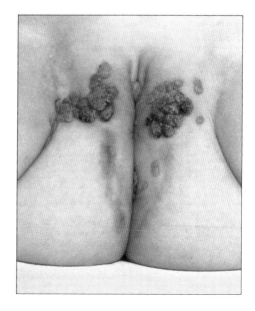

6.22 Anogenital warts (condylomata accuminata). The human papilloma virus causes anogenital warts. Intrapartum inoculation of virus from maternal genital lesions is responsible for the great majority of infections in children under three years. In older children, the possibility of sexual abuse should always be considered.

LICHEN STRIATUS

INCIDENCE / GENETICS
Over 50% of cases occur in children, usually between the ages of five and 15 years. Females are affected twice as often as males. Many affected patients are also atopic.

DIAGNOSIS
Biopsy and histology will establish the diagnosis, though this is rarely necessary.

CLINICAL PRESENTATION
This linear inflammatory dermatosis presents first as small, pink, lichenoid papules, initially discrete and then coalescent (**6.23**). The onset is sudden, and over the course of a week the lesions extend into a dull red, slightly scaly linear band, usually around 1 cm in width, and from a few centimetres to a limb length. It may be continuous or interrupted. In dark skin the lesion is invariably hypopigmented. Usually lichen striatus occurs on a single limb. The lesions may be pruritic. Extension may continue for up to four months.

AETIOLOGY / PATHOGENESIS
The reason for the linearity of the lesions is not known, but it is believed that this may reflect clonal predisposition.

TREATMENT
Treatment is usually unnecessary.

PROGNOSIS
Spontaneous recovery is usually complete within a year, though resolution may be followed by temporary hypopigmentation.

SEBACEOUS NAEVUS

INCIDENCE / GENETICS
Sporadic occurrence is the rule, but there have been occasional reports of familial cases. Sebaceous naevi may be found in 0.3% of all neonates in the UK.

AETIOLOGY / PATHOLOGY
The characteristic histopathological appearance showing an accumulation of mature sebaceous glands, associated with papillomatous hyperplasia of the overlying epidermis, is not seen until puberty. During earlier childhood, biopsies may be reported as showing no abnormality.

CLINICAL PRESENTATION
This lesion is a single round, oval or linear, well-circumscribed, slightly raised, pinkish-yellow, orange or tan plaque, with a smooth or velvety surface. The maximum dimension may vary from 1 to 10 cm. Sebaceous naevi most commonly occur as a single lesion, but may be multiple and extensive. The great majority occur on the head (**6.24**) and neck; in the scalp the lesions are devoid of hair. At puberty, the lesions become thicker and more elevated and, during adult life, they become progressively nodular.

Extensive sebaceous naevi may be associated with other developmental defects, mainly of the central nervous system, skeletal system and eyes.

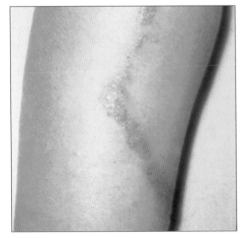

6.23 Lichen striatus. This is a curious acquired disorder in which a line of inflammatory papules develops in a child, at more or less any site. The cause is unknown and the condition resolves spontaneously after a period of months.

DIAGNOSIS

Diagnosis is usually made on clinical grounds. Histology may be used for confirmation.

TREATMENT

Lesions should be removed during childhood by excision with primary closure, mainly because their appearance deteriorates from adolescence, and because malignant change may occur in adult life.

PROGNOSIS

The development of benign tumours is considerably more common than malignant transformation, which is rare. Sebaceous naevi may be associated with intracranial hamartomatous malformations causing neurological symptoms, and other developmental abnormalities, particularly when they are extensive.

VERRUCOUS EPIDERMAL NAEVI

INCIDENCE

Prevalence is probably 0.1–0.5%, with an equal sex incidence. Patients who have multiple lesions with epidermolytic histopathology are likely to be mosaic for keratin gene mutations. This is of importance as it is clear that these patients may transmit bullous ichthyosiform erythroderma to their children.

AETIOLOGY / PATHOGENESIS

Verrucous epidermal naevi are circumscribed hamartomas comprised almost exclusively of keratinocytes. It is likely that all epidermal naevi reflect somatic mutations occurring in embryonic life. Naevi that demonstrate the histological change known as epidermolytic hyperkeratosis reflect mosaic mutations of the keratins 1 or 10, which, if generalized, cause bullous congenital ichthyosiform erythroderma.

Where a patient has multiple naevi of this type, there is a risk that germ-line mosaicism may also be present, with the risk of transmission of the mutant gene in full dose to the next generation. Transmission of mutant genes causing other types of verrucous epidermal naevi may prove lethal, but mosaicism can result in associated non-cutaneous developmental anomalies.

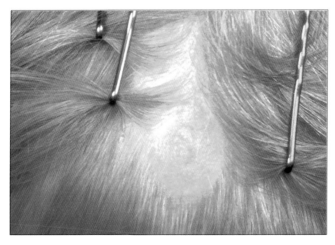

6.24 Sebaceous naevus. At birth, a well-demarcated, velvety yellow area of alopecia was visible in this child's scalp. It has remained unchanged since then. These lesions become more prominent at puberty because of activation of the sebaceous glands they contain and, over subsequent years, they tend to become nodular and may eventually be complicated by the development of a variety of low-grade malignant tumours. Surgical excision is therefore indicated in childhood.

CLINICAL PRESENTATION

Verrucous epidermal naevi may appear at any time during childhood. In the neonate, the lesions take the form of pink or slightly pigmented, velvety linear streaks or plaques. Later on they tend to darken and become keratotic (**6.25**). They may be almost any size, single or multiple, and at any site, though they are relatively uncommon on the face and head (where sebaceous naevi are common). Truncal lesions tend to be in transverse bands and do not cross the midline. Limb lesions tend to be linear.

Lesions in proximal flexures may become macerated and malodorous. Nail fold lesions may result in splitting or distortion of the nail plate and may cause recurrent paronychia.

DIAGNOSIS

Due to the genetic implications, a biopsy should be taken where several lesions are present, mainly to exclude epidermolytic hyperkeratosis.

TREATMENT

Cosmetically significant lesions may justify systemic retinoid therapy. Cryotherapy may help smaller lesions, but with a risk of recurrence. However, full-depth excision is the only reliable way of ablating lesions permanently. Malignant transformation is very rare.

PROGNOSIS

Until adolescence, verrucous epidermal naevi may increase in size and number, and in the degree of pigmentation and hyperkeratosis. Spontaneous resolution is very unusual. Nodules or ulcers may rarely develop in adult life, suggesting the development of tumours, which are usually benign or of low-grade malignancy.

A wide variety of developmental anomalies (CNS, skeletal, eye and dental) may be associated with all types of epidermal naevi, other than those demonstrating epidermolytic hyperkeratosis. This association is often termed the 'epidermal naevus syndrome'.

When epidermolytic hyperkeratosis is present, it is mandatory to warn the patient of the risk that any offspring may have bullous ichthyosis, though currently the risk cannot be quantified.

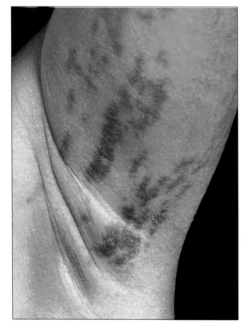

6.25 Verrucous epidermal naevi. This three-year-old Asian boy has warty, pigmented papules arranged in linear streaks in his left axilla. These were barely visible at birth and have developed gradually and progressively since.

LANGERHANS CELL HISTIOCYTOSIS (LCH)

See also 'Solid Tumours and Histiocytosis' chapter.

INCIDENCE / GENETICS

The incidence of LCH is unknown; many patients with mild single system involvement remain undiagnosed. The incidence is likely to be at least 4–6 per million.

AETIOLOGY / PATHOLOGY

The aetiology of LCH is unknown. Scientific evidence now suggests that it is a reactive condition, rather than a malignant disease. Phenotypic Langerhans cells accumulate in various tissues and cause damage, in part by cytokine production.

CLINICAL PRESENTATION

Langerhans cell histiocytosis (LCH) ranges from single-system (bone or skin) to multi-system disease. High mortality is associated with the more fulminant forms of LCH. In the skin, the most characteristic presentation is with scalp involvement; erythema and greasy scales may suggest seborrhoeic dermatitis (**6.26**). On the trunk, lesions are discrete yellow/brown scaly papules, often showing areas of purpura. Lesions may become nodular, crusted or eroded and ulceration may be seen, particularly in the anal and vulval areas. Chronic draining sinuses may develop over involved lymph nodes or cranial lesions.

DIAGNOSIS

Pathological diagnosis is essential since many diseases can clinically mimic LCH. In 1987 the Histiocyte Society recommended three levels of diagnostic confidence. A presumptive diagnosis is made when the histological appearance of the biopsy is consistent with the changes of LCH. Diagnostic confidence increases if marker studies are performed and lesional cells are found to be positive for S100 protein, peanut agglutinin or Alpha-D-mannosidase. If lesional cells are found to express the CD1 complex, or are shown on electron microscopy to exhibit Birbeck granules, this constitutes a definitive diagnosis.

TREATMENT

The appropriate therapy depends upon the extent and severity of the disease. Patients with single system, bone or skin disease have a good prognosis and often require no or only limited treatment. In symptomatic skin disease, topical nitrogen mustard (20%) is very effective. Psoralen photochemotherapy (PUVA) therapy may be useful if topical nitrogen mustard is not tolerated. Systemic chemotherapy may be indicated in multisystem disease.

PROGNOSIS

The three important prognostic indices in LCH are the age of the patient, the extent of the disease and the presence of vital organ failure.

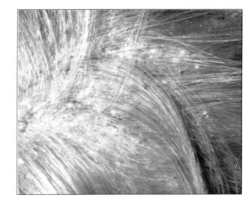

6.26 Langerhans cell histiocytosis. This child presented with gradually progressive brownish-yellow scaly papules on the scalp. The nappy area was also involved and, although the rash resembled seborrhoeic eczema, it was more persistent and refractory to treatment. The diagnosis was confirmed by skin biopsy.

INFANTILE ACNE VULGARIS

INCIDENCE / GENETICS
This condition mainly affects boys, starting at around three months of age. Untreated it may last until the age of five years.

AETIOLOGY / PATHOLOGY
It is thought that infantile acne results from trans-placental stimulation of the infant's adrenal glands, since most sufferers have elevated adrenal androgens. Infantile acne is rarely associated with systemic disease, but it can very occasionally be due to a virilizing tumour or congenital adrenal hyperplasia.

CLINICAL PRESENTATION
Acne in infants (**6.27**) is more localized than in older patients, but the entire acne spectrum may be seen, with pustules, comedones, nodules and even scarring.

DIAGNOSIS
No investigations are required for definitive diagnosis.

TREATMENT
Topical treatments for acne vulgaris tend to irritate the skin in infancy. Therefore it is probably best to avoid treating the mildest cases, as spontaneous improvement can be anticipated. Oral erythromycin may be given for six months if necessary. If the condition is severe and unresponsive, oral isotretinoin should be considered.

PROGNOSIS
Patients with infantile acne are more likely to develop severe acne later in life.

TUBEROUS SCLEROSIS

INCIDENCE
In the UK the incidence of TS is approximately 1 in 10,000 live births per year.

AETIOLOGY / PATHOGENESIS
TS is inherited as an autosomal dominant condition with variable penetrance. Mutations have been identified in two genes, TSC1 and TSC2 that map to chromosomes 9 and 16 respectively. Approximately 50% of cases are thought to be the result of a new mutation.

CLINICAL PRESENTATION
The characteristic components of the syndrome are skin lesions, learning difficulties and epilepsy, with wide variation in age of onset and in severity. Presentation before the age of five years, with cutaneous changes and/or epilepsy, is usual, but the disease may remain unrecognized until adolescence.

Skin lesions are found in 60–70% of cases. Lesions of five types are all pathognomonic:
1. Ovoid or ash-leaf shaped white macules, 1–3 cm in length are frequently present on the trunk and limbs. They may be found at birth or in early infancy, and are most easily detected by examination under Wood's light. Lesions may disappear in later childhood.
2. Angiofibromas appear between the age of three and ten years, and generally become more numerous at puberty. They are firm, discrete, reddish-brown telangiectatic papules, 1–10 mm in diameter, extending from the nasolabial folds to the cheeks and chin (**6.28**). They may be small in number, and overlooked, or numerous and conspicuous, occasionally forming large cauliflower-like masses.
3. The shagreen patch is an irregularly thickened, slightly elevated, soft, skin-coloured plaque, usually in the lumbosacral region.

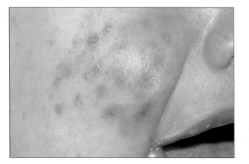

6.27 Infantile acne. This eight-month-old boy has multiple papules and comedones on the cheeks.

4. Fibrous plaques are common on the forehead and temple.
5. Periungual fibromas appear at, or after, puberty as smooth, firm, flesh-coloured excrescences emerging from the nail folds. They are usually 5–10 mm in length, but may be larger. This may be the only clinically evident abnormality. Other cutaneous manifestations include firm, fibromatous plaques, and pedunculated fibromas.

DIAGNOSIS

Difficulties in diagnosis may arise in infancy when the classic triad is not evident and there is no family history. DNA-based prenatal diagnosis is now available for some families where the mutation has been identified. In some cases, MRI scans or EEG may be necessary.

TREATMENT

Management usually involves a multidisciplinary approach, with care shared between paediatricians, dermatologists, clinical geneticists and neurologists. The cosmetic appearance may be improved by removing angiofibromas with laser therapy.

PROGNOSIS

For the severely affected infant, life expectancy is poor; 3% die in the first year, 28% before ten years of age and 75% before 25 years. Death is usually due to epilepsy. The prognosis for the older child with cutaneous stigmata and epilepsy is unpredictable. Each case must be investigated in detail and individually assessed.

JUVENILE DERMATOMYOSITIS

INCIDENCE / GENETICS

Approximately four cases per million per year are seen, with a male to female ratio of 1:2. Juvenile dermatomyositis affects all races. There is an increased incidence of HLA-B8 in Caucasian children.

AETIOLOGY / PATHOLOGY

A widespread vasculitis affects small arteries, capillaries and veins of the skin, muscle, subcutaneous tissue and gastrointestinal tract. The cause is unknown, though it seems likely that the disease is immunologically mediated. A significant relationship to preceding Coxsackie-B infection has been found.

CLINICAL PRESENTATION

The onset of this disease may be rapid, with characteristic erythematous and oedematous changes in the skin, particularly on the face (**6.29**), and most especially on the upper eyelids. Scaly erythematous plaques around the nails and over the knuckle joints (termed Gottron's papules) are characteristic, and dilated nail fold capillaries may be seen. Calcinosis is frequent in established cases. In addition to the weak and often painful proximal muscles, there may be difficulty with speech and swallowing.

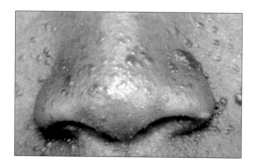

6.28 Tuberous sclerosis. The small reddish brown papules seen on the cheeks, nose and nasolabial folds are angiofibromas (formerly known as adenoma sebaceum). This adolescent did not have learning difficulties or epilepsy.

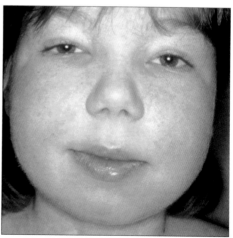

6.29 Juvenile dermatomyositis. This six-year-old girl recently developed muscular weakness, a dusky red facial rash and puffy facial oedema. The rash was also present on the knuckles, the elbows and knees.

DIAGNOSIS

Skin and muscle biopsy may be helpful, but disease activity may be patchy and histological changes may be easily missed. Electromyography may distinguish myopathy from a neuropathy, but the gold-standard investigation is an MRI scan, which clearly delineates areas of muscle inflammation and can be useful in directing biopsies. Radiology may show calcium deposits scattered throughout the muscles and soft tissues. Serum LDH (lactate dehydrogenate), creatinine kinase (CK) and transaminases are frequently but not invariably raised, but serial estimations of 24-hour urinary creatinine may provide the best index of disease activity.

TREATMENT

Rest is essential in the acute phase. Treatment with either prednisolone alone or in combination with an antimetabolite (azathioprine or methotrexate) may be required for some years, and the dosage reduced very gradually until the disease activity subsides. Ciclosporin may be added if the disease is unresponsive, and plasmapheresis may also be considered. Antimalarials may help a persistent rash. Physiotherapy is useful in preventing the development of contractures, and careful splinting may be required.

PROGNOSIS

The clinical course is variable; the condition may clear rapidly with steroids, or take many years to burn out. Although calcinosis is a good prognostic indicator for survival, gross disability may occur with contractures. Late recurrences are rare. There is a mortality rate of between 3 and 5%.

KLIPPEL–TRENAUNAY SYNDROME

INCIDENCE

Rare.

AETIOLOGY

Unknown.

PRESENTATION / DIAGNOSIS

Patients with this syndrome present with a limb, or part of a limb, which is increased in size and which bears a port wine stain (**6.30**). Associated venous varicosities confirm the diagnosis but these are often not present in the younger patient. Other types of vascular malformation may be present, such as superficial - lymphangiomas or angiokeratomas. Increased

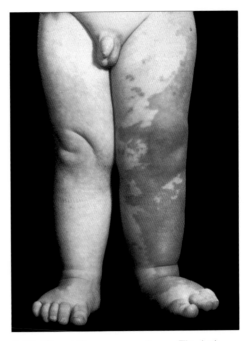

6.30 Klippel-Trenaunay syndrome. This little boy has an enlarged left leg. The bulk of the leg is increased, but its length is not measurably different from that of the right leg. There is extensive associated port wine staining of the affected leg. Ultimately, the leg will probably develop venous varicosities and there will be a risk of deep thrombosis and pulmonary embolus.

limb length implies bony hypertrophy; increased girth implies soft tissue overgrowth. Rarely there may be atrophy of the limb rather than hypertrophy. The affected limb may also be compromised by sympathetic overactivity with hyperhidrosis or vasoconstriction. Other developmental defects, such as polydactyly and syndactyly, may occur in the affected limb.

TREATMENT
The port wine stain and any associated superficial vascular naevi may be suitable for laser treatment.

Scoliosis and osteoarthrosis of knees and hips may occur secondary to a difference in leg length, and this should be looked for and appropriately corrected. Early on, the shoe on the shorter leg can be built up to compensate. Later, epiphysial stapling can be used to slow down growth in the longer leg. Amputation may be indicated if the enlarged limb, or part of it, is severely deformed.

Symptomatic patients with deep vein abnormalities are usually best treated with graduated compression stockings. Ligation and stripping of superficial venous varicosities may be surgically appropriate. Anti-thrombosis prophylaxis prior to any surgery should be considered because of the high rate of thrombo-embolic complications.

INCONTINENTIA PIGMENTI

INCIDENCE / GENETICS
It is inherited as an X-linked dominant trait that is usually lethal in males. More than 95% of the reported cases are females, the few males probably being the result of chromosomal anomalies such as 47XXY, or chromosomal mosaicism. The incontinentia pigmenti gene (NEMO) has recently been identified.

AETIOLOGY / PATHOGENESIS
This syndrome is not excessively rare.

CLINICAL PRESENTATION
Skin lesions are usually present at birth, and it is rare for them to make their first appearance more than a few days after birth. Three clinical stages are seen:
- The first stage comprises rather herpetiform groups of small bullae, usually containing clear fluid, often arranged in clearly linear or streaky patterns. These lesions can be seen at many sites. They may continue to occur in crops for several months (**6.31**). As the bullae resolve, they leave rather inflamed red plaques.

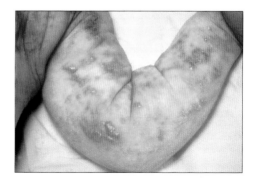

6.31 Incontinentia pigmenti. This one-week-old female infant presented with vesicles in a linear distribution on her lower limbs. A peripheral blood film showed eosinophilia. This was followed a few weeks later by warty lesions. She is now eight years old and has slate brown patches arranged in a swirl-like formation on her trunk. These lesions fade with time. Other systems which may be involved include the hair, nails, eyes and central nervous system.

- The second stage is not always seen. It is characterized by warty lesions, most often occurring on the dorsa of the hands and feet.
- The third stage is the residual pigmentation that develops at sites of earlier bullous lesions. The pigmentation is of rather greyish-brown colour and is arranged in streaks and whorls. It will not usually be present in the early weeks.

Inflammatory lesions are uncommon after six months of age but the pigmentation persists, slowly fading until it is often imperceptible by the second or third decade. There is frequently a more subtle fourth stage, of hypopigment-ation, which is often best seen on the lower leg; this feature can be important in detecting gene carriage in a mother.

Lesions in the scalp may lead to scarring alopecia and individual nails may be damaged. Hypodontia is very common in these patients. A small proportion of cases show ocular defects, including cataracts, uveitis and optic atrophy. Central nervous system involvement is an occasional complication; manifestations include mental retardation, developmental delay, spastic tetraplegia, microcephaly and epilepsy. Skeletal abnormalities are less common.

DIAGNOSIS

Eosinophilia up to 50% in the peripheral blood is usual when acute inflammatory skin changes are present.

Biopsy of the skin in the blistering phase can be helpful in establishing the diagnosis, with the presence of many eosinophils in the epidermis and dermis.

TREATMENT

No treatment, other than the control of secondary infection, is usually necessary. Skilled dental management can minimize cosmetic disability. Appropriate referrals to ophthalm-ologists and neurologists may be indicated. Genetic counselling should be offered.

EPIDERMOLYSIS BULLOSA

INCIDENCE / GENETICS

The overall incidence of all types of EB in the USA is approximately 1 in 50,000.

AETIOLOGY / PATHOGENESIS

Epidermolysis bullosa simplex is almost always inherited as an autosomal dominant trait. Junctional EB is usually inherited as an autosomal recessive trait. Dystrophic EB may be inherited either in an autosomal dominant (typically less severe) or in an autosomal recessive fashion (typically more severe).

Increasing numbers of genes are identified as causative for different EB subtypes. These genes encode for structural proteins of the basement membrane zone, hemidesmosomes and the keratin cytoskeleton of basal epithelial cells.

CLINICAL PRESENTATION

Epidermolysis bullosa is a broad term which incorporates a number of discrete disorders, which all have the common manifestation of skin fragility. In clinical practice, three subtypes are generally recognized, based on the level of the skin in which the split occurs. In epidermolysis bullosa simplex (EBS), the split is intraepidermal; junctional epidermolysis bullosa (JEB) has a characteristic split at the level of the dermo-epidermal junction within the basement mem-brane zone; and dystrophic epidermolysis bullosa (DEB) shows a split below the basement mem-brane zone.

Within each group there is a variety of disorders of highly variable severity. All forms of epidermolysis bullosa are characterized by the relatively ready development of blisters and ulceration at the site of various types of mechanical trauma. The skin and mucosae are both involved, to a variable degree. Onset is usually in the first year and, in most cases, within hours of birth. Intrauterine ulceration is common, resulting in areas of absent skin at birth. The most insidious common effect of mucosal involvement is faecal retention due to anal fissuring. The following features are relatively specific to each of these three groups:

- **Epidermolysis bullosa simplex (6.32).** Blisters heal without scarring. Mucosal involvement is less prominent. Main provocative trauma is rubbing from shoes and clothing. This condition is worse in hot environments. Involvement of the sole may be associated with hyperkeratosis.

- **Junctional epidermolysis bullosa (6.33)**. This is the form that is most often lethal in infancy, primarily because of failure to thrive (maybe due to intestinal involvement) and/or laryngeal involvement. Healing tends to be reluctant.
- **Dystrophic epidermolysis bullosa (6.34)**. Atrophic scarring leads to a variety of complications, including digital fusion, flexion deformity, oropharyngeal and oesophageal stricture formation.

DIAGNOSIS

Early skin biopsy is essential for accurate categorization and is available at specialist centres. Molecular genetic studies are also available.

TREATMENT

The management of epidermolysis bullosa involves a multidisciplinary approach and is usually coordinated at specialist centres. Children with more severe forms of EB will often require specialist nursing care, physiotherapy, hand surgery, occupational therapy and nutritional care, including gastrostomy feeding in some cases. In older patients with dystrophic EB the lifetime risk of squamous carcinoma is extremely high and patients require regular screening. Within the UK, the DEBRA association is a valuable patient help group and a strong supporter of patient care and research. Equivalent organizations exist in many countries.

Prenatal diagnosis is available in specialist centres and may be achieved by prenatal skin biopsy or, if the mutations are known, DNA-based diagnosis from chorionic villous biopsy or amniocentesis.

PROGNOSIS

Prognosis is highly variable, depending upon the precise type of epidermolysis bullosa. The most severe types are rapidly lethal; the mildest types are compatible with normal life expectancy and minimal impairment of quality of life.

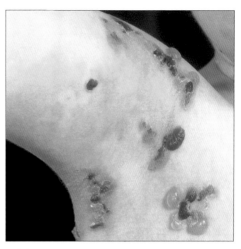

6.32 Epidermolysis bullosa simplex. In the Dowling-Meara form of EBS, grouped 'herpetiform' lesions are seen on the trunk and arms.

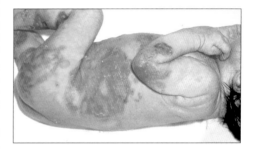

6.33 Junctional epidermolysis bullosa. This infant shows multiple areas of denuded skin. He presented at birth with two blisters. These rapidly progressed to extensive involvement of the skin and oral mucosa. He also developed a hoarse voice and failed to thrive. Hoarseness is a characteristic feature of this form of EB and is a useful clinical marker. He died aged six months. A non-lethal variant of JEB is recognized, but less common.

6.34 Dystrophic epidermolysis bullosa. This hand shows scarring, marked flexion contracture and early digital fusion. Soon after birth, the blisters appeared then ruptured, leaving raw areas of skin which healed with scarring. This can progress to encase the fingers in atrophic scarred skin. Corrective surgery is required if there is functional impairment. Involvement of the pharynx and oesophageal mucosa can lead to dysphagia. In adults, squamous carcinoma can develop.

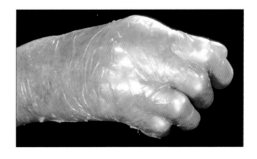

ACRODERMATITIS ENTEROPATHICA

INCIDENCE / GENETICS
Acrodermatitis enteropathica is a rare disease, transmitted as an autosomal recessive trait. The incidence in Denmark is approximately 1 in 500,000 live births.

AETIOLOGY / PATHOGENESIS
Acrodermatitis enteropathica is caused by a specific malabsorption of zinc (see also 'Gastroenterology' chapter).

CLINICAL PRESENTATION
This condition does not generally appear until a few weeks after weaning in the breast-fed, but often earlier in the formula-fed. An erythematous rash appears in a peri-orificial pattern in the napkin area (**6.35**) and around the mouth. The rash may be erosive or crusted, or it may be eczematous or psoriasiform. It tends to be highly symmetrical and gradually extends outwards without central clearing. The edge usually has a characteristic peeling character. This rash is highly refractory to standard treatments for napkin dermatitis, and this is an important diagnostic clue. At about the same time, it is very common for the infant to develop paronychia and, very often, fissures along the creases on the palm and the palmar aspects of the fingers.

Infants with acrodermatitis enteropathica are usually rather miserable. Despite the name of the condition, diarrhoea is uncommon in the earlier stages. Other characteristic late features include alopecia, failure to thrive and decreased resistance to infection.

DIAGNOSIS
The serum zinc level will usually, but not always, be low.

TREATMENT
An oral dose of zinc sulphate, 5 mg/kg per day, cures all clinical manifestations related to zinc deficiency within one or two weeks.

PROGNOSIS
Generally, lifelong therapy with zinc is required. Untreated, the disorder is lethal, though some affected children will survive for several years.

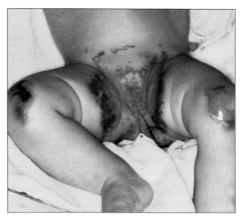

6.35 Acrodermatitis enteropathica. This four-month-old infant presented with an eczematous eruption around the orifices and extremities. She had been breast-fed for the first two months of life and subsequently changed to formula feeds. This is an autosomal recessive disorder caused by the intestinal malabsorption of zinc. The higher availability of zinc in breast milk is protective. Other features are diarrhoea, alopecia and stunted growth. The lesions cleared in two weeks with oral zinc. A similar appearance may be seen in acquired zinc deficiency in premature infants.

REFERENCES

General paediatric dermatology
Harper J, Orange A, Prose, N (eds). *Textbook of Pediatric Dermatology*. Oxford: Blackwell Science, 2000.

Viral warts
Fazel N, Wilcynsi S, Lowe L, Su LD. Clinical, histopathologic, and molecular aspects of cutaneous human papillomavirus infections. *Derm Clin* 1999; **17:** 521–536.

Atopic dermatitis
Holden C. Atopic Dermatitis. In: Champion RH, Burton JL, Burns DA, Breathnach SM (eds). *The Textbook of Dermatology*. Oxford: Blackwell Science, 1998: 681–708.

Williams H (ed). *The Epidemiology of Atopic Dermatitis*. Cambridge: CUP, 2000.

McHenry PM, Williams HC, Bingham EA. Management of atopic eczema. Joint Workshop of the British Association of Dermatologists and the Research Unit of the Royal College of Physicians of London. *BMJ* 1995; **310:** 843–847.

Scabies
Burns DA. Infestations. In: Champion RH, Burton JL, Burns DA, Breathnach SM (eds). *The Textbook of Dermatology* (6th edn). Oxford: Blackwell Science, 1998: 1458–1465.

Haemangioma
Atherton DJ. Haemangiomas. In: Champion RH, Burton JL, Burns DA, Breathnach SM (eds). *The Textbook of Dermatology* (6th edn). Oxford: Blackwell Science, 1998: 551–565.

Pityriasis rosacea
Parsons JM. Pityriasis rosea update. *J Am Acad Derm* 1986; **15:** 159–167.

Vitiligo
Gawkrodger DJ, Ravindran TS, Harper J. Forum on vitiligo. Royal College of General Practitioners: Member's reference book, 1995: 333–335.

Psoriasis
Camp R. Psoriasis. In: Champion RH, Burton JL, Burns DA, Breathnach SM (eds). *The Textbook of Dermatology* (6th edn). Oxford: Blackwell Science, 1998: 589–650.

Port wine stains
Atherton DJ. Port Wine Stains. In: Champion RH, Burton JL, Burns DA, Breathnach SM (eds). *The Textbook of Dermatology* (6th edn). Oxford: Blackwell Science, 1998: 569–576.

Eczema herpeticum
Atherton DJ, Harper J. Management of eczema herpeticum. *J Am Acad Derm* 1998; **18:** 757–758.

Epidermal naevi
Rogers M, McCrossin I, Commens C. Epidermal naevi and the epidermal naevus syndrome. J Am Acad Derm 1989; 20: 476–488.

Langerhans cell histiocytosis
Chu AC, D'Angio DJ, Favava B et al. Histiocytosis syndromes in children. *Lancet* 1987; **I:** 208–209.

Epidermolysis bullosa
Fine J-D, Bauer EA, McGuire J (eds). *Epidermolysis Bullosa: Clinical, Epidemiologic, and Laboratory Advances, and the Findings of the National Epidermolysis Registry*. Baltimore: Johns Hopkins University Press, 1999.

Uitto J. Molecular aspects of epidermolysis bullosa: novel pathomechanisms and surprising genetics. *Exp Derm* 1999; **8:** 92–95.

Atherton DJ. Epidermolysis Bullosa. In: Harper J (ed). *Inherited Skin Disorders*. Oxford: Butterworth-Heinemann, 1996: 53–68.

Ophthalmology
Ken K Nischal

ANATOMY OF THE EYE

See **7.1–7.3** for terminology of eye anatomy.

See **7.4** for description of eye movements.

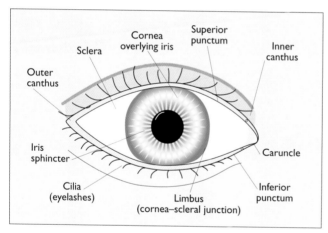

7.1 External landmarks of the eye and periocular region.

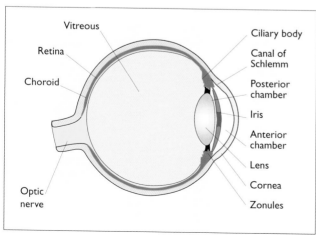

7.2 Cross-section of the globe.

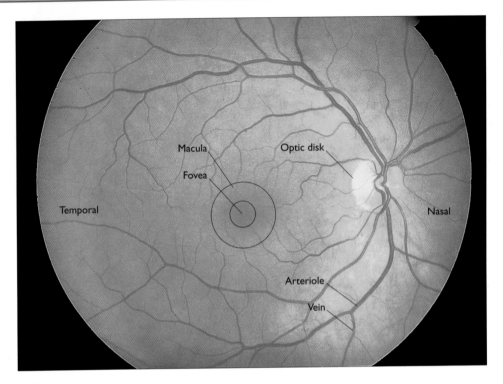

7.3 Fundus landmarks.

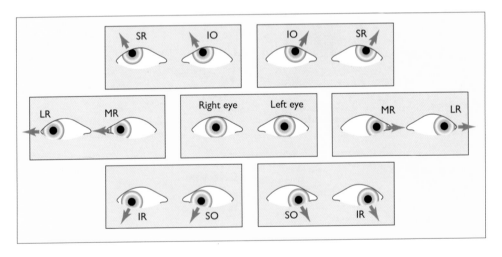

7.4 Schematic showing
the field of action of the
extraocular muscles.
SR = superior rectus
IR = inferior rectus
MR = medial rectus
LR = lateral rectus
IO = inferior oblique
SO = superior oblique

VISUAL DEVELOPMENT

VISUAL MILESTONES

It is essential to understand normal visual milestones: The chart (7.5) provides an easy guide to these. Delayed visual maturation may be seen in otherwise healthy children, which resolves by 6 months of age.

AMBLYOPIA

This is the commonest cause of decreased vision in childhood, affecting 2 to 3 in every 100 children. It occurs when the neural pathways between the affected eye and the brain fail to develop, usually due to lack of stimulation. The earlier the onset of amblyopia the greater the depth of the deficit. The critical period for visual development is probably between the first and eighth weeks of life; visual disruption during this period can cause dense amblyopia.

Amblyopia has numerous causes; the commonest are strabismus, visual deprivation (e.g. due to cataract or corneal opacification), significant difference between refractive error in the two eyes (anisometropic), significant bilateral refractive errors (ametropic) and significant astigmatism (meridional). Amblyopia is reversible by occlusion therapy of the better or good eye, with early detection and treatment offering the best outcome.

7.5 Observable visual behaviour
(after Blanche Stiff and Patricia Sonksen).

Behaviours	Neo	6wks	3m	4m	5m	6m	9m	12m
Blinks to flash	+	+	+	+	+	+	+	+
Turns to diffuse light	+	+	+	+	+	+	+	+
Fixes and follows near face	+ –	+ –	+	+	+	+	+	+
Watches an adult at 0.75m	+ –	+	+	+	+	+	+	+
F & F dangling ball at 6.5cm		+ –	+	+	+	+	+	+
Watches adult at 1.5m		+ –	+ –	+	+	+	+	+
Converges to 6.5cm			+ –	+	+	+	+	+
Fixates 2.5cm brick at 3.3m				+ –	+	+	+	+
Blinks to threat				+ –	+	+	+	+
Watches adult at 3m					+ –	+	+	+
Fixates 1.25cm sweet					+ –	+	+	+
Fixates 1.25mm sweet						+ –	+	+

☐ = upper limit of normal behaviour

LIDS

COLOBOMA
Definition
Incomplete formation of upper/lower lid(s).

Association
Goldenhar syndrome (upper lid), amniotic band syndrome and other clefting syndromes (usually lower).

Treatment
Lubrication in first instance to prevent exposure keratopathy. Early referral to oculoplastic surgeon to allow reconstruction of lid(s).

SYMBLEPHARON
Definition
Connection between lid and conjunctiva (**7.6**). Usually acquired but may be congenital.

Association
Acquired types are seen in Stevens-Johnson syndrome, toxic epidermolysis syndrome, alkali injuries to the eyes, ocular cicatricial pemphigoid and rarely, epidermolysis bullosa (recessive types usually).

Treatment
Prevention is the best approach in conditions where symblepharon may be acquired; topical lubrication and steroids may be needed but ophthalmic opinion must be sought early.

BLEPHARITIS
Definition
Inflammation of the eyelid margins (**7.7**), with or without chalazion (enlarged meibomian gland).

Association
Usually isolated but may be associated with acne rosacea. Abnormal meibomian glands may be seen in ectodermal dysplasia.

Treatment
Lid hygiene. Topical antibiotics may be needed and occasionally systemic antibiotics may be needed. Treatment is necessary to prevent corneal complications (vascularization/keratitis).

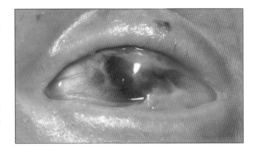

7.6 Neglected epidermolysis bullosa resulting in symblepharon of the lower lid and bulbar conjunctiva (see 'Dermatology' chapter). Also shown is keratinization and scarring of the cornea due to exposure keratopathy.

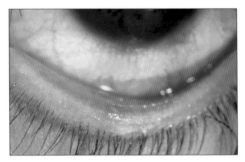

7.7 Blepharitis of the lower lid margin with phlycten (see page 175) of the lower limbus.

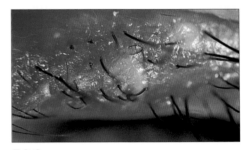

7.8 Stye.

STYE
Definition
This is an infected eyelash follicle (**7.8**).

Association
None.

Treatment
Removal of eyelash accelerates resolution. Occasionally topical antibiotics may be needed.

MOLLUSCUM CONTAGIOSUM
Definition
Common eyelid tumour (see also 'Dermatology' chapter) caused by a poxvirus. It is often situated on the lid margin and should be looked for in cases of follicular or chronic conjunctivitis. The lesions are small umbilicated nodules (**7.9**).

Association
Chronic or follicular conjunctivitis.

Treatment
Usually self-limiting but if conjunctivitis is troublesome then curettage of lid lesions may be needed.

CAPILLARY HAEMANGIOMA
Definition
Vascular anomaly (see Dermatology chapter) which histologically displays abundant endothelial cells with narrow vascular channels. They are the commonest tumours of eyelids or orbits in childhood.

Association
Dermal Kasabach-Merritt syndrome is thrombocytopenia due to platelet pooling within one or more large haemangiomas. Maffucci syndrome.

Treatment
The natural history of capillary haemangiomas is that they appear two or three weeks after birth, grow rapidly until 4 months of age and then stop growing by 6 months, regressing thereafter. The position of the haemangioma may result in visual deprivation by causing a ptosis, amblyopia from astigmatism or rarely compress the optic nerve if the haemangioma is intraconal in position. Treatment may involve intralesional and/or systemic steroids. Some cases demand surgical excision. Occlusion of the unaffected eye may be needed to prevent amblyopia developing in the affected eye.

PORT WINE STAIN
Definition
Dermal capillary vascular anomaly which may occur in the periocular region, (**7.10**); see also 'Dermatology' chapter.

Association
Ocular associations include episcleral haemangioma, iris heterochromia (affected iris darker than unaffected one), choroidal haemangioma and glaucoma. Systemic associations include Sturge-Weber syndrome and cutis marmorata telangectasia congenita.

Treatment
If periocular, there is increased risk of developing glaucoma and the child should be seen regularly to exclude this.

PTOSIS
Definition
Lowered upper lid margin position. May be measured in terms of palpebral aperture or marginal reflex distance. The latter is the distance of the upper lid margin to the central corneal reflection when using a torch as a target for the patient to look at. This should be 3.5–4.5 mm.

Association
Frequently seen in syndromes such as blepharophimosis, Noonan, Saethre-Chotzen, Freeman-Sheldon and Kabuki and in mitochondrial cytopathies (such as Kearnes-Sayre syndrome).

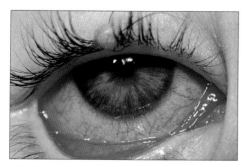

7.9 Molluscum contagiosum – raised papillomatous lesion with a central core containing virus particles.

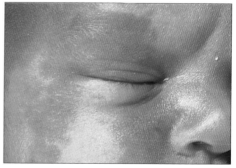

7.10 Port wine stain affecting periocular region.

Ptosis may be a presenting feature of myasthenia gravis or myotonic dystrophy.

Treatment

Ptosis may be due to dysfunction or absence of the levator palpebrae superioris muscle. Dysfunction may allow strengthening of the muscle while absence needs a frontalis sling (ie, attaching the lid to the frontalis muscle). Ptosis can cause amblyopia either because of stimulus deprivation (if severe ptosis) or astigmatism (mild to moderate ptosis). In any case, prompt ophthalmic referral is required.

LID RETRACTION
Definition
Usually retraction of upper lids (**7.11**).

Association
Thyroid eye disease (lid signs such as retraction and lid lag seen in 25–60% of paediatric cases), Parinaud syndrome, Marcus-Gunn jaw winking and primary congenital idiopathic lid retraction. Lower lid retraction is seen in cherubism (a rare, inherited condition characterized by fibro-osseous lesions of the maxilla and mandible recently localized to chromosome 4p16.3).

Treatment
No treatment is required except lubricating drops or ointment, used at night if there is evidence of lid lag and incomplete closure of the lids when asleep.

PRESEPTAL CELLULITIS
Definition
Infection of the lid without orbital involvement (**7.12**).

Association
In children, this is most commonly due to contiguous ethmoid sinusitis.

Treatment
Full ocular examination without dilation of pupils including visual acuity, eye movements, colour vision, pupil reactions and fundoscopy. Systemic antibiotics and referral to ENT team. Review to ensure no progression to orbital cellulitis (see later).

LID LAG
Definition
Delay or absence of normal downward excursion of upper lid on downgaze.

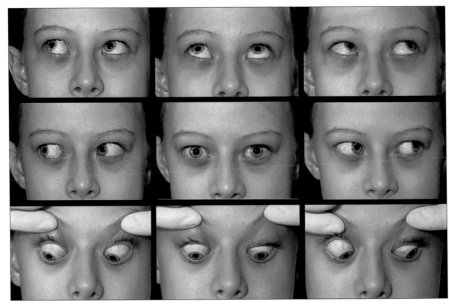

7.11 Lid retraction in thyroid eye disease. Eye movements are normal.

Association
Most commonly seen in congenital ptosis (usually unilateral) but also seen in thyroid eye disease and, rarely, polyneuritis.

Treatment
May need lubrication if incomplete eyelid closure at night

THE WATERING EYE
Epiphora (watering of the eye) is not uncommon and is due to a congenital blockage of the nasolacrimal duct. Lacrimal massage usually improves the situation but occasionally probing under general anaesthetic is needed. Very rarely, the lacrimal sac becomes expanded due to the distal blockage and the child presents with a dacryocoele (7.13). If this becomes infected it is termed a dacryocystitis.

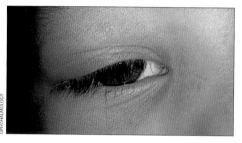

7.12 Preseptal cellulitis.

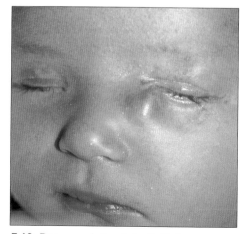

7.13 Dacryocoele in a baby. If this becomes infected it is termed dacryocystitis.

CORNEA

DEVELOPMENTAL DISORDERS

MICROCORNEA
Definition
Microcornea is an uncommon condition, defined as any cornea less than 10 mm in horizontal diameter.

Association
Hypermetropia, colobomas of the iris, corectopia, cataracts, microphakia, persistent hyperplastic primary vitreous, retinopathy of prematurity, angle closure glaucoma, infantile glaucoma, and chronic open angle glaucoma. Systemic associations include Ehlers-Danlos syndrome, Marfan syndrome, Rieger syndrome, Norrie syndrome, Trisomy 21 (Down syndrome), progeria, rubella, Turner syndrome, Waardenburg syndrome, Weil-Marchesani syndrome, Warburg micro-syndrome, cataract-microcornea syndrome and acro-reno-ocular syndrome.

CORNEA PLANA
Definition
Cornea plana is a flat cornea with a curvature of less than 43 diopters.

Associations
Ocular associations include sclerocornea, infantile glaucoma, angle closure glaucoma, chronic open angle glaucoma, retinal aplasia, anterior synechiae, aniridia, congenital cataracts, ectopia lentis, choroidal coloboma, blue sclera, iris coloboma, pseudoptosis, and microphthalmos. Systemic associations include osteogenesis imperfecta and epidermolysis bullosa (see 'Dermatology 'chapter).

Treatment
Review to exclude glaucoma and correct any refractive error.

MEGALOCORNEA
Definition
Megalocornea is a cornea with a horizontal diameter of more than 13 mm that is not progressive. If the cornea is enlarged in the presence of congenital glaucoma (7.14), it is not defined as megalocornea. Usually inherited as an X-linked recessive trait in most instances but maybe dominantly inherited.

Associations
Megalocornea most often occurs by itself, but other associated ocular conditions include anterior embryotoxon, mosaic corneal dystrophy, glaucoma. Systemic associations include Alport syndrome, craniosynostosis, dwarfism, Down syndrome, facial hemiatrophy, Marfan syndrome, Mucolipidosis type II and megalocornea –mental retardation syndrome.

KERATOCONUS
Definition
This disorder results in a central or paracentral thinning of the cornea, leading to poor visual acuity due to irregular and/or high astigmatism as the cornea bulges outward in a cone shape. Using direct ophthalmoscopy and a dilated pupil an oil droplet sign is seen. Other signs include scissoring of the light reflex on retinoscopy, slit lamp signs (Fleischer's ring, which is a brown deposition of iron in the epithelium at the base of the cone; Vogt's striae, which are small, thin, parallel striations in Descemet's membrane in the area of the cone, which with gentle pressure on the globe will momentarily disappear; prominent corneal nerves; endothelial guttata; and posterior shagreen). Rizutti's sign is that of a conical reflection nasally as a penlight is shone across the cornea from the temporal side. This tends to be a late sign of keratoconus, as is Munson's sign – a bulging of the lower eyelid anteriorly in down gaze, as a result of the cone pushing on the eyelid.

Associations
These include atopy, aniridia, blue sclera, congenital cataracts, ectopia lentis, microcornea, Leber's congenital amaurosis, retinitis pigmentosa, retinopathy of prematurity, and vernal conjunctivitis. Associated systemic conditions include Apert syndrome, atopy, brachydactyly, Crouzon syndrome, Down syndrome, Ehlers-Danlos syndrome type IV and VI, Raynaud syndrome, syndactyly, xeroderma pigmentosa and other connective tissue disorders.

Treatment
In mild to moderate cases contact lenses will correct the visual loss. In cases of acute hydrops, topical dehydrating, lubricating and steroid agents are needed. In severe cases, penetrating or deep lamellar corneal transplant is required.

SCLEROCORNEA
Definition
This is a congenital, non-inflammatory extension of opaque scleral tissue and fine vascular conjunctival and episcleral tissue into the peripheral cornea obscuring the limbus (7.15). Visual acuity is reduced only if the central cornea is involved. The severity of scleralization varies from mild to complete but is usually bilateral in 90% of cases. Cornea plana is concurrent in 80% of cases of sclerocornea.

Associations
These are common and include glaucoma, cataract, colobomas of the iris and choroid, blue sclera, cornea plana, aniridia, angle abnormalities, microphthalmos, and scleral

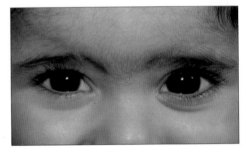

7.14 Bilateral congenital glaucoma with left eye bigger than right eye. Large corneas associated with congenital glaucoma are not termed megalocornea.

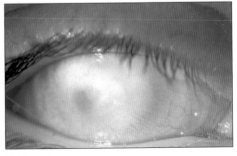

7.15 Sclerocornea.

perforations. Associated systemic abnormalities include spina bifida occulta, cerebellar abnormalities, cranial abnormalities, Hallermann-Streiff syndrome, Smith-Lemli-Opitz syndrome, osteogenesis imperfecta and hereditary osteonychodyplasias.

Treatment
Review to exclude glaucoma and cataract development. In bilateral total opacification, corneal transplant should be considered. Preoperative assessment with high frequency ultrasound is advisable to assess the presence of iridocorneal and keratolenticular adhesions.

PETERS' ANOMALY
Definition
Usually bilateral congenital central corneal opacity with defects in the posterior corneal stroma, Descemet's membrane, and endothelium with or without iridolenticular and/or keratolenticular adhesions.

Associations
Ocular associations include glaucoma, cataract, Axenfeld-Rieger syndrome, aniridia, microphthalmia, persistent hyperplastic primary vitreous (PHPV) and retinal dysplasia. Systemic abnormalities include craniofacial anomalies, central nervous system abnormalities, fetal alcohol syndrome, chromosomal abnormalities and **Peters plus syndrome** (rare autosomal recessive disorder comprising short-limbed dwarfism, cleft lip and/or palate, brachydactyly and learning difficulties.

Treatment
Review to exclude glaucoma and cataract. Treatment of glaucoma if present. If bilateral, corneal transplant should be considered.

CORNEAL DYSTROPHIES
See **Table 7.1** (next page). Only those dystrophies that commonly affect children are described.

POSTERIOR EMBRYOTOXON
A prominent, anteriorly displaced Schwalbe's ring seen only on slit lamp examination. Seen in up to 20% of normal population.

Association
Axenfeld-Rieger anomaly and Alagille syndrome (seen in 95% of cases).

Treatment
None.

CORNEAL DEPOSITS
Corneal deposition in the paediatric age group can vary from the simple deposition of iron in the epithelium, with no visual complications, to a full-thickness corneal opacification that can lead to profound amblyopia or even blindness. Proper diagnosis and management of these conditions is important in order to minimize or prevent profound complications.

Corneal deposition may be metabolic in origin or non-metabolic. The **metabolic** causes include the mucopolysaccharidoses (not MPS III – Sanfillippo), the mucolipidoses, glycogen storage disorders (namely Von Gierke's disease), sphingolipidoses (namely Fabry's disease), Gaucher's disease, gangliosidoses, cystinosis, Wilson's disease, tyrosinaemia type II, alkaptonuria, Niemann-Pick disease, LCAT deficiency and metachromatic leukodystrophy. **Non-metabolic** causes include corneal blood staining (seen after blunt trauma with blood in the anterior chamber), band-shaped keratopathy (**7.16**) (from calcium deposition in cornea), amyloid deposition, and neoplastic causes (i.e. monoclonal gammopathy).

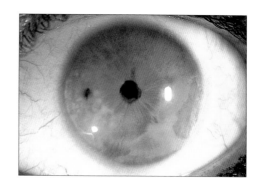

7.16 Band-shaped keratopathy, secondary to uveitis, in a patient with juvenile chronic arthritis. Note also a small, irregular pupil due to posterior synechiae (adhesions of the iris to the anterior capsule of the lens).

Table 7.1 Differential diagnosis of neonatal corneal opacity

Aetiology	Age of onset	Corneal signs	Other
INFECTIOUS DISEASE			
Herpes simplex (Type II)	4–10 days	Unilateral corneal ulcer, positive fluorescein staining, often in a geographic configuration	Viral culture for herpes
Rubella	Birth	Diffuse corneal oedema, often associated with cataracts	Serology including IgM
Neisseria gonorrhoeae	2–3 days	Diffuse punctate staining with possible corneal ulceration	Gram stain and culture
TRAUMA			
Tears in Descemet's membrane	Birth	Vertical corneal striae with oedema in the area of breaks in Descemet's membrane	History of forceps delivery often associated with soft tissue injury of the face
Corneal perforations with amniocentesis	Birth	Local corneal opacity with possible iris adhesions	Amniocentesis; traumatic cataract
DYSGENESIS SYNDROMES			
Peters' anomaly	Birth	Central corneal opacity may extend to the limbus; iridocorneal strands	60% with glaucoma
Sclerocornea	Birth	Peripheral corneal opacity associated with flattening of the cornea	May be associated with other anterior segment anomalies
Limbal dermoid	Birth	Limbal mass; yellow-white in appearance; may also have hair follicles	May be isolated or associated with Goldenhar syndrome
DYSTROPHIES			
Congenital hereditary endothelial dystrophy (CHED)	Birth to several months	Bilateral diffuse corneal oedema; corneal thickening; corneal diameter normal	Attenuated or absent endothelium; autosomal dominant or recessive
Posterior polymorphous dystrophy (PPD)	Infrequently at birth to first few years of birth	Deep linear opacities and thickening of Descemet's membrane (snail tracks); deep posterior vesicles; corneal oedema	Usually autosomal dominant
Congenital hereditary stromal	Birth	Diffuse, flaky stromal central anterior stromal haze with deeper involvement	
METABOLIC			
Mucopolysaccharidoses (Hurlers-MPS-IH most severe form)	Unusual at birth	Diffuse ground-glass appearance through all layers; bilateral and symmetrical	Urinary glycosaminoglycans; autosomal recessive
Mucolipidoses (Type IV)		Anterior and epithelial clouding	Autosomal recessive
Cystinosis (rare)	Rarely at birth, usually first year	White needle-like crystals within corneal stroma; ground-glass appearance	Renal impairment; crystals also in conjunctiva; glaucoma. Autosomal recessive
Tyrosinaemia	Neonate	Corneal epithelial deposits	Tyrosine in blood and urine; hyperkeratosis of skin
CONGENITAL			
Congenital glaucoma	Birth to first six months of life	Buphthalmos corneal oedema; Haab's striae (horizontal curvilinear breaks in Descemet's membrane due to stretch injury)	Increased ocular pressure; myopic shift; increased cupping

KERATITIS

Keratitis is an inflammation of the cornea. It may affect the epithelium, subepithelium or stroma. Most causes of keratitis are due to infection but there are non-infection-related causes.

INSUFFICIENT TEAR PRODUCTION (DRY EYE)

Definition

Insufficient production of aqueous tears leading to epithelial erosions, filamentary keratitis and secondary corneal vascularization.

Association

Riley-Day syndrome (familial dysautonomia), ectodermal dysplasia, keratoconjunctivitis sicca (KCS) usually due to primary or secondary Sjögren syndrome and radiation therapy.

Treatment

Adequate lubricating drops and in some cases temporary lacrimal punctal occlusion with silicone punctal plugs to decrease tear drainage.

NON-INFECTION-RELATED KERATITIS

Hereditary

Definition

Keratopathy (corneal erosions, epithelial defects) and corneal vascularization. The child is usually photophobic and has reduced visual acuity (7.17).

Association

Autosomal dominant keratitis (PAX 6, homeobox gene mutation), ectrodactyly, ectodermal dysplasia and cleft lip and palate syndrome (EEC), ectodermal dysplasia, keratitis-ichthyosis-deafness syndrome (KID), Riley-Day syndrome (familial dysautonomia), epidermolysis bullosa.

Treatment

Depends on cause, but lubrication is the mainstay of treatment.

Inadequate spreading of tears

Definition

Inadequate spreading of tears leads to epithelial erosions or dellen (area of corneal dessication).

Associations

Lid colobomas, corneal limbal dermoids (7.18 and 7.21) most commonly seen in Goldenhar syndrome, facial palsy, Moebius syndrome.

Treatment

Adequate ocular surface lubrication and removal of cause if possible (e.g. limbal dermoid removal or lid coloboma repair).

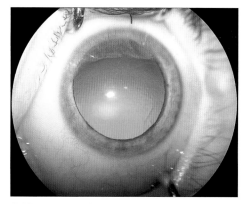

7.17 Keratitis affecting the superior half of the cornea. This was present from birth and progressive.

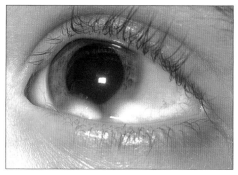

7.18 Limbal dermoids seen in a child with Goldenhar syndrome

Increased evaporation of tears
Definition
This is usually seen when there is proptosis or when the lids do not close adequately when the child is asleep.

Association
Craniosynostoses, lid colobomas, lagophthalmos, comatosed patients and lid ectropion (e.g. in cases of lamellar icthyosis).

Treatment
Eye ointment to exposed eyes when child asleep and regular daily lubrication. Tarsorraphy may be needed

Trauma (including corneal anaesthesia)
Definition
Repetitive trauma is the main cause of chronic keratitis and the presence of corneal hypo- or anaesthesia allows repetitive trauma. The accompanying reduced blink reflex reduces corneal wetting and exacerbates such a keratitis.

Associations
These may be congenital (familial dysautonomia, Goldenhar syndrome, oculofacial syndromes and leprosy) or acquired (damage to the trigeminal nerve due to herpes zoster, herpes simplex, intracranial tumours both pre and/or post surgery especially cerebellopontine angle tumours).

Treatment
Lubricating agents are needed. Tarsorraphy or botulinum toxin induced ptosis may be needed.

Avitaminosis A
Definition
Avitaminosis A is characterized by a thickening of the corneal epithelium, keratinization of the epithelium and a diffuse opacity. Secondary pannus and corneal vascularization can occur. In addition to corneal pathology, white foamy lesions of the temporal conjunctiva occur. These lesions are called Bitot spots and contain inflammatory cells and *Corynebacterium xerosis*.

Association
Malnutrition.

Treatment
The treatment is protein, calorie, and vitamin A replacement.

Vernal keratoconjunctivitis
Definition
Although seasonal allergic conjunctivitis is extremely common, vernal keratoconjunctivitis with corneal involvement is much less common. Mucoid discharge with lumps on the superior tarsal conjunctiva (papillae) (**7.19**) which cause trauma to the superior half of the cornea leading to corneal epithelial erosions, shield ulcers (5% of patients) and corneal vascularization (micropannus).

There may be limbal infiltration with the presence of Tranta's dots which are aggregates of eosinophils. Repeated such infiltration may leave a scar in the adjacent cornea in the form of a 'Cupid's bow', called a pseudogerontoxon. This is usually found superiorly and resembles an arcus senilis.

Treatment
Topical anti-allergic medication usually with topical steroid therapy and lubricating agents. Supratarsal steroid injection or topical cyclosporin drops may also be needed in severe cases.

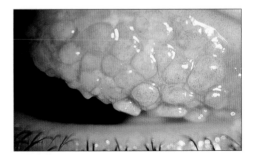

7.19 Giant papillae in vernal keratoconjunctivitis.

INFECTION-RELATED KERATITIS
Herpes simplex
Definition
Eye involvement occurs in 13% of newborns with systemic herpes simplex virus (HSV) infection. Herpes keratitis can occur at almost any age in children, as even neonates can become infected as they pass through the birth canal. Infections acquired at birth are usually of herpes simplex virus Type 2, while herpes contracted later in life is most often HSV Type 1. Primary herpes is the first exposure of the herpes virus to the patient. The hallmark sign of primary herpetic infection is conjunctivitis, which is accompanied by vesicles on the eyelids. Recurrent disease (secondary) can result in dendritic, disciform, or interstitial keratitis.

Association
Neonatal herpes simplex keratitis may be the only sign of systemic herpes simplex.

Treatment
Any child who will not open an eye should be considered to have either a foreign body or herpes simplex keratitis until proven otherwise. Examination under anaesthetic should be done in such cases.

Viral cultures from scrapings taken from the edge of any ulcer are necessary. However, PCR for HSV may be performed even on tears or conjunctival swabs from the affected eye.

Herpes simplex keratitis (epithelial) is treated with topical acyclovir while stromal and/or endothelial disease with intact epithelium is treated with topical acyclovir and topical steroids. Systemic acyclovir should be considered if systemic herpes simplex is a possibility.

Varicella-zoster
Definition
Corneal involvement is extremely rare, but ocular findings include swollen lids, vesicular lesions of the lids, and varying degrees of keratoconjunctivitis. Infrequently superficial punctate keratitis of the cornea occurs.

Associations
Immunodeficiency may be associated.

Treatment
Oral acyclovir, and topical cycloplegic drops for eye comfort.

Chlamydia trachomatis
Definition
Trachoma is a cause of blindness worldwide. The causative organism is *Chlamydia trachomatis*, an intracellular parasite. A chronic follicular conjunctivitis results from infection with secondary corneal scarring.

Action
Treat with topical and systemic tetracyclines if child with permanent dentition or with sulphonamides if not.

Bacterial
Definition
Usually stromal with accompanying hypopyon (pus in the anterior chamber).

Association
Bacterial keratitis in children is often the result of some type of predisposing factor such as: contact lenses, trauma, dry eyes, HSV, immunosuppression, immunodeficiency, or vitamin deficiency.

Treatment
Culture and Gram stain, followed by appropriate intensive topical antibiotics.

Fungal
Definition
Clinical suspicion should be raised if there are fuzzy borders of the infiltrate, an elevated infiltrate with initially intact epithelium, satellite lesions and pyramidal or convex hypopyon. Sometimes the infiltrate may be seen to develop pigmentation and this is suggestive of filamentous infection.

Association
The infection may be due to filamentous fungi such as *Aspergillus* or *Fusarium* spp.or to yeast-like fungi such as *Candida* spp. Most traumatic fungal ulcers are the result of filamentous organisms, while infection by yeasts are most common in patients with immunosuppression or dry eyes.

Treatment
Culture and Gram stain. Treat with systemic and topical anti-fungal agents.

CONJUNCTIVA

INFECTION-RELATED CONJUNCTIVITIS

NEONATAL CONJUNCTIVITIS
Definition
Conjunctival inflammation occurring during the first month of life (ophthalmia neonatorum – 7.20).

Association
Causes include chemical (relatively mild diffuse injection without discharge), gonococcal (copious purulent discharge which may be associated with membrane formations), herpes simplex type II, chlamydia and bacterial.

Action
This is a notifiable condition. Swabs and appropriate topical and if gonococcal or chlamydial, systemic antibiotics are needed.

BACTERIAL CONJUNCTIVITIS
Definition
Very common, usually, bilateral infection with mucopurulent discharge, conjunctival hyperaemia and, occasionally, membranes or pseudo-membranes.

Association
Commonest causes are *Staphylococcus aureus*, *Streptococcus pneumoniae*, and *Haemophilus influenzae*. Membranes and pseudo-membranes may be caused by haemolytic streptococci, gonococcus and *Corynebacterium diphtheriae*.

Treatment
Broad topical antibiotics. If membranes or pseudomembranes are present these should be physically removed and an anti-inflammatory topical drop added to the antibiotic.

Swabs should be taken if the discharge is copious or persistent despite topical antibiotics.

VIRAL CONJUNCTIVITIS
Definition
Common, contagious usually bilateral condition. Adenoviral conjunctivitis presents with watery discharge, conjunctival hyperaemia, follicular conjunctivitis, preauricular lymphadenopathy and pseudomembranes in severe cases.

Associations
Commonest causes are adenovirus, herpes simplex, enterovirus, and Epstein-Barr virus.

Treatment
Topical antibiotics to prevent secondary bacterial infections.

CHRONIC CONJUNCTIVITIS
Definition
This is usually unilateral but may be bilateral.

Associations
Molluscum contagiosum (molluscum eyelid lesions associated with ipsilateral follicular conjunctivitis), toxic conjunctivitis (aminoglycoside antibiotics, antivirals, glaucoma medication, eye makeup and preservatives) and Parinaud's oculo-glandular syndrome (follicular conjunctivitis and severe preauricular lymphadenopathy) most commonly caused by cat-scratch fever, tularaemia, sporotrichosis, tuberculosis, and coccidiodomycosis.

Treatment
Molluscum contagiosum is a self-limiting condition but if the conjunctivitis is too uncomfortable, the child should have an examination under anaesthetic and the eyelid lesion curettaged. For toxic conjunctivitis the offending topical medication should be discontinued if possible.

CHLAMYDIA CONJUNCTIVITIS
Definition
This usually unilateral condition causes a follicular conjunctivitis with preauricular lymphadenopathy.

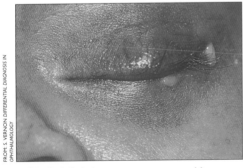

FROM: S. VERNON DIFFERENTIAL DIAGNOSIS IN OPHTHALMOLOGY

7.20 Ophthalmia neonatorum caused by chlamydia.

Associations
This condition may be sexually transmitted. Therefore in teenagers a history of sexual activity needs to be sought while in younger children the possibility of sexual abuse must be considered.

Treatment
Appropriate swabs. Treat with topical and systemic erythromycin, exclusion of pneumonitis and referral to genito-urinary medicine to exclude other sexually transmitted diseases.

NON INFECTION-RELATED CONJUNCTIVITIS

ALLERGIC CONJUNCTIVITIS
Definition
Very common, bilateral seasonal or perennial condition. There is chemosis (swelling of the conjunctiva), watery discharge and conjunctival hyperaemia.

Association
Hay fever.

Treatment
Topical anti-allergic medication.

ATOPIC KERATOCONJUNCTIVITIS
Definition
There is usually lid eczema, inflammation of the lid margins (blepharitis) and mucoid discharge.

Associations
Cataracts, keratoconus and retinal detachments may occur. Secondary glaucoma may occur if periocular steroids are used to treat skin.

Treatment
Lubricating agents and, if necessary, anti-allergy topical medication may be needed.

CONJUNCTIVAL PIGMENTATION

BENIGN MELANOSIS
Definition
Brown-black patches seen near the limbus and sometimes in the inter-palpebral bulbar conjunctiva. The patches move very easily over the globe and are most commonly seen in pigmented races.

Treatment
None needed as there is no risk of malignant change.

FLAT DEEP PIGMENTATION
Definition
This is due to unilateral subepithelial melanocytosis and as such the pigmentation cannot be moved over the globe. There is a slate-grey appearance, which may be isolated to the eye (melanosis oculi), isolated to the periocular skin (dermal melanocytosis), or involve both eye and skin (oculodermal melanocytosis or Naevus of Ota).

Associations
Naevus of Ota is associated with increased risk of glaucoma and increased risk of uveal melanoma. Oculo (dermal) melanocytosis is nine times more common in young patients with uveal melanoma than in the general population with uveal melanoma.

Treatment
Regular review.

ELEVATED CONJUNCTIVAL LESIONS

PIGMENTED NODULES
Naevus
Definition
Solitary, well-defined, slightly elevated lesion which moves freely over globe. Most – 75% – are pigmented. Naevi usually are present at the limbus, plica, caruncle and lid margin.

Association
Melanoma.

Treatment
Rapid growth may be seen around puberty; excisional biopsy may be needed to confirm diagnosis.

NON-PIGMENTED SMALL NODULES
Phlycten
Definition
Uncommon, straw-yellow, slightly elevated lesion usually at or near limbus, surrounded by hyperaemia (**7.6**).

Associations
Commonest cause is *Staphylococcus aureus* hypersensitivity seen in blepharitis. May also be caused by tuberculosis, herpes simplex and *Candida* infection.

Treatment
If associated with blepharitis then treat with topical antibiotic and topical steroid therapy.

NON-PIGMENTED LARGE NODULES
Epibulbar dermoid
Definition
Solid, elevated, congenital lesion usually located at the limbus. May have hairs on surface (7.21).

Associations
Ocular associations include lid coloboma, ocular coloboma, microphthalmos and aniridia, Goldenhar, Treacher-Collins and Franchescetti syndromes.

Treatment
If the lesion is very large or causing ocular surface wetting problems, it must be removed.

PLAQUE-LIKE CONJUNCTIVAL LESIONS
Pterygium
Definition
Wing-shaped, very common fleshy lesion usually at the nasal limbus. Seen in adults but may be seen in teenagers.

Association
Seen more commonly in equatorial regions.

Treatment
Rarely needed in teenagers but, in adults, if it encroaches on the corneal central axis it should be removed.

Bitot spot
Definition
Foamy plaques temporal to the limbus seen in avitaminosis A.

Treatment
Vitamin A replacement.

DIFFUSELY ELEVATED CONJUNCTIVAL LESIONS

LYMPHOMA
Definition
Diffuse subconjunctival fleshy lesion, which may be bilateral. Smaller patches have been termed 'salmon patches'.

Associations
Most commonly, Non-Hodgkin's or Burkitt's lymphoma.

Treatment
Excision biopsy followed by systemic therapy from oncology team.

PLEXIFORM NEUROFIBROMA
Definition
Diffuse, very smooth, elevated lesion extending from the lid to the superior bulbar conjunctiva.

Association
Neurofibromatosis 1.

Treatment
Usually none needed.

7.21 Very large limbal dermoid, causing difficulty in closure of the eyelids.

CONJUNCTIVAL TELANGIECTASIA

Definition
Dilated and tortuous bulbar conjunctival vessels are **not** normal.

Associations
Metabolic (Fabry disease, Fucosidosis, Galactosialidosis, GM1 gangliosidosis, multiple endocrine neoplasia IIa); haematological (dysproteinaemias, sickle cell anaemia); Louis-Bar (ataxia-telangiectasia) syndrome (**7.22**); Sturge-Weber syndrome; Rendu-Osler-Weber disease; capillary haemangioma, lymphangioma – conjunctival lesions are more saccular than true telangiectasia. (See also 'Neurology' and 'Immunology' chapters.)

7.22 Telangiectasia of the bulbar conjunctiva in a child with ataxia-telangiectasia.

SCLERA

PIGMENTATION OF THE SCLERA
Metabolic causes include alkaptonuria, haemochromatosis and jaundice while non-metabolic causes include osteogenesis imperfecta I, Marshall-Smith Russell-Silver, Roberts, and Ehlers-Danlos VI syndromes, all of which may be associated with blue sclera. May occasionally also be seen in Marfan, Hallermann-Streiff, Bloch-Sulzberger, Turner, Kabuki syndromes and in high myopia of any cause.

SCLERAL INFLAMMATION

EPISCLERITIS
Definition
Differentiated from scleritis because, unlike scleritis, it is not tender to the touch.

Associations
Simple episcleritis often follows a viral illness and is self-limiting. Nodular and diffuse may be associated with systemic lupus erythematosus, juvenile idiopathic arthritis, spondylo-arthropathy, inflammatory bowel disease, rheumatic fever, relapsing polychondritis, polyarteritis nodosa, and other systemic diseases.

Treatment
Topical mild steroid to treat episcleritis.

SCLERITIS
Definition
Inflammation of the sclera that is tender to touch. May be diffuse, nodular, or necrotizing.

Associations
Causes include idiopathic, infections, surgically induced (necrotizing or diffuse), rheumatic diseases, connective tissue disorders, enteropathies, vasculitides, granulomatous diseases, and certain skin disorders.

Treatment
Treat underlying condition and use nonsteroidal anti-inflammatory drugs systemically to treat eye initially.

DEVELOPMENTAL ANOMALIES OF THE GLOBE

NANOPHTHALMOS
Definition
The eye is small in its overall dimensions but is not affected by other gross developmental defects nor accompanied by other systemic congenital anomalies. There is high hypermetropia, with short axial length (16–18.5 mm), and a crowded anterior chamber predisposing to glaucoma.

Associations
Glaucoma occurs later in life, as do choroidal effusions because of the thickened inelastic sclera. Systemic associations include Kenny Caffey syndrome.

Treatment
Correction of refractive error and review for glaucoma and choroidal effusions.

SIMPLE MICROPHTHALMOS
Definition
This is the term used to describe an eye that is small but is otherwise essentially normal. It may be associated with systemic developmental anomalies in about 50% of cases. Since these eyes have a short axial length they are usually moderately hypermetropic. The corneal diameter can be normal, but cases associated with a systemic disorder can have microcornea. Most patients have a normal best-corrected vision for their age. The late ocular complications seen in nanophthalmos do not occur in simple microphthalmos.

Associations
These include fetal alcohol syndrome, diabetic embryopathy, myotonic dystrophy, achondroplasia, pseudotrisomy 18, neurodevelopmental delay, isolated growth hormone deficiency, mucopolysaccharidosis VI, and mucolipidosis III.

COMPLEX MICROPHTHALMOS
Definition
Cases tend to be bilateral, and the vision ranges from normal to no light perception, depending on the ocular malformation. Microphthalmos with coloboma is caused by incomplete closure of the embryonic fissure by the seventh week (7.23). Microphthalmos with cyst is a colobomatous malformation that results from a defective closure of the embryonic fissure. There is typically a protruding mass in the inferior orbit or lid associated with a severely malformed microphthalmic eye (7.24).

Associations
CHARGE syndrome (coloboma; heart defects; atresia choanae; retarded growth and development or central nervous system anomalies, or both; genital anomalies or hypogonadism, or both; and ear anomalies or deafness, or both). At least three of the features are necessary for the diagnosis. The heart defects may be lethal. Micro syndrome which comprises microphakia, microphthalmos, characteristic lens opacity, and atonic pupils, cortical visual impairment, microcephaly, and developmental delay. MIDAS (microphthalmia, dermal aplasia, and sclerocornea) syndrome. Oculodentodigital dysplasia. Multiple chromosomal abnormalities may be present.

ANOPHTHALMIA
Definition
Denotes cases where the eye appears to be absent. Primary anophthalmos due to failure of the outgrowth of the optic vesicle, unassociated with an abnormality of the neural tube, is the most common type. This must occur during the first two weeks of development and is usually bilateral (but asymmetric), sporadic, and, in most cases, the child is otherwise well-formed.

Associations
Patients with clinical anophthalmos have been shown to have a high incidence of developmental anomalies involving both eyes (88%), the brain (71%) and the body (58%) (7.25).

Treatment
The absence of a normal eye affects normal orbital growth and for this reason orbital expanders may be needed and referral to an oculoplastic surgeon is needed.

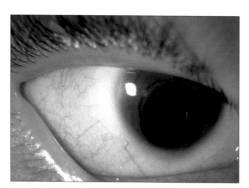

7.23 Microphthalmos with iris coloboma.

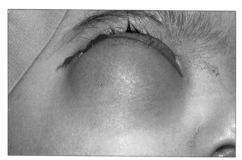

7.24 Microphthalmos with cyst. The cyst is bluish in colour and occupies the major part of the orbit.

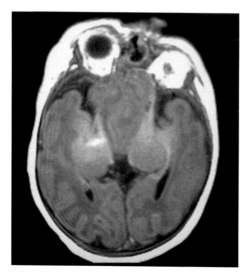

7.25 MRI of a child with clinical anophthalmos. Note the abnormal intracranial findings.

IRIS

CONGENITAL IRIS DEFECTS

IRIS COLOBOMA
Definition
Iris colobomas are classified as typical if they occur in the inferonasal quadrant and are due to non-closure of the embryonic fissure in the fifth week of gestation. Typical iris colobomas may involve the ciliary body, choroid, retina, and optic nerve.

Associations
Iris colobomas may be isolated or associated with ocular features such as retino-choroidal/optic nerve coloboma, microcornea, microphthalmos (**7.23**) or both or microph-thalmos with cyst. Nystagmus may be seen, as may cataracts. Although iris colobomas can be associated with almost any chromosomal abnormality they are frequently seen in branchio-oculo-facial, cat-eye, CHARGE, 13q deletion, Goltz, triploidy, Patau (trisomy 13), Wolf-Hirschhorn (4p-) and Walker-Warburg syndromes.

Treatment
Review for correction of refractive error and cataract progression if lens opacity is present.

ANIRIDIA
Definition
Aniridia (autosomal dominant) is a panocular, bilateral disorder. The most obvious presenting sign is absence of much or most of the iris tissue. In addition to iris involvement, foveal and optic nerve hypoplasia may be present, resulting in a congenital sensory nystagmus and leading to reduced visual acuity to 6/30 or worse. Anterior polar cataracts, glaucoma, and corneal opacification often develop later in childhood and may lead to progressive deterioration of visual acuity. Glaucoma occurs in up to half of all cases.

Associations
Wilm's tumour, genitourinary abnormalities and retarded growth or development (AGR triad) or both (WAGR) or associated with ataxia and neurodevelopmental delay (Gillespie syndrome).

Treatment

All children with sporadic aniridia should have repeated abdominal ultrasonographic and clinical examinations. One protocol advised that the child be seen every 3 months until the age of 5, every 6 months until the age of 10, and one a year until the age of 16. However, the examinations are best continued until chromosomal and then intragenic mutational analysis have confirmed a PAX6 mutation only. If chromosomal deletion is found, three-monthly scans should be performed and the child transferred to the care of a nephrologist.

IRIS TRANSILLUMINATION

The congenital causes of iris transillumination include albinism (both ocular and oculo-cutaneous) when it occurs because of absence of pigmentation in the posterior pigment epithelial layer (**7.26**). It may also be seen in the mid peripheral iris in female carriers of X-linked ocular albinism. Other causes include iris hypoplasia; X-linked megalocornea; Marfan's syndrome; ectopia lentis et pupillae; micro-coria. Small transillumination defects just visible near the iris root in blue-eyed children may be idiopathic with no clinical significance. Rarely, it occurs in association with congenital ocular fibrosis syndrome.

ACQUIRED IRIS DEFECTS

IRIS TRANSILLUMINATION

Causes include: iatrogenic – surgical or laser iridectomy or iridotomy respectively; pigment dispersion syndrome – may be seen in teenagers. It is thought to occur as a result of posterior bowing of the iris resulting in pigment dispersion from lens/iris pigment epithelium friction; herpes zoster ophthalmicus often results in sector iris atrophy; trauma – blunt injury may result in detachment of the iris root (iridodialysis) which results in pseudopolycoria.

CHANGES IN IRIS COLOUR

BENIGN PRIMARY IRIS TUMOURS
Brushfield spots

These occur in 38–90% of patients with Down syndrome. Very similar iris findings may occur in normal individuals (Wolfflin nodules).

SECONDARY TUMOURS
Juvenile xanthogranuloma
Definition

Iris involvement occurs almost exclusively in infants. Usually unilateral yellow nodules or diffuse infiltration may be seen.

Association

Spontaneous hyphaema (blood in the anterior chamber) and/or unilateral glaucoma may occur.

Treatment

All children with JXG should have ocular screening because even asymptomatic ocular lesions may be associated with glaucoma. Most ocular lesions will regress with topical steroids. Some cases may need systemic steroids and others a small dose of radiotherapy treatment.

LANGERHANS CELL HISTIOCYTOSIS

See also 'Solid Tumours and Histiocytosis' chapter.

Definition

Langerhans cell histiocytoses (eosinophilic granuloma, Letterer-Siwe, and Hand-Schuller-Christian disease), although similar to JXG, which is systemically benign, are systemic malignancies and need appropriate chemo-therapy.

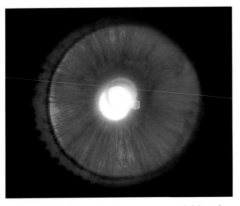

7.26 Iris transillumination seen in a child with ocular albinism.

Association
Usually limited to orbital involvement but iris nodules or choroidal involvement may rarely occur in Letterer-Siwe disease.

Treatment
Routine ophthalmic examination, treatment of underlying disease.

LEUKAEMIA / LYMPHOMA
See also 'Blood Diseases' chapter.

Definition
Leukaemia iris infiltrates, although rare, have been reported with most types of childhood leukaemia and lymphoma. Acute lymphoblastic leukaemia (ALL) is both the most common form of childhood leukaemia and the most likely to be associated with iris infiltration.

Association
Iris infiltration (nodules, spontaneous hyphema, heterochromia, pseudohypopyon with iritis, and/or acute glaucoma) is an ominous finding since the median time of survival after discovery of leukemic iris involvement is 3 months.

Treatment
Since these are immunocompromised patients anterior chamber aspiration or iris biopsy may be needed to exclude an infectious etiology. Chemotherapy may not be effective and low dose external radiation has been used successfully despite potential for cataract development.

HETEROCHROMIA IRIDES
The differential diagnosis of paediatric heterochromia irides (7.27) is extensive but may be classified on the basis of whether the condition is congenital or acquired and whether the affected eye is hypopigmented or hyperpigmented.

HYPOCHROMIC HETEROCHROMIA
Congenital causes
Horner syndrome; Waardenburg syndrome; piebaldism trait.

Acquired causes
Fuch's heterochromic cyclitis – rare type of unilateral iritis; nonpigmented iris tumours.

HYPERCHROMIC HETEROCHROMIA
Congenital causes
Iris mammillations – unilateral villiform protuberances that may cover the iris usually in association with oculodermal melanosis or neurofibromatosis; congenital iris ectropion (see page 179); unilateral iris coloboma (affected iris is darker); port wine stain.

Acquired causes
Cataract surgery in children – operated eye is darker in eyes operated early in life; topical medication (e.g. latanoprost, which is a prostaglandin analogue and causes darkening of the iris of the eye being treated); pigmented iris tumours; rubeosis iridis- iris neovascularization – causes include retinopathy of prematurity, retinoblastoma, Coats' disease, and iris tumours; siderosis – due to intraocular metallic foreign body.

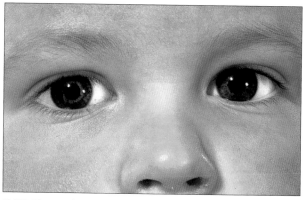

7.27 Heterochromia irides. This child had Waardenburg syndrome.

PUPIL ANOMALIES

LEUKOCORIA
Definition
A white pupil reflex.

Associations
Congenital cataract (may be unilateral or bilateral) (**7.28**). **Persistent hyperplastic primary vitreous** (a rare congenital, usually unilateral, condition). **Inflammatory cyclitic membrane**. **Retinal dysplasia** (very rare) may be associated with Norrie disease, Bloch–Sulzberger syndrome (incontinentia pigmenti), Warburg syndrome, Patau syndrome (trisomy 13) or Edward syndrome (trisomy 18).
Tumours and granulomas – retinoblastoma, retinal astrocytoma and toxocaral granuloma.
Retinal detachment – Retinopathy of prematurity, retinoblastoma, Coats' disease, toxocaral granuloma, and Stickler syndrome.
Miscellaneous – extensive retinal nerve fibre myelination and large chorioretinal coloboma.

DYSCORIA
Definition
An abnormality of the shape of the pupil.

Associations
Congenital causes are persistent pupillary membranes, iris coloboma, iris hypoplasia and ectopia lentis et pupillae (see later). Acquired causes – most commonly seen in iritis.

MIOSIS
Definition
A small pupil, usually less than 2 mm, which reacts poorly to dilating drops.

Associations
Congenital miosis (microcoria) may be due to an absence of the dilator pupillae muscle or fibrous contraction secondary to persistent pupillary membrane. It can be seen in congenital rubella syndrome, Marfan syndrome, in 20% of Lowe (oculocerebrorenal) syndrome and in ectopia lentis et pupillae.

MYDRIASIS
Definition
A large pupil, usually greater than 4 mm. May be true mydriasis or pseudo-mydriasis.

True mydriasis
Association
May be congenital but blunt trauma causing iris sphincter rupture, ciliary ganglionitis (unilateral most commonly after chicken pox – also known as Adie's pupil) or acquired neurological disease must be excluded, especially third nerve palsy.

Treatment
If there is ciliary ganglionitis, accommodation can be affected and the child will need a reading prescription.

Pseudo-mydriasis
Definition
Many cases of congenital mydriasis are actually part of the aniridia spectrum. Congenital iris ectropion is often mistaken as an enlarged pupil. Iris ectropion is eversion of the posterior pigment epithelium onto the anterior surface of the iris.

Association
Iris ectropion can occur as an acquired tractional abnormality, often in association with rubeosis irides or as a congenital non-progressive abnormality. Congenital iris ectropion may be associated with congenital and/or developmental glaucoma. Associated conditions include neuro-fibromatosis I, Prader-Willi syndrome and facial hemihypertrophy.

Treatment
Review to exclude glaucoma or association.

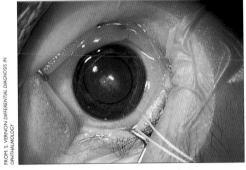

FROM: S. VERNON DIFFERENTIAL DIAGNOSIS IN OPHTHALMOLOGY

7.28 Leukocoria due to a congenital cataract, at operation.

CORECTOPIA

Definition

Refers to displacement of the pupil. Normally, the pupil is displaced inferonasally about 0.5mm from the centre of the iris.

Associations

Causes include sector iris hypoplasia, colobomas, ectopia lentis et pupillae, Axenfeld-Rieger anomaly, iridocorneal endothelium (ICE) syndromes. Intermittent corectopia, pupils shifting from central to eccentric positions, have been reported during coma and may represent a sign of rostral midbrain dysfunction.

Treatment

None.

ANISOCORIA

In this condition there is a difference in size between the two pupils. The three main causes in childhood that need to be considered are physiological, Horner syndrome, and Adie pupil (ciliary ganglionitis).

Treatment

The child should be examined in bright light and then in the dark. If the anisocoria is physiological then the difference will remain constant and will be no more than 2 mm. If the anisocoria is accentuated in bright surroundings this suggests that the larger pupil is at fault and cannot constrict. The commonest cause for this is ciliary ganglionitis (Adie's pupil). Examination by slit lamp to detect vermiform iris movements. If the anisocoria is accentuated in the dark, this suggests that the smaller pupil is at fault. The commonest cause for this is Horner syndrome.

Horner syndrome

Definition

Miosis, with ipsilateral ptosis and sometimes anhidrosis (7.29).

Associations

Congenital Horner syndrome is associated with hypopigmentation of the affected side. Acquired Horner syndrome may be due to: central (first order neurone) lesions; preganglionic (second order) lesions; postganglionic (third order) lesions; metastatic neuroblastoma perhaps causing a congenital Horner syndrome.

Pharmacologic testing

4% cocaine – one drop in each eye. The Horner pupil will NOT dilate. This confirms the presence of Horner syndrome. 24 hours later hydroxyamphetamine 1% can be used in each eye. If the lesion is preganglionic then BOTH pupils will dilate, but in a postganglionic one the Horner pupil will not. Alternatively, use 1:1,000 adrenaline into both eyes. In a preganglionic lesion NEITHER pupil will dilate but in a postganglionic one the Horner pupil will dilate.

Treatment

Even if there is heterochromia irides, metastatic neuroblastoma should be excluded. In an otherwise healthy child, at least a chest x-ray and spot urine VMA (vanylymandelic acid).

Adie syndrome

Definition

Mydriasis with vermiform iris movements on slit-lamp examination.

Associations

The commonest association is chicken pox infection but other viral infections may also cause ciliary ganglionitis.

Treatment

Accommodation is usually affected and the child may need reading spectacles.

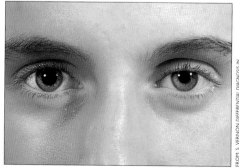

7.29 Left Horner syndrome with the left pupil slightly smaller and the left lid slightly ptotic (droopy).

FROM S. VERNON *DIFFERENTIAL DIAGNOSIS IN OPHTHALMOLOGY*

LENS ANOMALIES

APHAKIA

Definition
No lens.

Associations
The commonest cause is cataract extraction without lens implantation usually due to congenital cataracts. Rare causes are spontaneous resorption of a cataract (may be seen in Lowe syndrome and Hallerman-Streiff syndrome), congenital primary aphakia which is extremely rare (usually accompanied by other anterior segment anomalies) and spontaneous complete dislocation of the lens (either traumatic or related to already subluxed lens – see later).

Treatment
Refractive correction of aphakia. If iatrogenic surveillance to exclude glaucoma which can develop anytime in the patient's life.

ABNORMAL SHAPE

COLOBOMA
Definition
Rare, but may be associated with other colobomatous ocular defects.

LENTIGLOBUS
Definition
Rare unilateral condition which usually causes myopia.

Association
May be associated with posterior polar cataract.

ANTERIOR LENTICONUS
Definition
Rare bilateral condition with a conoid projection of the anterior surface of the lens centrally.

Association
Alport syndrome. Cataract may form later.

POSTERIOR LENTICONUS
Definition
Posterior conoid projection of the lens.

Association
Usually isolated but may be seen in Lowe syndrome.

DISLOCATED LENS

Ocular associations
Megalocornea (primary enlarged cornea), severe buphthalmos, very high myopia and aniridia. Familial ectopia lentis, ectopia lentis et pupillae and isolated familial microspherophakia. Ectopia lentis et pupillae is an autosomal recessive condition in which there is displacement of the pupil and lens in opposite directions.

Systemic associations
Marfan (**7.30**) (fibrillin gene mutation spectrum), Weil-Marchesani, Ehlers-Danlos, Stickler, Kniest syndromes, mandibulofacial dysostosis and osteogenesis imperfecta. Metabolic disorders include homocystinuria, hyperlysinemia and molybdenum cofactor deficiency (including sulfite oxidase deficiency)

Treatment
Exclude systemic association. Careful observation with refractive correction to ensure adequate visual development. May need lensectomy to improve visual function.

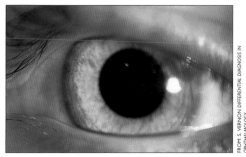

7.30 Dislocated lens in a child with Marfan syndrome.

LENS OPACITY

Lens opacities may be classified in terms of the age at which they occur or in terms of characteristic lens opacities for certain systemic associations.

CONGENITAL OR INFANTILE CATARACT
(See 7.28 and 7.31)

In the UK two-thirds are bilateral and one-third unilateral. 31% are associated with systemic disease (6% unilateral and 25% bilateral). 61% are associated with ocular disease (47% unilateral and 14% bilateral). No underlying cause or risk factor can be found in 92% of unilaterals and 38% of bilateral cases. Hereditary disease associated with 56% of bilateral and 6% of unilateral cases.

Therefore in all bilateral cases unless there is a hereditary risk or associated ocular disease the following investigations should be considered depending on the child's systemic condition.

Urine: reducing substances (galatosaemia), dipstick for proteinuria (Alport), amino acids (Lowe).

Serology: TORCH, red blood cell (RBC) galactokinase activity, RBC galactose-1-phosphate uridyltransferase activity, serum ferritin, karyotype, calcium, glucose, VDRL phosphorus, alkaline phosphatase.

Possible associations
- Hereditary
- Ocular: persistent hyperplastic primary vitreous, aniridia, iris coloboma, microphthalmos
- Systemic

Infection: intrauterine infection

Metabolic disease: galactosaemia, neonatal hypoglycaemia, hypocalcaemia

Renal disease: Lowe syndrome, congenital haemolytic syndrome

Chromosomal disorders: trisomy 13 (Patau syndrome) and 18 (Edward syndrome)

Neurological disease: Marinesco-Sjögren syndrome (ataxia), Smith-Lemli-Opitz , Zellweger and Sjogren-Larsson syndromes

Skeletal disorders: Conradi syndrome

Skin disorders: Ectodermal dysplasia, Rothmund-Thomson, incontinentia pigmenti and Cockayne syndromes

Miscellaneous: Norrie, Rubinstein-Taybi, Turner and Hallermann-Streiff syndromes.

Treatment

Lensectomy with sparing of the capsule for possible secondary implantation is one option, but lens removal with intraocular implantation has become more common. Amblyopia therapy with correction of the refractive state is essential.

JUVENILE CATARACT

Association
- Hereditary
- Ocular: coloboma, ectopia lentis, aniridia, retinitis pigmentosa, and posterior lenticonus.
- Systemic

Renal disease: Alport syndrome

Skeletal disease: Marfan syndrome

Skin disease: Atopic dermatitis, Marshall syndrome, lamellar icthyosis

Chromosomal disorders: Trisomy 21

Metabolic disease: Galactokinase deficiency, Fabry disease, Refsum disease, mannosidosis, diabetes mellitus, hypocalcaemia

Neurological disorders: Myotonic dystrophy, Wilson disease

Miscellaneous: Chronic uveitis, drug induced (steroids), neurofibromatosis II, Stickler syndrome.

Treatment

Lens aspiration with implantation is the usual method of treatment.

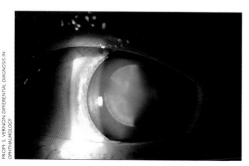

FROM: S. VERNON DIFFERENTIAL DIAGNOSIS IN OPHTHALMOLOGY

7.31 Congenital lamellar cataract.

RETINAL ANOMALIES

HAEMORRHAGES
Haemorrhages may be **pre-retinal**, **retinal** and **subretinal**.

Pre-retinal haemorrhages
Definition
The haemorrhage lies between the posterior vitreous face and the retina.

Association
Sickle cell retinopathy, trauma, subarachnoid haemorrhage (Terson syndrome), non-accidental injury (never seen in isolation; widespread retinal and subretinal haemorrhages also seen with or without retinal schisis).

Retinal haemorrhages
Definition
These may be flame shaped, dot and blot or Roth spots (superficial retinal haemorrhage with white centre)

Associations
Flame shaped haemorrhages are seen in retinal vein occlusions, acute papilloedema, optic disc drusen, acute hypertensive retinopathy, retinal perivasculitis (especially early CMV retinitis). Roth spots are seen in severe anaemias, leukaemia, bacterial endocarditis and may also be seen in trauma. Dot and blot haemorrhages may be seen in diabetes-mellitus-related retinopathy. The haemorrhage is full thickness in the retina. They may be seen in shaken baby syndrome in association with superfical and subretinal haemorrhages (**7.32**) (see 'Child Protection' chapter).

Treatment
Investigation to look for cause.

Subretinal haemorrhages
Definition
Red, raised area over which the retinal vessels are clearly visible.

Associations
Sickle cell anaemia, Coats' disease (retinal telangiectasia), trauma, shaken baby syndrome and, very rarely, choroidal neovascularization.

Treatment
Investigation to look for cause.

HARD EXUDATES
Definition
These are yellow waxy deposits which may be retinal (focal, diffuse or macular star) or subretinal.

Associations
Focal or diffuse hard exudates may be seen in diabetic retinopathy (unusual to see in children), old branch retinal vein occlusion, radiation retinopathy or retinal telangiectasia.

A macular star (stellate pattern of exudates centred on the macula) may be seen in malignant hypertension, papilloedema, neuro-retinitis and very rarely retinal angioma (Von-Hippel Lindau syndrome or idiopathic).

Subretinal exudates may be seen in Coats' disease (**7.33**) or rarely, with *Toxocara canis* retinochoroiditis.

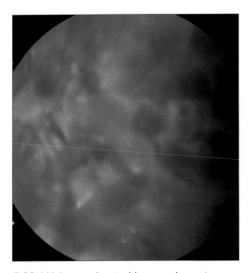

7.32 Widespread retinal haemorrhages in a proven case of shaken baby syndrome.

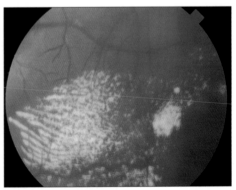

7.33 Hard exudates due to Coats' disease.

Retinopathy of prematurity

The international classification of retinopathy of prematurity is used to describe **location, extent** and **stage** of the disease. The **location** of ROP refers to the location relative to the optic nerve. This has been standardized by dividing the retina into three zones. Zone I is an area centered on the optic disc and extending from the disc to twice the distance between the disc and the macula. Zone II is a ring concentric to Zone I which extends to the nasal ora serrata (the edge of the retina on the side of the eye toward the nose). Zone III is the remaining crescent of retina on the temporal (toward the temple) side. The **extent** of ROP is described by how many clock-hours of the retina are involved. For example, if there is retinopathy extending from 1:00 around to 5:00, the extent of ROP is 4 clock-hours. Retinopathy of prematurity is a progressive disease. It begins with some mild changes in the vessels, and may progress on to more severe changes. The **stage** of ROP describes how far along in this progression the vessels have reached.

Stage 1 is characterized by a demarcation line between the normal retina nearer the optic nerve and the non-vascularized retina more peripherally.

Stage 2 ROP has a ridge of scar tissue and new vessels in place of the demarcation line.

Stage 3 ROP shows an increased size of the vascular ridge, with growth of fibrovascular tissue on the ridge and extending out into the vitreous (**7.34**, right).

Stage 4 refers to a partial retinal detachment. The scar tissue associated with the fibrovascular ridge contracts, pulling the retina away from the wall of the eye. Stage 4 is further categorized depending upon the location of the retinal detachment. In Stage 4A, the detachment does not include the macula, and the vision may be good. In Stage 4B, the macula is detached, and the visual potential is markedly decreased.

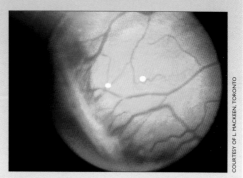

COURTESY OF L. MACKEEN, TORONTO

7.34 Stage III retinopathy of prematurity. There is a ridge, which has neovascularization on it. Distal to the ridge is an avascular zone.

Stage 5 ROP implies a complete retinal detachment, usually with the retina pulled into a funnel-shaped configuration by the fibrovascular scar tissue. Eyes with stage 5 ROP usually have no useful vision, even if surgery is performed to repair the detachment.

Plus disease implies dilation and tortuosity of the blood vessels near the optic nerve. It also includes the growth and dilation of abnormal blood vessels on the surface of the iris, rigidity of the pupil, and vitreous haze. The presence of plus disease suggests a more fulminant or rapidly progressive course. **Rush disease** is a term used to describe ROP in zone I with plus disease.

Risk factors
The lower the birthweight, prolonged supplemental oxygen, and respiratory distress syndrome have clearly been shown to be risk factors.

Treatment
If ROP does develop, it usually occurs between 34 and 40 weeks after conception, regardless of gestational age at birth. The laser treatment is applied to the retina anterior to the vascular shunt that does not yet have a blood supply. The purpose of the treatment is to eliminate the abnormal vessels before they lay down enough scar tissue to produce a retinal detachment. Other treatment options include cryopexy, scleral buckle, and vitrectomy. Treatment is initiated at threshold disease, which is Stage III for 5 contiguous clock hours or 8 non-contiguous clock hours.

COTTON WOOL SPOTS

Definition
These are small white lesions with fluffy edges which result from localised microvasculature occlusion resulting in ischaemia.

Associations
Retinal vein occlusion, acute hypertension, systemic vasculitides, HIV microvasculopathy, ocular ischaemic syndromes, haematological disorders (leukaemia, dysproteinaemias) trauma to chest and long bones (Purtscher retinopathy).

RETINAL NEOVASCULARIZATION

Definition
Retinal ischaemia may result in new vessel formation which can lead to retinal and vitreous haemorrhages as well as tractional retinal detachment. The new vessels may occur within the posterior pole or in the periphery.

Association
Posterior pole neovascularization – retinal vein occlusion, retinal vasculitis, retinal artery occlusion or radiation retinopathy. Peripheral neovascularization – retinopathy of prematurity, sickle cell disease, familial exudative vitreoretinopathy, incontinentia pigmenti or sarcoidosis.

Treatment
Laser treatment of the ischaemic retina is the principle of therapy.

RETINAL VASCULITIS

Definition
Inflammation around retinal veins (periphlebitis) or retinal arterioles (periarteritis).

Association
Periphlebitis: sarcoidosis, Behçet disease, cytomegalovirus retinitis, acute retinal necrosis, tuberculosis, frosted branch angiitis, or idiopathic. Periarteritis: systemic lupus erythematosus, dermatomyositis, polyarteritis nodosa or Wegener granulomatosis.

Treatment
Fundus examination to exclude retinal involvement.

MACULOPATHY

Definition
Abnormality of macula. This may be due to wrinkling, bull's eye appearance or crystalline deposits.

WRINKLED APPEARANCE OF THE MACULA

Definition
Striated appearance radiating out from the fovea which causes a drop in vision.

Association
Idiopathic is the commonest but may also be seen in juvenile retinoschisis, Bardet-Biedl syndrome, chronic intraocular inflammation.

BULL'S EYE MACULOPATHY

Definition
There is hyperpigmentation in the centre of the macula, surrounded by a hypopigmented zone, concentric to which is a final hyperpigmented zone.

Association
Long-term chloroquine use, some types of cone dystrophy (**7.35**), cone-rod dystrophy, rod-cone dystrophy, juvenile neuronal ceroid lipofuscinosis, benign concentric annular macular dystrophy (usually late onset) and Stargardt's disease (macular dystrophy starting in teens).

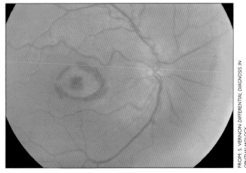

FROM: S. VERNON DIFFERENTIAL DIAGNOSIS IN OPHTHALMOLOGY

7.35 Bull's eye maculopathy seen in a case of cone retinal dystrophy.

COLOURED MACULAR LESIONS
Yellow lesions
Association

Best's vitelliform macular dystrophy is a very rare, dominantly inherited condition which starts in childhood. In the early stages there may be no lesion at the macula but usually there is an egg-yolk-like lesion at the macula (7.36 and 7.37).

Cherry-red spots
Definition

A change in the nerve-fibre layer surrounding the fovea, such as ischaemia or deposition of abnormal metabolic by-products, results in an accentuation of the normal deep red colour of the fovea, producing the typical cherry-red spot macula.

Associations

Central retinal artery occlusion, metabolic disorders such as Tay-Sachs disease, Sandhoff disease, Niemann-Pick disease, generalized gangliosidosis and sialidosis I and II.

PALE RETINAL LESIONS

Inflammatory lesions

Single focal lesions: These may be caused by toxoplasmosis (7.38), toxocariasis (7.39), candidiasis and cryptococcus.

Multiple focal lesions: These may be caused by candidiasis, sarcoidosis, Lyme disease, choroidal pneumocystosis, presumed ocular histoplasmosis syndrome, Behçet's disease, Vogt-Koyanagi-Harada (VKH) syndrome, sympathetic ophthalmitis and tuberculous choroiditis.

Diffuse lesions: These may be seen in CMV retinitis, acute retinal necrosis, herpes simplex retinitis and measles retinitis.

Treatment

In all the above cases appropriate serological investigations and radiological examinations need to be undertaken. Joint ophthalmic and rheumatological evaluation improves management of these cases.

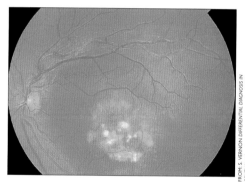

7.36 Yolk-like appearance of Best's disease.

7.37 Scrambled egg appearance of Best's disease.

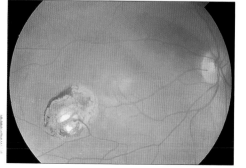

7.38 Extrafoveal toxoplasmosis scar.

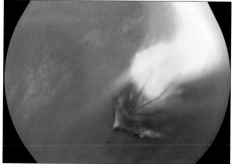

7.39 Peripheral *Toxocara* granuloma.

Non-inflammatory lesions

Focal pale lesions may be due to coloboma of the retina and choroid, 'polar bear tracks', retinal astrocytoma and retinoblastoma. Coloboma of retina and choroid (**7.40**): usually a circular or oval-shaped lesion which may be associated with a coloboma of the optic disc or iris. It is due to incomplete closure of the fetal ocular fissure. Retino-choroidal colobomas may be associated with a serous retinal detachment. Retinal astrocytoma: a hamartoma seen in 50% of patients with tuberous sclerosis. In children, a pale, almond-shaped lesion lies in the nerve-fibre layer. In adults it becomes calcified, showing a mulberry-like lesion. Usually unilateral. Early retinoblastoma: Small pale lesion, flat, elevated or nodular depending on how early it is detected.

Diffuse pale lesions
Non-hereditary

These include myelinated nerve fibres, high myopia, large coloboma of the optic disc and retina, retinal ischaemia and commotio retinae ('bruising' of the retina after blunt trauma).

Hereditary

These include albinism, and choroidal dystrophies such as choroideraemia and diffuse choroidal atrophy.

Multiple focal/discrete lesions
Hereditary

This includes typical retinitis pigmentosa, atypical retinitis pigmentosa, retinitis pigmentosa-like retinal dystrophy with systemic associations, female carriers of X-linked ocular albinism and female carriers of choroideraemia and angioid streaks. (See **Table 7.2**, page 203, for systemic associations of retinitis pigmentosa.)

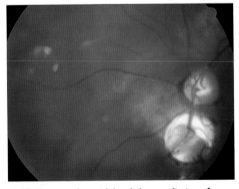

7.40 Retino-choroidal coloboma distinct from optic disc.

Other

This includes grouped congenital RPE hypertrophy ('bear tracks'), rubella retinopathy and congenital syphilis. Rubella retinopathy is a salt and pepper type pigmentary retinopathy where the vision is usually normal and is caused by congenital rubella (**7.41**). Congenital syphilis retinopathy varies from mild ('salt and pepper retinopathy') to severe pigment clumping, similar to retinitis pigmentosa.

Treatment

All cases need electrodiagnostic and visual field evaluation.

RETINAL DETACHMENT

This is an elevation of the neurosensory retina which may be **rhegmatogenous** (due to a retinal hole or tear), **exudative** (due to inflammatory exudate), **tractional** (due to traction on the surface of the retina – usually after trauma in children or as a result of untreated retinopathy of prematurity) or **solid** (due to a tumour). A choroidal detachment is most commonly seen in hypotony following intraocular pressure-lowering operations such as trabeculectomy. Here the choroid detaches with the retina still attached.

Treatment

In a child with high myopia and retinal detachment the possibility of Stickler syndrome must be excluded; vitreous anomalies seen on slit lamp examination can make the diagnosis.

FOLDS IN THE FUNDUS
Definition

These may be fine and multiple or large and single. Fine folds may be due to folds in the retina or the choroid or both. Chorioretinal folds are usually seen in the posterior pole and are usually horizontal. Large single folds are called falciform fold or ligament.

Associations

Chorioretinal folds: ocular hypotony, swollen optic discs, choroidal tumours, hypermetropia (long-sightedness, associated with a short ocular axial length), orbital pseudotumour or tumour (haemangioma or neoplasm). Falciform retinal folds: familial exudative vitreoretinopathy, Norrie's disease, retinopathy of prematurity and persistent hyperplastic primary vitreous (PHPV).

Treatment

Vitreoretinal evaluation is necessary.

THE OPTIC DISC

OPTIC DISC SWELLING
Unilateral
Association
Longstanding ocular hypotony (from any cause), uveitis, posterior scleritis, papillitis, neuroretinitis, acute phase of Leber's hereditary optic neuropathy, optic nerve glioma and other compressive lesion.

Bilateral
Association
Buried optic disc drusen (7.42 and 7.43), papilloedema (7.44), malignant hypertension, cavernous sinus thrombosis, and bilateral papillitis (7.45). In papillitis, vision is always affected but not in papilloedema unless it is chronic.

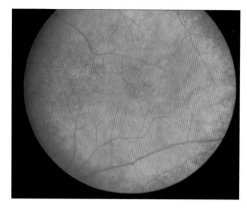

7.41 'Salt and pepper' retinopathy in a case of rubella retinopathy.

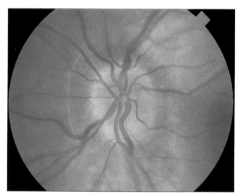

7.42 Swollen optic disc due to optic disc drusen; note the increased retinal vessels crossing the optic disc margins.

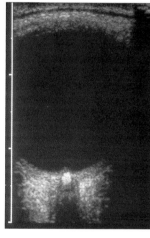

7.43 Ultrasound examination of case shown in 7.42. The optic disc drusen are shown as an increased echogenicity at the optic nerve head due to calcification.

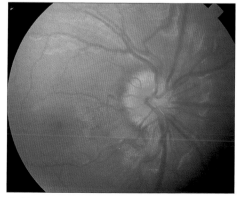

7.44 Papilloedema.

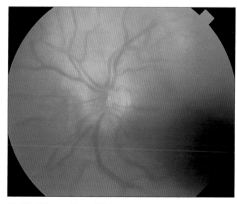

7.45 Bilateral papillitis.

OPTIC ATROPHY
Definition
Optic atrophy occurs due to loss of neuronal axons. It may be **primary, secondary, consecutive, primary hereditary, secondary hereditary**, or associated with contralateral optic disc swelling.

Primary optic atrophy
Primary optic atrophy is caused by any process affecting the visual pathways from the retro-laminar portion of the optic nerve to the lateral geniculate nucleus. Lesions affecting the anterior visual pathways from the globe to the chiasm will cause unilateral optic atrophy, whilst those affecting the optic chiasm or optic tracts will cause bilateral optic atrophy.

Association
Any tumour, but most commonly glioma in children.

Treatment
Neuroimaging is important. Surveillance with colour vision, visual field analysis, and electro-diagnostic testing may be necessary in cases of optic gliomas.

Consecutive optic atrophy
Definition
Consecutive optic atrophy is caused by diseases of the inner retina or its blood supply (**7.46**).

Associations
Retinitis pigmentosa (see Retina section) cone dystrophy, diffuse retinal necrosis (e.g. cytomegalovirus retinitis, acute retinal necrosis, and Behçet disease) cherry red spot at macula syndromes and mucopolysaccharidoses.

Secondary optic atrophy
Definition
Secondary optic atrophy is preceded by swelling of the optic nerve head (**7.47**) as a result of swelling, ischaemia, or inflammation – i.e. chronic papilloedema, papillitis.

Primary hereditary optic atrophy
Definition
Diffuse optic atrophy with visual loss.

Associations
Onset at 4 years (simple recessive type), onset at about 10 years (Kjer juvenile dominant type), onset between 5 and 14 years (recessive type) DIDMOAD – diabetes insipidus, diabetes mellitus, optic atrophy and deafness) and onset between 16 and 30 years (Leber's hereditary optic neuropathy).

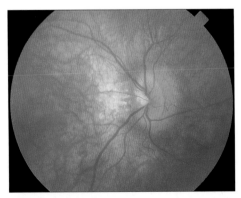

7.46 Retinal arteriolar attenuation in a case of cone dystrophy. The optic disc is tilted which is a normal variant.

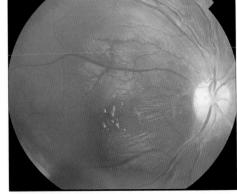

7.47 Optic atrophy following papilloedema.

Secondary hereditary optic atrophy

Definition
These are hereditary neurological disorders with optic atrophy which usually present during the first decade of life.

Associations
Behr (recessive), Friedreich ataxia (recessive), Charcot-Marie-Tooth disease (dominant, X-linked), adrenoleukodystrophies (two types – X-linked recessive and autosomal recessive), cerebellar ataxia type I (dominant).

SMALL OPTIC DISC

Definition
The optic nerve may appear small (hypermetropia) or actually be smaller than should be (tilted disc and optic nerve hypoplasia – 7.48).

Treatment
The possibility of endocrine dysfunction must be excluded in cases of optic disc hypoplasia.

LARGE OPTIC DISC

Definition
Seen in myopia, congenital optic disc pit, optic disc coloboma (7.49), and morning glory anomaly.

Treatment
Bilateral cases should be investigated with neuroimaging.

LARGE OPTIC DISC CUP

Definition
Most normal cups have a cup : disc ratio of 0.3 or less.

Associations
Physiological cupping (a cup : disc ratio greater than 0.7 is present in about 2% of the normal population) and glaucomatous cupping (7.50), where there is raised intraocular pressure, with or without increased corneal diameter, increased myopia, Haab's striae and increased axial length.

Treatment
This depends on severity of the glaucoma but varies from medical topical treatment to laser treatment or surgery.

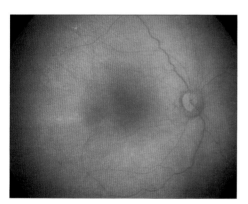

7.48 Optic nerve hypoplasia.

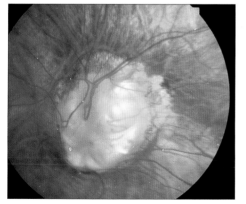

7.49 Marked optic disc coloboma.

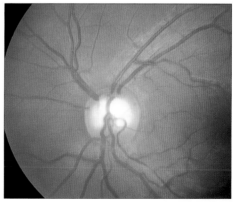

7.50 Optic disc cupping in juvenile glaucoma.

OPTIC DISC VASCULAR ABNORMALITIES

These may be **congenital** (prepapillary loop, Bergmeister papilla, persistent hyaloid artery, increased disc vessel numbers) or **acquired** (optic disc collaterals, neovascularization, optico-ciliary shunts, dragged optic disc vessels).

OPTIC DISC HAEMORRHAGES

Associations

Acute papilloedema, papillitis, infiltrative optic neuropathy, after optic nerve sheath decompression and optic disc drusen.

Treatment

Investigation to exclude early papilloedema are very important as is visual field analysis.

LESIONS OBSCURING THE OPTIC DISC

These include primary optic disc tumours such as capillary angioma (rare, **7.51**) and melano-cytoma; retinal turmours such as astrocytoma or combined hamartoma of the retina and RPE; infiltrative lesions due to leukaemia (**7.52**), TB granuloma or sarcoid.

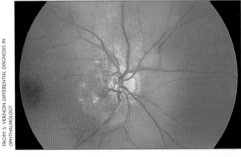

FROM: S. VERNON DIFFERENTIAL DIAGNOSIS IN OPHTHALMOLOGY

7.51 Retinal capillary angioma on the optic disc in a child with von Hippel-Lindau syndrome.

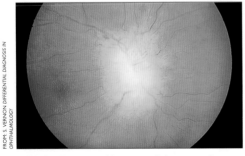

FROM: S. VERNON DIFFERENTIAL DIAGNOSIS IN OPHTHALMOLOGY

7.52 Leukaemic infiltration of the optic disc.

THE ORBIT

ABNORMALITIES OF GLOBE POSITION

Enophthalmos

Definition

The globe sits further back than normal giving the appearance that the eye on the affected side is smaller.

Associations

The commonest cause is trauma resulting in a blow out fracture, but it may be seen in microphthalmos and in self-induced orbital fat atrophy (caused by a child incessantly rubbing his or her eye[s]).

Treatment

Repair of orbital wall fracture is essential if it is the cause. In cases of microphthalmos a cosmetic shell can be applied.

Exophthalmos (proptosis)

Definition

In exophthalmos, the globe sits forward of its normal position. It is better described as prop-tosis which may be axial (forward without any displacement in any other direction) or non-axial (forward and, for example, down). Axial prop-tosis is caused by lesions within the cone of extraocular muscles, while non-axial proptosis is caused by lesions outside this cone. Rarely, proptosis may be intermittent (lymphangioma, capillary haemangioma), pulsatile (encephalo-coele, orbital roof fracture) or pulsatile with a bruit (congenital arteriovenous communication which may occur in isolation or as part of Wyburn–Mason syndrome).

Pseudoproptosis is caused by a large globe (e.g. high myopia, buphthalmos [congenital glaucoma]) lid retraction or contralateral enophthalmos.

Proptosis in neonates and infants

Tumours

These include capillary haemangioma (see Lids section and **7.53**), juvenile xanthogranuloma, teratoma, rhabdomyosarcoma, retinoblastoma (invading the orbit may very rarely present during infancy) and acute leukaemia.

Cystic lesions

These include microphthalmos with cyst, anterior orbital encephalocoele and posterior orbital encephalocoele which may be associated with neurofibromatosis I.

Shallow orbits

Shallow orbits are seen in patients with craniosynostoses such as Pfeiffer, Crouzon and Apert syndromes.

Proptosis in children
Inflammatory causes
These include:

Orbital cellulitis: usually secondary to ethmoiditis (**7.54**). In severe cases there may be visual compromise and/or development of cavernous sinus thrombosis. Orbital and brain imaging is essential. Treatment includes ENT assessment, intravenous antibiotics and abscess drainage.

Pseudotumour: idiopathic orbital inflammation which usually affects children between 6 and 14 years. If it is bilateral Wegener's granulomatosis must be excluded. Orbital imaging is essential.

Thyroid eye disease: may be seen in children and is associated with lid retraction. Surveillance for optic neuropathy is essential.

Benign tumours

Lymphangioma may present between the ages of 1 and 15 years (**7.55**). The lesion may remain stationary for long periods of time or it may suddenly enlarge either as a result of spontaneous bleeding (chocolate cyst) or in association with an upper respiratory tract infection.

Plexiform neurofibroma presents in patients with neurofibromatosis I between the ages of 2 and 5 years with non-axial proptosis.

Optic nerve glioma may be isolated or associated with neurofibromatosis I (**7.56**). Those associated with NF I tend to grow much less than those that are not. The eyeball is often turned down slightly as well as being proptosed. Monitoring with colour vision, electrodiagnostics and visual fields is important to evaluate visual function, while neuroimaging is needed to monitor growth of the tumour.

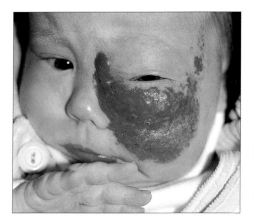

7.53 Left proptosis due to orbital and periorbital capillary haemangioma.

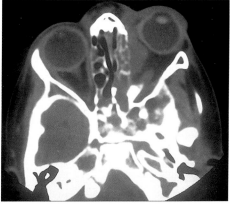

7.54 CT scan showing ethmoid sinusitis and contiguous orbital cellulitis with proptosis.

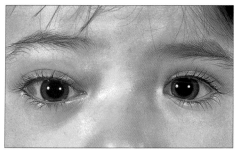

7.55 Proptosis due to orbital lymphangioma.

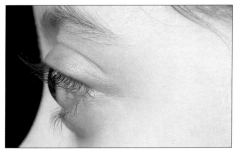

7.56 Proptosis due to optic nerve glioma.

Malignant tumours

See also 'Solid Tumours and Histiocytosis' chapter.

Rhabdomyosarcoma usually presents around the age of 7 years with proptosis, chemosis (swelling of the conjunctiva) and discomfort.

Metastatic neuroblastoma presents in a similar manner to rhabdomyosarcoma but usually at a younger age (under 5 years) with the primary tumour in the abdomen. Forty percent of metastases affect both orbits.

Langerhans cell histiocytosis. Orbital involvement may be seen and usually affects the superolateral quadrant of the orbit. CT scan shows soft tissue mass with adjacent bony lysis.

Acute leukaemia usually presents around 7 years of age with rapid onset proptosis, ecchymosis (bruising in the lids).

Retinoblastoma may occasionally present with proptosis but only in neglected cases.

Metastatic Ewing sarcoma is very rare but may present with rapid proptosis, ecchymosis, and chemosis.

Metastatic Wilms tumour may be associated with aniridia.

LACRIMAL GLAND ENLARGEMENT
Unilateral

Dacryoadenitis is usually caused by a viral infection of the lacrimal gland but may be associated with orbital pseudotumour. It is not usually associated with proptosis per se but causes the upper lid to develop an 'S' shape and is very tender to touch.

Dacryops is due to a dilatation of the major lacrimal ducts secondary to obstruction and again does not usually cause proptosis.

Pleomorphic adenoma. Very rarely this essentially 'adult' tumour presents in children with a painless, slowly progressive non-axial proptosis.

Bilateral

Physiological enlargement associated with shallow orbits (seen in Afro-Caribbeans).

Sarcoidosis may rarely cause bilateral firm enlarged lacrimal glands in children.

Acute leukaemia. In children: a form of acute myeloid leukaemia (chloroma) may cause bilateral lacrimal gland infiltration.

EYE MOVEMENT DISORDERS

See also 'Neurology' chapter.

These may be classified as disorders in primary position of gaze, anomalous eye movements and nystagmus. All cases should be referred for ophthalmic opinion.

OCULAR DEVIATION IN PRIMARY GAZE

If a deviation remains stable regardless of the position of gaze of the eyes it is called comitant. If it does change it is termed non- or in-comitant.

Esodeviation

This is a turning in of one or both eyes.

Pseudodeviation

Epicanthic folds: symmetric corneal reflexes confirm the absence of true esotropia.

Narrow interpupillary distance seen in hypotelorism.

True esodeviation
Comitant esotropia

Infantile esotropia (7.57) develops before the age of 6 months with a large and stable angle, cross-fixation (child uses right eye to look to left and vice versa as the eyes are so convergent), and normal refraction for age.

Non-accommodative esotropia: esotropia after 6 months of age with normal refraction.

Refractive accommodative esotropia: onset is usually between 2 and 3 years, associated with hypermetropia (long-sightedness).

Non-refractive accommodative esotropia: onset after 6 months but before 3 years. No significant refractive error but excessive convergence for near (called high accommodative convergence: accommodation ratio – AC/A ratio).

Sensory esotropia: due to reduction in vision with one eye much worse than the other, which disrupts fusion – e.g. in unilateral cataract.

Convergent spasm: intermittent esotropia with pseudomyopia and miosis due to accommodative spasm which may be seen after trauma or due to a posterior fossa tumour but usually has a functional element.

Incomitant esotropia

VI nerve palsy: may be congenital or acquired (associated with raised intracranial pressure). Esotropia gets worse when looking in the distance.

Möbius syndrome: bilateral gaze palsies, with esotropia in 50% of cases (due to superimposed VI nerve palsies). There is usually bilateral VII nerve palsies and may be associated V, IX, X, nerve palsies.

Duane syndrome: due to miswiring of the horizontal rectus muscles which leads to co-contraction of the medial and lateral recti. This leads to limited abduction with almost normal adduction (type I), or limited adduction with almost normal abduction (type II) or limited adduction and abduction in equal measures (type III). The eye movements are associated with widening of the palpebral fissure on abduction and narrowing on adduction. Types I and III may present with an esotropia in primary position of gaze. If a child has an abduction deficit but no esotropia in primary gaze, this cannot be a VI nerve palsy and must be Duane syndrome.

Exodeviation (the eyes diverge in primary position)

Pseudo-exodeviation

Hypertelorism: look for symmetry of corneal light reflexes.

True exodeviation

Comitant exotropia

Intermittent exotropia: common condition with exotropia more commonly present for distance than for near (**7.58**). In bright sunlight the child will characteristically close the diverging eye.

Sensory exotropia: much less common in children than sensory esodeviation.

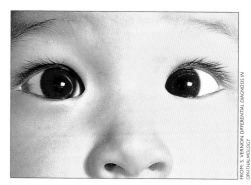

FROM: S. VERNON *DIFFERENTIAL DIAGNOSIS IN OPHTHALMOLOGY*

7.57 This child has epicanthic folds but the corneal light reflex on the right cornea is central, while the reflex in the left eye is off the pupil, indicating the presence of a left esodeviation.

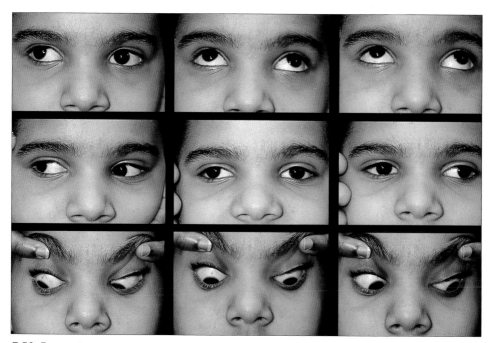

7.58 Exotropia.

Convergence insufficiency: usually seen in older children. Convergence exercises may help but there should be a low threshold to neuroimage if there are any neurological signs or worsening despite convergence exercises.

Incomitant exotropia
Congenital III nerve palsy: exodeviation and hypodeviation of the affected eye, with ptosis and miosed pupil. There is limitation of upgaze and adduction.

Acquired III nerve palsy (7.59): Rare. Same signs as congenital condition but pupil is dilated.
Duane Syndrome types II: see above.

ANOMALOUS EYE MOVEMENTS
Upshoots in adduction (on version testing)
Inferior oblique overaction: may be primary (usually bilateral and seen with esotropia but also with exotropia occurring in childhood) or secondary (to a superior oblique palsy) (7.60).

Duane syndrome I, II, III: see above. Upshoots occur due to a leash effect of a tight lateral rectus muscle secondary to co-contraction of the medial rectus muscle.
Dissociated vertical deviation: a bilateral condition most commonly seen in association with infantile esotropia. At moments of inattention the eye will move up and then move down to its original position while the fixating eye remains still. It differs from inferior oblique overaction in that the eye may elevate in any position of gaze.
Craniosynostoses (7.61): in the syndromic craniosynostoses – e.g. Apert, Pfeiffer, Crouzon: the extraocular muscles are excyclo-rotated such that the medial rectus now acts as an elevator as well as an adductor.

Downshoots in adduction (on version testing)
Duane syndrome I, II or III: see above.
Brown syndrome: this is not an uncommon condition where the tendon of the superior oblique muscle is unable to pass freely through its pulley (the trochlea, at the superomedial

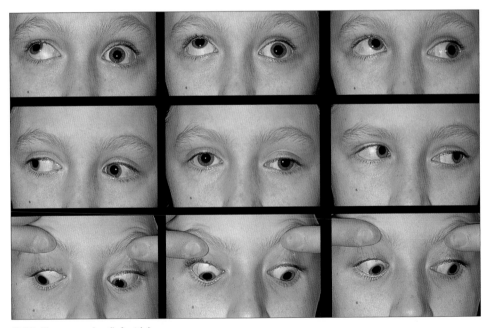

7.59 III nerve palsy (left side).

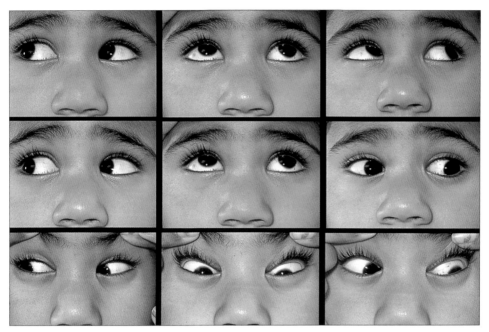

7.60 Right superior oblique palsy. The right eye does not depress in adduction as well as it should do. There is also a mild right inferior oblique overaction (there is a slight upshoot of the right eye in adduction).

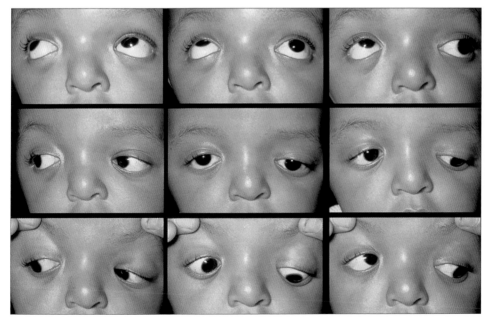

7.61 Child with Apert syndrome who shows anomalous eye movements with upshoots in adduction and coincident downshoots in abduction. This child also demonstrates a V pattern: when the child looks up, the eyes diverge, compared to when the child looks down. There is also a right depression deficit.

orbital rim). This results in restriction of elevation in upgaze usually just in the adducted position. As a result there may be a coincident downshoot in adduction on version testing. It is usually idiopathic but may be acquired due to inflammation at the trochlea or trauma.

Superior oblique overaction: which may be primary and usually seen with intermittent exotropia in older children (late teens).

Limitation of abduction

VI nerve palsy (7.62): there is always an esotropia in primary position of gaze. Duane I and II – there may not be an esotropia in primary position of gaze.

Any restrictive myopathy of the medial rectus: myositis, pseudo-tumour, and very rarely, thyroid eye disease.

Limitation of adduction

III Nerve palsy (7.59): may be congenital or acquired (see above).

Internuclear ophthalmoplegia (INO): a lesion in the medial longitudinal fasiculus leading to ipsilateral adduction limitation and contralateral eye abducting nystagmus.

Myasthenia gravis: very rare but may mimic adduction deficit.

Acute myositis: restriction of movement in direction of the field of action of the affected muscle.

Duane syndrome II and III.

Limitation of horizontal versions or gaze palsies

Any lesion of the PPRF (paramedian pontine reticular formation) causes ipsilateral gaze palsy.

One-and-a-half syndrome: a lesion of the PPRF/abducens nucleus and adjacent medial longitudinal fasiculus causing an ipsilateral gaze palsy and ipsilateral INO. A right-sided neurological lesion would lead to inability for either eye to look to the right, the right eye could not adduct (part of the INO) but the left eye could abduct but only with a nystagmus.

Bilateral pontine lesions result in total horizontal gaze palsies.

Fisher syndrome: rare variant of Guillain-Barré syndrome which may present in children with ophthalmoplegia, ataxia and areflexia, though the initial presentation may be one of horizontal gaze palsy or an INO.

Limitation of vertical eye movement
(one or both eyes)

Palsy of a muscle: superior rectus, inferior oblique (upgaze affected) and inferior rectus, superior oblique palsy (downgaze affected).

Orbital floor fracture: causing entrapped inferior rectus muscle and restriction of elevation.

Orbital space occupying lesion: such as capillary haemangioma, plexiform neurofibroma. Symblepharon – attachment of lid to globe will cause restriction of elevation or depression. This may be congenital and seen in clefting syndromes but also may be acquired, seen in epidermolysis bullosa, alkali injuries.

Brown syndrome: see above. Deficit in elevation.

Monocular elevation deficit: formerly called double elevator palsy. This may be due to idiopathic tightening of the inferior rectus muscle or idiopathic with no evidence of inferior rectus tightening.

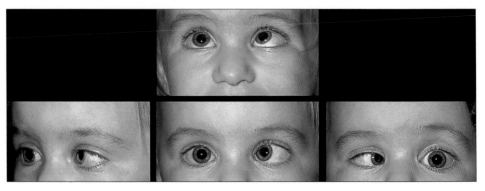

7.62 Left esotropia due to left VI nerve palsy (left abduction deficit).

Vertical gaze palsy

Parinaud syndrome: decreased upgaze, large pupils, convergence insufficiency and, convergence – retraction nystagmus. In children one of the commonest causes is a pinealoma.

Hydrocephalus: stretching of the posterior commissure results in loss of upgaze with or without tonic downward deviation of the eyes ('sunset' sign).

Metabolic causes: may affect vertical eye movements. Tay-Sachs disease may cause impairment of vertical and later horizontal gaze. Niemann-Pick variants may also cause vertical gaze anomalies.

Generalized limitation of ocular movements

This may be due to multiple ocular motor palsies or to other causes.

Due to multiple ocular motor palsies

Cavernous sinus lesions: very rare but may be a complication of orbital cellulitis. Tumours are very rare as are caroticocavernous fistula.

Superior orbital fissure lesion: rare but tumours of the orbit may cause problems here (e.g. leukaemia) or rarer infections (such as aspergilloma in immunocompromised children). Tolosa-Hunt syndrome (idiopathic granulomatous inflammation which is painful during the acute phase) may affect the superior orbital fissure or cavernous sinus.

Brainstem lesions: usually encephalitis but tumours of the brainstem (glioma) may also present with ophthalmoplegia.

Due to other causes

Chronic progressive ophthalmoplegia: may be associated with a mitochondrial cytopathy in which case it may be isolated or part of the Kearns-Sayre syndrome, oculopharyngeal dystrophy.

Myotonic dystrophy: may be seen in children either as the congenital variant or type I autosomal dominant variant which has demonstrated anticipation.

Drug toxicity: most commonly seen with phenytoin.

Acquired saccadic initiation failure (ocular motor apraxia): may be seen in lesions in the fronto-parietal cortex. Both vertical and horizontal saccades are affected. May be seen in Gaucher III. In congenital saccadic initiation failure, vetical saccades are unaffected.

Metabolic causes: Tay-Sachs disease, and occasionally other lipid-storage diseases.

Congenital fibrosis syndrome: familial condition which may affect all muscles. Often, however, the eyes are fixed in a downward position with bilateral ptosis and chin up head position.

ABNORMAL HEAD POSITIONS
Ocular causes

Nystagmus (7.63): a null position is a position of the eyes in the orbits where the nystagmus is most dampened; in this position the child sees better. The child adopts an abnormal head position so that the eyes are in the null position but the child is able to look straight ahead.

Unilateral ametropia (usually astigmatism): results in a head turn but rarely also a head tilt.

Strabismus: a child will usually develop an abnormal head posture to reduce the amount of diplopia. As a rule the head will turn or be moved in the direction of the underacting muscle(s). In order to see if the head posture is due to strabismic problems one eye should be patched; if it is strabismic in origin then the head posture will improve.

Types of abnormal head posture

Chin elevation: bilateral ptosis, any cause of elevation deficit (unilateral or bilateral – see above), nystagmus (null position with eyes in downgaze) and in certain types of horizontal strabismus (such as A or V pattern deviations where the eyes are almost straight in downgaze but either develop an esodeviation or exodeviation in upgaze).

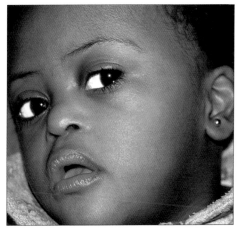

7.63 Child with nystagmus who adopts an abnormal head posture to improve vision by holding eyes in null position.

Chin depression: nystagmus with null position of eyes in upgaze, and A or V pattern deviations (with eyes straight in upgaze but not in downgaze).

Head tilt: may be caused by a superior oblique palsy (commonest cause – see **7.60**), Brown syndrome, and rarely posterior fossa tumour.

Head turn: lateral rectus or medial rectus palsy, Duane syndrome, nystagmus with null position in lateral gaze, manifest latent nystagmus (the nystagmus in the fixating eye dampens if that eye is adducted), homonymous hemianopia, unilateral deafness, and ametropia (see above).

NYSTAGMUS
Character of nystagmus

Horizontal jerk: combination of slow drift with fast corrective phase. The 'nystagmus' direction is the same as the fast corrective phase.

Pendular: nystagmus velocity is the same in both directions but on lateral gaze this usually develops a horizontal jerk component.

Oblique: due to a combination of horizontal and vertical directions of pendular nystagmus.

Early-onset nystagmus

Manifest nystagmus: is usually benign but may be acquired. It is uniplanar, dampens on convergence and worsens on eccentric fixation.

Latent nystagmus: no nystagmus with both eyes open but horizontal jerk nystagmus seen when one eye is covered. Most commonly seen with infantile esotropia but may be seen with other early onset deviations. The fast phase is towards the uncovered fixating eye.

Manifest-latent nystagmus: usually seen with infantile esotropia and dissociated vertical deviation. The nystagmus becomes worse when one eye is occluded.

Spasmus nutans: an early onset (3–18 months) unilateral or bilateral small amplitude high frequency horizontal nystagmus often associated with head nodding. Most often idiopathic with resolution by 3 years of age but it may be due to an optic pathway glioma.

Roving nystagmus: severe disruption of visual function may lead to this and the commonest causes are Leber's congenital amaurosis (severe retinal dystrophy) or optic nerve hypoplasia (bilateral).

Later-onset nystagmus

Coarse horizontal jerk nystagmus: usually seen in cerebellar disease, with fast phase ipsilateral to the lesion.

Torsional nystagmus: if pure then this is usually only seen in central vestibular disease such as syringomyelia or syringobulbia associated with Arnold-Chiari malformation, demyelination and very rarely, lateral medullary syndrome in children.

Downbeat nystagmus: usually seen in lesions at the craniocervical junction (e.g. Arnold-Chiari malformation), drug toxicity (phenytoin, carbamazepine), trauma, hydrocephalus, and demyelination.

Upbeat nystagmus: usually seen in cerebellar degenerations (e.g. ataxia telangiectasia) and encephalitis; in babies a retinal dystrophy should be excluded (especially cone dystrophy).

Gaze-evoked nystagmus: may be seen with lesions of the vestibulocerebellum axis, brainstem or cerebral hemispheres or after a gaze palsy or with drug toxicity (phenytoin and carbamezipine).

Periodic alternating nystagmus: the direction of the nystagmus reverses. May be congenital idiopathic but is usually seen with Arnold-Chiari malformation or cerebellar disease, trauma or demyelination.

Rebound nystagmus: attempt to maintain eccentric gaze results in gaze evoked nystagmus which dampens and sometimes reverses direction. On returning to primary gaze a transient nystagmus develops. Usually seen in cerebellar disease.

See-saw nystagmus: Pendular nystagmus in which one eye elevates and intorts while the other eye depresses and extorts and then the eyes reverse. The commonest cause is chiasmal or parasellar tumours but may also be seen in albinism as a transient finding, head trauma, and syringobulbia.

Internuclear ophthalmoplegia: the abducting eye has nystagmus (see above) and is due to a lesion in the medial longitudinal fasiculus.

Monocular nystagmus: may be seen in Spasmus nutans, unilateral deep amblyopia, superior oblique myokymia and optic nerve glioma.

Convergence-retraction nystagmus: seen in Parinaud syndrome (see above).

Ocular causes of nystagmus

Disruption of vision will lead to nystagmus. There may be obvious (usually bilateral) ocular disease such as corneal opacities, congenital cataract, microphthalmos, aniridia and oculocutaneous nystagmus or less obvious ocular disease such as retinal dystrophy (usually cone dystrophy or Lebers congenital amaurosis), ocular albinism, X-linked congenital stationary night blindness, optic nerve hypoplasia, and early onset optic atrophy.

Table 7.2 Systemic disorders associated with retinitis pigmentosa or retinal pigmentary retinopathy

1. Hearing difficulties

- **Usher syndrome**. USH 1: retinitis pigmentosa onset by age 10; cataract; profound congenital sensory deafness; labyrinthine defect. USH 2: retinitis pigmentosa onset in late teens; childhood sensory deafness. USH 3: postlingual, progressive hearing loss; variable vestibular dysfunction; onset of retinitis pigmentosa symptoms, usually by the second decade.
- **Alstrom syndrome:** retinal lesion causes nystagmus and early loss of central vision – in contrast to loss of peripheral vision first, as in other pigmentary retinopathies; dilated cardiomyopathy (infancy)/congestive heart failure; atherosclerosis; hypertension; renal failure; deafness; obesity; diabetes mellitus.
- **Infantile Refsum disease** (early onset): mental retardation; minor facial dysmorphism; retinitis pigmentosa; sensorineural hearing deficit; hepatomegaly; osteoporosis; failure to thrive; hypocholesterolemia.
- **Classical Refsum disease** (late onset): Cardinal clinical features of Refsum disease are retinitis pigmentosa, chronic polyneuropathy and cerebellar signs.
- **Cockayne** dwarfism: precociously senile appearance; pigmentary retinal degeneration; optic atrophy; deafness; marble epiphyses in some digits; photosensitivity; and mental retardation; subclinical myopathy.
- **Mucopolysaccharidosis** (MPS)
- **Kearns-Sayre** ophthalmoplegia: pigmentary degeneration of the retina. Deafness and cardiomyopathy are leading features.

2. Skin disorders
- **Refsum disease**
- **Cockayne syndrome**

3. Renal disorders
- **Senior-Loken syndrome:** renal dysplasia; retinitis pigmentosa; retinal aplasia; cerebellar ataxia; sensorineural hearing loss.
- **Rhyns syndrome:** retinitis pigmentosa; hypopituitarism; nephronophthisis; mild skeletal dysplasia.
- **Bardet-Biedl syndrome:** obesity; rod–cone dystrophy; onset by end of 2nd decade hypogonadism; renal anomalies; polydactyly; learning disabilities .
- **Cystinosis**
- **Alstrom syndrome**

4. Skeletal disorders
- **Bardet-Biedl syndrome**
- **Cockayne syndrome**
- **Jeune syndrome**: chondrodysplasia that often leads to death in infancy because of a severely constricted thoracic cage and respiratory insufficiency; retinal degeneration.
- **MPS 1H, 1S, 11,111**
- **Infantile Refsum disease**

5. Hepatic disorders
- **Zellweger syndrome**: hypotonia; seizures; psychomotor retardation; pigmentary retinopathy and cataracts.

6. Neurological/neuromuscular
- **Kearns-Sayre syndrome**
- **Chronic progressive external ophthalmoplegia**: retinitis pigmentosa and restricted eye movements.
- **Neuronal ceroid lipofuscinosis:** characterized by intralysosomal accumulations of lipopigments in either granular, curvilinear, or fingerprint patterns; progressive dementia, seizures and progressive visual failure.
- **Hallervorden-Spatz syndrome:** retinitis pigmentosa and pallidal degeneration.
- **Joubert syndrome:** hypoplasia of the cerebellar vermis; saccadic initiation failure; hyperpnea intermixed with central apnea in the neonatal period; retinal dystrophy.
- **Infantile Refsum disease**
- **Abetalipoproteinemia (Bassen-Kornzweig syndrome):** coeliac disease; pigmentary degeneration of the retina; progressive ataxic neuropathy; acanthocytosis.

SUGGESTED READING

Del Monte M, Archer S. *Atlas of Pediatric Ophthalmology and Strabismus Surgery*. Butterworth-Heinemann, 1993.

Friedman N, Pineda K, Kaiser PK. *Massachusetts Eye and Ear Infirmary Illustrated Manual of Ophthalmology*. Saunders, 2003.

Hartnett ME, Trese M, Capone A, Keats BJ, Steidl SM. *Pediatric Retina: Medical and Surgical Approaches*. Lippincott Williams and Wilkins, 2004.

Hertle RW, Schaffer DB, Foster JA. *Color Atlas and Synopsis of Pediatric Eye Care*. McGraw-Hill Education, 2001.

JJ Kanski. *Clinical Ophthalmology*. Butterworth-Heinemann, 2003.

Kaufman HE, Barron BA, McDonald MB (eds). *The Cornea: 2nd Edition*. Butterworth-Heinneman, 1998.

Taylor D. *Paediatric Ophthalmology*. Blackwell Science, 1996.

Tomsak RL.*Pediatric Neuro-Ophthalmology*. Butterworth-Heinneman,1995.

Wright KW, Spiegel PH. *Pediatric Ophthalmology and Strabismus (Requisites in Ophthalmology S.)*. Mosby, 1999.

Nelson LB. *Harley's Paediatric Ophthalmology*. Saunders, 1998.

Wright KW, Spiegel PH (eds). *Paediatric Ophthalmology and Strabismus: 2nd Edition*. Springer Verlag, 2002.

Online Mendelian Inheritance in Man.
http://www.ncbi.nlm.nih.gov/entrez/query.fcgi?CMD=search&DB=omim

Neurology
Fenella Kirkham

NEUROLOGICAL EXAMINATION: CRANIAL NERVES

Although neurological examination cannot always be performed in the correct order in young children, it is important to remember to perform the core components. Careful observation of the child's natural behaviour often gives diagnostic clues, but some areas (such as visual fields and acuity) must be formally tested.

THE EYE

See also 'Ophthalmology' chapter.

It is essential to examine visual fields to confrontation and visual acuity in every patient. In schoolchildren, visual fields can be compared to confrontation with the examiner's own (**8.1**). If this is not possible, a toy on a string is brought in from behind the child's head and a second examiner observes visual behaviour. Pendular nystagmus, or loss of the direct and consensual pupillary response to light, implies poor visual acuity. Visual acuity can be tested with a Snellen chart at 6 metres (20 feet) in children who can read letters.

From around the age of two, acuity can be tested with 5 or 7 letters by asking the child to match the letters they see at 6 metres and show them to a carer using a second chart. Under the age of two, a rapid screen of visual acuity can be conducted using small sweets or raisins and 'hundreds and thousands'. In formal testing, the infant's visual behaviour when shown two black and white grids of different spacing and width is observed; if he only looks at the larger it is assumed that he cannot see the smaller. Adequate fundoscopy often requires the pupils to be pharmacologically dilated.

Ptosis
Causes of unilateral ptosis

- Congenital – may be associated with dysmorphic features.
- Third nerve palsy. (**8.2**) The ptosis is usually severe. In a complete third nerve palsy, there is associated dilatation of the pupil and the eye will be 'down and out', due to involvement of the superior, inferior and medial rectus and the inferior oblique muscles. See 'Eye movements', page 208, for causes.
- Horner syndrome.

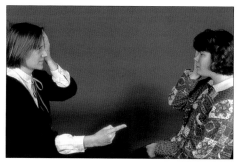

8.1 Visual field testing to confrontation. The patient is about 1 metre away and is looking at the examiner's nose. Both fields are tested together with the test object halfway between the patient and the examiner.

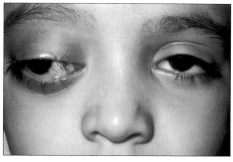

8.2 Right third nerve palsy and exophthalmos secondary to an orbital tumour. There is severe ptosis and the eye is 'down and out'; the pupillary dilatation cannot be seen.

Examination in Horner syndrome

- The ptosis is usually mild and is associated with constriction of the pupil, enophthalmos and decreased sweating (**8.3**).
- Look for lateral scar from cardiac operation.
- Examine the ipsilateral hand:
  – severe clawing in Klumpke's (**8.4**);
  – wasting of small muscles if T1 lesion alone (tumour in Pancoast region).
- Examine sensation in the arms:
  – syringomyelia – preserved position and vibration, reduced temperature and pain;
  – reduced sensation in T1 distribution in T1 lesion.
- Examine sensation in the face:
  – pain and temperature are distributed concentrically from around the mouth.
  – tactile sensation is distributed in the V_1, V_2 and V_3 distributions:
  – any abnormality in brain stem tumour;
  – dissociated in syringobulbia.

Causes of bilateral ptosis

- Congenital. (**8.5**) May have other dysmorphic features (sometimes associated with syndromes such as Noonan's).
- Myasthenia gravis. (**8.6**) The ptosis may be associated with involvement of the external ocular muscles leading to paralytic squint or complete ophthalmoplegia. Facial and bulbar weakness may also be prominent and there may be more generalized weakness. Look for evidence of fatiguability by asking the patient to look up, to sing a nursery rhyme, to chew or to hold their arms up.
- Neuromuscular diseases such as mitochondrial myopathy, dystrophia myotonica (see under chronic progressive weakness).

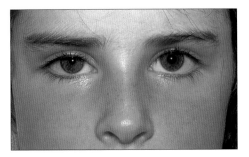

8.3 Right Horner syndrome with slight ptosis, enophthalmos, pupillary constriction and decreased sweating.

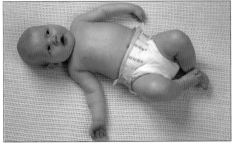

8.4 Left Klumpke's paralysis in a child with an ipsilateral Horner syndrome.

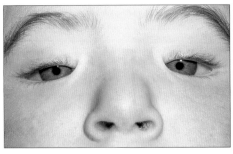

8.5 Bilateral congenital ptosis with abnormal epicanthic folds.

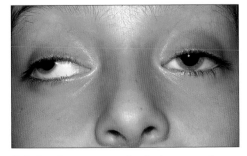

8.6 Autoimmune myasthenia demonstrating severe bilateral ptosis and partial opthalmoplegia with a right third nerve palsy.

MYASTHENIA

Neonatal myasthenia occurs in the infants of mothers with Acetylcholine receptor antibodies and is usually transient. Congenital myasthenic syndromes are inherited (usually recessively) and include:

- Acetylcholinesterase deficiency.
- Slow channel syndrome.
- Acetylcholine receptor deficiency.

Juvenile myasthenia gravis is similar to the adult autoimmune form, but young children may be Acetylcholine receptor antibody negative.

CLINICAL SIGNS

- Arthrogryposis at birth, which is often subtle (e.g. affecting only the hands).
- Repeated apnoeas.
- Frequent chest infections.
- Respiratory failure.
- Ptosis (may be subtle and unilateral).
- Ophthalmoplegia (often incomplete).
- Facial weakness.
- Bulbar weakness (e.g. on singing nursery rhymes).
- Generalized weakness.

DIAGNOSIS
Pharmacological

- Edrophonium (tensilon) – test dose 0.01 mg/kg; full dose 0.15 mg/kg.
- Atropine (0.1–0.4 mg) (must be drawn up before tests starts and should be given immediately if there is respiratory depression).
- Resuscitation trolley must be available and in working order before testing starts.
- Improvement in ptosis is usually the best end-point.
- Video monitoring of test is often useful as improvement is usually transient.
- A trial of a longer acting anticholinesterase may be helpful.

Electrodiagnostic studies

- Single fibre electromyography.
- Repetitive stimulation (but this is poorly tolerated in young children and may be falsely negative; it is occasionally performed under general anaesthesia if there is diagnostic difficulty).

Acetylcholine receptor antibodies

These may be negative in auto-immune myasthenia gravis in children.

The diagnosis of myasthenia in young children may be extremely difficult and if there is a high index of suspicion, testing may need to be repeated. Differentiation between congenital and juvenile (auto-immune) forms may be difficult as the age of onset overlaps and some young children with the auto-immune form are antibody negative. DNA testing will assume an increasing role in the diagnosis of the congenital myasthenic syndromes.

MANAGEMENT

- Awareness of the risk of respiratory insufficiency and cardiac dysrrhythmia in myasthenic crisis and the need for emergency ventilation, cardiac monitoring and sometimes pacing.
- Anticholinesterase drugs (e.g. pyridostigmine, neostigmine).
- Early thymectomy in severe cases of acetylcholine receptor antibody positive disease, especially if respiratory failure is prominent.
- Immunosuppression (e.g. with steroids for auto-immune form. Chronic high dose steroids should be avoided).
- Immunoglobulin or plasma exchange for acute exacerbations.

DISORDERS OF EYE MOVEMENT

See also 'Ophthalmology' chapter.

The mnemonic for innervation of eye muscles is LR_6 $(SO_4)_3$. Eye movement testing (see Ophthalmology chapter) is easy in young children if a puppet is used. The examiner should ask the child to follow eye movements horizontally to right and left and vertically in the midline and to each side. Nystagmus on lateral gaze is usually secondary to a cerebellar or brain stem lesion in childhood.

THIRD NERVE PALSY

At rest the eye is 'down and out', due to involvement of the superior, inferior and medial rectus and the inferior oblique muscles (**8.2**).

Causes of third nerve palsy

Space-occupying lesion in the orbit, e.g. tumour (**8.2**) or pseudotumour (which responds to steroids), pressure of the third nerve against the tentorium in uncal herniation (see under 'Coma' **8.102**), inflammation at base of skull (e.g. tuberculous meningitis), space-occupying lesion in the mid-brain (e.g. tumour – pyramidal tract signs usually present), and aneurysm of the posterior communicating artery (extremely rare in childhood).

FOURTH NERVE PALSY

This is extremely rare. It causes paralysis of the superior oblique muscle (SO_4). Head tilt is often prominent and the patient has difficulty in looking down (e.g. when walking down stairs). It is usually idiopathic but may be due to a pseudotumour of the orbit (see under 'Third nerve palsy').

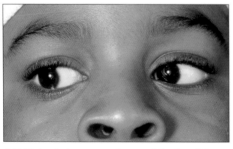

8.7 Right sixth nerve palsy as a false localizing sign in a boy with raised intracranial pressure.

SIXTH NERVE PALSY

The eye is unable to look laterally because of paralysis of the lateral rectus muscle (LR_6) (**8.7**).

Causes of sixth nerve palsy

False localizing sign in intracranial hypertension (see under 'Headache') (**8.7**) (e.g. tumour with hydrocephalus, pseudotumour cerebri – benign intracranial hypertension). There is papilloedema and other neurological signs may be present if there is a space-occupying lesion. Local causes in the orbit (e.g. tumour or pseudotumour – see 'Third nerve palsy'), and lesions in the nucleus in the pons (e.g. tumour) – the seventh nerve is usually involved as well.

OPHTHALMOPLEGIA

With involvement of third, fourth and sixth nerves.

Causes

Tumour or pseudotumour of the orbit (usually unilateral), myasthenia gravis (bilateral) – see under Ptosis, **8.6**, Miller-Fisher variant of Guillain-Barré syndrome (descending paralysis with prominent involvement of the cranial nerves) (bilateral) – see **8.35**, botulism and diphtheria.

LATERAL GAZE PALSY

The patient is able to look to one side but not the other. Convergence is preserved.

Causes

Frontal or brain stem lesion.

UPWARD GAZE PALSY

The patient is unable to look upwards. This implies pressure on the mid-brain.

Causes

Pinealoma or severe hydrocephalus (sun setting sign).

INVESTIGATIONS

Neuroimaging of the brain and orbits. If an orbital lesion is suspected, MRI is preferred because of the risk of radiation to the lens with CT and the higher diagnostic rate. For bilateral ophthalmoplegia, myasthenia must be excluded (see under 'Ptosis', page 205). Nerve conduction studies may be required to exclude the Miller-Fisher variant of Guillain-Barré syndrome (see under 'Acute weakness', page 221).

FACIAL PALSY

LOWER MOTOR NEURONE FACIAL PALSY

The child is asked to show his teeth, screw up his eyes against resistance, look surprised and blow his cheeks out. The facial expression (e.g. on smiling spontaneously) should also be noted.

A lower motor-neurone facial palsy presents as a very obvious weakness of the face with involvement of the eye. It may be unilateral (**8.8–8.10**) or bilateral.

Causes
Unilateral in the newborn (8.8)
- Trauma to the facial nerve (e.g. due to direct compression against the maternal sacrum or forceps delivery).
- Congenital peripheral (usually isolated) or nuclear (may be associated with other cranial nerve palsies) abnormalities.

Bilateral in the newborn
- Moebius syndrome (usually with bilateral sixth nerve and lower cranial nerve palsies).

MANAGEMENT
Clinically, it is important to distinguish between facial palsy and hypoplasia of the depressor angularis oris in asymmetric crying facies. EMG and nerve conduction studies may be needed to distinguish between a slowly resolving traumatic lesion and a congenital abnormality. Imaging of the base of the brain may be required. Occasionally, an injured facial nerve may require surgical repair if there is no recovery by three months. Cosmetic surgery usually offers a considerable improvement in facial appearance in congenital lesions, but may not be advisable until late childhood.

Unilateral in a previously well child (8.9)
- Acute otitis media.
- Viral – herpes simplex; herpes zoster including chicken pox (sometimes without vesicles); parvovirus B19.
- Lyme disease.
- Hypertension.
- Trauma.
- Kawasaki disease (see 'Infectious Diseases' chapter).
- Sarcoidosis (associated with parotitis).
- Tumour of the pons (patients usually also have a sixth nerve palsy)(**8.10**).
- Idiopathic (Bell palsy).

Bilateral in a previously well child
(Often associated with other lower cranial nerve signs – bulbar palsy (**8.15**, **8.16**).
- Guillain-Barré syndrome (see **8.35**).
- Myasthenia gravis (ptosis and ophthalmoplegia are usually also prominent, see 'Ptosis', **8.6**).
- Bell palsy may be bilateral.
- Brainstem lesion.

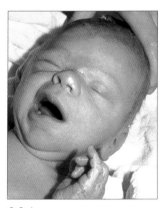 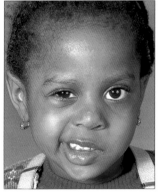 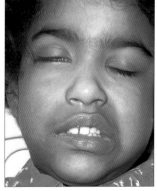

8.8 Lower motor neurone facial palsy in an infant. The involvement of the eye distinguishes this from asymmetric crying facies.

8.9 Lower motor neurone facial palsy in a child. Note the very obvious abnormality involving both upper and lower face.

8.10 Right facial nerve palsy in a child with a pontine glioma, who also had a right sixth nerve palsy (see 8.7) which was obvious when the eyelids were lifted.

MANAGEMENT

Lubricating eye drops and patching are important in preventing damage to the cornea. Antibiotics should be used for otitis media or if there is a suspicion of Lyme disease. Hypertension should be appropriately investigated and managed. Acyclovir should be considered if a viral aetiology is suspected and immunoglobulin is indicated for Kawasaki disease. Steroids are of no long-term benefit.

PROGNOSIS

There is usually a good recovery.

UPPER MOTOR NEURONE FACIAL PALSY

An upper motor-neurone facial palsy is often mild (**8.11**). The eye is usually not involved because of the bilateral innervation of the upper part of the face (**8.12**). The child usually smiles normally (**8.13**). Upper motor neurone facial palsies may also be bilateral (see **8.16**).

Unilateral
Causes

Involvement of the pyramidal tract above the facial nerve nucleus (usually in association with a hemiparesis). Lesion of the pons (in association with sixth nerve palsy). An apparently isolated upper motor neurone facial palsy is not uncommon in children with hippocampal sclerosis causing intractable epilepsy and may be a useful lateralizing sign.

Bilateral

Children with a spastic quadriparesis commonly have bilateral upper motor neurone facial weakness and bulbar palsy (**8.16**).

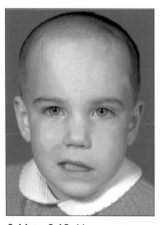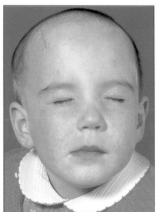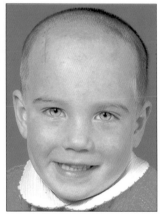

8.11 to 8.13 Upper motor neurone facial palsy in a child recovering from a cerebral abscess. The asymmetry of the lower face is obvious when the child is asked to show her teeth (**8.11**), the upper face is not involved, she is able to close both eyes normally (**8.12**) and there is only a mild palsy when she smiles (**8.13**).

LOWER CRANIAL NERVE ABNORMALITIES

PRESENTATION
Usually bilateral, almost always involving several cranial nerves with bilateral involvement of the seventh, ninth, tenth, eleventh and twelfth nuclei together. The weakness may be upper or lower motor neurone. Sucking, swallowing and speech are commonly affected. There may be deviation of the uvula in a unilateral lesion (**8.14**) causing oromotor dyspraxia.

CAUSES
Lower motor neurone (bulbar palsy, **8.15**) – as for bilateral lower motor neurone facial weakness. Upper motor neurone (pseudobulbar palsy, **8.16**) – as for bilateral upper motor neurone facial palsy. The Worster-Drought syndrome is a form of cerebral palsy involving predominantly the bulbar muscles.

TREATMENT
Management of feeding and speech difficulties.

PROGNOSIS
The problems often improve with careful management and with time but there are usually residual difficulties.

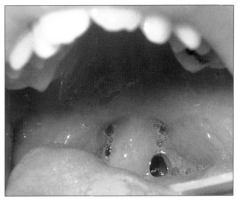

8.14 Deviation of the uvula in a child recovering from a bulbar palsy.

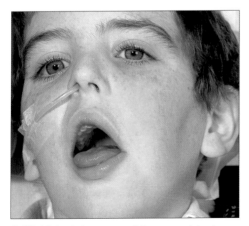

8.15 Multiple lower cranial nerve palsies in a child with a cerebellar infarct. There is a bilateral fifth cranial nerve motor weakness evident in the slack jaw, bilateral facial palsy, bulbar palsy (evidenced by the feeding tube) and flaccid tongue weakness.

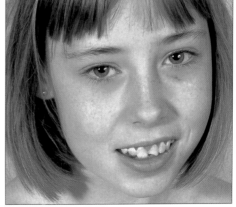

8.16 Bulbar palsy in a child with upper motor neurone cerebral palsy. She had early feeding difficulties and now has bilateral facial weakness and dysarthria.

WILSON'S DISEASE

See also 'Metabolic Diseases' chapter.

INCIDENCE
One in 30,000.

GENETICS
Autosomal recessive; ATP78 gene on 13q. Age of onset: between four and 50 years (neuro-logical presentation is rare under eight years, but possible in patients over four years of age).

CLINICAL SIGNS
- Facial immobility.
- Rigidity.
- Dysarthria.
- Dysphagia.
- Tremor, especially of the wrist and shoulder (usually pill-rolling).
- Behavioural difficulties with aggression, euphoria, immaturity.
- Kayser-Fleischer ring at limbus cornea (always in patients with neurological presentation) (**8.17**).
- Liver disease. Haemolytic anaemia.

INVESTIGATIONS
- Serum copper <7.8 mmol/L and caeruloplasmin <100 mg/L.
- 24 hour urinary copper >100 mg.
- Liver biopsy if high clinical index of suspicion and above investigations normal.
- Neuroimaging may show low density in deep grey matter.

TREATMENT
- D-penicillamine (start slowly, as clinical deterioration is common at the start of treatment), Trientine.
- Pyridoxine and zinc supplementation.
- Steroids may be useful if the patient has mild symptoms of hypersensitivity on penicillamine.

SYDENHAM'S CHOREA

CLINICAL SIGNS
- Behavioural abnormalities – obsessive-compulsive, emotional lability (PANDAS – Paediatric Autoimmune Neuropsychiatric Disorders Associated with Streptococcal infections).
- Chorea, usually bilateral, and often involving the face.

INVESTIGATIONS
- Anti-streptococcal titre, anti DNAase B, anti basal ganglia antibodies.
- ECG and echocardiogram.

TREATMENT
- Long-term penicillin.
- Carbamezepine.
- Haloperidol.

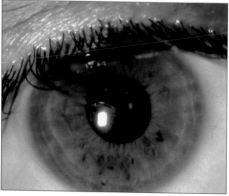

8.17 Wilson's disease. Kayser-Fleischer ring in a child.

MOTOR SYSTEM

In a child, examination of the motor system is usually performed in the following order:

1. **General observation:** e.g. for tics, abnormal facial movement, wasting (**8.18**), fasciculation.

2. **Gait:** habitual; stressed by walking on the toes or heels or running; heel-to-toe along a line to bring out ataxia.
   The following are common:
   - Hemiplegia, with circumduction of foot and often increasing dystonic posturing of hand. (**8.18**)
   - Diplegia (**8.19**).
   - Ataxia (see pages 216–218).

3. **Posture:** ask the child to stand with his feet together, to stretch his arms out with his fingers stretched wide apart and to keep his eyes closed. The following may be observed:
   - Drift downwards of one arm in a unilateral pyramidal lesion (spastic hemiparesis).
   - Dystonic posturing, including athetoid writhing (**8.20**).
   - Chorea.
   - Tremor.
   - Inability to maintain posture in patients with loss of position sense.

4. **Finger-to-nose testing:** to bring out ataxia (with past pointing) or dystonia (usually terminal shake with no past pointing) (**8.21**). Also heel-to-shin testing.

5. **Formal examination of all four limbs:** examining for asymmetry, wasting, fasciculation, tone, power, co-ordination and reflexes.

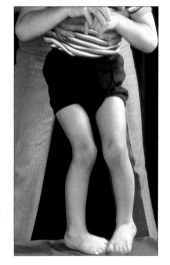

8.18 Congenital hemiparesis. Wasting and dystonic posturing of the hand in a child.

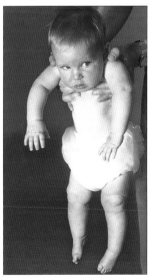

8.19 Diplegia in a child, demonstrating weakness and abnormal posture.

8.20 Severe dystonia in a child with damage to the basal ganglia (left).

8.21 Dystonic posturing in an infant (right).

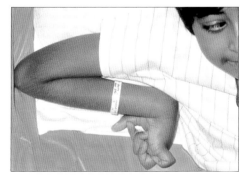

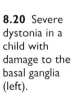

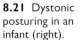

PYRAMIDAL DISORDERS

In a long-standing pyramidal disorder, there is 'clasp-knife' rigidity accompanied by increased tendon reflexes and upgoing plantar responses. For further details, see under Cerebral palsy (page 227) – spastic hemiplegia and quadriparesis. Acutely, hypotonia and hyporeflexia are characteristic (see under Stroke, page 249, and Spinal cord disorders, page 224).

EXTRAPYRAMIDAL DISORDERS

The diagnosis of an extrapyramidal disorder is often made simply by observing the posture of the child at rest. Extrapyramidal disorders improve during sleep and examination under anaesthesia may be required to assess whether or not a deformity is fixed.

The slow writhing movements of athetosis are a form of dystonia and may be distinguished from the rapid movements of chorea, although the two may occur together. There may be more difficulty in distinguishing some of the other movement disorders (see **Table 8.1**).

Table 8.1 Distinguishing between movement disorders

		Tremor	Chorea	Dystonia	Tics	Myoclonus	Ataxia
Action	Rest	+	(+)	(+)	+	(+)	
	Action		+	+		+	+
Speed	Fast	+	+		+	+	
	Slow			+			+
Complexity	Simple	+			+	+	+
	Complex		+	+			
Site	Proximal	+	+	+	+	+	
	Distal		+		+	+	+
Type	Stereotyped	+			+	+	+
	Variable		+	+			

Treatable causes of extrapyramidal abnormalities

Condition	Diagnostic test	Treatment
Wilson's disease	Plasma copper, caeruloplasmin	Penicillamine
Sydenham's chorea	Antistreptococcal titre, anti DNAase B	Penicillin
Segawa syndrome	Trial of L-DOPA, Guanosine triphosphate cyclohydrolase I gene	L-DOPA
Systemic lupus erythematosus	Antinuclear antibodies, anti-double-stranded DNA autoantibodies	Immunosuppression
Moyamoya (see 'Stroke')	MR angiography	Revascularization
Arteriovenous malformation	Contrast CT, MRI, conventional arteriography	Surgery, embolization, radiotherapy
Tumour	Neuroimaging	Radiotherapy
Glutaric aciduria type I	Urinary organic acids	Protein restriction Carnitine
Homocystinuria	Plasma total homocysteine, methionine	Pyridoxine Methionine restriction Betaine
Infections	Mycoplasma, CMV, HIV	Antimicrobials
Drugs and toxins	Urine and blood screening	Withdrawal
Hysteria	Exclusion of alternatives, observation	Rehabilitation
Sandifer syndrome (reflux)	pH studies, barium swallow	Omeprazole, Nissen fundoplication

SEGAWA SYNDROME (DOPA-RESPONSIVE DYSTONIA)

GENETICS
Autosomal-dominant with reduced penetrance. Mutation in gene coding for guanosine triphosphate cyclohydrolase I, rate-limiting step for tetrahydrobiopterin (co-factor for phenyl-alanine, tyrosine and tryptophan, mono-oxygenases).

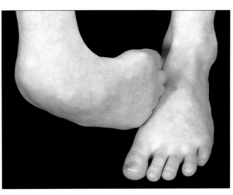

8.22 Dystonia of the foot.

CLINICAL
- Dystonia, often worse in the evening (**8.22**).
- Equinovarus posturing of foot.
- Gait disturbance.
- Ankle clonus (unsustained).
- Extensor posturing of big toe.
- Spasticity.

INVESTIGATIONS
Exclude alternative causes, especially Wilson's. DNA. Trial of levodopa.

TREATMENT
Levodopa/carbidopa (Sinemet) in doses of up to 100/25 mg tds.

Some other causes of dystonia and/or chorea
- Hypoxic-ischaemic damage (may be delayed or worsen after initial stability).
- Bronchopulmonary dysplasia.
- Post cardiopulmonary bypass.
- Trauma (may be delayed).
- Ataxia-telangiectasia (see under 'Ataxia', **8.25**).
- GM1 and GM2 gangliosidoses.
- Mitochondrial disease (e.g. Leigh's syndrome).
- Hallervordan-Spatz disease.
- Huntington's chorea.

Management
- **Clinical:** prepare an accurate description of movement disorder and any associated behavioural manifestation (video and further opinions may be helpful); slit lamp examination by ophthalmologist for Kayser-Fleischer rings.
- **Initial investigations:** neuroimaging (may include MRA), plasma copper and caeruloplasmin, ASOT, plasma amino acids, urine organic acids, plasma lactate, alpha fetoprotein. May need CSF lactate, white cell enzymes, pH studies and barium swallow, DNA testing for Huntington's chorea or Ataxia-telangiectasia if clinically indicated.
- **Long-term:** appropriate treatment of underlying cause, trial of levodopa for dystonia, anticholinergics (e.g. benzhexol). In severe extrapyramidal disorders, appropriate seating and treatment of Sandifer syndrome, i.e. gastroesophageal reflux, may produce improvement and diazepam may reduce dystonic spasms..

ATAXIA

Although ataxia implies a cerebellar lesion, it may be very difficult to distinguish cerebellar ataxia from a peripheral neuropathy, action myoclonus or dystonia in a young child. Horizontal nystagmus and past pointing suggest involvement of the cerebellum, whereas areflexia indicates a peripheral neuropathy (see also extrapyramidal disorders).

Causes of acute ataxia
- Posterior fossa space-occupying lesion (may be accompanied by head tilt (**8.23**):
  - tumour (e.g. medulloblastoma, **8.24**);
  - extradural or subdural haematoma;
  - cerebral infarction (**8.109**).
- Acute cerebellitis (e.g. mycoplasma).
- Post-infectious cerebellitis (e.g. chicken pox).
- Guillain-Barré syndrome (see under 'Acute weakness' page 221).
- Drugs and toxins (e.g. phenytoin, carbamezepine, lead).

Causes of non-progressive chronic ataxia
- Cerebellar malformations.
- Ataxic cerebral palsy (often accompanied by epilepsy and parietal lesions on neuroimaging).

Other causes of progressive ataxia
- Hereditary sensory and motor neuropathy (see also chronic progressive weakness).
- Ataxia-telangiectasia (AT) (**8.25**).
- Ataxia-oculomotor apraxia (also abnormality of AT gene).
- Friedreich's ataxia (FA-abnormality of Frataxin gene) (**8.26**).
- Early onset ataxia with preserved deep tendon reflexes (also abnormality of Frataxin gene).
- Metachromatic leukodystrophy, other leukodystrophies.
- GM1 and GM2 gangliosidoses.

Investigations
- Neuroimaging. This should be urgent if there is reduced visual acuity (secondary to raised intracranial pressure), vomiting or headache. It should be avoided if the patient is areflexic and clinically has a peripheral neuropathy or telangiectasia in view of the chromosomal fragility in AT.
- Nerve conduction studies to diagnose peripheral neuropathy and to distinguish hereditary sensory and motor neuropathies from Friedreich's ataxia.
- Alpha-fetoprotein and immunoglobulins to screen for ataxia-telangiectasia.

Treatable causes of intermittent or progressive ataxia		
Condition	**Diagnosis**	**Treatment**
Posterior fossa tumour	Neuroimaging	See under 'Brain Tumours'
Drugs and toxins	Urine drug screen	Stop drugs
Hartnup disease	Urine amino acids	Nicotinamide
Maple syrup urine disease	Urine amino acids	Thiamine
Biotinidase deficiency (see under 'Epilepsy')	Urine organic acids Plasma biotinidase	Biotin
Hereditary paroxysmal cerebellar ataxia	Gene on 19q	Acetazolamide
Refsum disease	Plasma phytanic acid	Dietary
Pyruvate dehydrogenase complex deficiency	Plasma/CSF lactate Enzyme assay Gene on Xp22	Thiamine may help
Primary Vitamin E deficiency	Plasma vitamin E	Vitamin E
Secondary Vitamin E deficiency Abetalipoproteinaemia Hypobetalipoproteinaemia	Plasma vitamin E Acanthocytosis Plasma triglycerides Plasma lipoproteins	(+A+K)
Alpha-tocopherol transfer protein	Gene probe	
Glucose transporter deficiency	Low CSF glucose	Ketogenic diet

- White blood cell chromosome fragility (AT), DNA if high index of suspicion of AT or FA; urine amino and organic acids, plasma amino acids; plasma and CSF lactate, biotinidase; phytanic acid; triglycerides and lipoproteins; white cell enzymes.

ATAXIA-TELANGIECTASIA

(See also 'Immunology' chapter.) Autosomal recessive. ATM gene on 11q22-23. ATM protein required for DNA repair. Protein similar to mammalian phosphatidylinositol-3' kinase.

Clinical features
- Oculomotor apraxia.
- Telangiectasia – conjunctiva (**8.25**) and upper face.
- Truncal ataxia due to loss of Purkinje cells.
- Dysarthria.
- Choreoathetosis/dystonia.
- Thymic hypoplasia with low IgA, IgG and IgM.
- Recurrent chest infections, bronchiectasis.
- Lymphoma, leukaemia.
- Premature senescence.
- Insulin-resistant diabetes.

Diagnosis
- High alpha-fetoprotein.
- Immunoglobulin deficiency.
- White blood cell chromosome fragility.
- ATM gene on 11q22-23.
- MRI shows cerebellar degeneration; may show leukodystrophy.

Management
- Antibiotics for infections.
- Avoidance of radiation for diagnosis or treatment of neoplasia.

Prognosis
Depends on frequency of infections and/or occurence of neoplasia.

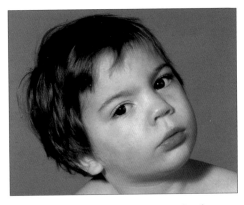

8.23 Head tilt may suggest a posterior fossa tumour and a careful examination should be performed to look for evidence of nystagmus, ataxia and cranial nerve signs.

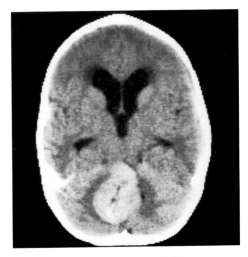

8.24 CT scan showing a medulloblastoma.

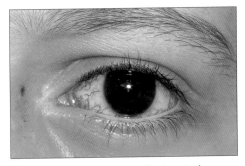

8.25 Ataxia-telangiectasia. Conjunctival telangiectasia.

FRIEDREICH'S ATAXIA

Prevalence
1 in 8,000.

Genetics
Autosomal recessive. Reduplication of GAA sequence in intron 1 of Frataxin gene on 9q. Reduplication reduces Frataxin: protein associated with mitochondrial membranes and crests; may reduce oxidative stress by preventing iron accumulation. Size of expansion (120–1,700 repeats) is related to the patient's age at onset.

Clinical signs
- Ataxia – mixed sensory and cerebellar.
- Speech – scanning dysarthria, then slurred.
- Intention tremor, clumsiness of hands.
- Nystagmus (relatively rare).
- Fatigue.
- Cardiac symptoms secondary to cardiomyopathy.
- Pes cavus (**8.26**).
- Loss of position and vibration sensation, particularly in legs.
- Loss of tendon jerks (classically absent at ankle, brisk at knee).
- Extensor plantars (pyramidal involvement, as for brisk knee jerks).
- Scoliosis.
- Diabetes.
- Optic atrophy.
- Deafness.

Diagnosis
- ECG, echocardiography.
- Nerve conduction – reduced amplitude sensory nerve action potential; reduced velocity motor and sensory conduction.
- Frataxin gene on 9q.

Management
Multidisciplinary, treating cardiomyopathy, scoliosis, motor disorder and diabetes.

Prognosis
Death in early or middle adult life.

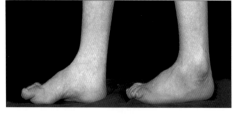

8.26 Friedreich's ataxia. Pes cavus.

HYPOTONIA IN INFANCY

Clinical signs
History of maternal illness (e.g. myasthenia gravis), other family, pregnancy and birth history, and fetal movements. Examination of infant with typical facial appearance, posture (**8.27**), degree of truncal, limb and facial weakness, reflexes, tongue fasciculation in Werdnig-Hoffman syndrome. Examination of parents, especially the mother, for dystrophia myotonica (ability to bury eyelashes), myotonia exacerbated by cold, myasthenia (ptosis and weakness).

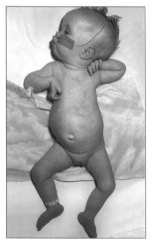

8.27 Infant with hypotonia and abnormal posturing of the hands secondary to a cervical cord lesion.

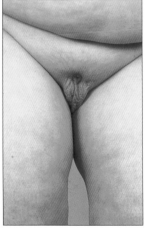

8.28 Small genitalia and obesity in an older child with Prader-Willi syndrome.

Investigations

- Molecular genetic studies for characteristic condition, (e.g. Prader-Willi – **8.28**, dystrophia myotonica – **8.30**).
- Creatine phosphokinase (CPK).
- Echocardiography (e.g. for Pompe's).
- X-ray of the knee to look for patellar calcification/stippling in peroxisomal disorders.
- Appropriate biochemistry for metabolic condition (e.g. very long chain fatty acids for peroxisomal disorders or plasma/CSF lactate for mitochondrial disease).
- Electromyography (EMG) and nerve conduction studies. Single fibre or repetitive stimulation for myasthenia.
- Neuroimaging of brain to exclude structural brain abnormality, either isolated or in association with muscle disease (e.g. white matter abnormality in Fukuyama congenital muscular dystrophy).
- Muscle biopsy may be justified in the neonate if diagnosis cannot be secured by an alternative method.
- Stool for clostridium botulinum.

DYSTROPHIA MYOTONICA

Incidence
One in 7,500.

Genetics
Autosomal dominant; inherited from mother if neonate affected, expansion of a triplet repeat (CTG) in the 3'-untranslated region of the myotonin protein kinase gene on chromosome 19q13, disruption mRNA metabolism.

Causes of weakness in infancy

- Dystrophia myotonica (**8.30**)
- Congenital muscular dystrophy
- Myopathies:
  - Pompe's disease (Glycogen storage disease type II)
  - Nemaline myopathy
  - Myotubular myopathy
- Spinal muscular atrophy type I (Werdnig-Hoffman) (**8.32**)
- Congenital and neonatal myasthenia (page 207)
- Botulism
- Peripheral neuropathies
- Spinal cord disease:
  - Trauma (**8.27**)
  - Congenital malformation
- Central
  - Chromosomal
    - Down syndrome
    - Prader-Willi (**8.28**)
      - Genomic imprinting with interstitial deletion in paternal 15q1.1-1.3
  - Metabolic
    - Peroxisomal
      - Zellweger syndrome (**8.29**)
      - Neonatal adrenoleukodystrophy
    - Amino acidurias
    - Organic acidurias
    - Mitochondrial disorders
  - Structural brain malformation
  - Cerebral haemorrhage
  - Sepsis

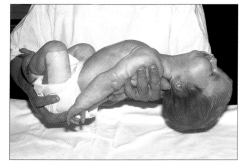

8.29 Zellweger disease. Infant showing profound hypotonia and characteristic facies.

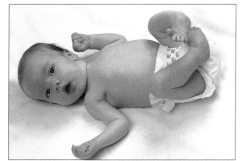

8.30 Infant with dystrophia myotonica with characteristic fish-shaped mouth, decreased tone and bilateral talipes. Mother cannot bury her eyelashes. (The ward setting is often too warm to demonstrate difficulty in releasing.)

Presentation

Often mild distal limb weakness (**8.30**) with characteristic facial weakness (inability to bury eyelashes) and myotonia – worse in cold weather (demonstrated by percussion of muscle or by shaking hands as the patient has difficulty in releasing), early cataracts, frontal balding, testicular atrophy, cardiac arrhythmias (paternal > maternal inheritance). May present in the neonatal period with severe weakness, respiratory insufficiency, arthrogryposis (talipes equinovarus is particularly common) and facial weakness with characteristic 'fish-shaped' mouth (maternal inheritance).

Diagnosis

Molecular genetic studies in characteristic cases. EMG shows myopathic features with myotonic discharges ('dive bomber') in older children and adults.

HEREDITARY MOTOR AND SENSORY NEUROPATHY TYPE I (CHARCOT-MARIE-TOOTH DISEASE)

PREVALENCE

1 in 26,000.

GENETICS

Usually dominant. Recessive and X-linked forms may be clinically similar. Commonly 1.5 megabase duplication within band 17p11.2 on chromosome 17. Reduplication leads to three copies of gene encoding peripheral myelin protein 22 (PMP-22). Occasionally point mutation in PMP-22 gene. Other loci include chromosomes 1 and 8 and the X chromosome.

CLINICAL

Usually presents <10 years, with gait disturbance – instability, high-stepping, difficulty in running, frequent falls; also pes cavus (the patient may also have hammer toe), pes planus and valgus deformity, symmetrical wasting of the peroneal muscles, calves or lower thighs (**8.31**), reduced or absent reflexes, subtle sensory abnormalities.

DIAGNOSIS

- Nerve conduction: motor and sensory conduction velocities <50% normal. Increased distal latencies.
- Molecular genetic studies.

MANAGEMENT

Often none is needed. Occasionally deterioration may respond to steroids. High-dose ascorbic acid is being explored.

PROGNOSIS

Compatible with normal lifespan, the patient is often ambulant throughout.

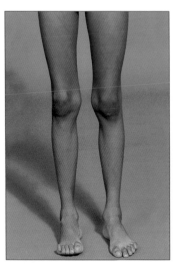

8.31 Charcot-Marie-Tooth disease. Wasting of the lower legs.

SPINAL MUSCULAR ATROPHY TYPE I (WERDNIG–HOFFMAN DISEASE)

INCIDENCE
One in 20,000.

GENETICS
Autosomal recessive. Deletion of exon 7 of the survival motor neuron (SMN) gene on chromosome 5q13 in 95% of cases. Up to 55% also have deletions in the adjacent neuronal apoptosis inhibitory protein (NAIP) gene. Pathologically there is loss of anterior horn cells.

PRESENTATION
Progressive proximal weakness of the limbs from birth or soon afterwards (**8.32**). Paralysis of the intercostal muscles leads to narrowing of the chest and abdominal breathing. Clinical features of small chin, fasciculation of the chin and tongue, preserved eye and facial movements and areflexia.

DIAGNOSIS
EMG shows neurogenic pattern with reduced activity during maximal effort, increased duration and amplitude of motor unit potentials and increased numbers of polyphasic potentials. DNA testing.

PROGNOSIS
Death by 18 months as, at present, there is no effective treatment; respiratory support may prolong life.

ACUTE GENERALIZED WEAKNESS IN A PREVIOUSLY WELL CHILD

INVESTIGATIONS
Creatine phosphokinase (CPK) to diagnose dermatomyositis or viral myositis. Nerve conduction to diagnose Guillain-Barré (may be normal in initial phase of illness); CSF is usually unnecessary as the protein is not raised until a few days after onset in Guillain-Barré; other conditions (e.g. botulism) may have characteristic neurophysiological features. Exclusion of myasthenia (see under Ptosis). MRI cervical spine if suspicion of cord lesion (e.g. if there is bladder involvement – **8.33**).

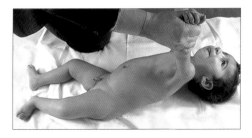

8.32 Infant with spinal muscular atrophy to show truncal and limb hypotonia, bell-shaped chest, frog-legged posture and preserved facial movement with alert expression.

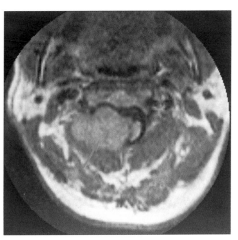

8.33 A neurofibroma at C1 pushing the cord over. This type of lesion can occasionally cause a flaccid quadriparesis and if there is any doubt about the diagnosis of Guillain-Barré, MRI of the neck should be considered, especially if there is bladder involvement.

MANAGEMENT

- Assessment of respiratory function and reserve. Vital capacity using a spirometer should be performed regularly if the patient is unventilated and can co-operate.
- Ventilation if there is evidence of increasing respiratory failure, rapid general deterioration, or signs likely to be associated with respiratory failure (e.g. bilateral facial weakness in Guillain-Barré syndrome – **8.35**).
- Treatment of cause (e.g. surgery for spinal cord tumour, immunosuppression for dermatomyositis, immunoglobulin (and/or plasmapheresis) for Guillain-Barré if continuing to deteriorate and/or respiratory compromise).
- Physiotherapy and occupational therapy.

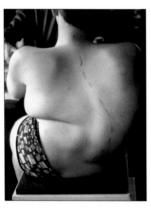

8.34 Asymmetrical flaccid weakness leading to scoliosis in a boy who had previously had polio.

Causes of acute generalized weakness in a previously well child

- Guillain-Barré syndrome (**8.35**).
- Dermatomyositis (**8.36–8.38**).
- Viral myositis.
- Myasthenia (see under 'Ptosis', **8.6**).
- Cervical cord lesion (e.g. acute disseminated encephalomyelitis, trauma, tumour – **8.33**).
- Botulism. Associated with fixed, dilated pupils.
- Other toxins (e.g. lead, vincristine).
- Poliomyelitis (**8.34**) (including vaccine-associated). Usually asymmetrical weakness.
- Other enteroviruses, Japanese B encephalitis virus.
- Acute presentation of chronic weakness (e.g. hereditary sensory motor neuropathy – **8.31**).

GUILLAIN–BARRÉ SYNDROME

INCIDENCE
0.6-1.1/100,000 children

PATHOLOGY
Inflammatory demyelinating polyradiculoneuropathy in most patients. Preceding infections include Campylobacter, cytomegalovirus, Epstein-Barr virus.

CLINICAL SYMPTOMS AND SIGNS
These include pain, ascending weakness, ataxia, respiratory weakness, bulbar weakness, bilateral facial weakness, and ophthalmoplegia (**8.35**).

MANAGEMENT
Admission and close observation, particularly of respiratory and cardiac function (see above). Intravenous immunoglobulin if there is rapid deterioration, the patient is not walking or is likely to require ventilation. Plasmapheresis if immunoglobulin does not arrest deterioration or lead to improvement. Ventilation for respiratory failure. Pacing for cardiac dysrrhythmias. Physiotherapy to prevent contractures and aid mobilization during recovery.

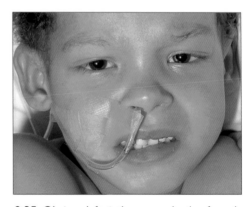

8.35 Obvious left sixth nerve palsy (on formal testing of eye movements, patient had more extensive ophthalmoplegia), bilateral facial nerve weakness and bulbar palsy – requiring nasogastric feeding, in a child recovering from Guillain-Barré syndrome.

DERMATOMYOSITIS

PRESENTATION
General misery, generalized weakness and pain, heliotrope rash over eyelids (**8.36**), elbows, and knees. Calcinosis over joints (e.g. the elbow in chronic cases) (**8.37**). Collodion patches over extensor surface of fingers (**8.38**).

INVESTIGATIONS
ESR. Creatine phosphokinase. Muscle biopsy shows increased class I antigen expression. Inflammatory changes may be patchy.

MANAGEMENT
Immunosuppression with oral steroids, aza-thioprine and cyclosporin A. Intravenous immunoglobulin.

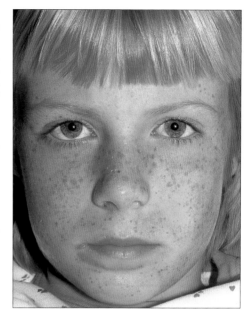

8.36 Dermatomyositis. Heliotrope rash in a child. Note the characteristic serious expression.

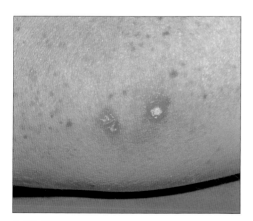

8.37 Dermatomyostis. Nodular calcification of the skin over the elbow.

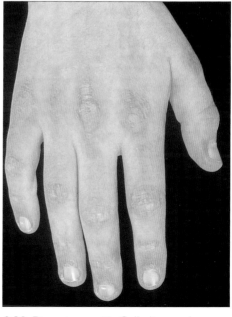

8.38 Dermatomyositis. Collodion patches over the finger joints.

SPINAL CORD DISORDERS

Acute spinal cord injury usually occurs in the context of trauma. High dose methyl prednisolone is neuroprotective and should be given as soon as possible after injury. As there may be no bony injury, all children involved in significant trauma should be nursed flat and in a stiff collar until they are conscious enough to confirm that there is no pain in the neck or back indicative of ligamentous injury and instability.

Chronic spinal cord injury may occur in children with skeletal deformities and may present with the insidious onset of pyramidal and/or lower motor neurone and sensory signs (**8.39–8.41**). Tumours may present with pain, stiffness, focal neurological deficit or bladder symptoms. Diagnosis is usually made with MRI of the spine, which is indicated urgently in a unit where the child can be surgically decompressed if there is recent deterioration. Transverse myelitis may be clinically similar, but can be distinguished on MRI. Methyl prednisolone should be given as soon as possible as there is evidence for improved outcome compared with historical controls.

Predisposing syndromes
- Down syndrome
- Mucopolysaccharidoses
- Achondroplasia
- Goldenhar syndrome
- Klippel-Feil syndrome
- Conradi syndrome
- Coffin-Lowry syndrome

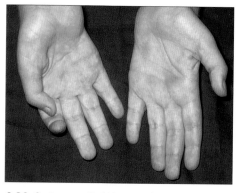

8.39 Syringomyelia. Wasting of the small muscles of the hands, worse on the right.

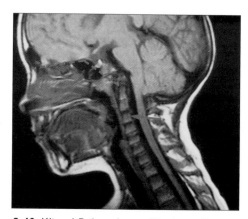

8.40 Klippel-Feil syndrome. Platybasia (flat skull base – dotted line) and basilar invagination (top of 2nd vertebra moved up – arrow) in a child with pyramidal signs in all four limbs.

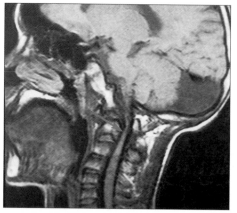

8.41 Conradi syndrome. Thinning of the cord in the high cervical region in a child.

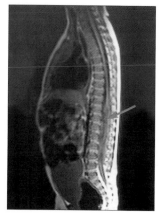

8.42 Cord tumour, probably ependymoma.

CHRONIC AND PROGRESSIVE WEAKNESS IN THE OLDER CHILD

Clinical signs

History of weakness, family history, and associated features (e.g. learning difficulties, cardiac manifestations). Examination includes Gower's manoeuvre (**8.43**) to demonstrate proximal weakness, distribution of weakness, facial involvement, ptosis (**8.6**), presence or absence of muscular hypertrophy (**8.44**), additional features including scoliosis (**8.34**), cardiac involvement, learning difficulties. Examination of family members (e.g. both parents in HMSN I) (**8.31**).

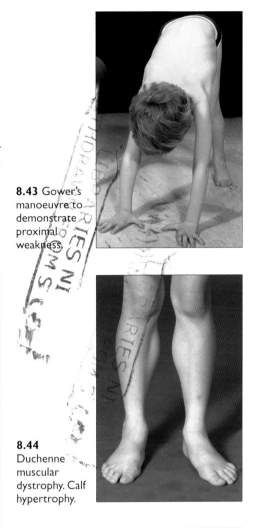

8.43 Gower's manoeuvre to demonstrate proximal weakness.

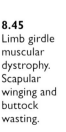

Causes of chronic and progressive weakness in the older child

Spinal disorders

Muscle disease
Dystrophies
  Duchenne and Becker forms (**8.44**)
    X-linked recessive
    Dystrophin gene on X chromosome
    Majority of boys with dystrophy have abnormality dystrophin
    Affected girls
      Manifesting carriers
      Translocations
  Limb girdle (**8.45**)
    Abnormalities of sarcoglycans (a, b, g, d), calpain 3
  Fascioscapulohumeral
  Emery-Dreifuss
Dystrophia myotonica (see page 219, **8.30**)
Myopathies
  Nemaline
  Central core
  Minicore

Myasthenia (see under Ptosis, **8.6**)

Anterior horn cell disease
Kugelberg-Welander form of spinal muscular atrophy

Neuropathies
Hereditary sensory and motor neuropathy type I (HMSN I) (Charcot-Marie-Tooth) (**8.31**)
HMSN II

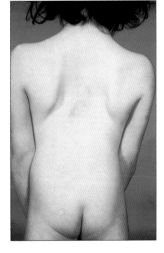

8.44 Duchenne muscular dystrophy. Calf hypertrophy.

8.45 Limb girdle muscular dystrophy. Scapular winging and buttock wasting.

Investigations

Creatine phosphokinase. Edrophonium test and acetylcholine receptor antibodies if myasthenia likely. Molecular genetic studies: Duchenne – dystrophin deletion on X chromosome; Dystrophia myotonica – CTG expansion on chromosome 19. HMSN I – Duplication of 1.5-Mb region of chromosome 17 including the peripheral myelin protein 22 gene. Electromyography and nerve conduction studies. May need to include single fibre studies and repetitive stimulation if initial studies are not diagnostic and myasthenia is likely. ECG and echocardiogram. Muscle biopsy to include appropriate stains, including dystrophin. MRI spine.

Management

For management of myasthenia, see under 'Ptosis', page 205. Unfortunately, no curative treatments exist for the muscular dystrophies or the hereditary neuropathies. Physiotherapy to strengthen muscles and reduce contracture formation; maintenance of ambulation with ischial weight-bearing calipers and knee/ankle/foot orthoses; treatment of scoliosis by maintaining ambulation, standing, the use of appropriate seating, a well-fitting, comfortable polypropylene jacket, and surgical stabilization.

DUCHENNE / BECKER MUSCULAR DYSTROPHY

Incidence

Duchenne 1 in 3,500; Becker 1 in 30,000 of male births.

Genetics

X-linked, large gene on Xp21 produces protein, dystrophin, located on muscle membrane. **Duchenne** (severe): 'nonsense' mutations terminating triplet 'reading frame', therefore no functional dystrophin. **Becker** (mild): 'missense' mutations disrupting triplet 'reading frame', therefore reduced quantities of abnormal but partially functional dystrophin produced. The majority affected are boys, although girls may have translocation involving Xp21, Turner's syndrome or be manifesting carriers.

Presentation

Abnormal gait aged 3–4 years, unable to run, sometimes with language delay and other cognitive problems. May later develop cardiomyopathy (Becker).

Duchenne: relentless progression, loss of ambulation by 8 to 12 years, death by early twenties.

Becker: may present later, slower progression, often normal lifespan.

Management

Physiotherapy to maintain full range movements. Night ankle/foot orthoses to prevent tendoachilles shortening. Ischial weight-bearing calipers for ambulation. Jacket/spinal surgery usually necessary to treat scoliosis once chairbound. Steroids appear to provide some short-term benefits if prescribed early at a dose of 0.75 mg/kg/day. Because of concern about the long term side-effects, intermittent dosing. e.g. 10 days per month, is being explored.

CEREBRAL PALSY

See also 'Orthopaedics and Fractures' chapter.

A nonprogressive movement disorder, caused by an insult to the immature brain occuring prenatally, perinatally or in the first few years of life.

INCIDENCE
One in 500 live births in Westernized countries.

TYPES OF CEREBRAL PALSY
- Spastic: hemiparesis; diplegia; quadriparesis.
- Dystonic/dyskinetic: quadriparesis with dystonia or chorea; hemiparesis; diplegia.
- Ataxic: relatively rare; must exclude inherited conditions (see under ataxia).
- Mixed types: commonly spastic and dystonic.

AETIOLOGY OF CEREBRAL PALSY
Prenatal factors
Predisposing risk factors
- Low birth weight for gestational age (dyskinetic; spastic quadriplegia). May explain effect of parity, social class, poor reproductive performance.
- Sex: M >F.
- Race: White > Black.
- Multiple birth, twin death, prematurity.
- Complications: bleeding, infection, pre-eclampsia.
- Genetic predisposition (e.g. Factor V Leiden).

Specific causes
- Genetic (e.g. arginase deficiency [diplegia]). Also ataxic cerebral palsy (see under Ataxia).
- Structural brain malformation (e.g. microcephaly, agenesis corpus callosum, Sturge-Weber syndrome).
- Ischaemia (e.g. porencephaly – often middle cerebral artery, 'fetal stroke', periventricular leukomalacia).
- Teratogens (e.g. alcohol – 8.3% of fetal alcohol sydrome have cerebral palsy).
- Deficiencies (e.g. iodine [New Guinea]), magnesium.
- Infections (e.g. rubella, cytomegalovirus, toxoplasma).

Non-motor features associated with cerebral palsy
- Microcephaly
- Learning difficulties
- Speech disorders
- Epilepsy
- Disorders of vision and/or hearing
- Squint
- Sensory loss
- Impaired growth – local or general
- Contractures and deformities

Perinatal factors
- Prematurity. (**uncomplicated**: diplegia; **complicated**: severe, mixed). Intraventricular and intracerebral haemorrhage. Periventricular leukomalacia.
- Jaundice (dyskinetic). Kernicterus now very rare in term infants but hyperbilirubinaemia is a risk factor in the premature.
- Asphyxia (dystonic quadriparesis +/– deafness; spastic quadriparesis +/– dystonia, +/– complications, e.g. learning difficulties, epilepsy).

Prenatal factors, especially fetal leanness, are an important risk factor for perinatal asphyxia and CP.

Postnatal factors
- Infection – meningitis, encephalitis, gastroenteritis with dehydration.
- Head injury – car accidents, non-accidental injury.
- Hypoxic-ischaemic encephalopathy – near miss sudden infant death syndrome, near drowning, postoperative (e.g. cardiopulmonary bypass).
- Status epilepticus – may be followed by hemiseizure/hemiplegia/epilepsy.
- Cerebrovascular accident (see under Stroke).

MANAGEMENT OF CEREBRAL PALSY

Therapy team: physiotherapist; occupational therapist; speech therapist; social worker; community nursing team; community paediatrician. Responsible for:

1. Assessment and management of feeding difficulties (the patient may need nasogastric feeding or gastrostomy if the problem is severe); gastroesophageal reflux; management of drooling (hyoscine patches, reimplantation salivary ducts).
2. Diagnosis and management of epilepsy (see under 'Epilepsy', page 240).
3. Management of hydrocephalus (see under 'Hydrocephalus', page 232).
4. Managing motor disorder and its potential consequences: seating to prevent hip dislocation and scoliosis (8.46); standing frame to prevent hip dislocation (8.47); walking aids (e.g. K-walker); postural management (e.g. discouraging children with diplegia from sitting between their legs); stretching exercises to keep full range of movement; ankle-foot-knee orthoses (8.48) (day and/or night) to keep full range of movement; botulinum toxin to encourage full range movement and prevent shortening; regular x-rays of hips (to exclude dislocation, 8.49) and spine; orthopaedics or gait laboratory.
5. Language difficulties: comprehension; expression (children with dysarthria may benefit from communication aids); support for family and child; education.

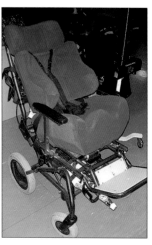

8.46 Appropriate seating for a child with cerebral palsy who is at risk of complications such as hip dislocation and scoliosis. It can be adjusted to correct posture and prevent permanent deformity.

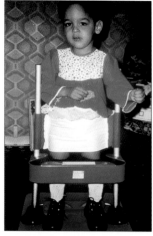

8.47 Child in a standing frame. Putting weight through the legs encourages the correct formation and orientation of the head of the femur and the acetabulum, making dislocation less likely.

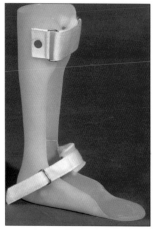

8.48 Ankle-foot orthosis which may be used to prevent shortening of the tendo-achilles in growing children.

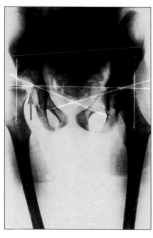

8.49 X-ray showing right hip dislocation. The lines drawn on the x-ray allow serial comparison to determine whether the hip is progressively dislocating.

SPINA BIFIDA

See also 'Orthopaedics and Fractures' and 'Neonatal and General Paediatric Surgery'.

INCIDENCE
Approximately 1 in 500, but very variable geographically. Reduced incidence since antenatal diagnosis with α-fetoprotein and ultrasound.

AETIOLOGY
Genetic factors are important. The risk of having a further affected child if one is already affected is 1 in 30. The risk of having a third child if two are affected is 1 in 6. Environmental factors are also important, particularly poor intake of folic acid in the first trimester.

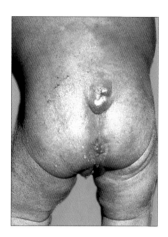

8.50
Myelocoele.

DEFINITIONS
- Meningocoele: cord usually normal, lesion covered with skin.
- Myelocoele or myelomeningocoele (**8.50, 8.51**): cord exposed and abnormal, only thin covering if any; risk of neurological impairment very high.
- Spina bifida occulta: spinal cord covered with bone and skin, but usually marked with hairy patch or lipoma. Children usually present later with bladder problems or minor gait disorders.

SITE
Most commonly in the lumbo-sacral area, less commonly in the dorsal region, uncommonly in the cervical region. Ten percent of lesions affect the skull (encephalocoeles).

8.51 Myelo-meningocoele.

MANAGEMENT
- Early closure of the spinal defect. Today this is done in the majority of instances although in some children with extensive neurological damage or severe hydrocephalus surgical treatment may not be appropriate.
- Management of hydrocephalus: a shunt will usually be inserted.
- Management of the bladder: it is essential that the child has regular urine specimens performed and has a urodynamic study to examine the nature of the neuropathic bladder. Intermittent catheterization is usually used to improve continence and prevent infection. Children will need regular urines performed and adequate treatment of the urinary tract infections. With careful management, it is now unusual for children to go into chronic renal failure.
- Physical management: many children with flaccid limbs can be given appropriate calipers and can walk. Other children may be wheelchair bound. It is important to prevent kyphoscoliosis with an appropriate jacket.

Complications of spina bifida

- **Loss of sensation:** Sensory loss in the skin can lead to ulceration (**8.52**) as the child may not know that he has burnt or cut himself. The ability to recognize a full rectum or bladder may also be lost.
- **Bladder problems:** Most children with lumbo-sacral myelomeningocoeles are incontinent to a degree. The bladder sphincters are often innervated abnormally and this may lead to a neuropathic bladder, which does not empty properly. The pressure inside the urinary tract may be high because of this and the child is also subject to frequent urinary tract infections. This combination can lead to chronic renal failure in the long term.
- **Hydrocephalus:** usually secondary to Arnold Chiari malformation of the brain stem. Occurs in patients with high lesions – e.g. thoracolumbar myelomeningocoele.
- **Paralysis:** With a lumbo–sacral lesion, the legs will be partially paralyzed to an extent dependent on the site of the lesion and the degree of damage to the spinal cord. Secondary syringomyelia (**8.53**) may lead to deterioration.
- **Limb deformities:** If the limbs are partially paralysed, there will be muscular imbalance and limb deformities may be present from birth or develop at a later stage.
- **Kyphoscoliosis:** The vertebral column may be abnormal and children are at high risk of kyphoscoliosis.

HEADACHES

Headache is common in children and only rarely signifies serious intracranial pathology. However, brain tumour is the second commonest form of cancer in childhood and a delay between the onset of symptoms and diagnosis has significant influence on the prognosis. It is impossible to be absolutely certain of the aetiology of a child's headache on the basis of one consultation.

History taking
- Headache: timing, site, severity, nature.
- Associated symptoms (e.g. nausea, visual disturbance).
- Snoring, apnoea, recurrent tonsillitis, allergic rhinitis, sinusitis.

Indications for neuroimaging
- Nocturnal or early morning headaches.
- Headaches associated with nausea or vomiting.
- Any neurological signs.
- Age <6 years or learning difficulties.
- Inability to reassure child and family.

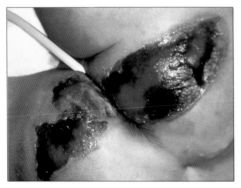

8.52 Spina bifida. Pressure sores secondary to poor sensation. Patients do not now normally have indwelling catheters.

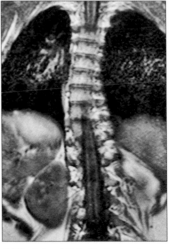

8.53 Spina bifida. Syrinx and scoliosis.

MIGRAINE

Clinical criteria

Paroxysmal headache separated by free intervals, with at least two to four of the following: unilateral pain; nausea; visual aura; family history in parents or siblings.

Prevalence

The overall prevalence of migraine in childhood is 4%. A family history is common.

Characteristic features of migraine

- Periodic throbbing, severe headaches .
- Gastrointestinal symptoms.
- Visual phenomena (e.g. photophobia or scotomata).
- Pallor, malaise.
- Desire to lie down in a darkened room/ inability to continue tasks.

Occasional features of migraine

- Hemiplegia (hemiplegic migraine) (see under 'Motor system', page 213).
- Aphasia.
- Visual field defects (see under 'Cranial nerves', **8.1**).
- Third nerve palsy (ophthalmoplegic migraine) (see under 'Cranial nerves', **8.2**).

Management

Full neurological and general examination on two occasions. Reassurance and removal of triggers (e.g. lack of regular food or sleep) with relaxation techniques to combat stress and psychological support. A diet free of chocolate, cheese and oranges (including juice) works for the majority of children. A simple analgesic can be prescribed as soon as the child knows the migraine is starting. Other medications include pizotifen (but this causes weight gain), propranolol (contraindicated in asthma) and clonidine. Flunarizine or Verapamil may help those with hemiplegic migraine.

PSYCHOGENIC HEADACHES

The distinction between psychogenic (tension) headaches and common migraine is blurred, but psychogenic headaches are typically continuous.

Characteristic features of psychogenic headaches

- Continuous pressure like a tight band or an aching.
- A precipitating cause, such as a family problem or examination pressure.

Management

Full neurological and general examination on two occasions. Reassurance and removal of triggers, relaxation and psychological support as for migraine.

Examination of a child with headache

- Level of consciousness
- Neck stiffness
- Measure height and weight (?craniopharyngioma)
- Measure child's head circumference
- Blood pressure with a paediatric cuff
- Skin for café au lait spots of neurofibromatosis
- Visual acuity (reduced in papilloedema, craniopharyngioma, optic glioma)
- Visual fields (**8.1**) (bitemporal loss in cranio- pharyngioma, homonymous in temporal/ parietal/occipital lesions)
- Fundi (for papilloedema)
- Cranial nerves (?brain stem involvement), nystagmus (?posterior fossa lesion)
- Gait – habitual, on toes, on heels, heel to toe (?ataxia, ?hemiparesis)
- Finger-to-nose testing or building tower for younger children (?ataxia)
- Arms outstretched, eyes closed (?pyramidal drift, ?extrapyramidal movements)

Causes of headache

Monophasic illnesses associated with headache

- Headache associated with acute infections in childhood:
  Usually not serious: associated with fever caused by e.g. otitis media, tonsillitis
  Potentially serious: neck stiffness (?meningitis, subarachnoid haemorrhage)
- Headache after head injury:
  Usually benign
  Occasionally associated with microscopic damage to the brain
  Migrainous – may be associated with hemiplegia or cortical blindness

Recurrent headaches

- Migraine
- Tension
- Intracranial hypertension – space occupying lesion; pseudotumour cerebri (benign intracranial hypertension)
- Sleep-disordered breathing

INTRACRANIAL HYPERTENSION

Characteristic features of intracranial pressure

- Nocturnal, waking the child from sleep.
- Early morning.
- Associated with nausea and/or vomiting.
- Focal signs if space-occupying lesion.

Occasional features of intracranial pressure

- Continuous headache.
- Headache later in the day.
- Headache increasing in frequency.

Management

Immediate referral for neuroimaging and possible neurosurgical intervention, especially if visual acuity is reduced (see under 'Cranial nerves').

Causes

- Hydrocephalus.
- Tumours.
- Other space occupying lesions (e.g. abscess, haemorrhage).
- Venous sinus thrombosis (**8.54**).

HYDROCEPHALUS

The presence of an increased amount of cerebrospinal fluid (CSF) under increased pressure, with enlargement of the ventricular system.

ANATOMY

See **8.55**. CSF is produced by the choroid plexuses of the lateral ventricles and circulates through the foramina of Monro, the third ventricle, the aqueduct of Sylvius and the foramina of Luschka and Magendie at the exit of the fourth ventricle, entering the subarachnoid space in the cisterna magna, which is continuous with the spinal subarachnoid space. The fluid passes via the basal and ambiens cisterns to reach the subarachnoid space over the surface of the cerebral hemispheres and the spinal cord, where it is absorbed through the arachnoid villi or granulations into the cerebral venous sinuses.

AETIOLOGY

Obstruction to the flow of CSF at any point, failure of CSF absorption or over-production of CSF.

DEFINITIONS

Communicating hydrocephalus implies that there is no obstruction to CSF flow, but there is either a failure of reabsorption, which is common (e.g. secondary to meningitis or subarachnoid bleeding), or overproduction of CSF (e.g. choroid plexus tumour).

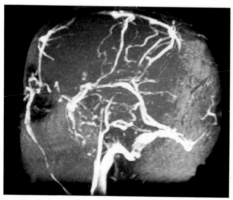

8.54 MR venogram showing sagittal sinus thrombosis in a child with chronic headache on waking. The arrow points to absent flow in the sagittal sinus.

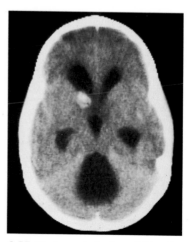

8.55 Hydrocephalus in a child with tuberous sclerosis. All four ventricles are demonstrated.

Non-communicating or obstructive hydro-cephalus is a term used for hydrocephalus due to mechanical obstruction, occasionally at the foramina of Monro, more commonly at the aqueduct of Sylvius, or at the foramina of Luschka and Magendie.

SPECIFIC CAUSES
Congenital malformations
- Congenital aqueduct stenosis. Usually sporadic, occasionally X-linked with adducted thumbs.
- Chiari or Arnold Chiari malformation (8.56). Downward displacement of the medulla and cerebellar tonsils through the foramen magnum, usually associated with open spina bifida.
- Dandy-Walker Syndrome (8.57): The cause is the obstruction of the foramina of Luschka and Magendie during early cerebral development. The cerebellum is hypoplastic and there is a greatly distended fourth ventricle.

Tumours
- Tumours can block the CSF flow at any point, most commonly at the aqueduct of Sylvius, in the fourth ventricle, or at the foramen of Monro.

Inflammation
- Infection. Hydrocephalus may occur after severe meningitis, which can cause adhesions, particularly in the subarachnoid space, thus blocking the reabsorption of CSF. Organisms include bacteria (e.g. *Pneumococcus, Haemophilus influenzae, Mycobacterium tuberculosis* and *Toxoplasma*).
- Bleeding. Hydrocephalus is common after intraventricular bleeding in preterm babies, either secondary to blockage at the aqueduct of Sylvius or to blockage of the absorption channels in the subarachnoid space. Hydrocephalus also occurs after subarachnoid bleeding in older children.

CLINICAL PRESENTATION
- Fetus: obstructed labour
- Neonate: increasing head circumference, separation of the sutures, sunset sign (8.58).
- Older child: symptoms of raised intracranial pressure; night-time or early morning headache; early-morning vomiting; poor visual acuity; papilloedema (see 'Ophthalmology' page 191); ataxia, deterioration in school performance.

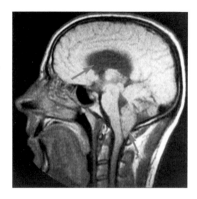

8.56 Chiari malformation with cerebellar tonsillar herniation (lower arrow) and hydrocephalus (upper arrow).

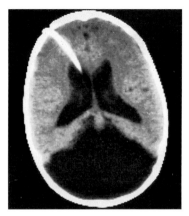

8.57 Dandy-Walker malformation with cerebellar hypoplasia, an enlarged fourth ventricle, and hydrocephalus drained by a shunt (arrow).

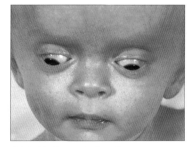

8.58 Hydrocephalus showing 'sunsetting' in an infant.

INVESTIGATIONS

Skull x-ray and shunt series (**8.59**). CT scan. MRI scan for aqueduct anatomy.

MANAGEMENT

- Medical: osmotic diuretics such as isosorbide or acetazolamide are of no benefit and may be harmful.
- Shunt procedures: various types of shunt have been designed, the majority allowing drainage of CSF from the lateral ventricles via a piece of tubing passed underneath the skin into the peritoneum.
- Third ventriculostomy.

SHUNT COMPLICATIONS

- Infection. Low grade pathogens such as *Staphylococcus epidermidis* commonly colonize the shunt during insertion. They continue to divide very slowly and become protected from the natural host defences and from antibiotics by secreting a slime. Children may present years after the original insertion of the shunt with fever, vomiting, headache and symptoms of shunt blockage.
- Blockage. The shunt may block either because it is infected, or because the child has grown so much that the tubing no longer reaches the atrium or the peritoneum.

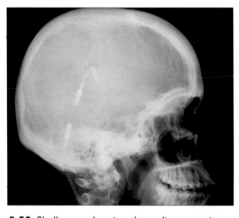

8.59 Skull x-ray showing shunt disconnection.

BRAIN TUMOURS

INCIDENCE

One in 27,000 children. This is the second commonest form of cancer in childhood.

SITE OF TUMOUR

55% are infratentorial (cerebellum or brain stem) in children under 12.

PRESENTATION

Raised intracranial pressure

- Headache (classically in the early morning and often mild).
- Vomiting (classically in the early morning).
- Reduced visual acuity (for methods of testing, see under 'Cranial nerves', page 205).
- Papilloedema (see 'Ophthalmology' chapter, page 191).

Symptoms and signs directly referable to the tumour

- Reduced visual acuity (optic nerve or chiasm glioma; craniopharyngioma [**8.60**]).
- Visual field defect (craniopharyngioma; occipital glioma).
- Ataxia (posterior fossa tumour – truncal suggests medulloblastoma (**8.24**) or brain stem glioma; unilateral suggests cerebellar astrocytoma (**8.61**).
- Head tilt (**8.23**) (posterior fossa tumour).
- Cranial nerve signs (brain stem glioma, VI+VII –(**8.10**) diffuse fibrillary pontine glioma: lateral gaze palsy – pilocytic pontine lesion).
- Hemiplegia (thalamic glioma; cortical glioma; brain stem glioma).
- Epilepsy (supratentorial astrocytoma, oligodendroglioma, ependymoma).
- Parinaud syndrome (tumour in the pineal region) – upgaze paralysis, retraction nystagmus, dissociation pupillary response to light and accommodation.
- Diencephalic syndrome (**8.62**) (hypothalamic glioma) – emaciation, accelerated skeletal growth, hypotension, hypoglycaemia, hyperactivity.
- Precocious puberty (hypothalamic glioma).
- Diabetes insipidus (craniopharyngioma [**8.60**]).

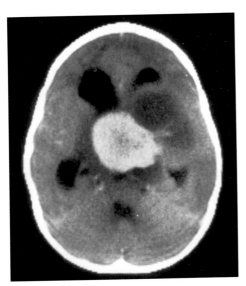

8.60 CT scan showing craniopharyngioma.

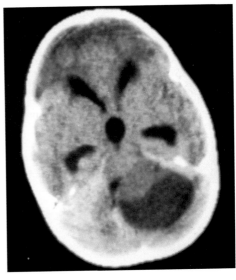

8.61 CT scan showing a cystic astrocytoma in one lobe of the cerebellum.

MANAGEMENT

- Surgery: is always undertaken if possible – total excision, partial excision, or biopsy. It may be impossible if the site of the lesion means that surgery would cause extensive brain damage.
- Radiotherapy – local, or whole craniospinal axis. This is usually avoided if the patient is under the age of three years because of the neurodevelopmental sequelae.
- Chemotherapy is useful for very malignant tumours, because drugs kill rapidly growing cells (e.g. medulloblastoma and malignant astrocytoma of the cerebrum). It is used as an adjunct to surgery and radiotherapy if excision is incomplete or there is a relapse. It is also used in the very young (<3 years) to postpone or avoid the need for radiotherapy.

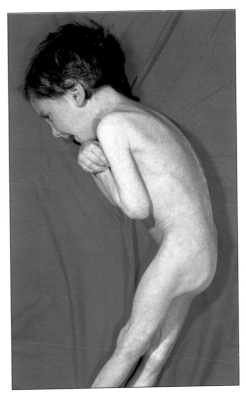

8.62 Extreme wasting in the diencephalic syndrome.

COMMON BRAIN TUMOURS IN CHILDREN

See also 'Solid Tumours and Histiocytosis' chapter.

INFRATENTORIAL (see 'Ataxia' page 216)

Medulloblastoma (8.24)

A mid-line tumour presenting with truncal ataxia and signs and symptoms of raised intracranial pressure. It seeds down the neuraxis via the CSF, so there may be spinal cord dysfunction at presentation. The five-year survival rate with surgery, radiotherapy and chemotherapy is about 55%..

Astrocytoma (8.61)

Arises in the mid-line of the cerebellum but usually extends into the cerebellar hemisphere on one side. On imaging, the majority have a cyst with a tumour nodule in the wall; histologically these are pilocytic (benign). Management is mainly surgical and prognosis is usually good, with 94% 25-year survival in one series. Diffuse or fibrillary tumours have a less good prognosis and require radiotherapy.

Ependymoma

Arises from the lining of the ventricle, histology variable. May spread along CSF pathways and occasionally outside the CNS. Treated with surgery alone if possible; radiotherapy is required if excision is incomplete or tumour is malignant.

Brain-stem glioma

The prognosis for diffuse fibrillary glioma is very poor indeed, with survival usually less than one year. Radiotherapy and chemotherapy offer palliation. Focal pilocytic glioma may be cured by resection.

SUPRATENTORIAL

Craniopharyngioma (8.62)

Arises from the Rathke's pouch (buccal epithelium). Often solid and cystic components. Tumour is slow growing but may be diagnosed late if visual acuity and fields are not tested in children with headache. Surgical excision is curative if the tumour not large; radiotherapy is required if complete excision would jeopardize carotid arteries, optic nerves or hypothalamus. Survival is excellent if total removal is achieved, but children often have endocrine sequelae (e.g. diabetes insipidus, hypothyroidism or inadequate corticosteroid production, requiring appropriate replacement.

Optic glioma (8.63)

Thirty to forty percent of patients have neurofibromatosis type 1. Treatment is controversial. Surgery is usually required for anterior optic nerve tumours with complete visual loss. A conservative approach is warranted if visual loss is minimal. Radiotherapy and/or chemotherapy are then instituted if vision deteriorates.

Glioma

Surgery alone is sufficient if it is pilocytic (benign) and accessible; radiotherapy and/or chemotherapy if it is fibrillary (malignant) or in eloquent territory (e.g. the thalamus, **8.64**).

Primitive neuroectodermal tumours

These are highly malignant, with a tendency to seed (similar to infratentorial medulloblastoma) and usually present under the age of 5 years (see 'Urology' chapter). Treatment is usually radical surgery plus chemotherapy with or without radiotherapy.

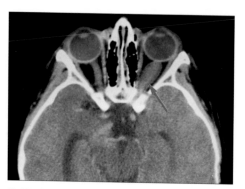

8.63 Optic glioma. CT scan.

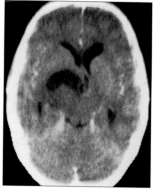

8.64 Thalamic glioma. CT scan.

PROGNOSIS

This depends on the site of the lesion, its histology and on whether or not total excision can be performed. Over half of children with brain tumours survive for more than five years and are considered to be cured.

The quality of life is often compromized by learning difficulties following radiotherapy as well as neurological disability (most commonly ataxia, visual impairment or epilepsy). Endocrine deficits may be the result of tumour, surgery and/or radiotherapy. Abnormalities such as growth hormone deficiency and hypothyroidism may be late effects; careful long-term monitoring is essential.

MACROCEPHALY

CAUSES

- Familial.
- Ex-premature infant.
- Hydrocephalus (**8.55–8.59**).
- Subdural haemorrhage or effusion (**8.65**).
- Glutaric aciduria type I.
- Degenerative (**8.66**):
  – Alexander's disease;
  – Canavan's disease (N-acetylaspartic aciduria).

PSEUDOTUMOUR CEREBRI (BENIGN INTRACRANIAL HYPERTENSION)

CLINICAL FEATURES

Features include headaches characteristic of intracranial hypertension and papilloedema (not essential for diagnosis) (see under Ophthalmology). There can be reduced visual acuity (in association with papilloedema) and smell, as well as visual field abnormalities (enlarged blind spot, reduced nasal field with papilloedema) and VI palsy (not essential for diagnosis) (**8.7**, page 208).

MANAGEMENT

Neuroimaging to exclude space-occupying lesion and venous sinus thrombosis. Lumbar puncture under sedation to measure pressure and remove CSF to reduce it. Medical treatment includes steroids and acetazolamide, as well as anticoagulation for venous sinus thrombosis. Frequent ophthalmological/ neurological follow-up. ICP monitoring for decision on Lumboperitoneal shunting if headaches are intractable. Optic nerve fenestration may be required if there is visual deterioration.

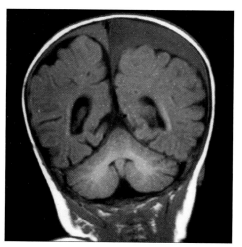

8.65 MRI showing bilateral subdural effusions and communicating hydrocephalus in a baby who was non-accidentally shaken. Cranial ultrasound is not sufficient to exclude this diagnosis. The advantage of MRI over CT is that the likely number and timing of injury/ies may be established, as effusions of different ages have different densities on the scan.

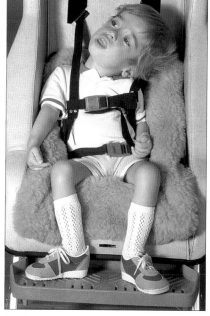

8.66 Macrocephaly in a child with progressive disease.

LEARNING DIFFICULTIES

The majority of children with learning difficulties make steady progress through their developmental milestones but at a slower speed than normal. Developmental slowing, arrest or regression is more likely to be caused by a treatable condition (e.g. epilepsy, hydrocephalus, or sleep apnoea) than by a degenerative disease, although it is important to take a careful history and to perform a full physical examination to exclude the latter.

A detailed developmental assessment should be undertaken to determine the cognitive profile, as the causes of specific learning difficulties (for example, in language) may be different from those causing global delay. In some cases the cognitive profile may be specific for the underlying diagnosis (e.g. relatively well-preserved verbal ability in children with Williams syndrome, **8.67**). Parents may find the associated behavioural difficulties (e.g. hyperactivity or behaviour within the autistic spectrum) more difficult to deal with than the learning difficulties.

Certain children with learning difficulties may have cerebral palsy (see page 227), with implications for aetiology and therapy. Serial measurement of head circumference is important from the diagnostic point of view, as microcephaly recognized at birth is very likely to be recessively inherited (see appropriate section), while acquired microcephaly may be due to birth asphyxia (**8.68**) or Rett syndrome (**8.69**).

Some children with learning difficulties have dysmorphic features (**8.70 – 8.73**), which may be diagnostic. Those with neurocutaneous stigmata (see sections on Neurofibromatosis, Tuberous sclerosis, Epilepsy) may have other associated problems, such as epilepsy or the risk of malignancy. Epilepsy should be managed carefully, as frequent fits may reduce the child's potential for learning.

ESSENTIAL INVESTIGATIONS

Chromosomes (**8.74**), including fragile X. If a diagnosis (e.g. Angelman syndrome – see under Epilepsy, **8.83**) is considered likely clinically, more specific genetic investigation is often appropriate. Metabolic investigations suggested by clinical features (e.g. mucopolysaccharides – **8.75**). EEG if epilepsy. Neuroimaging has a low yield unless there is epilepsy or a specific syndrome (e.g. Joubert – **8.76**).

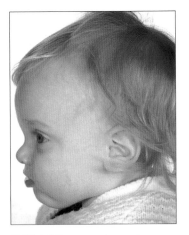

8.67 Williams syndrome in an infant.

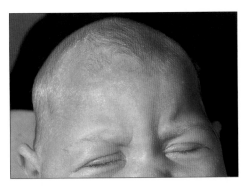

8.68 Acquired microcephaly in a child asphyxiated at birth.

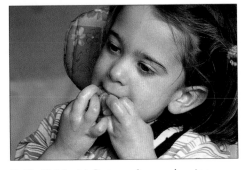

8.68 Child with Rett syndrome, showing characteristic hand involvement.

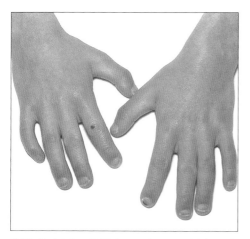

8.70 Smith-Lemli-Opitz syndrome, with broad space between thumb and first finger.

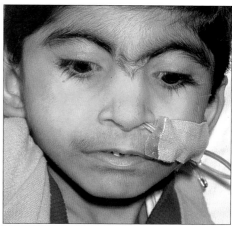

8.71 Cornelia de Lange syndrome with prominent eyebrows.

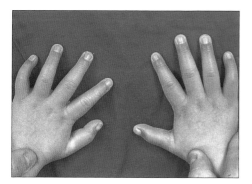

8.72 Coffin-Lowry syndrome with tapering fingers.

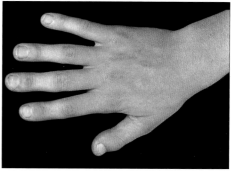

8.73 Rubinstein-Taybi syndrome with broad thumbs.

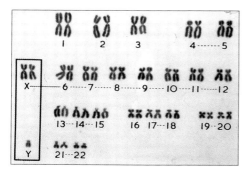

8.74 Klinefelter syndrome. Chromosomes showing an extra X chromosome in a boy who presented with language delay.

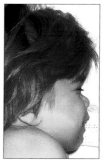

8.75 Hurler syndrome with coarse hair.

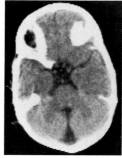

8.76 Joubert syndrome (abnormal eye movements, intermittent hyperpnoea and apnoea, hypotonia, ataxia). CT shows cerebellar vermis agenesis.

EPILEPSY

PREVALENCE
Affects 1/200 children; up to 25% intractable.

CAUSES
Neonate
Hypoglycaemia; hypocalcaemia; hyponatraemia; hypernatraemia; infection – meningitis, systemic; birth asphyxia; birth trauma; intraventricular haemorrhage; drug withdrawal; stroke – venous sinus thrombosis, arterial; structural brain malformations (e.g. lissencephaly), cortical dysplasia; metabolic conditions (e.g. hyperglycinaemia); pyridoxine deficiency/dependency); biotinidase deficiency (see 'Metabolic Diseases' chapter); peroxisomal disorders; mitochondrial disorders; Menkes' kinky hair disease (**8.77**).

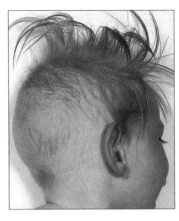

8.77 Menkes' kinky hair disease.

Child
Primary/secondary tumour – glioma; dysembryoblastic neuroepithelial tumour (**8.78**); structural brain malformation – neuronal migration defects, such as lissencephaly, double cortex, polymicrogyria, or hemimegalencephaly – hippocampal sclerosis (**8.79**), tuberous sclerosis (see 'Genetics' chapter), or other neurocutaneous syndromes such as hypomelanosis of Ito (**8.80**), linear sebaceous naevus, or incontinentia pigmenti (**8.81**); Sturge-Weber syndrome (**8.82**); genetic syndromes (e.g. Angelman – **8.83**); metabolic (e.g. mitochondrial, glucose transporter deficiency).

CLASSIFICATION OF SEIZURES
- Focal.
- Generalized: absence/tonic-clonic/tonic/akinetic/myoclonic.
- Unclassified.

It is usually important to classify syndrome as well as seizures in children (see table).

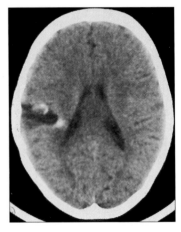

8.78 CT scan showing dysembryo-plastic neuroepithelial tumour in a child presenting with complex partial seizures. Although there was no increase in the size of the lesion on serial neuroimaging, it was removed after workup for epilepsy surgery and the patient became seizure-free.

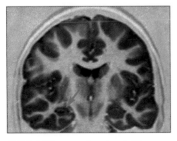

8.79 MRI scan showing R hippocampus with signal change and atrophy compatible with hippocampal sclerosis (arrow). Around 70% are seizure-free after surgery.

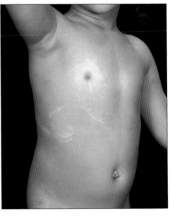

8.80 Hypomelanosis of Ito.

Common seizures syndromes in childhood

Name	Age onset	Seizures	EEG	Treatment
Febrile convulsions	6m–5y	Generalized tonic-clonic	Not necessary	Rectal diazepam only
Childhood absence	3–12y	Absence+/-automatism	3Hz spike + wave	Ethosuximide, Valproate
Myoclonic absence	1–12y	Absence+myoclonic jerk	3Hz spike + wave	Valproate, Lamotrigine
Absence + eyelid myoclonia	2–5y	Absence+myoclonia eyelid	High amplitude spikes/slow	Valproate+ ethosuximide
Juvenile myoclonic epilepsy	3-18y	Absence, myoclonic jerks, generalized tonic-clonic	Multi-spike with fragmentation	Valproate, Lamotrigine, Topiramate
Benign Rolandic	1–12y	Focal motor with oro-pharyngeal manifestation	Rolandic spikes	Carbamezepine
Benign occipital	1–10y	Nocturnal vomiting, eye deviation, coma	Occipit. paroxysms high amp spike/wave	Carbamezepine
Infantile spasms	3–18m	Brief spasms in runs – awake	Hypsarrythmia	Steroids, Vigabatrin
Severe myoclonic of infancy	3–12m	Early, prolonged, lateralized febrile convulsions, myoclonic, absence		Valproate, Clobazam Stiripentol
Landau-Kleffner	2–5y	Loss comprehension, occasional seizures	Generalized abnormality asleep	Prednisolone Valproate
Lennox-Gastaut	2–5y	Absence, akinetic, tonic, generalized tonic-clonic	1–2.5Hz spike + wave	Valproate, Lamotrigine, Topiramate
Myoclonic-astatic	2–4y	Absence, akinetic	2.5–3Hz spike + wave	Valproate, Lamotrigine

8.81 Incontinentia pigmenti in an older child who had blisters in the neonatal period.

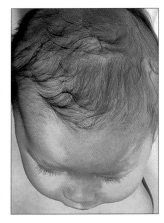

8.82 A capillary haemangioma in the ophthalmic division of the fifth cranial nerve; Sturge-Weber syndrome is diagnosed when there is underlying pial angioma over the surface of the brain. this may lead to epilepsy, contralateral hemiparesis and learning difficulties. Epilepsy surgery (e.g. hemispherectomy) may improve behaviour and learning as well as seizures if epilepsy is severe.

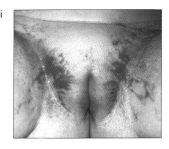

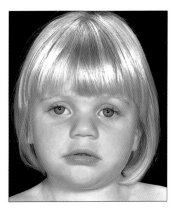

8.83 Angelman syndrome.

CLINICAL EXAMINATION

- History taking to establish seizure type and seizure syndrome, family history, pregnancy and birth, development, and progress at school.
- Examination, particularly looking for abnormal head size, neurocutaneous syndromes, focal signs (e.g. mild upper motor neurone VII – see under 'Cranial nerves'), or mild hemiparesis (see under 'Motor system').
- EEG – initially while the patient is awake and, if this is not diagnostic, sleep-deprived or asleep. Video telemetry may be required for surgical candidates, patients who may have non-epileptic seizures and in other cases where the diagnosis of epilepsy is uncertain; seizures may then be documented synchronously on EEG (**8.84**) and video.
- Neuroimaging is unnecessary if the patient has easily-controlled primary generalized epilepsy or a clinical history and an EEG compatible with a benign partial epilepsy syndrome. Magnetic resonance imaging (MRI) (**8.79**) is usually preferred as the diagnostic rate is much higher; specific sequences may be required, such as coronal cuts through the temporal lobes (**8.79**). Computed tomography (CT) is occasionally useful to demonstrate calcification, for example in tuberous sclerosis or Sturge-Weber syndrome. Positron emission tomography (PET) and single photon emission tomography (SPECT) (**8.85**) are usually reserved for patients who are surgical candidates.
- CSF for glycine, lactate and glucose.

MANAGEMENT

- No regular treatment, e.g. for occasional generalized tonic-clonic seizures, but a benzodiazepine, e.g. buccal midazolam, should be available.
- Anticonvulsants.
- Ketogenic diet.
- Surgery. Resection for focal lesions (e.g. temporal lobectomy or amygdalo-hippocampectomy to remove dysplastic and/or scarred tissue, removal of cortical dysembryoplastic neuroectodermal tumour, hemispherectomy). Corpus callosotomy is usually reserved for intractable drop attacks.
- Vagal nerve stimulation.
- Appropriate education and family support.

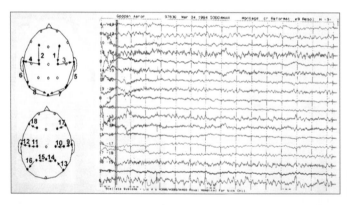

8.84 EEG at the onset of a seizure.

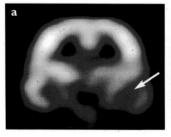
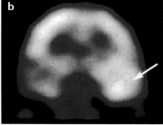

8.85 Interictal **(a)** and ictal **(b)** SPECT scans showing relative hypoperfusion in the temporal lobe interictally and hyperperfusion ictally.

NEUROLOGICAL AND COGNITIVE DETERIORATION

The majority of children who deteriorate neurologically and cognitively do not have a recognizable degenerative disease.

LIKELY CAUSES

- Epilepsy, either clinically obvious or unrecognized (see 'Epilepsy', page 240). May be associated with cognitive deterioration, aphasia (Landau-Kleffner syndrome), autistic regression, or hemiparesis.
- Hydrocephalus. May be associated with cognitive deterioration and/or ataxic diplegia.
- Malnutrition.
- Sleep apnoea
- Psychosocial deprivation.
- Physical or sexual abuse.

CAUSES IN SPECIFIC CONDITIONS

- Sickle cell disease. Subclinical infarction (8.86, 8.87). See 'Stroke', page 249.
- Cerebral palsy. Epilepsy, hydrocephalus, cervical cord damage (causes deteriorating pyramidal function), or vertebrobasilar dissection (causes recurrent strokes) in athetoid cerebral palsy with constant head movement.

Tests for children with progressive conditions

- Sleep study
- EEG (awake and asleep)
- Urine for metachromatic granules
- Blood film to look for evidence of storage in lymphocytes
- CT and/or MRI head and ?spine, MRA, MRV
- Plasma lactate
- Plasma amino acids
- Urine organic acids
- Plasma ammonia
- CSF lactate, glucose, measles antibodies, neurotransmitters
- Electroretinogram, visual evoked potentials
- Nerve conduction
- Very long-chain fatty acids
- White cell enzymes
- Skin biopsy
- DNA for the appropriate mutation

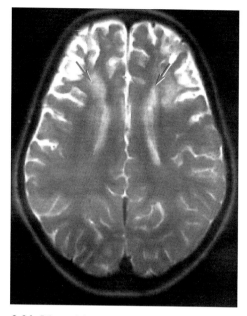

8.86 Bilateral frontal infarction in a child with sickle cell disease.

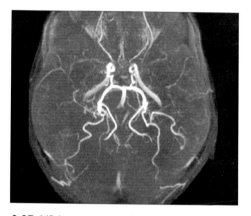

8.87 MRA arteriogram showing bilateral occlusion of the distal internal carotid arteries in a child with sickle cell disease. Moyamoya collateral is not obvious on this scan but may be seen on MRA or conventional angiography in patients with severe stenosis or occlusion.

COMMON CONDITIONS WITH NEUROLOGICAL DETERIORATION

MULTIPLE SCLEROSIS (MS)

MS is rare in childhood, and uncommon in adolescence (2.7% of all cases present <16 years). Although usually relapsing–remitting, it is occasionally chronic progressive. Presents with sensory symptoms, optic neuritis (but most cases of optic neuritis do not have MS), diplopia and motor disturbance. MS has an unpredictable course.

Diagnosis

MRI abnormality (**8.88**). CSF oligoclonal bands in 85% of cases. Abnormal evoked potentials. Elevated myelin basic protein.

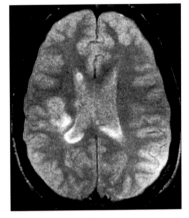

8.88 Multiple sclerosis: demyelination.

Treatment

Steroids improve the recovery rate after a relapse. β-interferon decreases the frequency of attacks in relapsing-remitting MS.

ADRENOLEUKODYSTROPHY

X-linked gene at Xq28 coding for peroxisomal membrane protein. Onset commonly between the ages of four and eight years. Deterioration in gait with cognitive decline and pyramidal, extrapyramidal and cerebellar signs. Adrenocortical insufficiency in about 10% of cases (pigmentation is very rare, **8.89**).

Diagnosis

Neuroimaging – white matter abnormality (**8.90**). Elevated very long-chain fatty acids. DNA testing.

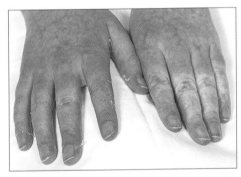

8.89 Adrenoleukodystrophy: pigmentation of the hands.

Management

Steroid replacement therapy for adrenal insuffiency. Dietary manipulation for asymptomatic patients (under investigation). Bone marrow transplant for early symptomatic (but there is 30% mortality). Symptomatic management for those with advanced neurological manifestations.

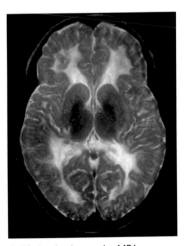

8.90 Leukodystrophy. MRI showing abnormal white matter in a child with a progressive movement disorder.

KRABBE'S (GLOBOID CELL) LEUKODYSTROPHY

Autosomal recessive gene on 14q coding for β-galactocerebrosidase. The infantile form is commonest but it may present at later ages. Clinical signs include restlessness, irritability, progressive pyramidal and extrapyramidal hypertonia and reduced reflexes.

Diagnosis

High CSF protein and prolonged nerve conduction velocities. Neuroimaging often non-specific (usually not white matter abnormality). β-galactosidase is present in white cells.

METACHROMATIC LEUKODYSTROPHY

Autosomal recessive gene on 22q coding for cerebroside sulfatase. There are infantile and juvenile forms:

- Infantile (0–25 months): irritability; gait disturbance; spasticity in legs; reduced tendon reflexes.
- Juvenile (4–10 years):mental regression; movement disorder (mixed pyramidal and peripheral neuropathy (**8.91**); seizures.

Diagnosis

Urinary metachromatic granules. Nerve conduction velocities prolonged. High CSF protein. Neuroimaging shows periventricular white matter abnormality. Low arylsulfatase A in white cells.

CEROID LIPOFUSCINOSES (INFANTILE – SANTAVOURI)

Affects infants aged from 6 to 12 months, causing developmental regression and ataxia. The patient has stereotyped hand movements, with progressive microcephaly, and optic atrophy.

Diagnosis

Extinguished ERG. Progressive slowing and flattening on EEG. Cerebral atrophy on neuroimaging. Autosomal recessive CLN1 gene on chromosome 1p coding for palmitoyl protein thioesterase.

CEROID LIPOFUSCINOSES (LATE INFANTILE – JANSKI-BIELSCHOWSKY)

Affects children between 18 months and 4 years, causing developmental regression, ataxia, and eventually epilepsy and macular and retinal degeneration.

Diagnosis

EEG shows spike in response to photic stimulation synchronous with flash. ERG extinguished (not necessarily at presentation). Skin shows curvilinear bodies in cytosomes. Autosomal recessive CLN2 gene on chromosome 11 codes for a lysosomal peptidase

CEROID LIPOFUSCINOSES (JUVENILE – BATTEN'S)

Affects children between 4 and 7 years of age, causing progressive visual loss and behavioural disturbance, with slow cognitive deterioration. Dysarthria, and extrapyramidal, pyramidal and cerebellar signs gradually supervene.

Diagnosis

Vacuolated lymphocytes in peripheral blood. EEG shows pseudoperiodic bursts of slow waves. ERG and VEP decreased. Atrophy and calcification on neuroimaging. Skin shows fingerprint profiles. Autosomal recessive gene on chromosome 16 coding for a novel protein.

Management of all ceroid lipofuscinoses

Seizure control (lamotrigine, sodium valproate). Management of progressive movement disorder (see under 'Cerebral Palsy'), visual loss and behavioural problems.

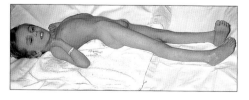

8.91 Metachromatic leukodystrophy. Quadriparesis in a child with peripheral neuropathy.

TAY SACH'S DISEASE

Autosomal recessive gene on chromosome 15 causing hexosaminidase A deficiency. Common in Ashkenazi Jews.

Clinical signs

The patient is startled by loud noises, with developmental regression, hypotonia, then hypertonia and seizures. A cherry-red spot at the macula is a characteristic early sign (**8.92**).

Diagnosis

White cell hexosaminidase A.

NIEMANN–PICK DISEASE TYPE C

Autosomal recessive (95% are homozygous for NCP1 gene on chromosome 18); lysosomal cholesterol storage.

Clinical signs

Poor school progress, ataxia, hepatomegaly, vertical gaze palsy (**8.93**).

LEIGH'S DISEASE

Mitochondrial disorders (pyruvate carboxylase deficiency, pyruvate dehydrogenase deficiency, respiratory chain enzyme deficiencies).

Clinical signs

Progressive movement disorders, usually extra-pyramidal. Ptosis and ophthalmoplegia. Seizures.

Diagnosis

Neuroimaging shows low density in putaminae and caudate (**8.94**). Raised blood and CSF lactate. Blood for mitochondrial mutations. Open muscle biopsy for respiratory chain enzymes. Skin biopsy for pyruvate dehydrogenase deficiency and respiratory chain enzymes.

COMA AND ACUTE ENCEPHALOPATHIES

CAUSES

- Accidental head injury: extradural haematoma (**8.95**); intracerebral haematoma; penetration (e.g. gunshot wound); diffuse brain oedema (**8.96**).
- Non-accidental injury: subdural haemorrhage/effusion (see under 'Macrocephaly', **8.65**); stroke – spontaneous intracerebral haemorrhage; hemispheric ischaemia secondary to carotid occlusion; posterior fossa stroke; venous sinus thrombosis (**8.97**) diffuse brain oedema.
- Infections: meningitis – *pneumococcus, haemophilus, meningococcus,* tuberculous (**8.98**); encephalitis – herpes simplex, enteroviruses, mycoplasma; cerebral abscess (**8.99**); cerebral malaria (**8.100**).

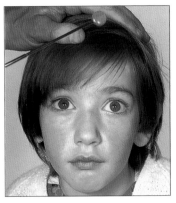

8.93 Difficulty in looking up in a patient with Niemann-Pick type C.

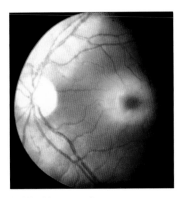

8.92 Cherry-red spot.

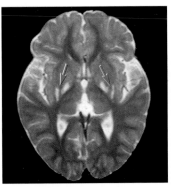

8.94 Leigh's disease. MRI.

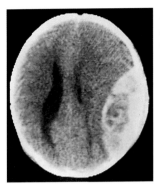

8.95 CT scan showing L extradural haematoma.

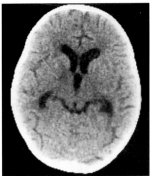

8.98 CT scan showing characteristic hydrocephalus and small right internal capsule lesion (arrow) in a child with tuberculous meningitis and a hemiplegia.

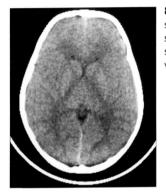

8.96 CT scan showing brain swelling with small ventricles.

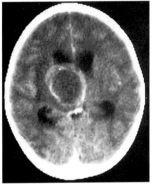

8.99 Contrast CT scan showing ring enhancement in cerebral abscess.

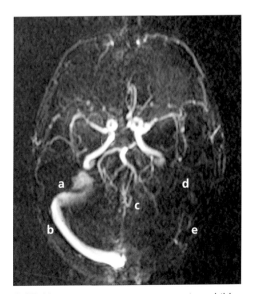

8.97 Magnetic resonance venogram in a child with sickle cell disease, presenting with seizures and coma after two weeks of headache and vomiting. The right sigmoid (a) and transverse sinus (b) can be clearly seen, while the straight sinus (c) and left sigmoid and transverse sinuses (d, e) have been obliterated.

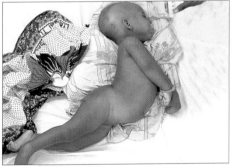

8.100 Extensor posturing in a child with cerebral malaria.

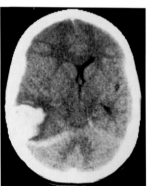

8.101 Purpuric rash in meningococcal septicaemia.

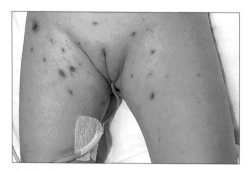

8.102 Hypertensive fundus with a macular star and papilloedema.

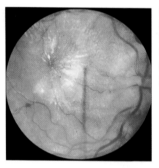

8.103 CT scan showing intracerebral haemorrhage with midline shift.

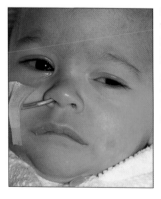

8.104 Left third nerve palsy with ptosis and eye 'down and out' in an infant with left hemispheric swelling.

- Shock: meningococcal sepsis (**8.101**); toxic shock syndrome (staphylococcus); haemorrhagic shock/encephalopathy.
- Diabetic encephalopathy – ketotic. Diffuse brain oedema may worsen after treatment.
- Drug-induced coma/poisoning.
- Status epilepticus.
- Hypertensive encephalopathy (**8.102**) – preceded by visual symptoms and seizures.
- Hypoxic–ischaemic encephalopathy.
- Hepatic encephalopathy. Mild encephalo-pathy accompanied by foetor/flap. Viral hepatitis.
- Space-occupying mass: spontaneous intracerebral haemorrhage (**8.103**); arterial stroke – large hemispheric or brainstem; venous sinus thrombosis; tumour.

EMERGENCY MANAGEMENT

- Secure airway, treat shock, measure and maintain blood pressure, stop seizures.
- Assess level of consciousness using paediatric modification of Glasgow coma scale (main differences from adult version are in verbal scale).
- Patient should be ventilated electively if Glasgow coma score <12 or deteriorating level of consciousness or signs of central or uncal herniation.
- Assess brain stem function for signs of central or uncal herniation: posturing – extensor (**8.100**) or flexor; pupillary size, symmetry, reaction to light; oculocephalic (Doll's eye) reflex (provided there is no neck trauma); oculovestibular (caloric) reflex; unilateral ptosis and/or eye down and out and/or large fixed pupil and/or contralateral hemiparesis suggests uncal herniation (**8.104**).
- Immediate investigations include blood glucose, chemistry including liver function tests, ammonia, full blood count, blood cultures, urine drug screen.
- Immediate treatment may include antibiotics if fever, aciclovir particularly if there are seizures.
- Emergency neuroimaging and referral to neurosurgical unit if there is a space-occupying lesion.

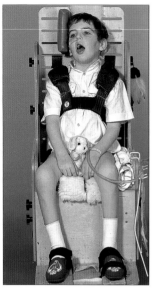

8.105 Flaccid quadriparesis and locked-in state in a child recovering from coma. CT scan showed cerebellar and occipital infarction. He appeared to be locked in for 6 months but eventually recovered, although he had a visual field deficit.

STROKE

INCIDENCE
One in 15,000 children (half haemorrhagic, half ischaemic).

CONDITIONS PREDISPOSING TO ARTERIAL STROKE
These include sickle cell disease (**8.86**, **8.87**), cardiac disease, and homocystinuria (**8.106**).

Approximately 50% of children have no previously diagnosed underlying condition. Fifteen percent of children presenting with acute focal neurological signs suggestive of arterial ischaemic stroke have alternative aetiologies, e.g. cerebral venous sinus thrombosis (**8.54**, **8.99**), hemiplegic migraine, metabolic disease (e.g. mitochondrial cytopathy or ornithine carbamoyl transferase deficiency).

- Establish cause if CT normal. It is safer to delay lumbar puncture if patient is deeply unconscious (Glasgow coma score <12) or has signs suggesting cerebral herniation. Bacterial meningitis may be diagnosed by rapid antigen screening at delayed lumbar puncture after antimicrobial therapy; tuberculous meningitis is usually accompanied by communicating hydrocephalus (**8.97**) but must be excluded (Ziehl-Nielsen, polymerase chain reaction) or treated.
- Continue fluids – maintenance post-resuscitation; avoid hypo osmolar fluids and fluid restriction. Mannitol may be given if patient is not shocked or dehydrated and does not have an intracranial haemorrhage.

PROGNOSIS
This may be extremely difficult to predict accurately (**8.105**) and should only be attempted by experienced doctors with as many ancillary investigations as possible. Although improving level of consciousness and preserved EEG do not guarantee a good outcome, prolonged deep coma with a low amplitude EEG almost always predicts severe handicap, persistent vegetative state or death.

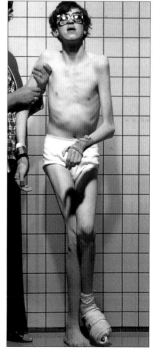
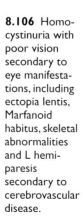

8.106 Homocystinuria with poor vision secondary to eye manifestations, including ectopia lentis, Marfanoid habitus, skeletal abnormalities and L hemiparesis secondary to cerebrovascular disease.

RISK FACTORS FOR ISCHAEMIC STROKE IN CHILDHOOD

Infection (chickenpox, tonsillitis, *Mycoplasma* or *Chlamydia*); head or neck trauma (arterial dissection) (**8.107**, **8.108**); hyperhomocysteinaemia; prothrombotic disorders (e.g. Factor V Leiden, antiphospholipid syn drome – more evidence for role in venous thrombosis); hyperlipidaemia – cholesterol or lipoprotein (a); hypoxaemia and reactive polycythaemia in sickle cell disease and cyanotic congenital heart disease; immunodeficiency (e.g. HIV).

CLINICAL SIGNS

History – rapidity of onset (sudden suggests embolus, stuttering suggests thrombotic occlusion of underlying cerebrovascular disease), known medical conditions, recent illnesses (e.g. chickenpox, recent head trauma major or minor – predisposes to arterial dissection), family history. Examination – level of consciousness (see under coma), distribution and severity of weakness, facial involvement, associated features.

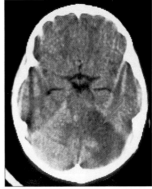

8.109 CT scan of a patient presenting in coma (8.105), illustrating the left cerebellar infarct.

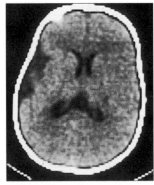

8.110 Residual cortical damage in a child who presented with stroke in the neonatal period.

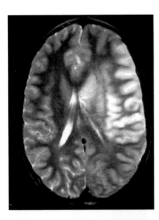

8.107 Large infarct with midline shift in the right middle cerebral territory in a child who sustained a carotid dissection (see also 8.108, 8.113).

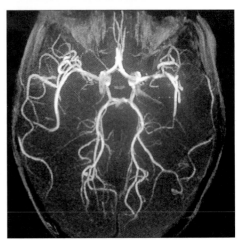

8.111 MRA showing turbulence in the proximal middle cerebral artery (arrow), probably secondary to chicken pox.

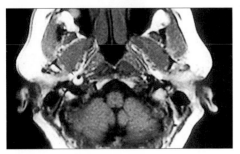

8.108 Axial fat saturated T'-weighted MRI of the neck shows blood in the wall (arrow) characteristic of dissection.

INVESTIGATIONS

- Neuroimaging. Haemorrhage must be excluded by CT, (**8.102**) which may demonstrate infarction (**8.107**, **8.109**), or MRI. MRI detects smaller ischaemic lesions in symptomatic and asymptomatic high risk patients (**8.86**) and is particularly useful for separating ischaemic stroke from alternative pathologies. MR angiography (MRA) allows diagnosis of some of the possible underlying cerebrovascular abnormalities (e.g. demonstrating turbulence or occlusion in the distal internal carotid or proximal middle cerebral arteries (**8.87**, **8.111**). MR venography may demonstrate occlusion of the large venous sinuses (e.g. in sagittal or straight sinus thrombosis) (**8.54**, **8.99**). Arteriography may be used to diagnose arteriovenous malformations (**8.112**) or aneurysms in patients with haemorrhage or to delineate the cause of stroke in ischaemic cases if MRA is normal or not diagnostic (e.g. in arterial dissection (**8.113**) or small vessel vasculitis).
- ECG and echocardiography, although relatively few children with stroke have previously unrecognized cardiac abnormalities.
- Screening for underlying prothrombotic and metabolic disorders which might predispose to recurrent stroke (activated protein C resistance; DNA testing for factor V Leiden, thermolabile methylene tetrahydrofolate reductase and prothrombin 20210; plasma total homocysteine; anticardiolipin antibodies and lupus anticoagulant; cholesterol; immunodeficiency, nocturnal hypoxaemia). There is little important evidence for a link between deficiencies of protein C, protein S, antithrombin III, heparin cofactor II or plasminogen and arterial stroke in childhood, but the tests may be worth doing in patients with cerebral venous sinus thrombosis

MANAGEMENT

- Acute presentation. Urgent transfer to a centre with neurosurgical and paediatric neurological facilities enables rapid decompression of haemorrhage or massive cerebral infarction if necessary and may also allow emergency management of ischaemic stroke in selected patients after MR imaging (e.g. anticoagulation for venous sinus thrombosis or arterial dissection). Aspirin reduces early recurrence in arterial stroke in adults and at low dose (5 mg/kg), the risk of Reye syndrome is less than the risk of recurrence, although there are no data on efficacy in childhood. Thrombolysis improves outcome for arterial stroke in adults if commenced within three hours and may be worth considering for stroke occuring in hospital (e.g. in the context of congenital heart disease) although a recent procedure is a contraindication.

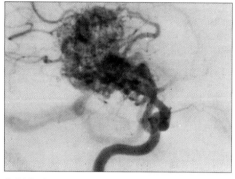

8.112 Arteriogram showing arteriovenous malformation in a child with an acute spontaneous intracerebral haemorrhage.

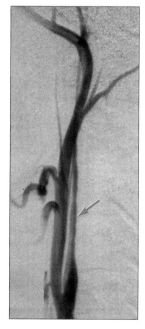

8.113 Arteriogram showing the typical 'rat-tail' dissection of the internal carotid artery in a child who presented in a coma with a very large right middle cerebral artery territory infarct. He had a previous history of hemiplegic migraine but developed this episode of hemiparesis a few days after falling from his skateboard. Fat-saturated MRI of the neck may demonstrate the additional lumen in this condition.

- Prevention of recurrence. Although there are no population-based data, recurrent stroke occurs in at least 10% of hospital based series of paediatric ischaemic stroke. Folate, B_6 and B_{12} supplementation may reduce homocysteine levels, carries no known risk and is probably a reasonable addition to low dose aspirin prophylaxis. Anticoagulation with warfarin for 3–6 months should be considered for those with venous sinus thrombosis, arterial dissection or, more controversially, for the relatively few children with Factor V Leiden, prothrombin 20210, anti-cardiolipin antibodies >100 international units or lupus anticoagulant. Regular transfusion to maintain the haemoglobin S percentage below 30% is the only evidence-based method of preventing recurrent stroke in sickle cell disease, and appears to have a role in primary prevention, although it is often poorly tolerated by the patient. Increasing fruit/vegetable intake and exercise, and correction of chronic hypoxaemia (e.g. corrective surgery for cyanotic congenital heart disease, adeno-tonsillectomy or oxygen supplementation for those with sleep-disordered breathing – for example, patients with sickle cell disease) may be important.

REFERENCES

Aicardi J, Gillberg C, Ogier H, Bax M. *Diseases of the Nervous System in Childhood* (3rd edition). London: MacKeith Press 2005.

Aicardi J, Arzimanoglou A, Guerrini R. *Aicardi's Epilepsy in Children*. Lippincott Williams and Wilkins 2003.

Alper G, Narayanan V. Friedreich's ataxia. *Pediatr Neurol.* 2003; **28**: 335–341.

Brewer GJ, Askari FK. Wilson's disease: clinical management and therapy. *J Hepatol.* 2005; **42** Suppl(1): S13–21.

Callenbach PM, van den Maagdenberg AM, Frants RR, Brouwer OF. Clinical and genetic aspects of idiopathic epilepsies in childhood. *Eur J Paediatr Neurol.* 2005; **9**: 91–103.

Cohen ME, Kressel P. *Weiner and Levitt's Pediatric Neurology* (House Officer Series) .

Dubowitz V. *A Colour Atlas of Muscle Disorders in Childhood*. London: Wolfe Medical Publications Ltd, 1989.

Eyre JA. *Coma*. Baillière's Clinical Paediatrics. London: Baillière Tindall 1994.

Guerrini R. Genetic malformations of the cerebral cortex and epilepsy. *Epilepsia.* 2005; **46** Suppl 1: 32–7.

Ganesan V and Kirkham F. *Stroke and Cerebrovascular Disease in Childhood*. London International Review of Child Neurology (MacKeith Press) 2006.

Kirkham FJ. Stroke in childhood. *Archives of Diseases in Childhood* 1999; **81**: 85–89.

Kirkham FJ. Non-traumatic coma. *Archives of Diseases in Childhood* 2001; **85**: 303–312.

Kirkham FJ, Ganesan V. *Neurology. Paediatric Investigations* (ed J Stroobant and D Field). Churchill Livingstone 2002; chapter 12 pp 331–381.

Levene M, Chervenak F, Whittle M, Bennett M, Punt J. *Fetal and Neonatal Neurology and Neurosurgery* (3rd edition). London: Churchill Livingstone 2001.

Maria BL. *Current management in child neurology* (3rd edition). Hamilton, Ontario: BC Decker Inc 2005.

Machuca-Tzili L, Brook D, Hilton-Jones D. Clinical and molecular aspects of the myotonic dystrophies: a review. *Muscle Nerve* 2005; **32**: 1–18.

McKinnon PJ. ATM and ataxia telangiectasia. *EMBO Rep.* 2004; **5**: 772–776. Review.

Ryan MM, Ouvrier R. Hereditary peripheral neuropathies of childhood. *Curr Opin Neurol.* 2005; **18**: 105–110.

Segawa M, Nomura Y. Rett syndrome. *Curr Opin Neurol.* 2005; **18**: 97–104.

Jan MM. Misdiagnoses in children with dopa-responsive dystonia. *Pediatr Neurol.* 2004; **31**: 298–303.

Royal College of Physicians Intercollegiate Stroke Working party. *Stroke in childhood: clinical guidelines for diagnosis, management and rehabilitation.* www.rcplondon.ac.uk/pubs/books/childstroke/childstroke_guidelines.pdf

Segawa M, Nomura Y, Nishiyama N. Autosomal dominant guanosine triphosphate cyclohydrolase I deficiency (Segawa disease). *Ann Neurol.* 2003; **54** Suppl 6: S32–45.

The National Institute for Health and Clinical Excellence (NICE). *The diagnosis and care of children and adults with epilepsy*. www.nice.org.uk/page.aspx?o=227586

The Paediatric Accident and Emergency Research Group. The management of decreased conscious level in children – an evidence-based guideline. www.nottingham.ac.uk/paediatric-guideline

Tidball JG, Wehling-Henricks M. Evolving therapeutic strategies for Duchenne muscular dystrophy: targeting downstream events. *Pediatr Res.* 2004; **56**: 831–841.

van de Warrenburg BP, Sinke RJ, Kremer B. Recent advances in hereditary spinocerebellar ataxias. *J Neuropathol Exp Neurol.* 2005; **64**:171–180.

Walker DA, Perilongo G, Punt JAG, Taylor RE. *Brain and Spinal Tumours of Childhood*. London: Arnold Publishers 2004.

Gastroenterology
Susan Hill

CLINICAL PRESENTATION

ACUTE GASTROENTERITIS
Incidence
One of the most common childhood diseases with 0.3–0.8 episodes per child per year world-wide. The commonest cause for hospitalization is diarrhoea in infants aged from 6–24 months.

Aetiology/pathogenesis
An acute infectious disease that is usually viral in developed countries. The most common virus is rotavirus (**9.1**). Other causes include adenovirus, astrovirus, calicivirus and small round viruses (**9.2, 9.3**). Infects the small intestine and destroys enterocytes.

Presentation
Acute onset of vomiting then diarrhoea, often with abdominal pain and possible pyrexia. Incubation period 2–7 days.

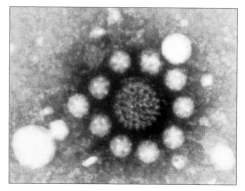

9.1–9.3 Acute gastroenteritis. Electron microscope appearance of enteric viruses (all named after their electron microscope appearances).
9.1 Acute gastroenteritis. Rotavirus (centre) and astrovirus (surrounding).

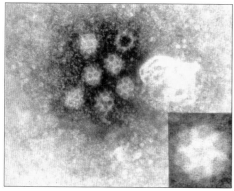

9.2 Acute gastroenteritis. Calicivirus.

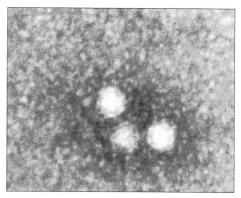

9.3 Acute gastroenteritis. Small round virus.

Table 9.1. Clinical features of dehydration

Percentage weight loss	Severity	Clinical	Signs
<5%	Mild	Not unwell	Dry mucous membranes, thirst
5–10%	Moderate	Apathetic, unwell	Sunken eyes and fontanelle (infants)
			Reduced skin turgor, oliguria, tachypnoea
10–15%	Severe	Shocked	Poor peripheral circulation, hypotension, tachycardia
>15%	Critical	Moribund	Severely shocked

Diagnosis

History of frequency, volume and content of diarrhoea and vomitus. Fluid balance (with record of recent fluid intake and urine output) and clinical examination are required to assess risk and current state of dehydration. Clinical examination to assess state of hydration (**Table 9.1**).

Treatment

The mainstay of treatment is oral rehydration solution (water with electrolytes and carbohydrate). Give in small quantities as often as possible (even every 15 or 30 minutes). May need nasogastric tube. If possible avoid intravenous fluids (enteral fluids are less likely to cause fluid/electrolyte imbalance). Best absorbed immediately after a vomit. Give only commercially available solutions (approximately one teaspoon sugar, and one teaspoon of salt to a pint of water), and avoid home-made preparations. Flat Coca-Cola may be given to the older child.

Food should be continued as tolerated, particularly if the patient is malnourished.
NB: Highly contagious. Careful hand-washing is most effective way to prevent spread.

Prognosis

Full recovery usually within 24–36 hours, but symptoms can persist for 10–14 days. The patient can excrete the virus and remain infectious even after clinical recovery. In the immunocompromised, symptoms may persist for more than two weeks. Rarely, symptoms persist and children develop more chronic diarrhoea (post-enteritis syndrome) from cow's milk protein. A suitable vaccine for rotavirus is being sought.

FAILURE TO THRIVE
Presentation

Failure to gain weight at the expected rate/ according to the weight percentile (**Table 9.2**). Below the 0.4 centile for weight (and possibly height), not explained by parental size (**9.4**).

A child whose parents claim they have not gained weight or grown for several months. Weight more than 2 centiles below height centile.

Diagnosis

History of feeding, diet, stool, family, behaviour. Investigations as guided by clinical presentation.

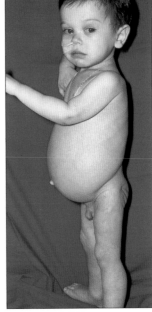

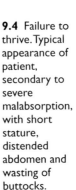

9.4 Failure to thrive. Typical appearance of patient, secondary to severe malabsorption, with short stature, distended abdomen and wasting of buttocks.

CONSTIPATION
Incidence/genetics
Common. There is evidence of an inherited predisposition, and a family history of atopy when associated with food intolerance.

Aetiology
There may be an anal stricture or tightening in infancy obstructing defaecation, or poor fluid and/or calorie intake resulting in a small amount of hard stool. Later in infancy a relatively low fibre/high milk intake can lead to painful, hard stool (possibly with an anal fissure adding to the pain). Infants may then strain to hold stool in to avoid pain when they next sense defaecation. If constipation persists in the older child a megarectum (with poor faecal sensation) and retained faecal mass and overflow faecal incontinence may develop. Psychological factors such as fear, confusion, shame, guilt, anger, despair, withdrawal, dissociation and abdication of responsibility may ensue.

Patients with a personal or family history of atopy may have an allergic colitis with an eosinophilic infiltration of colonic mucosa. There is abnormal colonic motility with constipation and/or diarrhoea.

Table 9.2. Gastrointestinal causes of failure to thrive

- Poor calorie intake
  - Protein-calorie malnutrition
  - Feeding problems

- Vomiting
  - Gastro-oesophageal reflux

- Malabsorption
  - Small intestinal enteropathy
    - a Coeliac disease
    - b Food sensitive enteropathy
    - c Small intestinal Crohn's disease
    - d Eosinophilic gastroenteropathy
    - e Autoimmune enteropathy
    - f Other less common enteropathies
    - g Protein losing enteropathy
    - h Lymphangiectasia
  - Pancreatic insufficiency
    - a Shwachman syndrome
    - b Cystic fibrosis

- CHO intolerance
  - Lactose

Presentation/diagnosis
Constipation can be defined as delay or difficulty in defaecation that is severe enough to cause significant distress to the patient.
- Abnormally hard stool with increased length of time between defaecation episodes causing distress to the child when bowels are opened.
- Soiling – escape of stool into underclothing.
- Encopresis – passage of normal stools in abnormal places.
- Examination of spine, sacrum and lower limb reflexes to exclude neuropathic bowel.
- Abdominal x-ray with radio-opaque tubing swallowed on three consecutive days, cut into a different shape each day, and x-rayed on the fifth day (**9.5**) to estimate transit time.
- Rectal biopsy (full thickness – histological appearance of excess of acetylcholinesterase-positive nerves and absence of ganglion cells) is necessary to exclude Hirschsprung's disease (see 'Neonatal and General Paediatric Surgery' chapter). Hirschsprung's may be present with delayed passage of meconium beyond 48 hours of age.
- Blood RAST (specific IgE) and skin-prick tests for cow's milk, egg, wheat and soya, if the child is atopic with suspected food intolerance.
- Colonoscopy with histological examination of mucosal biopsies in atopic children may demonstrate underlying eosinophilic/allergic colitis.
- Blood tests to exclude hypothyroidism and hypercalcaemia may be indicated.

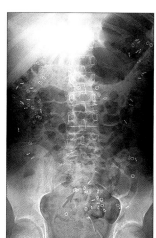

9.5 Abdominal x-ray demonstrating faecal loading and presence of three types of radio-opaque markers, that have been ingested to measure transit time.

Differential diagnosis
Some healthy breast-fed babies may pass infrequent stools. Poor fluid intake and/or calorie intake may lead to infrequent hard stools in infancy and older children.

Treatment
Multidisciplinary approach.
- Dietary: improved fluid and fibre intake may cure milder cases at any age. A six- to eight-week trial of cow's milk and egg-free diet, that should be continued if there is clinical improvement.

Initial medical treatment:
- Softening retained faeces using lactulose and, if extensive, hard faecal loading, docusate.
- Evacuation of retained faeces if softening stool alone does not work. Initially use senna, and add in sodium picosulphate if needed.
- Polyethylene glycol solution can be given orally or via nasogastric tube for more resistant cases.
- Micro or phosphate enemas are often effective in evacuating rectal masses, but the child needs to understand and cooperate with treatment or fear and discomfort of defaecation may be heightened.

Maintenance drug treatment
- This may be added, initially with lactulose (5–10ml t.d.s.) or methylcellulose tablets for an osmotic effect along with a stimulant laxative such as senna (infants and older children). Docusate added from pre-school age to soften stool with intermittent sodium picosulphate elixir as a stimulant providing an osmotic load if maintenance laxatives fail (may be regularly given at weekends in school age child).
- Once-daily senna to prevent reaccumulation of faeces (effect for 12–14 hours post dose).
- Parallel psychological treatment for both the child and family is needed for school age children (around 50%).
- Appropriate dietary exclusions for food-sensitive colitis (See under 'Food-sensitive enteropathy' page 263).

Prognosis
Treatment with stimulant laxatives should be continued for about 12 months in order to prevent relapse. Lifelong problems may ensue if treatment fails.

INFANTILE COLIC
Incidence
Common.

Aetiology
Cow's milk intolerance is associated in some patients.

Presentation/diagnosis
Excessive crying in a healthy, thriving infant. The crying usually starts from about four weeks of age and ceases by about four or five months. It usually occurs in the evening and persists for more than three hours a day. Check that there are no other causes such as too hot, too cold, inappropriate feeding or discomfort.

Treatment
Reassure parents. Try exclusion of cow's milk from the diet. Give hypoallergenic formula as milk substitute. Many infants are or become symptomatic with soya milk as well. If infant is breast-fed, mother can exclude milk from her diet and should have a calcium supplement. It is also helpful to reduce stimulation.

Prognosis
Resolves.

RECURRENT ABDOMINAL PAIN
Incidence
Affects up to 1 in 10 children.

Aetiology
Improvement in gastrointestinal investigation techniques has led to more frequent organic diagnoses. Gastro-oesophageal reflux (see page 277) possibly underlying in up to 50% of cases. Food-allergic colitis (in association with diarrhoea or constipation) and gastritis and duodenitis also fairly common. Almost any disorder that can cause abdominal pain, including pancreatic and gall bladder disease.

Diagnosis
More than three attacks of abdominal pain over more than three months, sufficiently severe to interfere with normal activities. A thorough clinical history and examination are essential to check for non-specific presentations of a range of diseases. Investigations depend on symptoms. It is helpful to see the patient during an attack. Initial investigations: urine culture, full blood count and ESR, stool microscopy and culture and faecal occult blood may be helpful. If pain persists and is not resolving, upper gastro-intestinal endoscopy and/or a 24-hour

oesophageal pH study should be carried out. Colonoscopy is performed if colitis suspected.

Treatment
As for underlying cause.

Prognosis
Long-term follow-up indicates improvement with age, although a high proportion of patients report symptoms continuing into adult life.

TODDLER'S DIARRHOEA
Incidence/genetics
Common. Affects males more than females. Familial predisposition, with a parent with a history of irritable bowel or sibling with similar symptoms in about 80%.

Aetiology
Excessive intake of fruit juice, such as apple juice, may cause diarrhoea due to the osmotic effect of high sugar content. An underlying allergic colitis, particularly if mucus and/or blood in the stool.

Diagnosis
Loose, frequent, foul-smelling, daytime stool (usually with mucus) in children from one to about six years of age. Specific IgE (RAST tests) to test for possible food intolerances in atopic children. If blood is present, colonoscopy to exclude a polyp and mucosal biopsies for histological examination for allergic/eosinophilic colitis is mandatory. Plasma IgA to look for associated deficiency.

Treatment
Dietary review by a paediatric dietician and appropriate manipulation – for example, advice on reducing intake of fruit juices if excessive. If there is a positive RAST test or eosinophilic colitis, exclude the relevant food from the diet (see allergic colitis). Trial of a cow's milk, egg and wheat (the most common offending foods) free diet may be tried without initial colonoscopy. May respond to treatment with a 5-aminosalicylate prepartion or oral disodium cromoglycate

Prognosis
Improves with age.

CHRONIC INTRACTABLE DIARRHOEA
Incidence/genetics
Rare. Familial occurrence with apparent X-linked inheritance in some cases.

Aetiology
Can be divided into three groups:
- Those with a specific diagnosis, but no known therapy (microvillus atrophy, phenotypic diarrhoea, and epithelial dysplasia or 'tufting' disease) (**9.6**).
- A specific diagnosis, but partial resistance to therapy (some cases of autoimmune enteropathy and immunodeficiency).
- No specific diagnosis.

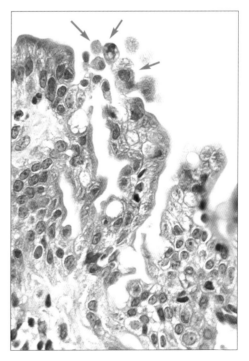

9.6 Tufting enteropathy. Histological appearance of small intestine with 'grape-like' tufts at villus tip (x25).

Diagnosis

Symptoms are four or more loose stools per day for more than two weeks, with associated failure to thrive (**9.7**, **9.8**) and at least three negative stool cultures . Watery stool may be mistaken for urine. Termed **intractable** if prolonged, despite extensive hospital investigation. Essential investigations include stool for malabsorption: fat globules, alpha-1 antitrypsin (protein loss), reducing substances and sugar chromatography (osmotic diarrhoea). Stool electrolyte levels: Na >80mmol/l if secretory diarrhoea. Stool elastase to screen for pancreatic insufficiency (beware of false positive results with watery diarrhoea).

Upper and lower intestinal endoscopy with mucosal biopsies for histological examination (to detect possible enteropathy and colitis) with periodic acid Schiff (PAS) staining to detect abnormal brush border in microvillus atrophy (**9.9**, **9.10**). Electron microscopy of mucosal biopsies to detect microvillus involutions and inclusion bodies in microvillus atrophy (**9.11**, **9.12**, **9.13**). Peripheral blood immune studies to detect an associated systemic immunodeficiency that might also involve the intestine. Immunological staining of intestinal mucosa if inflammatory infiltrate in lamina propria.

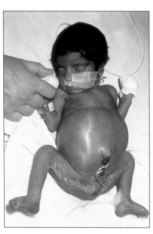

9.7 Neonate presenting with severe, intractable, watery diarrhoea and failure to thrive, with abdominal distension and excoriation of nappy area.

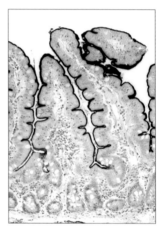

9.9 Brush border of normal small intestine stained with PAS (x40).

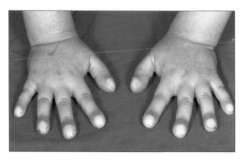

9.8 Anaemia and clubbing of fingers in a child with chronic intractable diarrhoea and malabsorption, with underlying tufting enteropathy.

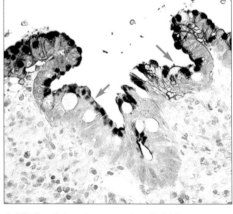

9.10 Brush border stained with PAS in microvillous atrophy, illustrating disruption of the microvilli (x100).

Treatment

Immunoglobulin replacement therapy in immunodeficiency.

Trial of immunosuppressive treatment if excessive inflammatory cells in intestinal mucosa. Gradual reintroduction of enteral feed as tolerated, usually as semi-elemental continuous feed but may need elemental or modular feed. Supportive with parenteral nutrition. Long-term home parenteral nutrition by parents is the best option if the child fails to respond adequately to treatment. A multidisciplinary ethical review with parents, before deciding whether to commence long-term home parenteral nutrition, is helpful (especially when a paediatrician with ethical training is involved) to establish appropriate treatment regime. Intestinal transplant is still experimental.

Prognosis

Recovery unlikely. Patients with microvillus atropy usually develop liver failure by 2 years of age. Little improvement with age. Risk of inducing suffering with no eventual recovery needs to be assessed prior to sending home on treatment with parenteral nutrition, particularly if child also has failure of another major organ.

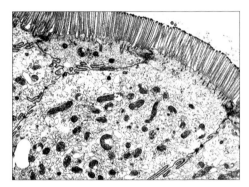

9.11 Electron microscope appearance of normal microvilli on small intestine enterocyte (×13,000).

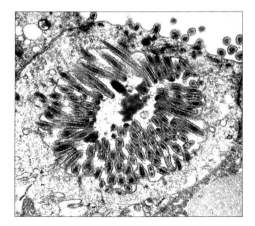

9.12 Electron microscope appearance of distorted microvilli within and on enterocyte surface in microvillous atrophy (×13,000).

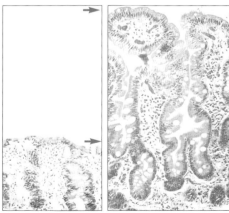

9.13 Histological appearance of subtotal villous atrophy (severe enteropathy) compared with normal small intestine.

CHRONIC INTESTINAL FAILURE
Aetiology/pathogenesis
The three major causes are:
- A severe enteropathy (see intractable diarrhoea).
- A major abnormality of the intestinal neuromusculature.
- Short intestine.

Diagnosis
Inability to maintain weight or grow despite adequate nutrition. May present with chronic diarrhoea with or without vomiting. Essential investigations are shown in **Table 9.3**.

Treatment
There are two main aims:
- To make the best possible use of any intestinal absorptive capacity.
- To maintain normal weight gain and growth with parenteral nutrition (see treatment for short bowel syndrome).

A small intestinal transplant with or without liver transplant is currently reserved for patients with less than six months of life expectancy (usually due to liver failure or lack of venous access). Major problems with lymphoproliferative disease; maintaining long-term graft viability and infection limit the two-year survival rate to less than 70% and graft survival to about 50%.

Prognosis
Dependent on careful administration of parenteral nutrition by parents at home with support from a specialist gastrointestinal and nutrition team. Fewer complications of parenteral nutrition at home (less frequent septicaemic episodes).

Improvement in the outcome of intestinal transplant would make this option feasible.

Table 9.3 Essential investigations for chronic intestinal failure

- Stool microscopy and culture.

- Stool-reducing substances and sugar chromatography for sugar malabsorption (osmotic diarrhoea).

- If liquid stool, check sodium content (>80mmol/l secretory diarrhoea).

- Upper and lower gastrointestinal endoscopy with mucosal biopsies for histological examination for mucosal inflammation.

- Barium meal to detect structural abnormalities and, if previous intestinal resection, length of remaining small and large intestine.

- If there is evidence of abnormal intestinal motility, investigate transit time with marker (such as carmine red dye) or radiopaque pellets (see constipation), and intestinal motility studies to detect abnormal peristalsis (initially an electrogastrogram – EGG).

- Trial of gradual introduction of appropriate enteral feeds (elemental or semi-elemental liquid feeds) administered in the most appropriate manner (taken orally, via a nasogastric tube or gastrostomy directly into the stomach, or via a jejunostomy or nasojejunal tube into the jejunum).

GASTROINTESTINAL DIAGNOSES

FABRICATED AND INDUCED ILLNESS

Incidence
Males and females equally affected.

Aetiology
The reason for the perpetrator's actions is often poorly understood. Many are lonely and isolated. Up to half have nursing training or some extra medical knowledge (such as medical receptionist), and some have a previous history of falsifying symptoms about themselves. It is most commonly the mother.

There are several degrees of manifestation of the syndrome. At its least severe, the perpetrator embellishes a history in the hope that the child will have more medical attention. The next stage is the perpetrator who simulates illness without harming the child (for example by contaminating specimens). At its most severe, the perpetrator directly harms the child, for example sabotaging the central line or giving harmful treatment, such as laxatives when the child already has diarrhoea, or adding excessive salt to infant feeds (**9.14**).

Diagnosis
Common gastrointestinal symptoms are vomiting, diarrhoea and gastrointestinal bleeding. There is usually a mild underlying gastrointestinal disorder (for example atopic associated cow's milk protein intolerance) with worsening of existing symptoms and development of new symptoms when mother is with the child. The mother usually appears appreciative, cooperative and pleasant, is close to the child, reluctant to leave the hospital and, whenever possible, forms close relationships with the professional staff caring for the child. The father is usually distant (although the syndrome has been described in fathers). The average time from onset to diagnosis is 15 months.

The closest possible observation of mother and child is necessary, usually with a nurse 'specialing' (24-hour individual observation) the patient. There is controversy over the use of video surveillance. All staff must meticulously record all observations (**9.15**). Toxic screening of urine and vomit specimens and blood group of blood specimens are necessary. A multidisciplinary team should be involved, including a social worker and psychiatrist.

Treatment
If the mother is unwilling to confess when presented with all the evidence, she may need to be directly confronted. She should be told that the paediatrician and child psychiatrist are trying to help her and that the social worker has legal responsibilities.

Prognosis
There is a mortality rate of about 9% with the greatest risk among children under three years old. Child victims may become perpetrators themselves. Often more than one child in a family is affected at different times.

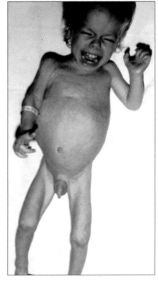

9.14 Induced illness on presentation, aged 20 months, with severe wasting and developmental delay due to starvation. The mother claimed the child had an enormous appetite.

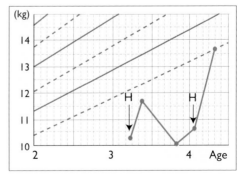

9.15 Weight plotted on weight centile chart for a child aged 3–4 who gained weight when in hospital (H) and failed to thrive at home.

COELIAC DISEASE
Incidence/genetics
Coeliac disease is a chronic small intestinal enteropathy associated with ingestion of gluten that resolves on exclusion of gluten from the diet. It occurs in at least 1 in 2,000 Caucasians, among populations with a high wheat intake, such as Europeans, North and South Americans, Australians and in the Punjab region of India, with a particularly high frequency of 1 in 300 in Western Ireland. Most patients are HLA-DQ, DQ2 or DQ8 positive.

Aetiology
Coeliac disease is an autoimmune disease. Tissue transglutaminase (t Tg) has been identified as the major autoantigen. Ingestion of wheat, barley, rye or oats initiates immunologically mediated tissue injury. This injury is stimulated in subjects with particular MHC genes (see above).

Diagnosis
Common symptoms and signs are anorexia, vomiting, abdominal distension, diarrhoea, irritability and failure to thrive, buttock wasting, and in the older child, short stature (**9.16**, **9.17**). Constipation may occur. Onset is from a few weeks after introducing wheat to the diet in infancy, but can be at any age throughout life. Autoimmune diseases such as diabetes mellitus and thyroid disease are associated, and it occurs with increased frequency in Down and Turner syndromes. In adults, dermatitis herpetiformis, splenic atrophy and neoplasia (in particular, T cell lymphoma of the small intestine) may develop.

The definitive diagnosis is made by a minimum of two proximal small intestinal biopsies according to the ESPGHAN criteria. Biopsy on a wheat-containing diet reveals a subtotal villous atrophy (**9.18**). When rebiopsied after several weeks on a gluten-free diet, the intestinal mucosa appears normal (**9.19**). If there is full clinical remission when gluten is excluded from the diet, it is only necessary to take one biopsy on presentation. More than one biopsy is required if:
- At presentation the child is under 2 years old.
- There is an atypical histology.
- Teenagers wish to re-introduce gluten into their diet.

The proximal small intestine, where gluten is largely absorbed, is most severely affected.

Detection of plasma tissue transglutaminase (t Tg) and/or endomysial antibodies is good evidence for coeliac disease, but not diagnostic. IgG and IgA anti-gliadin, and IgA anti-reticulin antibodies, are associated. Persistently positive antibodies, or their reappearance, indicate gluten ingestion.

Iron-deficiency anaemia, low red cell and serum folate, low plasma albumin and globulins (due to low circulating IgG and IgM) and prolonged prothrombin time are non-specific and usually secondary to malabsorption.

Pathology
Major histological features of jejunum are hyperplastic subtotal villous atrophy, with increased numbers of lamina propria plasma cells and increased ratio of intraepithelial lymphocytes to surface epithelial cells.

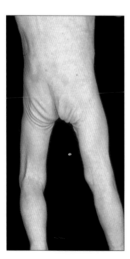

9.16 Coeliac disease, showing severe wasting of buttocks and thighs.

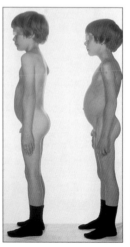

9.17 Coeliac disease. The twin on the right shows the signs of distended abdomen and short stature.

Immunological abnormalities include an increased proportion of intraepithelial lymphocytes with gamma/delta T cell receptors, reduced lamina propria suppressor cell numbers and increased antibody (including anti-gliadin antibody) production. Gluten-specific CD4 positive T cells are restricted by the HLA-DQ DQ2 heterodimer. There is aberrant HLA-DR expression by immature crypt enterocytes, reduced enterocyte survival time and increased intestinal permeability.

Differential diagnosis
Wheat-sensitive enteropathy, which is usually transient, atopic-associated wheat intolerance. It is commonest in infants and pre-school children, with currently an increasing incidence in older children (see 'Food-sensitive enteropathy').

Treatment
Dietary exclusion of gluten in wheat, rye, barley and oats. Some children may tolerate oats. Reintroduction of oats can be tried after 1 year if child is well, but should be excluded again if any symptoms develop.

Prognosis
Almost certainly lifelong, but fully controlled with a gluten-free diet. There is an association with small intestinal lymphoma in later life, possibly more common in patients who are on a normal gluten-containing diet.

FOOD-SENSITIVE ENTEROPATHY
Incidence/genetics
A fairly common disorder, usually associated with a family and/or personal history of atopic disease, or immunodeficiency. Gastrointestinal symptoms precipitated by cow's milk may affect 1 in 200 infants.

Aetiology/pathogenesis
Food-sensitive enteropathy occurs when there is a lack of tolerance of a food by the intestinal immune system. Patients usually have a major or minor (often atopic-associated) immunodeficiency. IgA deficiency is common. The enteropathy most frequently occurs with cow's milk (the major dietary constituent in bottle-fed infants), also with egg, soya and wheat or almost any food; rice, chicken and fish intolerance have been described. The enteropathy is of variable severity and rapidly resolves when the offending food is excluded from the diet.

Food sensitivity may develop when intestinal immunity is low, during acute gastroenteritis or due to a long-term immunodeficiency allowing excessive antigen absorption.

Diagnosis
Usually associated with vomiting, diarrhoea, failure to thrive, irritability and abdominal pain. Children usually dislike the offending food. For example, children with associated cow's milk intolerance may only take milk on cereal, in tea or as milkshakes.

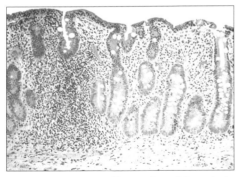

9.18 Coeliac disease. Proximal small intestinal histology (x 400). Subtotal villous atrophy with villous shortening, crypt hypertrophy, increased numbers of intraepithelial lymphocytes and lamina propria plasma cells.

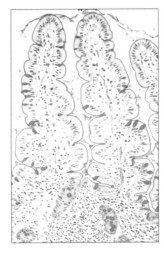

9.19 Histological appearance of normal small intestine.

The diagnosis may be made when symptoms resolve on excluding the offending food from the diet for 6–8 weeks. If dietary exclusion fails or is inappropriate, upper intestinal endoscopy with duodenal mucosal biopsy should be done (**9.20**). There is thinning of intestinal mucosa with a patchy, partial villous atrophy and increased lamina propria cellularity (**9.21**). There may be an eosinophilic infiltration of the small intestinal lamina propria. Food specific IgE antibodies in peripheral blood (RAST test) and skin prick test for dietary allergen may be positive. The definitive diagnosis is made if a repeat small intestinal biopsy is histologically normal after a minimum of eight weeks dietary exclusion (**9.22**) – not usually necessary.

Differential diagnosis

Food-sensitive enteropathy should be distinguished from immediate hypersensitivity, IgE mediated, allergic response to food, in which there is usually a reaction to the food within an hour and no underlying enteropathy. The enteropathy is less severe than in coeliac disease.

Treatment

Removal of the offending food from the diet for a minimum trial period of 6–8 weeks, with advice from a dietitian, simultaneously treats the patient and confirms the identity of the offending food or foods. Long-term total exclusion is not essential in all older children who may tolerate certain foodstuffs with traces of the offending food. If it is not possible to detect an offending food, give oral disodiumcromoglycate (up to 60 mg/kg/d) and immunosuppressive treatment in more resistant cases. The patient is not challenged with an offending food, as early reintroduction can cause more severe symptoms and even anaphylaxis. Gradual reintroduction can take place after several weeks or months of full health.

Prognosis

Food-sensitive enteropathies usually improve as the gut matures from about 18 months to two years of age or later, but can persist throughout childhood. Partial intolerance to a food may continue into adult life; for example, some children with cow's milk intolerance never drink milk but can tolerate milk in cooking.

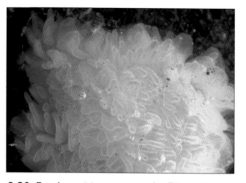

9.20 Food-sensitive enteropathy. Dissecting microscope appearance of normal small intestine showing villi when on appropriate diet.

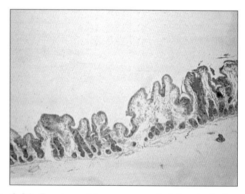

9.21 Food-sensitive enteropathy. Histological appearance of proximal small intestinal biopsy in food-sensitive patient, showing partial villous atrophy with mucosal thinning (x 250).

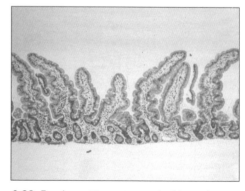

9.22 Food-sensitive enteropathy. Normal mucosa on exclusion diet.

AUTOIMMUNE ENTEROPATHY

Incidence/genetics

A rare disorder, recognized in European, Arab, North American and Japanese children. There is evidence of a genetic predisposition with both a high incidence of autoimmune disease in first degree relatives and, in some families, apparent X-linked, recessive inheritance (overall male: female ratio 2:1).

Aetiology/pathogenesis

The enteropathy is of variable severity, with lymphocytic infiltration of the lamina propria. The three main immunological features are:
- Circulating enterocyte antibodies.
- In some patients, antibodies have been shown to fix complement.
- Aberrant HLA-DR staining of enterocytes in affected small intestine.

Diagnosis

Protracted diarrhoea with failure to thrive usually commences in infancy after the neonatal period, or, less commonly, at any age throughout childhood. The onset often appears to be after acute infectious gastroenteritis with rapid resolution of symptoms in other affected family members. Associated with organ specific autoimmune diseases of the thyroid, parathyroid, liver, kidney and pancreas. Peripheral blood should be tested for anti-enterocyte antibodies. There should be histological examination of a small intestinal mucosal biopsy and colonoscopy as well, if there are colitic symptoms or persistent unexplained diarrhoea after the treatment of enteropathy.

Treatment

Dietary antigen ingestion should be reduced, with specific dietary exclusions. May require liquid enteral tube feeds and in severe cases, parenteral nutrition. Patients who do not respond to dietary management are treated with immunosuppressive agents. In most patients prednisolone and azathioprine are effective and, in others, ciclosporin and tacrolimus have been of benefit.

Prognosis

Ranges in severity from a protracted episode of diarrhoea that resolves spontaneously over a few weeks to a relentless disease process with intestinal failure and survival dependent on parenteral nutrition. Patients may require immunosuppressive treatment for months or years.

EOSINOPHILIC GASTROENTEROPATHY

Incidence

Rare

Aetiology

Probable allergic reaction to specific foods. Symptoms depend on underlying disease, which may be:
- Mucosal with malabsorption.
- Muscle layer disease affecting intestinal motility.
- Subserosal disease with eosinophilic ascites.

There is usually a family history of atopy.

Diagnosis

The patient suffers from abdominal pain, nausea, vomiting, poor weight gain and diarrhoea. Symptoms of intestinal pseudo-obstruction and ascites may develop. Essential investigations include endoscopy with mucosal biopsy of stomach and small intestine. The oesophagus and colon may also be involved. Histologically there is an eosinophilic infiltration of affected mucosa/submucosa/muscle layer. Plasma albumin, globulins and Hb may be low. There is often a peripheral blood eosinophilia.

Treatment

Exclusion of offending foods from diet. Immunosuppression, initially with trial of prednisolone.

Prognosis

Good if symptoms are controlled with treatment.

CLASSIC INFLAMMATORY BOWEL DISEASE

Crohn's disease and ulcerative colitis are termed classic inflammatory bowel disease (IBD) (**Table 9.4**). They are chronic inflammatory disorders of unknown aetiology, primarily involving the gastrointestinal tract, but with some systemic features. The major features distinguishing ulcerative colitis from Crohn's disease are the site and type of inflammation and histology. Ulcerative colitis usually affects the colon and is limited to the mucosa. Crohn's disease may affect any area of the gastrointestinal tract from the mouth to the anus and involves the full thickness of the bowel wall. Immunological mechanisms are important in the pathogenesis of both diseases.

ULCERATIVE COLITIS

Incidence/genetics

Ranges from 1 in 25,000 to 50,000 in childhood. Fifteen percent have an affected first degree relative. Association with HLA-DR2 has been recognized and weak association with HLA-B27 and HLA-Bw35 in Caucasians. However, affected patients in the same family may be of different HLA types, and monozygotic twins are usually discordant for the disease.

Table 9.4 Extraintestinal manifestations of classic IBD

- Growth failure
- Arthritis and arthralgia
  - 20–25% ulcerative colitis and 11% Crohn's
- Sacroilitis and ankylosing spondylitis associated with HLA-B27
- Erythema nodosum in approximately 5% of patients with Crohn's (commoner in Crohn's)
- Pyoderma gangenosum in 0.5–5% of ulcerative colitis and 0.1% of Crohn's
- Liver disease
  - sclerosing cholangitis
  - chronic active hepatitis and cholelithiasis may rarely occur and can be severe
- Ocular manifestations
  - uveitis is acutely symptomatic in less than 3% of patients
  - episcleritis and conjunctivitis may develop
- Renal manifestations
  - usually formation of calcium oxalate stones in up to 5% of children with Crohn's disease (associated with ileal disease)

Aetiology/pathogenesis

The aetiology is unknown, but appears to be multifactorial. Immunological mechanisms are involved. Autoimmunity is a feature and in 80% of cases there is an IgG1 antibody to a colonic polypeptide, specific to ulcerative colitis. Positive perinuclear anticytoplasmic antibody (p-ANCA) is associated with an increased risk of developing primary sclerosing cholangitis and 'pouchitis'.

Inflammation is confined to the intestinal mucosa. The colon is affected most severely. There can be associated gastric and/or small intestinal disease. The lesion is continuous with macroscopically a granular haemorrhagic appearance, friability and loss of vascular markings (**9.23**). Histologically there is vascular congestion, crypt branching and abscesses, loss of goblet cells and Paneth cell metaplasia with mucosal inflammatory cell infiltration.

Diagnosis

Most commonly presents with bloody diarrhoea and mucus. Other features are lower, colicky abdominal pain, anorexia, weight loss, and urgency of stool. Ten percent present with fulminating colitis, often with toxic megacolon when vomiting, pyrexia, tachycardia and severe abdominal pain; distension and tenderness may occur with reduced bowel sounds and bloody diarrhoea (>5 stools over 24 hours). Extra-intestinal manifestations include arthralgia and arthritis, delayed growth and sexual maturation (less severe than in Crohn's disease) and, rarely, liver disease (in particular primary sclerosing cholangitis). Essential investigations are the same as those for Crohn's disease.

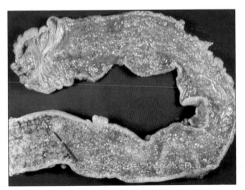

9.23 Ulcerative colitis showing extensive colonic involvement with inflammation and bleeding.

Treatment

With a 5-aminosalicylate preparation. Patients frequently also require immunosuppressive treatment with prednisolone, then azathioprine as well if steroid-dependent (for steroid-sparing effect). Ciclosporin has been effective in resistant disease. May need nutritional supplements and, in severe disease, parenteral nutrition. Surgery/total colectomy with ileostomy for up to six months, then ileoanal pull-through, is indicated for severe colitis (i.e. colitis that fails to respond to aggressive immunosuppressive therapy along with antibiotics and parenteral nutrition) and for uncontrolled bleeding. Yearly colonoscopy, if pancolitis continues for over ten years, as surveillance for possible malignancy.

Prognosis

Chronic relapsing disease course. Most children lead a normal lifestyle, but up to 20% have incapacitating disease. The risk of colonic malignancy increases if there is active pancolitis or left-sided colitis for ten years or more. The disease can be cured by total colectomy, but inflammation or pouchitis of the surgically-fashioned ileal pouch occurs in at least one-third of patients.

CROHN'S DISEASE
Incidence/genetics

The incidence of Crohn's disease has increased since the 1950s to approximately 1 in 25,000 children. Almost one-third of patients present in late childhood. Both sexes are affected equally. North Europeans, Anglo-Saxons and European and North American Jews classically develop the disease. It is more common in urban dwellers. Approximately 35% of patients have a first-degree relative affected by Crohn's or ulcerative colitis. An increased incidence of HLA-DR1, HLA-DQw5 and HLA-DR2 has been found in Caucasians, along with concordance in mono- but not di-zygotic twins.

Aetiology/pathogenesis

There is no proven aetiology. Infection is probably important at the onset of symptoms (for example, atypical mycobacterium may be involved in a small minority of cases) with immunological imbalances leading to inflammation, perpetuating the disease. Dietary and microbial antigens are probably involved. Symptoms are exacerbated by smoking.

Immunological abnormalities include an increase in CD4 and CD8 T cells with increased numbers of activated cells, abnormal T cell cytotoxicity, reduced suppressor T cell

activity detected in remission (which may fail to 'switch off' normal mucosal immune responses), increased circulating soluble interleukin-2 receptors in proportion to disease activity, increased numbers of monoclonal B cells and increased serum levels of pro-inflammatory cytokines, such as interleukin-1 and tumour necrosis factor-alpha.

Diagnosis

Insidious onset with loss of appetite, weight loss, abdominal pain, diarrhoea and poor growth. Can present as short stature, delayed puberty or with an abdominal mass, perianal inflammation, aphthous mouth ulcers and extra-intestinal problems, such as fever, arthritis, uveitis, erythema nodosum and liver disease. Over 50% of cases have an ileocolitis; at least 30% have small bowel disease alone and 10–15% colonic disease alone. The disease may affect any part of the gastrointestinal tract (**9.24–9.26**).

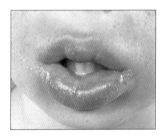

9.24 Crohn's disease of the lip.

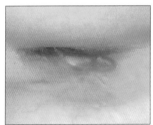

9.25 Crohn's disease affecting the perianal region.

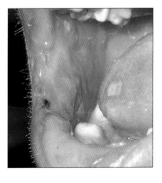

9.26 Crohn's disease. Aphthous ulceration of the mouth.

Colonoscopy with biopsy of terminal ileal and colonic mucosa should be carried out, along with upper intestinal endoscopy. Macroscopically at colonoscopy there is patchy inflammation with aphthous ulceration, sometimes with 'snail track' ulcers and 'cobblestone' appearance (**9.27**). The presence of non-caseating epitheloid granulomata on histological examination is diagnostic. The mucosal inflammatory infiltrate consists of monocytes, macrophages, lymphocytes and plasma cells with neutrophils when acutely inflamed.

Blood platelet and haemoglobin level, ESR/CRP and plasma albumin are used for monitoring disease activity. Technetium-labelled white cell scan can detect active disease in both small intestine and colon (**9.28**). Barium contrast studies (**9.29**) are used to investigate for strictures (and mucosal oedema and ulceration). Liver enzymes, bone age and density should be checked.

Treatment

- Diet: preferred treatment is with liquid enteral feeds and withdrawal of normal food for 6–8 weeks or longer. Elemental and polymeric feeds are both effective with full (over two thirds of cases) or partial remission while enabling 'catch up' weight gain and growth.
- Immunosuppression: prednisolone, adding in azathioprine (for a steroid-sparing effect if steroid-dependent disease), or other immune-suppressive drug (if resistant to treatment) can be used along with/instead of dietary treatment, (e.g. mercaptopurine, methotrexate, ciclosporin). Thalidomide is proving effective in some resistant cases.
- Biological therapies such as infliximab (anti-tumour necrosis factor [TNF] antibody) infusion. Used for fistulae repair and disease resistant to other treatment.
- 5-aminosalicylic acid derivative is given to treat colitis.
- Antibiotic treatment: metronidazole and ciprofloxacin for perianal disease.
- Surgery should be reserved for acute emergencies or chronic strictures.

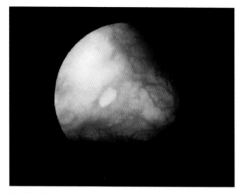

9.27 Crohn's disease. Appearance of the colon at colonoscopy, showing aphthous ulceration and loss of normal vascular pattern.

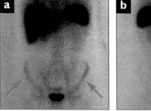
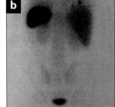

9.28 Crohn's disease. Technetium white cell scan showing (**a**) abnormal uptake in intestinal inflammation in Crohn's disease and (**b**) the normal appearance, with no uptake in the intestine.

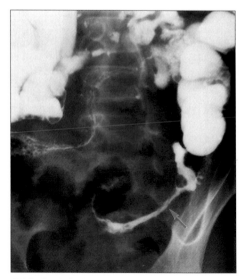

9.29 Crohn's disease. Radiological contrast studies demonstrating intestinal stricturing.

Prognosis
There is usually a chronic relapsing disease course. If the disease is controlled with aggressive medical treatment, there is a reduced need for surgery. About 5% of children have an initial presentation, then remain in remission, and about 5% have disease that is resistant to treatment, requiring aggressive medical treatment and possible surgery.

ALLERGIC COLITIS
Incidence/genetics
The commonest cause of non-infectious diarrhoea in infancy. Higher incidence in males. Family history of atopy, particularly in mother. Increasingly recognized in older children.

Diagnosis
Onset of diarrhoea, often with blood and mucus in the neonatal period or infancy in an otherwise healthy, thriving baby. Occurs in breast-fed as well as bottle-fed babies. May present as toddler's diarrhoea (see page 257). Investigations include colonoscopy (**9.30**) with mucosal biopsies. Macroscopically, there is colonic erythema (often patchy) and, histologically, an inflammatory infiltrate of the colonic lamina propria with eosinophils and plasma cells. Specific IgE radioabsorbent (RAST) tests for specific foods, and skin-prick tests for allergens, may indicate offending foods. Plasma immunoglobulin levels may demonstrate immunodeficiency, most commonly a low IgA and/or IgG subclass levels.

Treatment
Dietary exclusion of offending foods. Cow's milk, soya, egg and wheat are most common, but many other foods have been implicated, including fish, pork and beef.

Prognosis
Improves with age, but there is often persistent intolerance to a large amount of the offending food. Most children cannot drink cow's milk, but may tolerate it in cooking or when boiled.

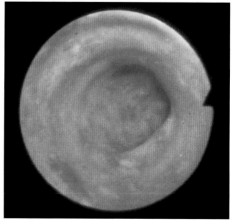

9.30 Allergic colitis. Macroscopic appearance of colon at colonoscopy: patchy erythema.

LYMPHANGIECTASIA
Incidence
Rare.

Diagnosis
Oedema and diarrhoea, usually in child less than three years old, but can develop in adolescence. Associated failure to thrive. Increased frequency of infections.

May develop secondary to elevated lymphatic pressure in congestive heart failure. Small intestinal mucosal biopsy should be carried out, with histological examination for dilated lacteals and distorted villi. Plasma lymphocytes $<1.5 \times 10^9/l$.

Treatment
Low-fat, high-protein, medium-chain triglyceride diet. Fat-soluble vitamin supplements. If a limited area is affected, surgical resection should be considered.

Prognosis
Severity in proportion to extent of intestinal disease.

ULCERS
Gastric ulcer
Incidence
Rare.

Aetiology
Usually secondary to other disorders, such as acute stress, including burns, intracranial pathology, salicylates and other non steroidal anti-inflammatory drugs in children under 10 years old. It is still not certain whether *Helicobacter pylori* is associated with gastric ulcer in children.

Diagnosis
Peptic ulcers in the neonatal period commonly present with life-threatening haemorrhage or perforation and secondary ulcers in older children frequently present in a similar manner. Abdominal pain may occur in older children. Gastroscopy should be carried out (**9.31**).

Treatment
H_2 receptor antagonists or proton pump inhibitors.

Prognosis
Secondary ulcers usually resolve completely after the acute episode.

Duodenal ulcer
Incidence
As for *Helicobacter pylori* (see page 272).

Aetiology
Associated with *H pylori* infection.

Presentation/diagnosis
Clinically there is usually episodic epigastric pain, often awakening the patient at night. Associated with recurrent vomiting; haematemesis may occur. Endoscopy should be carried out, with mucosal biopsy for histological examination. Mucosal sections should be stained with a substance, such as Giemsa, to detect *H pylori*.

Treatment
As for *H pylori*.

Prognosis
Excellent, with lack of recurrence if *H pylori* is eradicated.

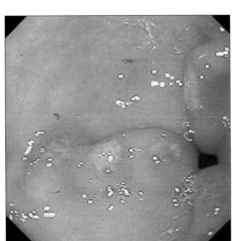

9.31 Endoscopic appearance of gastric ulcers and erosions adjacent to pylorus.

POLYPS
Isolated inflammatory / juvenile polyp
Incidence/genetics
One percent of pre-school/school age children. Predominantly male.

Aetiology
Inflammatory colonic polyp, with more than one in over 50% of cases. May occur in any area of the colon. About 60% of polyps are proximal to the sigmoid colon.

Diagnosis
Painless rectal bleeding (frank blood passed with or without faeces) in 90%. Also abdominal pain, rectal or polyp prolapse via rectum, pruritus, pain after defaecation, rectal mucus, diarrhoea or constipation. Colonoscopy with polypectomy and histological examination should be conducted (**9.32**). Macroscopically, polyps are rounded with a slender stalk; histologically, they are hamartomatous.

Treatment
Endoscopic polypectomy via colonoscope.

Prognosis
Low recurrence. No subsequent problems.

Juvenile polyposis syndrome
Incidence/genetics
May be familial or sporadic. If there are more than ten polyps it is more likely to be a syndrome.

Aetiology
Multiple inflammatory polyps occur throughout the colon. The stomach and small intestine may be affected as well. Histologically polyps are hamartomatous.

Diagnosis
Most commonly patients present with painless rectal bleeding and prolapse. The rectal haemorrhage is rarely life-threatening and can be asymptomatic. Failure to thrive, diarrhoea and intussusception may occur. Symptoms usually start from five years of age in sporadic cases and from nine years in familial cases. Colonoscopy with polypectomy and histological examination of polyp should be conducted.

Treatment
Polypectomy at colonoscopy. Regular colonoscopic surveillance.

Prognosis
In generalized juvenile polyposis there is an increased incidence of gastric, duodenal, pancreatic and colonic adenomata and adenocarcinoma (usually in adult life) which has not been seen when polyps are limited to the colon.

Familial polyposis coli and Gardner syndrome
Incidence/genetics
Autosomal dominant. Familial polyposis coli affects about 1 in 8,000. Gardner syndrome is rare.

Aetiology
Multiple (thousands) of adenomatous colonic polyps (**9.33**). Gastric and small intestinal polyps also occur in Gardner syndrome.

Diagnosis
Diarrhoea, abdominal pain, rectal bleeding from about ten years of age. Patients with Gardner syndrome also develop bony abnormalities (particularly osteomas of frontal and

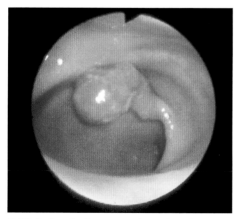

9.32 Isolated inflammatory/juvenile polyp.

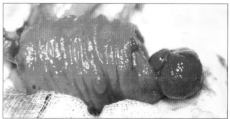

9.33 Colon showing multiple polyposis.

mandibular bones), dental abnormalities, central nervous system and thyroid tumours and, in over 90% of cases, hypertrophy of retinal pigment epithelium. Colonoscopy should be carried out, with polypectomy of larger polyps and histological examination.

Treatment
Regular endoscopic examination and eventual colectomy.

Prognosis
100% malignancy risk with time.

Peutz-Jegher syndrome
Incidence/genetics
Autosomal dominant.

Aetiology
Hamartomatous polyps of the small intestine and, in some cases, the colon.

Diagnosis
Abnormal pigmentation of lips, extending onto the facial skin and in the buccal mucosa (**9.34**). Most common symptom is abdominal pain due to intussusception/mechanical intestinal obstruction by a polyp. May present with iron-deficiency anaemia due to bleeding from an intestinal polyp. Investigations: a small intestinal barium study and colonoscopy. Video-capsule examination if suspected polyp not detected with other investigations.

Treatment
Conservative. Removal of those polyps causing excessive bleeding or intussusception by endoscopy (or via an enterotomy at laparotomy if otherwise inaccessible).

Prognosis
Usually good, but a few patients develop intestinal and, rarely, gastric malignancy.

INFECTIONS AND INFESTATIONS

HELICOBACTER PYLORI
Incidence
H pylori infection is rare in children under 14 years in developed countries, but common worldwide.

Pathogenesis
H pylori is a gram-negative, spiral, motile organism (**9.35**). It produces a large amount of urease; this may lead to gastritis by producing ammonia which may be toxic to the gastric mucosa. It is probable that spread is by person to person.

Diagnosis
May present with symptoms of duodenal ulcer, epigastric pain and vomiting, often waking the patient at night. Infection with *H pylori* is associated with gastritis, but the gastritis is often asymptomatic. Gastrointestinal symptoms, such as recurrent abdominal pain, are not associated with an increased incidence of *H pylori* gastritis. Upper gastrointestinal endoscopy with biopsy should be conducted. Gastric antral colonization can be detected on histological appearance (with special staining, such as Giemsa), urease testing and culture.

Treatment
A two-week course of triple therapy with an H_2 receptor antagonist or proton pump inhibitor, plus antibiotics such as metronidazole and amoxicillin (or clarithromycin).

Prognosis
Duodenal ulcers do not recur after eradication of *H pylori*.

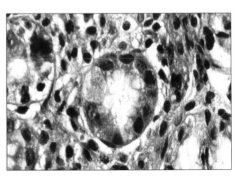

9.35 *Helicobacter*-like organisms within gastric glandular epithelium in sagittal and cross section.

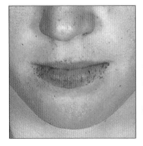

9.34 Peutz-Jegher syndrome, showing brown pigment-ation of lips and surrounding facial skin.

CAMPYLOBACTER JEJUNI

Incidence/aetiology

Usually sporadic and the source is not identified, but can be transmitted from undercooked chicken and other meat, and untreated water. Currently, it is the most frequently reported cause of acute bacterial diarrhoea in the UK.

Diagnosis

Onset with malaise, headache and fever and, within 24 hours, nausea, abdominal pain and diarrhoea. The diarrhoea may be mild, profuse and watery or bloody (especially in young children). Associated with Guillain-Barré syndrome. Stool culture in a low oxygen and high carbon dioxide environment will detect the presence of typical gram-negative curvilinear rods.

Treatment

Usually self-limiting. Erythromycin if severe or persistent infection, or patient is under two years old.

CLOSTRIDIUM DIFFICILE

Aetiology

C difficile and toxin can be detected in the healthy newborn and 10–50% of asymptomatic infants but less than 5% by one year of age. It is a gram-positive anaerobic bacterium that produces a cytotoxin and an enterotoxin.

Diagnosis

Acute or chronic mild diarrhoea, or severe pseudomembranous colitis. Stool testing for cytotoxin, toxigenic *C difficile* or toxin A should be conducted. Colonoscopy will reveal raised, adherent yellow-white mucosal plaques and erythematous friable colonic mucosa (**9.36**).

Treatment

Stop any antibiotic the patient is taking when diagnosed. Treat with vancomycin or metronidazole.

SALMONELLA

Incidence

Peak incidence in infancy and early childhood.

Aetiology

Gram-negative, motile, aerobic bacilli (**9.37**), acquired from contaminated food or drink. There are three types of *Salmonella*: *enteritides* (described here) *choleraesius*, and *typhi* (typhoid fever).

Diagnosis

Salmonella enteritides: incubation period is usually 12–72 hours (longer periods have been described in neonates). Onset is usually accompanied by nausea and fever, then diarrhoea, which can be watery or bloody. Bacteraemia and systemic infection with meningitis, osteomyelitis and pneumonia is most common in infancy.

Treatment

The mainstay of treatment is replacement of fluid and electrolyte losses by oral therapy if possible and, if not, intravenous fluids. Antibiotics are not recommended, except in infants under three months of age or those who are bacteraemic.

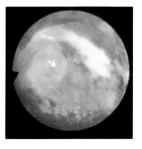

9.36 Macroscopic colonic appearance at colonoscopy in pseudomembranous colitis, demonstrating severe erythema and yellow-white plaques.

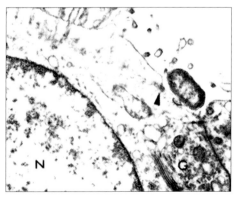

9.37 Electron microscopic appearance of *Salmonella* infection (×15,000).

PATHOGENIC ESCHERICHIA COLI

Incidence
A common, worldwide problem, particularly in developing countries.

Aetiology
Faecal–oral transmission. *E coli* are gram-negative motile bacilli which are some of the most common flora of the healthy large intestine. The pathogenic organisms each have one of four properties that the organisms in the normal flora do not possess. These are intestinal wall invasion, enterotoxin and cytotoxin production, or adherence to the bowel wall.

- Enterotoxin producing *E coli* (ETEC) produce heat labile (similar to cholera toxin) and heat stable toxins which result in profuse diarrhoea.
- Enteroinvasive *E coli* (EIEC) produce the same toxin as the shiga toxin from *Shigella dysenteriae*. They are spread through contaminated food and water, but can also pass from person to person.
- Enterohaemorrhagic *E coli* (EHEC) such as *E coli* 0157 produce cytotoxin. They are transmitted from cattle, and are often acquired from undercooked fast food.

Diagnosis
There are at least four different mechanisms of virulence (see aetiology above), each of which presents in a different way.

- Enterotoxigenic *E coli* (ETEC) – 'traveller's diarrhoea', nausea, vomiting, cramping abdominal pain and watery diarrhoea.

9.38 Renal biopsy of haemolytic uraemic syndrome showing microthrombi, swelling and destruction of glomerular capillaries.

- Enteroadherent (EPEC) *E coli* infection presents with a fever and a more prolonged illness, which can persist for many weeks in children, with the same symptoms as ETEC.
- Enteroinvasive *E coli* (EIEC) presents with fever and bloody diarrhoea that is clinically indistinguishable from *Shigella*.
- Enterohaemorrhagic *E coli* (EHEC) causes bloody diarrhoea with haemolytic uraemic syndrome often developing about a week after the onset, particularly in young children (**9.38**). Thrombocytopenic purpura may also develop.

Investigations should include stool culture and antibiotic sensitivities of organisms. In severe infection in small children, monitor for possible haemolytic uraemic syndrome (if 0157:H7 infection) or thrombocytopenia.

Treatment
Rehydrate and maintain hydration (see 'Acute gastroenteritis', page 253). Give appropriate antibiotic if severe infection, immunosuppressed or in infancy.

Prognosis
Full recovery can be expected with appropriate treatment. Recovery is less good if haemolytic uraemic syndrome is present.

GIARDIA LAMBLIA

Incidence
A flagellate protozoan, which infects in cyst form and becomes a motile trophozoite. Occurs virtually world-wide. Childhood prevalence increases with age.

Pathogenesis
Food and water, and person-to-person spread occur and may be transmitted by animals. Infects the small intestine and may cause an enteropathy of variable severity.

Diagnosis
Acute infection may present as watery diarrhoea, anorexia and abdominal distension. More frequently chronic diarrhoea develops with nausea, foul tasting flatulence, poor appetite and malabsorption (steatorrhoea). Essential investigations: microscopy of stool detects only some 80% of cases, even when several specimens are investigated (**9.39**). Can be detected on microscopy of duodenal fluid and/or proximal small intestinal mucosal biopsy.

Treatment
Metronidazole, 30 mg/kg/day as single dose for 3 days, or a single dose of tinidizole, 30 mg/kg.

Prognosis
Chronic infection is associated with immuno-globulin deficiency. If *Giardia* remains untreated, growth may be impaired.

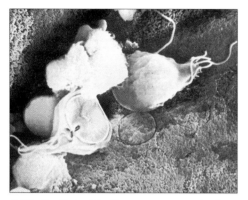

9.39 *Giardia lamblia.* Electron micrograph of trophozoites in the small intestine.

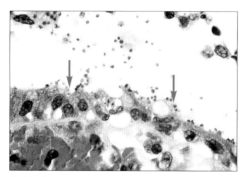

9.40 Cryptosporidiosis: intestinal specimen. (×250).

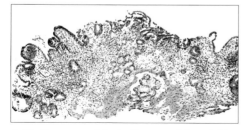

9.41 Cryptosporidiosis: *Cryptosporidium* visible on small intestinal mucosa. (×16)

YERSINIA ENTEROCOLITICA
Aetiology
Outbreaks from contaminated milk and food.

Diagnosis
Most commonly, acute self-limiting diarrhoea. Can cause fever and cramping abdominal pain, mimicking acute appendicitis. Ultrasound examination can differentiate between them. Chronic diarrhoea may ensue, possibly with erythema nodosum and arthritis. May mimic Crohn's disease. Isolation of *Yersinia* has been difficult, but a polymerase chain reaction-based assay may be feasible. Colonoscopy findings may mimic Crohn's disease with mucosal thickening of the terminal ileum, aphthous ulcers and nodularity.

CRYPTOSPORIDIUM
Incidence
A coccidian parasite that becomes incorporated in the intestinal epithelial cell, but outside the cytoplasm. Distribution is worldwide with 10% or more prevalence in developing countries. Spread by water and person-to-person contact.

Pathogenesis
May be due to disruption of microvillous membrane. An enteropathy of variable severity may develop. *Cryptosporidium* may infect small and/or large intestine (**9.40**, **9.41**). It reproduces both sexually and asexually.

Diagnosis
Acute, watery diarrhoea with fever, nausea, vomiting and abdominal discomfort after incubation period of one to seven days. May cause prolonged symptoms in immunodeficiency. The stool should be examined for oocytes, which can also be detected in duodenal juices and sputum with suitable staining techniques.

Treatment
Partial response to macrolide antibiotics (erythromycin, azithromycin, spiramycin, clindamycin). Hyperimmune bovine colostrum may reduce symptoms in the immunocompromised.

ASCARIS LUMBRICOIDES (ROUNDWORM)

Incidence

Ascaris lumbricoides is one of the commonest human parasitic infections worldwide. It is not common in the UK.

Aetiology

Larvae hatched from ingested eggs enter the venous system and migrate through the lungs to the oesophagus. Fertilized eggs from adult worms in the intestine are passed with faeces to contaminate soil; the cycle recurs when they, in turn, are ingested.

Diagnosis

Most infected people are symptom-free. Respiratory symptoms (cough, wheeze), fever and eosinophilia occur during the pulmonary phase. Anorexia, abdominal cramps and even intestinal obstruction may occur with heavy infestation. Worms can migrate to obstruct the biliary system (causing jaundice), pancreatic ducts (causing pancreatitis), appendix (causing appendicitis), and lead to volvulus, intussusception, intestinal perforation and peritonitis. The faeces should be examined microscopically for ova and adult worms, and sputum and gastric washings should be used to detect larvae.

Treatment

Mebendazole, albendazole, flubendazole or piperazine. Endoscopy to relieve biliary and pancreatic duct obstruction. Intestinal obstruction may be relieved by antihelminthic drug with intravenous fluids and nasogastric suction, but surgery may be necessary.

ENTEROBIUS VERMICULARIS (THREADWORM) (9.42)

Incidence

Most common in temperate and cold climates, but also occurs worldwide. Particularly affects children, but may be transmitted to other family members.

Diagnosis

Anal pruritis, particularly at night when the adult female lays eggs in the perianal region. Rarely, other symptoms may develop; for example, symptoms of appendicitis when worms enter the appendix lumen or if adult worms migrate through the intestinal wall to invade other organs. The 'Sellotape test' involves placing a piece of clear adhesive tape over the perianal region at night, then removing it in the morning and examining it for small white specks/ova.

Treatment

Mebendazole is the drug of choice (except for children under 1 year of age, for whom it is not recommended), or piperazine. The whole family should be treated and treatment repeated two to four weeks later to eradicate any worms hatched since first treatment.

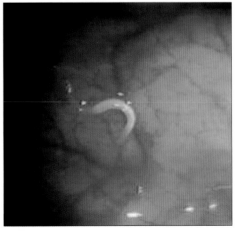

9.42 *Enterobius vermicularis* (threadworm) seen on colonic mucosa at colonoscopy.

FEEDING PROBLEMS

INCIDENCE
Common.

AETIOLOGY
May be caused by poor feeding technique, incorrect feed (for example, powdered milk made up to wrong strength) or inappropriate type of feed. Gastro-oesophageal reflux is an extremely common underlying disorder. There may be a food intolerance (see page 263), or psychosocial deprivation. It frequently becomes a secondary behavioural problem which may persist even if the underlying aetiology has resolved or improved. Poor feeding may also occur with neuromuscular disease, cardiac, respiratory, renal or hepatic failure and intercurrent infection. A child who has had a prolonged period of parenteral or enteral feeding may have lost or never developed feeding skills.

DIAGNOSIS
The infant is unwilling to ingest sufficient calories for normal weight gain and growth. Affected children often gag on food or fluids. There is food refusal, with the child turning their head away from the spoon or teat when fed, vomiting and poor weight gain. There should be close observation of feeding by an experienced nurse (e.g. a health visitor) and appropriate advice may resolve the problem. If the problem continues, the patient should have a careful medical examination (to look for evidence of underlying organ failure as in aetiology) and have possible underlying infection excluded (urine culture essential). If it still persists, there should be investigation as for gastro-oesophageal reflux.

TREATMENT
Advice should be given by specialist feeding nurse, speech therapist or other professional with specialist feeding knowledge. A child unable to feed orally needs cautious stimulation to 'desensitize', initially just touching the face around the mouth, then introducing a variety of shapes and textures to suck and mouth.

Treat any associated disease. If unable to ingest sufficient calories despite appropriate treatment, the child may benefit from overnight continuous feeds via an artificial feeding device with pump or daytime bolus feeds, while the underlying aetiology is investigated and treated.

Artificial feeding devices used are:
- Initially nasogastric tube.
- Gastrostomy may be inserted if support will be needed for several months or years (**9.43**).
- Naso-jejunal tube if the patient is unable to tolerate feeding via the stomach
- Gastro-jejunostomy
- Jejunostomy for longer-term small intestinal feeding

Problems with artificial feeding include infections with gastrostomy or jejunostomy devices; dislodgement is also common with gastro-jejunostomy and a naso-jejunal tube.

PROGNOSIS
As for underlying cause. If there is a significant underlying medical disorder the child may need continuous overnight feeds for months or years. Psychological dependence on an artificial feeding device commonly occurs. It is important to 'wean off' the device as soon as possible.

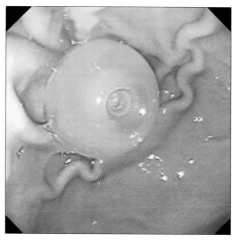

9.43 Endoscopic view of gastrostomy water inflated balloon *in situ*.

GASTRO-OESOPHAGEAL REFLUX

INCIDENCE
Commonest cause of chronic vomiting in infancy. Also presents in pre-pubertal children prior to their growth spurt when they have gained weight but not grown.

AETIOLOGY
Common problem in cerebral palsy. Increased frequency in children with other GI disease.

DIAGNOSIS
Excessive regurgitation/posseting, oesophagitis or respiratory disease. Poor feeding, poor weight gain, prolonged crying/colic and nocturnal screaming may develop. Onset is usually in the neonatal period, with excessive posseting and vomiting of milk after and be-tween feeds. The vomit does not contain bile, but can be bloodstained (due to oesophageal excoriation). If reflux is severe there may be associated apnoeic episodes. Older infants are reluctant to ingest lumpy food and may have gagging and choking episodes. Symptoms in the older child include epigastric pain, dys-phagia (may chew food for a prolonged length of time and be reluctant to swallow) and small appetite (frequently doesn't finish meals). Investigations:

- 24-hour repetition oesophageal pH study with pH microelectrode placed in the lower oesophagus.
- Barium swallow and meal in more severe cases (to exclude underlying structural disorder, such as malrotation). If reflux is seen on barium study, a pH study may be unnecessary if there is good response to treatment.
- Sputum microscopy: fat-laden macrophages present if aspiration has occurred.
- Upper gastrointestinal endoscopy if anaemic (possible oesophagitis) or failure to thrive not resolving with treatment (**9.44, 9.45**). Mucosal biopsy of oesophagus to detect oesophagitis, stomach for gastritis, or small intestine to investigate for enteropathy.
- Six-week trial of cow's milk exclusion, if appropriate, or investigate for possible underlying food-sensitive disease (see Food-sensitive enteropathy, page 263).

DIFFERENTIAL DIAGNOSIS
- Hypertrophic pyloric stenosis, urinary tract or other infection.
- Feeding mismanagement.
- Cow's milk protein intolerance/other food intolerance is frequently associated (particularly in atopic families).

TREATMENT
- Place infant prone or on side with head elevated.
- Thickened feeds with carobel or vitaquik (to supplement calorie intake if failing to thrive).
- Gaviscon
- Prokinetic agent to improve gastric emptying (e.g. domperidone).
- H_2 antagonist (e.g. ranitidine – withdraw when reflux is well controlled with prokinetic agent).
- Proton pump inhibitor if poor response to H_2 antagonist.
- Manage associated disease, for example exclude offending food(s) from diet (see Food-sensitive enteropathy, page 263).
- Surgery only when maximal medical treatment fails, a stricture has developed, or chronic oesophagitis causes chronic anaemia.
- Early fundoplication for infants with clearly documented apnoeic or cyanotic episodes due to reflux (near-miss cot deaths).
- Earlier surgery for the neurologically impaired child who fails to respond to medical treatment.

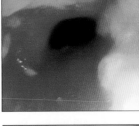

9.44 Endoscopic appearance of oesophagitis.

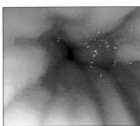

9.45 Endoscopic view of normal lower oesophageal sphincter, demonstrating mucosal 'Z' line.

PROGNOSIS

Symptoms resolve in most patients during the second year of life. In some cases more prolonged medical treatment is necessary.

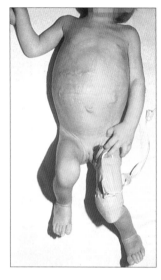

9.46 Intestinal pseudo-obstruction. Abdominal distension and failure to thrive.

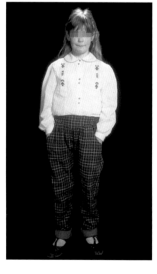

9.47 Intestinal pseudo-obstruction. The same child as in 9.46 growing and developing normally, solely on parenteral nutrition.

INTESTINAL PSEUDO-OBSTRUCTION

INCIDENCE / GENETICS

Very rare. Some cases may be X-linked or autosomal recessive.

AETIOLOGY

Lack of normal intestinal motility due to an abnormality of the intestinal neuromusculature (either nerves or muscles). Autoimmune disease in some patients. Hollow visceral myopathy is a myopathic variant that affects the urinary tract as well as the intestine.

DIAGNOSIS

Abdominal distension, constipation, vomiting, failure to thrive (**9.46**). Intermittent more severe obstructive episodes. There should be histological examination of full thickness intestinal biopsy to assess abnormalities of intestinal smooth muscle and nerve plexuses, and intestinal manometry should be carried out.

TREATMENT

Supportive. May need overnight continuous liquid enteral feeds to absorb sufficient nutrients. The most severely affected patients require parenteral nutrition (**9.47**).

PROGNOSIS

Chronic relapsing disorder.

SHORT BOWEL SYNDROME

INCIDENCE

Malabsorption, in the presence of a shortened small intestine. The condition is increasing in frequency, with improved survival in neonates' post-intestinal resection for severe necrotizing enterocolitis.

AETIOLOGY

Most patients are anatomically normal at birth and acquire the syndrome, most commonly following intestinal resection in infancy (usually necrotic intestine in necrotizing enterocolitis removed from premature infants), or resection of necrotic bowel following volvulus (usually with associated malrotation) at any age. Rarely, congenital short bowel occurs, usually in association with other congenital abnormalities, such as gastroschisis, or multiple small intestinal atresias resulting in 'apple peel' or 'Christmas tree' deformities.

DIAGNOSIS

Diarrhoea and failure to thrive. There is usually watery, osmotic stool due to sugar malabsorption, and steatorrhoea may occur. Symptoms can be exacerbated if there is loss of the ileo-caecal valve, which acts as a barrier preventing colonic bacteria invading the small intestine and a brake for the passage of fluid from the small to large intestine.

Investigations:

- Barium meal and follow-through to look for anatomical abnormalities (strictures, malrotation) and estimation of small intestinal length (if not already done at laparotomy).
- Intermittent monitoring for bacterial overgrowth which is particularly important if there is loss of the ileocaecal valve. Microscopy of stool and duodenal juices and indirect evidence from detection of bacterial matabolites in urine or hydrogen breath test.
- Nutritional investigations, plasma electrolytes and urea (low if poor protein intake), trace elements (including zinc, copper, selenium), fat soluble vitamins, A, E (most likely to be low) and K (prothrombin time) and haemoglobin, ferritin and folate.

- Vitamin B_{12} deficiency is particularly likely to develop subsequent to terminal ileal resection. Investigate with Schilling test (page 293).
- Trace elements and fat soluble vitamins need to be checked every three months if the patient is stable on long-term parenteral nutrition.

TREATMENT

Immediately post-resection, total parenteral nutrition is necessary to replace all nutrient and fluid losses. Enteral feeds should be added as soon as possible to maintain intestinal and liver function. The longer term management is to gradually reduce the volume of parenteral nutrition, with a corresponding increase in enteral feeds as adaption occurs.

Once the patient is established on a reasonable volume of enteral feed, it is best given continuously overnight with daytime boluses. Once about 50% of nutrition is tolerated enterally, an attempt can be made to reduce the number of nights per week on parenteral feeds. If long-term parenteral nutrition is required, management at home by parents should be organized (less complications than in hospital). The patient may require regular vitamin B_{12} injections.

PROGNOSIS

Neonatal short bowel syndrome continues to improve over the first four or five years. Adaption is often sufficient for parenteral nutrition to be withdrawn, providing there is about 25-30 cm of small intestine. The patient is unlikely to cope without parenteral nutrition if still receiving it at 5 years, despite good management.

If less than 30 cm of small intestine remains, many patients die during the first two years of life with liver failure. If they survive, they continue to be dependent on parenteral nutrition for normal growth (they have short stature (**9.48**) if parenteral nutrients are withdrawn). Small intestinal transplantation may be a reasonable alternative in the future, but up to now there has been a two-year survival of less than 70% (with intestinal graft survival about 50%).

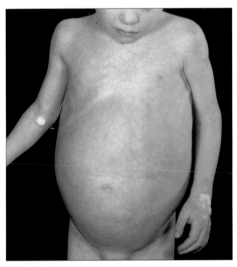

9.48 Child with short bowel subsequent to neonatal resection (see scar) of necrotic intestine due to volvulus (and malrotation), now presenting with short stature and abdominal distention due to malabsorption.

CONGENITAL AND INHERITED DISORDERS

CONGENITAL CHLORIDE DIARRHOEA

Incidence/genetics
Rare (1 in 43,000 in Finland) autosomal recessive disease.

Aetiology
Selective defect in intestinal chloride transport.

Diagnosis
Maternal polyhydramnios (**9.49**), often premature birth, lack of passage of meconium (instead watery stool often mistaken for urine) with distended abdomen. Rapid hyponatraemic, hypochloraemic dehydration with mild metabolic alkalosis (and hypokalaemia). May lose more than 10% of birth weight in 24 hours. May be referred to renal unit with secondary pre-renal renal failure. There should be investigations of plasma electrolytes and acid:base balance.

Treatment
Sodium, chloride and potassium replacement (may need 6 mmol/kg chloride, less with increasing age, with ratio of Na:K Cl 2:1 in infancy and 6:5 in older children).

Prognosis
If diagnosed early in neonatal life and adequately treated, there will be normal growth and development.

GLUCOSE–GALACTOSE MALABSORPTION

Incidence/genetics
Rare. Autosomal recessive gene on chromosome 22.

Aetiology
A selective defect in the intestinal glucose and galactose/sodium cotransport system. The gene, SGLT1 is on chromosome 22.

Diagnosis
Severe osmotic diarrhoea from birth. Stool sugar chromatography.

Treatment
Exclude glucose and galactose from the diet, substituting a fructose-based feed. In older children and adults a certain amount of glucose and galactose can be tolerated and dietary intake is altered according to symptoms.

Prognosis
Tolerance of offending carbohydrates improves with age. If diagnosed and treated early, normal growth and development.

SUCROSE–ISOMALTASE DEFICIENCY

Incidence/genetics
A rare condition that is inherited as an autosomal recessive trait.

Aetiology
Total or almost complete lack of sucrase activity with reduced maltase activity on small intestinal brush border.

Diagnosis
Frothy, watery diarrhoea, possibly with secondary dehydration, malnutrition, some vomiting and even steatorrhoea. Onset of symptoms when sucrose added to diet – for example, when the breast-fed baby commences solids.

Treatment
During the first year of life, diet excludes sucrose, glucose polymers and starch. The patient can usually tolerate starch after the age of 2 or 3 years.

Prognosis
Adult patients adjust their diets according to symptoms.

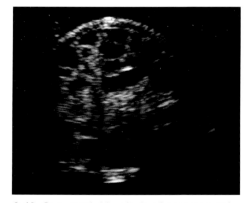

9.49 Congenital chloride diarrhoea: antenatal ultrasound for polyhydramnios showing dilated loops of bowel due to *in utero* diarrhoea.

LACTOSE MALABSORPTION

Incidence
In most of the world's population, lactose intolerance develops in adult life; it does not, however, affect most Caucasians.

Aetiology
Low or absent mucosal lactase is normal in non-Caucasians over five years old, with activity falling to 5–10% of the childhood level (**9.50**, **9.51**). Secondary lactose intolerance may occur when the small intestinal enterocyte brush border is damaged during infectious gastroenteritis.

Diagnosis
Loose, watery, frothy stools following ingestion of milk, with perianal excoriation. May develop following an acute infectious episode of gastroenteritis. Stool sugar chromatography to identify lactose in the stool.

Treatment
Avoidance of the offending sugars. Non-Caucasian adults avoid symptoms with a low-lactose diet.

Prognosis
Low lactase following infectious gastroenteritis usually rapidly resolves. Congenital deficiencies are a lifelong problem, but are asymptomatic if an appropriate diet is adhered to.

CYSTIC FIBROSIS
See also 'Respiratory Medicine' chapter.

Incidence/genetics
A disorder of epithelial cell chloride transport. At 1 in 2,000 to 3,000 live births, cystic fibrosis is the commonest autosomal recessive disease in Caucasians. Carrier frequency about 5%. The cystic fibrosis gene was discovered in 1989 and over 400 mutations are known. Disease severity correlates with mutation type; there is concordance for disease severity within families. The $\Delta F508$ mutation (a severe mutation) accounts for about 70% of cases in Caucasians. Patients with two 'severe' mutations have worse pancreatic failure.

Aetiology
Cystic fibrosis is caused by mutations in the transmembrane conductance regulator protein (CFTR) gene on chromosome 7, which encodes a cyclic-AMP regulated chloride channel protein.

Defective CFTR leads to altered electrolyte transport in epithelial cells of the gastrointestinal tract and tracheobronchial tree. The major gastrointestinal defect is malabsorption due to steatorrhoea, because of greatly reduced pancreatic exocrine secretions. Liver disease develops due to damage to intrahepatic biliary epithelial cells.

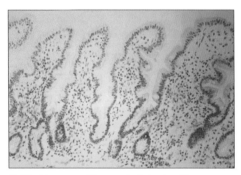

9.50 Absence of lactase in inherited lactose intolerance. Note histologically normal small intestine (x40).

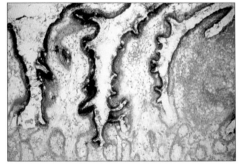

9.51 Normal small intestinal mucosa with positive brush border staining for lactase.

Diagnosis

Variable. May present in the neonatal period or later in childhood with failure to thrive and/or recurrent chest infections. Gastrointestinal abnormalities involve the intestine, pancreas and liver:

- Over 85% of patients have fat malabsorption and failure to thrive. They may present in infancy with oedema, hypoalbuminaemia and anaemia. Patients have a large appetite (unless severe chest disease or other disorder such as gastro-oesophageal reflux has developed) in association with poor weight gain.
- Meconium ileus occurs in ± 10% of cases.
- Distal intestinal obstruction syndrome (DIOS) affects about 10% of cases. Patients have intermittent episodes of intestinal obstruction with inspissated faecal contents (meconium ileus equivalent) in the terminal ileum and right colon. Intussusception may occur.
- Rectal prolapse occurs in up to 20% of cases (in 10% prior to diagnosis). Onset is from one to two-and-a-half years of age and spontaneous remission usually occurs by the age of five years.
- Cow's milk protein intolerance occurs in about 8% of patients under 3 years old.
- 20–25% of patients develop liver disease, progressing to cirrhosis in about 5% (see page 286–288).
- Virtually all males are infertile.

Investigations
- Sweat test: pilocarpine iontophoresis of small area on forearm to induce sweating and analysis for chloride and sodium content.
- Serum trypsinogen: high level in early infancy. Manifestations of the disease are largely due to sticky, inspissated, dehydrated secretions.
- Plain abdominal x-ray in meconium ileus: ground-glass appearance (air bubbles trapped in meconium). Intraperitoneal calcification if meconium peritonitis.
- Barium enema in meconium ileus: microcolon (**9.52**).
- Stool elastase: screening test for pancreatic insufficiency.
- Pancreatic function tests: low volume of secretions with low bicarbonate and relatively normal enzyme levels.
- Genetic markers include the ΔF508 gene mutation.
- Nutritional monitoring: include serum fat soluble vitamin levels (particularly vitamin E).

Treatment

- High calorie intake, including increased fat, should be encouraged. Pancreatic enzyme (enteric-coated) and fat-soluble vitamin supplements should be given to all patients.
- Meconium ileus intestinal obstruction treated with a hypertonic enema (gastrografin or hypaque) with intravenous fluid support.
- Distal intestinal obstruction syndrome can be relieved with a mild laxative (if mild), oral N-acetylcysteine, gastrografin enema or intestinal lavage. Ensure appropriate dose of pancreatic supplements is prescribed.
- Psychological support needed.
- Combined heart-lung transplants have been given with a similar success rate to transplants given for other diseases.
- Preliminary gene therapy studies are in progress using viral vectors to introduce normal CFTR DNA.

Prognosis

Morbidity and early mortality are usually secondary to chronic pulmonary disease. The median survival for females is about 28 years and for males about 32 years. If a patient has a less severe genetic mutation with relatively good pancreatic function (hence less steatorrhoea and a better nutritional state), presentation is later and prognosis better.

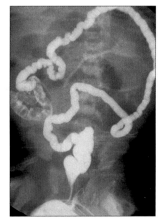

9.52 Cystic fibrosis. Barium study showing extensive micro-colon in a child presenting with meconium ileus.

PANCREATIC DISEASE

SHWACHMAN–DIAMOND SYNDROME

Incidence
Rare, but probably the second most commonly diagnosed cause of exocrine pancreatic insufficiency in childhood. Probable autosomal recessive inheritance with equal male : female incidence.

Aetiology
The pathogenesis is unknown, but a fetal insult in the fifth month of gestation, when both the exocrine pancreas and myeloid bone marrow are developing, would explain their association (**9.53**).

Diagnosis
Feeding difficulties with failure to thrive, diarrhoea and recurrent infections usually develop within the first few months of life. There is exocrine pancreatic insufficiency associated with bone marrow and haematological abnormalities.
Investigations:
- Pancreatic function tests: reduced lipase, trypsin and amylase secretion, with relative normal fluid volume and bicarbonate level in comparison to cystic fibrosis.
- Ultrasound: may demonstrate a small pancreas. The main pancreatic ducts are normal.
- Pancreatic histology: pancreatic acini are replaced by fat, while islet cells remain normal.

- Haematology: cyclical neutropenia and neutrophil mobility tests demonstrate an abnormal response to standard bacterial stimulation in over 90% of all cases. A cyclical thrombocytopenia occurs in two thirds and anaemia in 50% of patients.
- Bone marrow aspiration: may demonstrate marrow replacement by fibrous tissue or fat or myeloid arrest.
- Skeletal x-rays: metaphyseal chondrodysplasia of the femoral neck, short ribs with anterior flaring, vertebral wedging, clinodactyly and long bone changes.
- Hepatomegaly may occur and raised serum aminotransferase levels.
- Rarely, cardiac, respiratory, renal and testicular abnormalities may occur.

Differential diagnosis
Cystic fibrosis can be excluded with a sweat test, as patients with Schwachman syndrome have normal sweat electrolytes. Other causes of malabsorption, such as food-sensitive enteropathy or coeliac disease, are excluded with small intestinal biopsy (histologically-normal small intestinal mucosa in Shwachman-Diamond). Other immunodeficiencies not associated with pancreatic insufficiency and bony abnormalities.

Treatment
Pancreatic enzyme replacement. Prophylactic antibiotics may reduce the frequency of intercurrent infections. Severe haematological manifestations may warrant bone marrow transplantation.

Prognosis
The majority of patients enjoy relatively good health. Poor growth persists, despite pancreatic enzyme replacement. Recurrent infections continue and were the cause of death in up to 20% of cases in the past. Cases of leukaemia have been reported.

9.53 Shwachman syndrome. Chest deformity.

ACUTE PANCREATITIS

Incidence/genetics

Inflammation of the pancreas. Uncommon. Acute pancreatitis may develop after penetrating abdominal injury.

Aetiology

About 30% of cases are associated with severe multisystem disease, such as sepsis, shock, systemic infection, collagen vascular diseases, inflammatory bowel disease, Reye's syndrome. About 25% are related to trauma (blunt abdominal injury, including child abuse) or mechanical obstruction, others to metabolic disorders (hyperlipidaemia, hypercalcaemia, cystic fibrosis, malnutrition, renal disease, hypothermia, diabetes mellitus, organic acid-aemias). In up to 25% of cases there is no known predisposing factor.

Pathology

Poorly understood. Pancreatic inflammation can be induced by overstimulation of the gland, obstruction, increased permeability or overdistension of the duct, drugs, toxins and certain metabolic abnormalities.

Diagnosis

Abdominal pain of sudden onset, usually epigastric, with increasing severity over a few hours and continuing for just a few hours or as long as several weeks (average four days). In about a third of cases, pain radiates – usually through to the back. Attacks can be pain free. Also, frequently vomiting, particularly with food, anorexia, and may develop greasy stool. Investigations:

- Contrast-enhanced CT scan is the most useful investigation. It can be normal in mild pancreatitis. Abnormalities include changes in pancreatic size and texture, and visualization of complications such as pseudocyst, abscesses, calcification, duct enlargement, oedema, exudate and bowel distension.
- Serum amylase: raised level for 2–5 days.

Diagnostic if amylase level is raised to more than three times normal, but may not be increased at all. Serum lipase remains elevated for longer.

- Abdominal ultrasound may demonstrate an enlarged pancreas with reduced echogenicity.

Differential diagnosis

Other causes of abdominal pain and vomiting; for example, food sensitivity, intestinal malrotation, hepatitis.

Treatment

Supportive, according to symptoms and complications. If severe, full monitoring in intensive care is necessary. The aim is to rest the pancreas, but controlled trials have not usually demonstrated benefit. The usual treatment is to stop oral intake, give intravenous fluids, jejunal feeds (i.e. beyond the pancreatic duct) or parenteral nutrition, analgesia and antibiotics if infection suspected (**9.54**, **9.55**).

Prognosis

Variable, ranging from mild self-limiting abdominal discomfort to fulminant disease, progressing to multiorgan failure and, in some cases, a fatal outcome in hours or days.

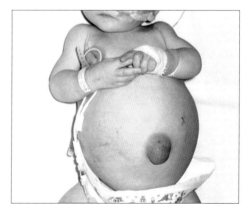

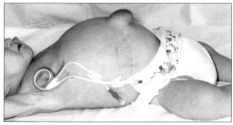

9.54, **9.55** Acute pancreatitis: abdominal distension of the abdomen with blood stained ascitic fluid, positive Cullen's sign (bruising around the umbilicus); management, including parenteral feeding with nasogastric drainage.

CHRONIC / HEREDITARY PANCREATITIS
Incidence/genetics
Autosomal dominant trait with variable penetrance (40–80%).

Diagnosis
Usually starts around ten years of age, but can begin from one year. Episodes of abdominal pain occur from monthly to yearly and last from two days to two weeks. Can be precipitated by large, fatty meals, alcohol and stress. Frequency of attacks usually decreases with age. There is severe epigastric pain that may radiate to the back and is lessened by adopting the fetal position. Epigastric tenderness and, in some cases, reduced bowel sounds and abdominal distension occur (**9.55, 9.56**).

Treatment
Symptomatic and supportive treatment (see acute pancreatitis above). Pain relief can be difficult even with strong analgesics. Somatostatin, oral pancreatic supplements and daily vitamin A and E can be helpful. Surgical treatment if intractable pain or complications.

Prognosis
Long-term complications such as pancreatic exocrine insufficiency or diabetes mellitus may develop. If pancreatic duct is dilated or pseudocyst or pancreatic ascites develops, pancreaticojejunostomy is beneficial. Other patients lead normal lives without surgery.

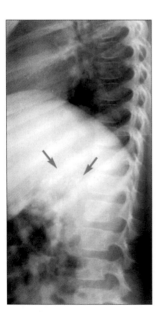

9.56 Chronic pancreatitis: lateral x-ray of abdomen and chest demonstrating pancreatic calcification.

LIVER DISEASE

SCLEROSING CHOLANGITIS
Incidence/genetics
Rare, but increasingly recognized with improved investigatory techniques. Family history of autoimmune disease. Can be hereditary, presenting in the neonate.

Aetiology
Most commonly associated with ulcerative colitis in adults and occurs with other autoimmune disease (including autoimmune enteropathy), or may develop with immunodeficiency, cystic fibrosis, psoriasis, reticulum cell sarcoma, sickle cell disease.

Pathogenesis
Poorly understood. Chronic inflammation and fibrosis with beading (dilatation) and stenosis of affected intra- and/or extra-hepatic bile ducts. Obliteration of peripheral ducts.

Diagnosis
Insidious onset with intermittent jaundice, pruritis, hepatomegaly, pyrexia, weight loss. Essential investigations: cholangiography to discover any bile duct changes (**9.57**); non-organ-specific autoantibodies are associated (antinuclear antibody, ANA and antineutrophil cytoplasmic antibodies, ANCA).

Treatment
Response to immunosuppressive therapy if autoimmune associated. Disease usually progresses with eventual liver failure and need for transplant.

Prognosis
Progresses to liver failure over about ten years.

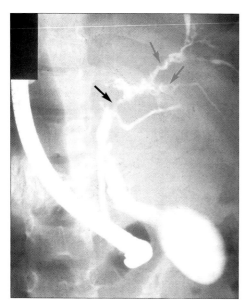

9.57 Sclerosing cholangitis. Endoscopic retrograde cholangiogram (ERCP) demonstrating dilatation, stenosis (black arrow) and irregularity of bile ducts (red arrows).

CHRONIC HEPATITIS

May present either when jaundice continues for more than three months after an acute hepatitis or develops insidiously. Classically, histologically divided into two groups:
• Chronic persistent hepatitis
• Chronic active hepatitis
Currently moving toward aetiological classification.

Incidence
Rare.

Aetiology
A: Hepatitis surface antigen-positive hepatitis
B: Hepatitis surface antigen-negative hepatitis
• Viral infection
    Hepatitis C (HCV),
    Cytomegalovirus,
    Epstein-Barr virus.
• Autoimmune chronic hepatitis
    Primary biliary cirrhosis.
• Metabolic/genetic abnormalities
    Wilson's disease,
    Alpha-1 antitrypsin deficiency,
    Cystic fibrosis.
• Drugs such as isoniazid.

Chronic persistent hepatitis
Diagnosis
Persistently elevated liver transaminase levels following an episode of acute hepatitis. In other patients, gradual onset of fatigue, malaise, anorexia and right upper quadrant discomfort. The diagnosis is made on the histological appearance of tissue obtained at percutaneous liver biopsy. There is normal hepatic lobular architecture, with an infiltration of monocytes in portal areas. Elevated plasma transaminase levels (with normal prothrombin time, alkaline phosphatase, albumin, globulin and gamma glutamyltransferase).

Treatment
Observation only; monitor transaminase levels.

Prognosis
Excellent (except may rarely progress to chronic active hepatitis or cirrhosis, if hepatitis B surface antigen-positive).

Chronic active hepatitis
Pathogenesis
Autoimmune damage to the liver with defective supressor 'T' lymphocytes.

Diagnosis
Acute onset of jaundice in most patients. May present insidiously with malaise, fatigue, anorexia, nausea. Hepatosplenomegaly in up to 80% of patients. May develop symptoms secondary to other organ-specific autoimmune disorders (see 'Autoimmune enteropathy', page 265) or inflammatory bowel disease.

Diagnosis is made on the histological appearance of percutaneous liver biopsy. Patchy hepatocellular necrosis with destruction of lobular architecture and regenerating hepatocytes with multiple nuclei are all seen.

Raised serum transaminases and bilirubin almost always occur. Frequently there are several other circulating autoantibodies, including antinuclear (ANA) in up to 75% of cases, with smooth muscle (SMA) or liver/kidney microsomal antibodies and multiple organ-specific autoantibodies.

Treatment
Immunosuppressive therapy with prednisolone and azathioprine for autoimmune disease. Interferon therapy if there is hepatitis B.

Prognosis

Usually a good response to immunosuppressive therapy (usually prednisolone then agathioprine), preventing progression to serious liver damage and cirrhosis.

ACUTE HEPATITIS
Aetiology

Viral infection such as hepatits A, B,C, D, E, cytomegalovirus, Epstein-Barr virus. May be drug-related.

Diagnosis

Usual onset is with flu-like symptoms. Jaundice, nausea, vomiting, loss of appetite, fever, tenderness in the right hypochondrium, muscle and joint pain, and pruritis with erythmatous macular rash, may also occur. Investigations include viral screening and liver function tests.

Treatment

Withdraw any drug treatment that may cause hepatitis.

Prognosis

Prognosis depends on aetiology. There is full recovery in the vast majority of cases. Approximately 5% of cases of hepatitis B and 50% of hepatitis C develop chronic disease.

ALAGILLE SYNDROME
Incidence/aetiology

The major inherited biliary disorders are those affecting the intrahepatic ducts. Alagille syndrome is the most common. It is a rare, autosomal-dominant multisystem disorder, characterized by reduced bile duct number and function.

Diagnosis

Intrahepatic bile duct paucity. Vascular anomalies. Other abnormalities may occur in the development of the heart, liver, eyes, vertebrae and the craniofacial region.

Treatment

Low fat diet with increased intake of medium-chain triglycerides and best possible carbohydrate and protein intake. Fat-soluble vitamin supplements.

Prognosis

High risk of bleeding. Over 30% of deaths maybe related to vascular anomalies. Other causes of death are end-stage liver disease, cardiac/renal disease and intercurrent infection. Liver transplant may be required.

MINERAL DEFICIENCIES

ZINC DEFICIENCY
Incidence/genetics

Rare. Acrodermatitis enteropathica is an autosomal recessive disorder due to a selective defect in the intestinal absorption of zinc (see also 'Dermatology' chapter).

Aetiology

May also develop in protein-energy malnutrition, short bowel syndrome and other malabsorptive states.

Diagnosis

Scaly, erythematous skin rash with bullae and pustules develops around mouth and anus. May occur symmetrically in interdigital areas and over buttocks, hands, feet and elbows. Also alopecia, dystrophic nails, photophobia, conjunctivitis and glossitis (**9.58–9.61**). Diarrhoea with malabsorption, psychological and behavioural disturbances and susceptibility to infection may develop. Investigations: plasma zinc level; copper and zinc levels are inversely proportional to each other; other trace elements may also be deficient.

Treatment

Oral zinc supplementation. If possible, treat underlying malabsorptive disorder.

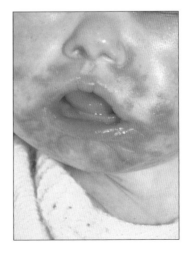

9.58 Zinc deficiency affecting perioral area and face.

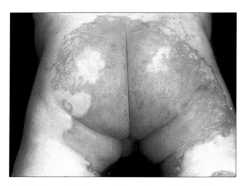

9.59 Zinc deficiency. Skin rash on buttocks.

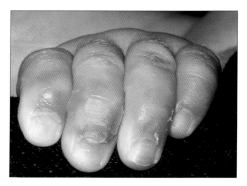

9.60 Zinc deficiency affecting the fingers.

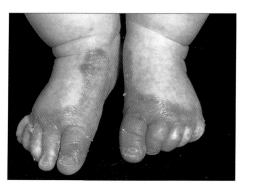

9.61 Zinc deficiency. Appearance of feet.

IRON DEFICIENCY

Incidence
Common in infancy. Increased frequency in Asian children, vegetarians and vegans. Also increased frequency in toddler and adolescents.

Aetiology
Poor intake, malabsorption or excessive losses. Poor nutritional intake in the pre-school child, particularly if a high milk intake. Secondary to overt or occult gastrointestinal or other blood loss. For example, severe gastro-oesophageal reflux, gastritis or ulcerative colitis.

Diagnosis
Lethargy with poor exercise tolerance. Pica, poor appetite and poor concentration span. Also, lowered resistance to infection and poor thermoregulation. Anaemia. Investigations: haemoglobin; haematocrit; red blood cell indices demonstrate a normocytic, or microcytic, hypochromic anaemia; rarely, a bone marrow aspirate required. Plasma ferritin level indicates adequacy of iron stores.

Treatment
Improved diet or treatment of the underlying cause of blood loss. Oral iron supplements may also be required.

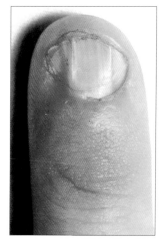

9.62 Trophic nail changes associated with iron deficiency, showing flattening and concavities (koilonychia).

COPPER DEFICIENCY

Incidence/genetics
Rare. Menke's disease is an X-linked recessive disease with poor copper absorption and metabolism, affecting 1 in 50,000 to 100,000.

Aetiology
Unsupplemented, long-term, total parenteral nutrition, severe malabsorption or administration of high dose zinc.

In Menke's disease, defect of intracellular copper transport.

Diagnosis
Anaemia and neutropenia. Bony abnormalities and skeletal fragility. Skin depigmentation.

Microscopically, pili torti of hair is seen in Menke's disease (**9.63**).

Treatment
Copper supplements. Parenteral supplements in Menke's disease.

COPPER EXCESS: WILSON'S DISEASE

Incidence/Genetics
Rare autosomal recessive disorder. 1 in 10,000 to 30,000 worldwide. Carrier frequency of 1 in 90. Gene identified on chromosome 13.

Aetiology
Disorder of copper balance in which there is inadequate biliary excretion of copper.

Diagnosis
Hepatic disease: from five years of age, variable manifestation ranging from an acute self-limiting hepatitis with full recovery, to fulminant hepatic failure. Chronic liver failure and cirrhosis in older patients.
Central nervous system: from six years of age, but more commonly in teens and 20s. Motor, not sensory disease. Initially tremor, incoordination, dystonia, fine motor difficulties. Later drooling, dysarthria, gait disturbance.
Ophthalmological: Kayser-Fleischer rings (**9.64**).
Psychiatric: poor school performance, anxiety, depression, compulsive behaviour, even psychosis.
Cardiac: arrythmia, myocardial disease.
Renal: proximal tubular dysfunction. Renal stones are common.
Investigations: increased 24-hour urinary copper excretion, usually decreased caeruloplasmin level.

Treatment
See 'Neurology' chapter, page 212.

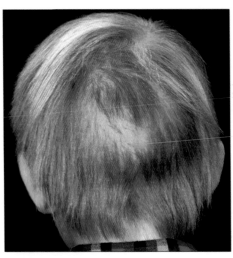

9.63 Menke's disease: pili torti.

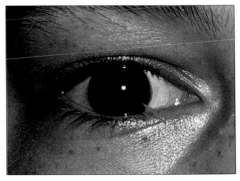

9.64 Wilson's disease: jaundice, faint Kayser-Fleischer ring (arrow) and spider naevi.

SELENIUM DEFICIENCY

Incidence
Rare.

Aetiology
Occurs in children on unsupplemented long-term parenteral nutrition or with severe malabsorption.

Diagnosis
Cardiomyopathy, myositis, macrocytic anaemia. Measurement of plasma level and glutathione peroxidase activity.

Treatment
Supplement enteral/parenteral nutrition.

VITAMIN DEFICIENCIES

Vitamins are organic food substances. They are not synthesized by the body. Small amounts are essential for normal body metabolism. The B group vitamins and vitamin C are water soluble. Vitamins A, D, E and K are fat soluble.

SCURVY, VITAMIN C / ASCORBIC ACID DEFICIENCY

Incidence
Rare, in famines.

Aetiology
Citrus fruit and green vegetables contain ascorbic acid. It is essential for collagen synthesis for bone, cartilage and dentine. An important antioxidant. Required for adrenal gland function and iron absorption.

Diagnosis
Bleeding of gums and around hair follicles and capillaries. Irritability and painful limbs causing 'pseudoparalysis'. Investigations: response to supplements; plasma and white cell ascorbic acid level; bone x-ray: calcificaton of sub-periosteal haematoma with 'ground-glass' appearance of metaphyses and dense rim, 'smoke-ring' of cortical bone around epiphyses.

Treatment
Ascorbic acid 500 mg per day for a week, and investigate dietary source.

Prognosis
Treat immediately or the patient is at risk of sudden death. There is a rapid response to treatment, apart from bone remodelling, which takes some months.

BERIBERI, VITAMIN B$_1$, THIAMIN DEFICIENCY

Diagnosis
Manifests in two forms – 'wet' and 'dry' beriberi.

- India and the Far East: 'Wet' beriberi with acute high output cardiac failure, in breast-fed infants of mothers with a diet of polished rice. Coughing, choking and aphonia with laryngeal oedema. Drowsiness and meningism.
- Developed countries and older children: 'Dry' beriberi/Wernicke's encephalopathy presents as encephalopathy in children on long-term total parenteral nutrition. In older children with a diet based on polished rice, presents with sensory and motor neuropathy.

Patients can become comatose just two weeks after stopping vitamin supplements in parenteral nutrition, if there is no oral intake. Investigations: trial of supplements. Examine blood for transketolase activity.

Treatment (9.65)
Parenteral (intravenous or intramuscular) vitamin B (50–100 mg) preparation, then oral supplements. Dietary intake of nuts, peas, beans, pulses, brewer's yeast. Enrich rice with thiamin.

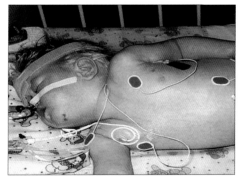

9.65 Beriberi coma reversed within three hours of intravenous dose B-group vitamins.

PELLAGRA / NIACIN DEFICIENCY
Incidence
Endemic in parts of Africa, where diet is based on maize.

Aetiology
Poor bioavailability of nicotinic acid in maize and low in tryptophan. Pyridoxine deficiency may also result in pellagra – essential cofactor for nicotinic acid synthesis from trypyophan.

Diagnosis
- Skin: photosensitive dermatitis with scaling and pigmentation (**9.66**).
- Gut: angular stomatitis and diarrhoea.
- Neurological: depression, dementia, delerium, peripheral neuropathy.

Investigations: there is a rapid response to supplements. Urine, N1methyl nicotinamide and pyridone derivative.

Treatment
Orally, parenteral vitamin B (100 mg) preparation, four-hourly. Add pulses, wholemeal cereals, meat or fish to diet.

RIBOFLAVIN / VITAMIN B$_2$ DEFICIENCY
Aetiology
Pyridoxine is antagonized by isoniazid, hydralazine, penicillamine and oestrogens.

DIAGNOSIS
Cheilosis, magenta coloured tongue (**9.67**) and nasolabial seborrhoea. If deficient, *in vitro* addition of flavin adenine dinucleotide increases erythrocyte glutathione reductase activity by more than 30%.

TREATMENT
Riboflavin 20 mg/day. Add milk, eggs, liver, pulses or legumes to diet.

PYRIDOXINE / VITAMIN B$_6$ DEFICIENCY
Diagnosis
Convulsions, depression and peripheral neuropathy. Investigations: rapid response to supplements; serum pyridoxal 5-phosphate; *in vitro* increase in red cell aspartate and alanine aminotransferases in presence of pyridoxal 5-phosphate.

Treatment
Oral pyridoxine 10 mg/day. Whole grains, bananas, liver and peanuts are dietary sources.

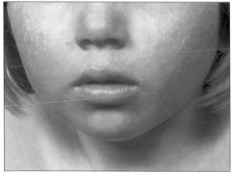

9.66 Pellagra patient showing associated dermatitis.

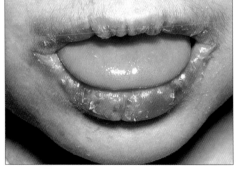

9.67 Angular stomatitis and cheilosis (inflammation and cracking of the lips) and magenta tongue with B-group vitamin deficiency.

CYANOCOBALAMIN / VITAMIN B$_{12}$ DEFICIENCY

Incidence
Rare.

Aetiology
Ileal resection, vegan diet or intrinsic factor deficiency or abnormality. B$_{12}$ is derived solely from animal products.

Diagnosis
Anaemia, yellow tint to skin, glossitis, paraesthesia, ataxia and dementia. Investigations: Schilling test – give radioactive isotope of vitamin B$_{12}$ orally, then intramuscular dose (not radioactive). Collect urine for 24 hours. If less than 10% of oral dose detected there is malabsorption. Repeat the same test with intrinsic factor to exclude intrinsic factor deficiency as the cause for malabsorption.

Treatment
Vitamin B$_{12}$ 1,000 μg twice-weekly until normal Hb, then every six weeks.

VITAMIN K / NAPHTHOQUINONE DEFICIENCY (9.68)

Incidence
Rare

Aetiology
Newborn infants and in children with fat malabsorption.

Diagnosis
Coagulopathy or haemorrhagic disease of newborn. May affect bone formation. Prothrombin time prolonged. The normal intestinal flora can manufacture quinones with vitamin K activity. Antibiotics may suppress their manufacture and lead to deficiency.

Treatment
Vitamin K 5 mg, as required.

RETINOL / VITAMIN A DEFICIENCY

Incidence
Rare.

Aetiology
Poor intake or secondary to fat malabsorption.

Diagnosis
Xerophthalmia: conjunctival xerosis with Bitot spots, keratinization and necrosis of cornea (**9.69, 9.70**). Vitamin A blood level <200 μg/l.

Treatment
Vitamin A 150 mg orally and 150 mg intramuscular for 3 days, then 9 mg/day for 2 weeks. Dietary intake of yellow or orange fruit and green leafy vegetables, liver, milk, butter, cheese, eggs.

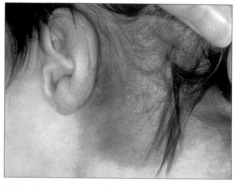

9.68 Unusual site of bleeding seen in vitamin K deficiency.

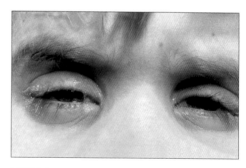

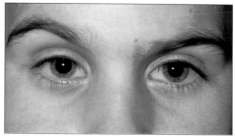

9.69, 9.70 Vitamin A deficiency in a child with short gut and steatorrhoea, before treatment (above) and after (below).

TOCOPHEROL / VITAMIN E DEFICIENCY

Incidence
Rare.

Aetiology
Fat malabsorption. This is the most common vitamin deficiency in children with long-term intestinal failure.

Diagnosis
Presents with steatorrhoea and haemolysis in premature neonates. Neurological changes: wide-based gait, spinocerebellar degeneration, ocular palsy. Investigations: serum vitamin E level or red cell susceptibility to haemolysis by hydrogen peroxidase.

Treatment
Oral or intramuscular tocopherol supplements.

VITAMIN D DEFICIENCY

Incidence/genetics
Vitamin D-dependent rickets is autosomal recessive. Hypophosphataemic rickets is X-linked dominant.

Aetiology
- Poor dietary intake or renal disease (low 1,25 dihydroxy vitamin D – the most active form).
- Vitamin D deficiency in absence of metabolic defect may develop in children who are not exposed to sunlight (such as institutionalized children).
- Children with fat malabsorption may develop rickets due to vitamin D and calcium malabsorption. Black children are most susceptible.
- Anticonvulsants induce hepatic enzymes; give 10 µg/day vitamin D.

Diagnosis
- Rickets: genu valgum, epiphyseal swelling (especially distal radii) and growth retardation.
- Skull: craniotabes, delayed closure of fontanelles and bossing of frontal and parietal bones.
- Chest: 'pectus carinatum' (**9.71**), rickety rosary (enlarged costochondral junctions) and Harrison's sulci (rib cage depression where diaphragm inserted)
- Teeth: delayed dentition.

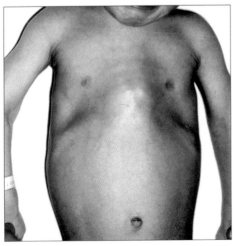

9.71 Nutritional rickets. Pectus carinatum and Harrison's sulci.

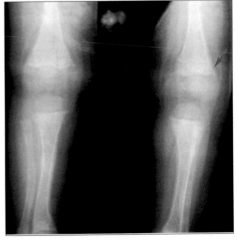

9.72 Rickets. X-ray of knee demonstrating splaying (arrow) and irregularity of femoral and tibial metaphyses.

- Additionally, irritability, hypotonia, respiratory failure, tetany, laryngospasm, convulsions, aminoaciduria.

Investigations: blood – plasma alkaline phosphatase raised with low phosphate and/or calcium; x-ray – wide metaphyseal plate and concave diaphyseal ends (**9.72**); plasma vitamin D level. The severity of rickets is proportional to the amount of specific vitamin D metabolites and calcium and phosphate ion product.

Treatment

Vitamin D 1,000 to 5,000 µg IV/day until normal alkaline phosphatase is achieved, then 10 µg/day and 500 ml/day of milk for calcium requirements. Expose to sunlight (ergocalciferol is the most important source). Dietary source: oily fish, fortified margarine.

REFERENCES

Acute gastroenteritis
Walker-Smith JA, Sandhu BK, Isolauri E et al. ESPGAN Working Group on Acute Diarrhoea. Recommendations for feeding if childhood gastroenteritis. *J Paed Gastroenterol Nutr* 1997; **24**: 619–620.

Infantile colic
Lucassen PLB, Assendelft WJ, Gurtels JW *et al.* Effectiveness of treatment for infantile colic: systematic review. *BMJ* 1998; **316**: 1563–1569.

Constipation
Clayden GS. Personal practice: management of chronic constipation. *Arch Dis Child* 1992; **67**: 340–344.

Recurrent abdominal pain
Stordal K, Nygaard EA, Bentsen B. Organic abnormalities in recurrent abdominal pain in children. *Acta Paediatr* 2001; **90**: 638–642.

Toddler's diarrhoea
Fenton TR, Milla PJ. The Irritable Bowel Syndrome. In: Milla PJ, Muller DPR (eds). *Harries' Paediatric Gastroenterology*. London: Churchill Livingstone, 1988: 272–285.

Intractable diarrhoea
Cuenod B, Brousse N, Goulet O *et al.* Classification of intractable diarrhoea in infancy using clinical and immunohistological criteria. *Gastroenterol* 1990; **99**: 1037–1043.

Chronic intestinal failure
Vanderhoof JA. Preliminary experience with intestinal transplantation in infants and children. *Pediatrics* 1996; **97**: 583–584.

Fabricated and induced illness
Meadow R. Management of Munchausen syndrome by proxy. *Arch Dis Child* 1985; **60**: 385–393.

Coeliac disease
Walker-Smith JA, Guandalini S, Schmitz J, Schmerling DH, Visakorpi JK. Revised criteria for diagnosis of coeliac disease. Report of working group of European Society of Paediatric Gastroenterology and Nutrition. *Arch Dis Child* 1990; **65**: 909–911.
Rossi TM, Tjota A. Serological indicators of celiac disease. *J Ped Gastroenterol Nutr* 1998; **26**: 205–210.
Schmitz J. Lack of oats toxicity in coeliac disease. *BMJ* 1997; **314**: 159.

Food-sensitive enteropathy
Hill DJ, Hosking CS. Cow's milk allergy in infancy and early childhood. *Clin Exp Allergy* 1996; **26**: 243–246.

Autoimmune enteropathy
Hill SM, Milla PJ, Bottazzo GF, Mirakian R. Autoimmune enteropathy and colitis: is there a generalised autoimmune gut disorder? *Gut* 1991; **32**: 36–42.

Eosinophilic gastroenteropathy
Byrne WJ. Gastroenterologic Disorders. In: Stiehm ER., Fulganti VA (eds). *Immunologic Disorders in Infants and Children*. Philadelphia: Saunders, 1980: 492–517.

Crohn's disease
Hyams JS. Crohn's disease in children. *Ped Clin N Am* 1996; **45**: 255–277.

Ulcerative colitis
Kirschner BS. Ulcerative colitis in children. *Paed Clin N Am* 1996; **43**: 235–254.
Sugita A, Sachar DB, Bodian C, Ribeiro MB, Aufses AH Jr, Greenstein AJ. Colorectal cancer in ulcerative colitis. Influence of anatomical extent and age at onset on colitis-cancer interval. *Gut* 1991; **32**: 167–169.

Allergic colitis
Hill SM, Milla PJ. Colitis caused by food allergy in infants. *Arch Dis Child* 1990; **65**: 132–133.

Duodenal ulcer
Sherman PM. Peptic ulcer disease in children. Diagnosis, treatment and the implication of *Helicobacter pylori*. *Gastroenterol Clin N Am* 1994; **23**: 707–725.

Juvenile polyposis syndrome
Woodford-Richers K, Bevan S, Churchman M et al. Analysis of genetic and phenotypic heterogeneity in juvenile polyposis. *Gut* 2000; **46**: 656–660.
Winter SW. Intestinal Polyps. In: Walker WA *et al* (eds). *Pediatric Gastrointestinal Disease* (2nd edn). St Louis: Mosby, 1996: 891–907.

Peutz-Jeghher's syndrome
Winter SW. Intestinal Polyps. In: Walker WA *et al* (eds). *Pediatric Gastrointestinal Disease* (2nd edn). St Louis: Mosby, 1996: 891–907.

Familial *polyposis coli* and Gardner's syndrome
Winter SW. Intestinal Polyps In: Walker WA *et al* (eds). *Pediatric Gastrointestinal Disease* (2nd edn). St Louis: Mosby, 1996: 891–907.

Lymphangiectasia
Shmitz J. Protein Losing Enteropathies. In: Milla PJ, Muller DPR (eds). *Harries' Paediatric Gastroenterology*. London: Churchill Livingstone, 1988: 260–271.

Helicobacter pylori
Drumm B, Koletzko S, Oderda G. *Helicobacter pylori* infection in children: a consensus statement. European Paediatric Task Force on Helicobacter pylori. *J Pediatr Gastroenterol Nutr* 2000; **30**: 207–201.

Campylobacter jejuni
Blaser MJ. Bacterial gastrointestinal infections. *Gastroenterol Ann* 1986; 3: 317–340.

Clostridium difficile
Wilkins TD. Role of *Clostridium difficile* toxins in disease. *Gastroenterology* 1987; **93**: 389.

Salmonella.
Laney DW, Cohen MB. Approach to the pediatric patient with diarrhoea. *Gastroenterol Clin N Am* 1993; **22**: 499–516.

Pathogenic *Escherichia coli*
Cantey JR. *Escherichia coli* diarrhoea. *Gastroenterol Clin N Am* 1993; **22**: 609–622.

Yersinia enterocolitica
Black RE, Slome S. Yersinia enterocolitica. *Infec Dis Clin N Am* 1988; **2**: 625–641.

Giardia lamblia
Farthing MJG. Parasitic and Fungal Infections of the Digestive Tract. In: Walker WA *et al* (eds). *Pediatric Gastrointestinal Disease* (2nd edn). St Louis: Mosby1996: 664–676.

Cryptosporidium
Farthing MJG. Parasitic and Fungal Infections of the Digestive Tract. In: Walker WA *et al* (eds). *Pediatric Gastrointestinal Disease* (2nd edn). St Louis: Mosby1996: 664–676.

Enterobius vermicularis **(threadworm)**
Burns DA. Infestations in school children. *Prescriber's J* 1988; 2: 80–87.

Ascaris lumbricoides **(roundworm)**
Pawlowski ZS. Ascariasis. In: Pawlowski ZS (ed). Clinical Tropical Medicine and Communicable Diseases. London: Ballière Tindall, 1987: 595.

Gastro-oesophageal reflux
Hillemeier AC. Gastroesophageal reflux. *Ped Clin N Am* 1996; **43**: 197–212.

Intestinal pseudo-obstruction
Rudolph CD, Hyman PE, Allschuler SM *et al*. Diagnosis and treatment of chronic intestinal pseudo-obstruction in children: report of consensus workshop. *J Pediat Gastroenterol Nutr* 1997; **24**:102–112.

Short bowel syndrome
Vanderhoof J. A., Langnas AN. Short bowel syndrome in children and adults. *Gastroenterol* 1997; **113**: 1767–1778.

Congenital chloride diarrhoea
Holmberg C, Perheentupa J, Launiala K, Hallman N. Congenital chloride diarrhoea: clinical analysis of 21 Finnish patients. *Arch Dis Child* 1977; **52**: 255–267.

Glucose galactose malabsorption
Desjeux JF. Congenital Transport Defects. In: Walker WA *et al* (eds). *Pediatric Gastrointestinal Disease* (2nd edn). St Louis: Mosby, 1996: 792–816.

Sucrase-isomaltase deficiency
Auricchio S. Genetically Determined Disaccharidase Deficiencies In: Walker WA *et al* (eds). *Pediatric Gastrointestinal Disease* (2nd edn). St Louis: Mosby, 1996: 761-785.

Cystic fibrosis
Shalon BS, Adelson JW. Cystic fibrosis: gastrointestinal complications and gene therapy. *Pediatr Clin N Am* 1996; **43**: 157–196.

Shwachman-Diamond syndrome
Smith OP. *Seminars in Haematology* 2002; **39**: 95–102.

Acute pancreatitis
Weizman Z, Durie PR. Acute pancreatitis in childhood. *J Pediatr* 1988; **113**: 24–29.

Chronic/hereditary pancreatitis
Moir CR, Konzen KM, Perrault J. Surgical therapy and long-term follow up of childhood hereditary pancreatitis. *J Pediat Surg* 1992; **27**: 282–287.

Chronic active hepatitis
Gupta SK, Fitzgerald JF. Chronic hepatitis. In: Walker WA *et al* (eds). *Pediatric Gastrointestinal Disease* (2nd edn). St Louis: Mosby, 1996:1320–1329.

Vitamin K/naphthoquinone deficiency
Hey E, Vitamin K–what, why, and when. *Arch Dis Child Fetal Neonatal Ed.* 2003; **88**: 80–3.

Renal Diseases

Rose de Bruyn • Sally Feather
Chula Goonasekera • Sarah Ledermann
Stephen Marks • Margot Nash
Lesley Rees • Sushmita Roy
Neil Sebire • Richard Trompeter
William van't Hoff • Paul Winyard

HAEMOLYTIC URAEMIC SYNDROME (HUS)

INCIDENCE AND AETIOLOGY

One of the commonest causes of acute renal failure in childhood.

Classified into diarrhoea-associated (D+ HUS) or typical HUS, and non-diarrhoea associated (D– HUS) or atypical HUS:

- D+ HUS occurs mainly in childhood, sporadically in summer months or in epidemics. Infective causes vary across the continents but *Escherichia coli* 0157 (H7 and other serotypes) and *Shigella dysenteriae* type 1 are the commonest aetiological organisms.
- D– HUS accounts for 10% of cases, affects all ages without seasonal pattern. Infective causes are neuraminidase-producing *Streptococcus pneumoniae* and HIV (human immunodeficiency virus). Other causes include defects in complement factors such as factor H.

Nomenclature is sometimes confusing, since diarrhoea is not always absent in D- HUS. 'Idiopathic HUS' has replaced 'atypical HUS', with inherited forms of HUS accounting for a large proportion of these cases: increasing genetic advances in delineating autosomal dominant or recessive forms (including factor H deficiency and inborn errors of cobalamin metabolism).

Drug-induced causes of HUS with calcineurin inhibitors (ciclosporin and tacrolimus), chemotherapeutic agents, antiplatelet agents and oral contraceptive pills. Other causes include transplantation (bone marrow and solid organ), malignancy, pregnancy, systemic lupus erythematosus, and glomerulonephritis.

CLINICAL PRESENTATION

HUS should always be considered in children who present with diarrhoea (often bloody), vomiting and severe abdominal pain. They may have pallor, lethargy, jaundice, petechiae, bleeding, oliguria, anuria, fluid overload, oedema, hypertension, convulsions, coma, pancreatitis and pneumonia.

DIFFERENTIAL DIAGNOSIS

There is an overlap with thrombotic thrombocytopenic purpura (TTP) which is also characterized by thrombocytopenia, microangiopathic haemolytic anaemia and abnormalities in renal function. Neurological symptoms and signs, and associated fever, are much more prominent, however, in TTP.

DIAGNOSIS

Triad of Coombs' negative microangiopathic haemolytic anaemia (**10.1**) with fragmented red cells, thrombocytopenia and acute renal failure. Investigations include FBC, differential white cell count, blood film, reticulocyte count, ferritin, Coombs' tests, group and save, urea, creatinine, serum electrolytes, glucose, amylase, lipase, LDH, haptoglobin, liver function tests, serology, Thomsen-Friedenreich antigen (T-Ag), anti-streptolysin O titre (ASOT), urinalysis, stool culture, renal ultrasound and percutaneous renal biopsy (not routinely indicated in D+ HUS but may show predominant glomerular or arteriolar involvement and acute cortical necrosis).

TREATMENT

Overall treatment of HUS is similar to any cause of acute renal failure therapy, with optimal fluid and electrolyte management, diuretic therapy, other anti-hypertensive agents and dialysis. There is no role for antibiotics, except when there is proven streptococcal infection, which may exacerbate HUS. Peritoneal dialysis is the preferred renal replacement modality. Consideration for plasma infusions and/or exchange in patients with idiopathic HUS (**10.2**). In poorly responsive or resistant forms of idiopathic HUS, treatments with steroids, intravenous immunoglobulin, vincristine, splenectomy and bilateral nephrectomies are anecdotally advocated, although there are conflicting results in different case series.

PROGNOSIS

D+ HUS results in complete recovery in the majority of cases, with no relapses. There is reduced morbidity and mortality during epidemics by prompt recognition, identification and isolation of individuals to prevent spread, and elimination of the source with removal of contaminated food and water. The prognosis in D– HUS is worse, with a progressive course and 25% relapse rate.

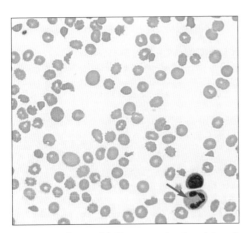

10.1 May Grunwald-Giemsa stained peripheral blood smear showing a reactive lymphocyte above a neutrophil (arrow) with evidence of microangiopathic haemolytic anaemia. There are numerous red blood cell fragments, thrombocytopenia, few spherocytes and polychromasia in a case of diarrhoea-associated haemolytic uraemic syndrome.

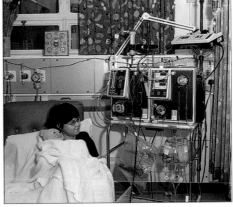

10.2 This patient is receiving treatment with plasma exchange, which can be used for many renal conditions, including atypical haemolytic uraemic syndrome and the glomerulonephritides (either primary renal diseases such as membranoproliferative glomerulonephritis and idiopathic, rapidly progressive glomerulonephritis, or secondary to vasculitis or systematic lupus erythematosus).

NEPHROTIC SYNDROME

INCIDENCE

The nephrotic syndrome (NS) consists of heavy albuminuria, hypoalbuminaemia and oedema (**10.3**). It may be primary or secondary to an overt systemic disorder. In children the commonest variety of NS is characterized by minimal histological changes in the glomeruli (minimal change – MCNS (**10.4**) and response to corticosteroid therapy (steroid-responsive – SRNS) (**Table 10.1**).

INCIDENCE OF MCNS

MCNS has a median age of onset of 2.5 years. It is commoner in boys than girls, and in Asian than Caucasian children. It is associated with atopy. There is heavy, highly selective proteinuria which responds to corticosteroid therapy. Microscopic haematuria may be present, (but not macroscopic haematuria) (**Table 10.2**).

10.3 Nephrotic oedema in an infant of 3.5 years of age. In NS the oedema is dependent, accumulating in low pressure areas around the eyes, in the legs, and as ascites.

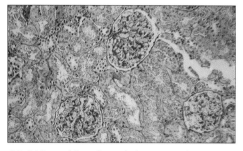

10.4 Minimal histological changes in the glomeruli.

Table 10.1 Glomerular histology in primary NS in children

Glomerular histology	Children (n)	Steroid-responsive (n)
Minimal change (MCNS)	98 (78% of total)	93 (95% of MCNS)
Focal segmental glomerulosclerosis (FSGS)	12	2
Proliferative glomerulonephritis		
Membranoproliferative	6	1
Diffuse mesangial	4	3
Crescentic	4	0
Membranous nephropathy	2	0
Chronic glomerulonephritis	1	0
Total	**127**	**99**

Table 10.2 Clinical and laboratory features in children with primary nephrotic syndrome

Percentage of cases:	MCNS	FSGS	MPGN
Age <8 years	80	50	3
Male	60	69	36
Systolic BP >95th centile	21	49	36
Urine RBCs >10^5/ml	23	48	51
Plasma C3 <90 mg/dl	1	4	74
IgG/transferrin clearance ratio <10% (highly selective)	53	13	10
Plasma creatinine >98th centile	33	41	50

DIAGNOSIS

Hypoalbuminaemia causes oedema because of a disturbance of the Starling equilibrium in the capillary bed, and rapid albumin loss results in hypovolaemia with abdominal pain, shock, and risk of thrombosis. Venous thrombosis is multi-factorial, with sluggish peripheral circulation, relative polycythaemia, hyperlipidaemia, platelet hyperaggregability, hyperfibrinogenaemia and loss of control proteins such as antithiombin-III, all contributing to the procoagulant state. Loss of IgG and complement components, particularly Factor B of the alternative pathway, predisposes to infection, typically pneumococcal septicaemia and peritonitis.

TREATMENT

The initial treatment is corticosteroids (**Table 10.3**). Renal biopsy should be considered at presentation if the child is <1 or >12 yr of age, has macroscopic haematuria, or has renal impairment or hypertension; and at any stage if the child is steroid resistant (**Table 10.4**). If the child is steroid sensitive, minimal change histology can be presumed and does not need to be confirmed by biopsy. Prophylactic penicillin is also mandatory when nephrotic.

PROGNOSIS

One-third of children with MCNS have only a single episode, one-third relapse occasionally, and one-third become steroid-dependent frequent relapsers. Relapses eventually cease; the development of steroid resistance is unusual, and end-stage renal failure almost never occurs.

Table 10.3 Levels of treatment

Level	Relapse	Treatment
1	Initial episode	Prednisolone 60 mg/m^2/day for 28 days
2	First two	Prednisolone 60 mg/m^2/day until remission
3	Frequent	Prednisolone 0.5–1.0 mg/Kg alternate days
4	On prednisolone 0.5–1.0 mg/kg/alt day	Levamisole 2.5 mg/kg/alt day
5	On levamesole	As levels 2 and 3
6	On prednisolone 0.5–1.0 mg/kg/alt day	Cyclophosphamide 3 mg/kg/day for 8 weeks
7	Post-cyclophospharnide	As levels 2 and 3
8	On prednisolone 0.5–1.0 mg/g/alt day	Cyclosporin A commence at 5 mg/kg/day in 2 doses for one year (monitor CyA level)
9	On cyclosporin A	Add alternate day maintenance prednisolone
10	On CyA + pred >0.5 mg/kg/alt day	Consider chlorambucil

Table 10.4 Definitions

1	Nephrotic syndrome	Oedema; plasma albumin <25 g/l; proteinuria> 40mg/m^2/hr
2	Remission	Proteinuria <4 mg/m2/hr or Albustix 0/trace for 3 consecutive days
3	Relapse	Proteinuria >40 mg/m2/hr or Albustix ≥2+ for 3 consecutive days
4	Frequent relapses	≥2 relapses in 6 months
5	Steroid sensitive	Remission achived with steroid therapy within 28 days
6	Steroid resistance	No remission in spite of >4 weeks prednisolone >60 mg/m^2/day
7	Steroid dependence	Relapse on or within 2 weeks of steroid therapy

POLYCYSTIC KIDNEY DISEASES

CLASSIFICATION AND GENETICS

- Autosomal recessive polycystic kidney disease (ARPKD). Caused by mutations in PKHD1 on 6p21.
- Autosomal dominant polycystic kidney diseases (ADPKD). Commonest mutation is in PKD1 on 16p13. The gene codes for a cell signalling molecule. A minority of ADPKD cases are caused by PKD2 on 4q, which encodes a calcium channel.
- Glomerulocystic disease. Autosomal dominant but detailed genetics unknown.
- Tuberous sclerosis. Autosomal dominant, with mutations of TSC2 on 16pl3 (adjacent to PKD1).
- von Hippel-Lindau disease. Autosomal dominant inheritance with mutation of gene on 3p25-26.
- Oro-facio-digital syndrome type 1. X-linked dominant.
- Acquired polycystic kidney disease. Secondary to chronic hypokalaemia or uraemia.

INCIDENCE

Considering all ages, the incidence of ARPKD is 1 in 10,000 and of ADPKD 1 in 1,000. The former accounts for the majority of cases in childhood but it is increasingly recognized that ADPKD is not uncommon in paediatric practice. Other causes listed above are rare.

PRESENTATION

ARPKD may present antenatally, with abnormal renal ultrasound, or neonatally with nephromegaly and renal failure. Less severe cases have renal impairment and hypertension in infancy whereas, in later childhood, mild renal disease can coexist with liver fibrosis and portal hypertension. ADPKD can present with loin pain, urinary infection, mild renal impairment or hypertension in childhood but it is generally clinically silent until adulthood. There is a rare and severe early onset variety of ADPKD with contiguous mutations of PKD1 and TSC2.

DIAGNOSIS

Prenatal genetic diagnosis of ADPKD or ARPKD is feasible, especially if DNA from affected relatives is available. Severe ARPKD may be detected in the last trimester by ultrasound scan showing enlarging kidneys and oligohydramnios. If renal failure is not severe, an intravenous urogram postnatally shows characteristic dilatation of the medullary collecting ducts in ARPKD.

Ultrasound scans (**10.5**) do not reliably distinguish between ARPKD and early ADPKD but cysts enlarge considerably in the course of the latter disorder. Renal cysts are seen well on CT scan (**10.6**) but this is not superior to the less costly and less invasive ultrasound. Always investigate the parents with renal ultrasound scans; one will be affected in ADPKD and new mutations are unusual. In ARPKD, periportal liver fibrosis can be diagnosed by biopsy or suggested by isotope (HIDA) scans; in ADPKD, liver cysts may be present.

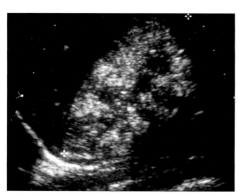

10.5 Ultrasound scan image demonstrating large bright kidney of ARPKD.

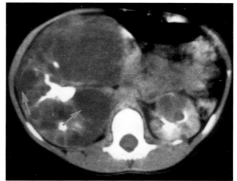

10.6 Computerized tomography scan of ADPKD. Note the asymmetrical involvement with visible cysts (arrows).

PATHOLOGY

ARPKD cysts arise from collecting ducts while ADPKD cysts arise from all nephron segments. There are aberrations of cell proliferation, apoptosis, epithelial cell polarity and the extracellular matrix.

In addition, PKHD1 and PKD182 all expressed in the primary cilium. OFD1 protein is expressed in the centrosoma/basal body of the primary cilium.

TREATMENT

Controlled trials in adults with ADPKD show that low protein diets, control of hypertension and cyst surgery have little, if any, significant influence on progression to renal failure. However, hypertension in PKD should be vigorously treated to reduce cardiovascular damage and possibly slow progression. Renal transplantation is effective, although native nephrectomy may be required for nephromegaly or recurrent urinary infections. Portal hypertension in ARPKD and liver cysts and Berry aneurysms in ADPKD also need treatment in their own right.

PROGNOSIS

A significant proportion of ARPKD patients develop renal failure soon after birth and a small subset of ADPKD patients have a severe infantile presentation. Half of ARPKD patients develop end-stage renal failure by adolescence, whereas only half of ADPKD patients develop uraemia in a lifetime. The rate of disease progression is highly variable even in single PKD kindreds.

VESICO-URETERIC REFLUX AND ITS NEPHROPATHY

See also 'Urology' chapter.

CLASSIFICATION

Vesico-ureteric reflux (VUR) is the retrograde passage of urine from the bladder into the ureter and/or the renal pelvis, calyces and collecting ducts. It can be secondary to high bladder pressure due either to anatomical lesions of the urethra (e.g. posterior urethral valves) or to neuromuscular incoordination of bladder emptying (e.g. neurogenic bladder). 'Reflux nephropathy' describes the presence of primary VUR when associated with renal disease: these kidneys can be either malformed during development or damaged postnatally by pyelonephritis associated with reflux of infected urine.

GENETICS

Isolated primary VUR is an autosomal dominant disorder with incomplete penetrance and variable expression; the genetic defect is unknown. Rarely primary VUR can be inherited (although several candidate loci have been defined) as part of a syndrome (e.g. with optic nerve colobomas, in which case mutations of PAX 2 have been defined).

INCIDENCE

Estimates of the incidence of VUR in children range between 1 in 50 to 200. The risk of primary VUR in a sibling approaches 50% when screened with a micturating cystourethrogram (MCUG) before the age of 2 years.

PRESENTATION

When VUR is associated with other abnormalities the clinical presentation is determined by the primary disease (e.g. poor urinary stream with posterior urethral valves). Primary VUR may be clinically silent and many of the milder cases regress over years. The commonest presentation is with urinary tract infection (UTI) and indeed VUR is frequently diagnosed when investigating children for UTI. Recurrent pyelonephritis in the first years of life may lead to hypertension or chronic renal failure in later childhood or adulthood.

DIAGNOSIS

Severe prenatal VUR can be detected as hydronephrosis on ultrasound scanning in the second trimester. In this case, a MCUG soon after birth will confirm the presence and define the extent of VUR, and will also diagnose any coexisting urethral pathology. In younger children with UTI, MCUG is the investigation of choice to detect VUR (**10.7**), while in older children VUR can be diagnosed by indirect radionucleotide cystogram (**10.8**). In addition, the kidneys should always be imaged to assess the presence of coexisting renal malformations (by ultrasound scan) or scarring (by DMSA isotope renography). Given the high familial incidence of primary VUR, screening of young siblings of index cases is recommended.

PATHOLOGY

In primary VUR there is an anatomical defect in the uretero-vesical junction. In 'reflux nephropathy' renal histopathology reveals either immature tissues (dysplasia) or scarring (chronic interstitial fibrosis) – i.e. not acquired postnatally.

TREATMENT

All neonates with severe antenatal hydro-nephrosis should be commenced on prophy-lactic antibiotics pending definitive diagnosis. Posterior urethral valves should be resected and other associated defects treated. Management of primary VUR aims to prevent recurrent pyelonephritis, achieved in most children by long-term antibiotic prophylaxis. Antireflux surgery is an alternative but, as yet, there is no evidence of its superiority to medical management.

PROGNOSIS

The long-term prognosis of primary VUR depends on the presence and severity of the associated nephropathy.

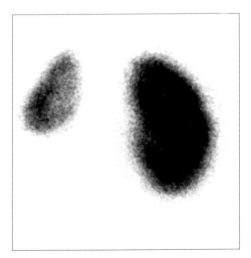

10.7 DMSA isotope is taken up by functional kidney tubules. In this posterior view, the left kidney is small after scarring from pyelonephritis.

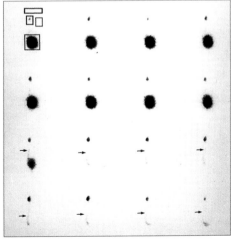

10.8 Indirect radionucleotide cystogram shows a small amount of isotope in the left kidney after injection of MAG3, which is filtered by the glomerulus. On sequential views, the urinary bladder empties upon voiding with reflux of isotope up the left ureter (arrows).

HENOCH–SCHÖNLEIN PURPURA

INCIDENCE / AETIOLOGY

Relatively common small vessel vasculitis peaking at 4–6 years. Often preceded by upper respiratory infection. Cause is unknown; rarely associated with underlying C2 or C4 deficiency. Pathology is leukocytoclastic vasculitis, with IgA deposition. Renal biopsies are consistent with IgA nephropathy.

CLINICAL PRESENTATION

Rash (required for diagnosis) – typically symmetric and gravity dependent, especially on forearms, legs and buttocks (**10.9**). Petechial or purpuric, often palpable, non-blanching and evolving colours (pink, yellow, green and then brown). Rash may be macular or urticarial initially. May have oedema, especially of hands, feet, face and/or scrotum. Gastrointestinal tract involvement is present in 65% of cases, with bowel wall haemorrhage causing dull peri-umbilical abdominal pain, vomiting, and tenderness.

May have melaena or intussusception. Typical 'thumb-printing' on barium enema. Transient arthritis (in 65% of cases) in multiple joints, especially knees and ankles (see also 'Rheumatology' chapter). Renal involvement (in 50% of cases) – any type but commonly haematuria. May have nephrotic syndrome, hypertension, rapidly progressive renal failure with crescentic glomerulonephritis. Also malaise, fever, headaches.

DIFFERENTIAL DIAGNOSIS

Consider low platelets (sepsis, leukaemia, idiopathic thrombocytopenic purpura, haemolytic uraemic syndrome) and vasculitis (SLE, microscopic polyarteritis, polyangiitis nodosa, acute post-streptococcal glomerulonephritis).

DIAGNOSIS

FBC and clotting (to exclude thrombocytopenia and coagulation abnormalities); urea; creatinine; electrolytes; urinalysis (to detect significant renal involvement). If renal involvement is severe, consider C3, C4, anti-nuclear antibody (ANA), anti-neutrophil cytoplasmic antibody (ANCA), anti-streptolysin O titre (ASOT), renal ultrasound and biopsy. If intussusception is suspected, abdominal ultrasound should be performed.

TREATMENT

Symptomatic pain relief, explanation, re-assurance. If prolonged, watch nutrition. Prednisolone 1–2 mg/kg/day for severe gut involvement (has also been suggested for severe joint or skin involvement), and NSAIDs for joint pain.

Consider plasma exchange, cyclophosphamide, methylprednisolone, oral prednisolone, dipyridamole, aspirin for rapidly progressive glomerulonephritis. Follow-up for renal problems, hypertension and proteinuria for at least 1 year, or longer if these problems persist.

PROGNOSIS

Very good. Usually self-limited with complete resolution by a mean of one month, but can recur, more rarely after years. Microscopic haematuria may persist, or macroscopic episodes occur after URTIs. One to five percent have long-term renal problems, with hypertension or impaired function. This is more likely if there has been hypertension, significant proteinuria, or crescentic/ rapidly progressive glomerulonephritis at presentation. It uncommonly recurs in renal transplants.

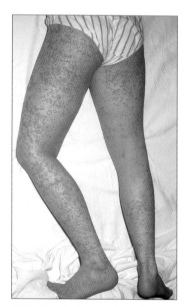

10.9 Classical purpuric rash on bilateral lower limbs of patient with Henoch-Schönlein purpura.

RENAL AGENESIS AND DYSPLASIA

CLASSIFICATION / GENETICS

Renal agenesis and dysplasia represent malformations in which the fetal organs have failed to undergo a normal pattern of differentiation. In renal agenesis, no kidney tissue can be detected. Dysplastic kidneys contain undifferentiated and metaplastic elements, while multicystic dysplastic kidneys contain large cysts; their excretory function is often absent or considerably reduced. Most are sporadic, although some are associated with other defects in multiple organs (e.g. CHARGE and VACTERL associations).

Rarely, families have been reported with definite inheritance of agenesis or dysplasia. These can occur in isolation or be syndromal (e.g. X-linked Kallmann syndrome with renal agenesis and infertility; autosomal dominant branchio-oto-renal syndrome with renal dysplasia and deafness; renal cysts and diabetes syndrome).

INCIDENCE

The incidence of bilateral renal agenesis is highly variable, depending on the study. Unilateral disease is often clinically silent and the estimated incidence is 1 : 1,000 to 10,000. The incidence of multicystic and bilateral renal dysplasias is about 1 : 5,000.

PRESENTATION

Unilateral multicystic dysplastic kidneys classically present as an abdominal mass in infancy although, increasingly, these malformations are detected by antenatal ultrasound scanning. About 20–30% of such children have contralateral abnormalities, including pelviureteric or ureterovesical obstruction. Bilateral renal malformations can result in oligohydramnios, premature delivery and the Potter sequence (oligohydramnios, oliguria, pulmonary hypoplasia and limb deformities). Renal dysplasia is very commonly associated with abnormalities of the lower urinary tract including obstructive lesions (e.g. posterior urethral valves in boys and ureteroceles in girls).

DIAGNOSIS

Renal dysplasia is suggested on ultrasound scanning by the visualization of irregular-shaped organs with loss of corticomedullary differentiation (**10.10**). Cysts, where present, can be identified but these cases need to be distinguished from polycystic kidney disease or hydronephrosis.

Technically, the diagnosis of dysplasia can only be made by histology but this is rarely clinically indicated. If ultrasound suggests unilateral agenesis, a DMSA isotope renogram can be performed to exclude the possibility of an ectopic kidney.

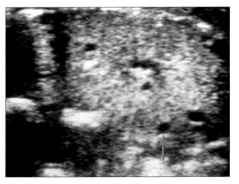

10.10 Renal ultrasound scan shows loss of corticomedullary differentiation in a dysplastic kidney. Note the small subcortical cysts (arrow).

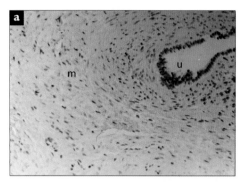

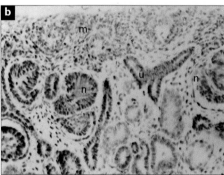

10.11 The upper panel (**a**) shows histology of a dysplastic kidney. Note the lack of tissue differentiation versus a human fetal kidney (**b**) which contains primitive nephrons (n) in addition to mesenchyme (m) and branches of the ureteric bud (u).

PATHOLOGY

Dysplastic kidneys contain immature ducts which are considered to be branches of the ureteric bud surrounded by fibromuscular and undifferentiated cells (**10.11**). There may also be metaplastic tissue including cartilage.

TREATMENT

When bilateral malformations are associated with severe oligohydramnios, termination should be considered due to the poor prognosis associated with pulmonary hypoplasia. A subgroup with large bladders and urinary obstruction have been treated with vesico-amniotic shunts. Although this procedure may increase the amount of liquor, it is unproven whether lung growth is accelerated. Those with bilateral dysplasia require lifetime follow-up for the detection and treatment of chronic renal failure.

Unilateral multicystic dysplastic kidneys probably do not require any specific treatment, but prophylactic antibiotics are indicated until associated urological contralateral abnormalities can be excluded. There is evidence that many of these organs involute spontaneously over months or years (**10.12**). Some authorities, however, recommend removal of these kidneys because of a (disputed) risk of renal malignancy and hypertension.

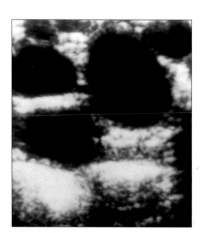

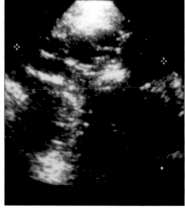

10.12 This multicystic dysplastic kidney partially involuted over two years.

PROGNOSIS

Bilateral agenesis or severe dysplasia may cause neonatal death if associated with pulmonary hypoplasia. With advances in dialysis and transplantation, renal failure can be adequately treated although some of these children die in the first year from malformations of other organs (e.g. lung, heart, brain and gut). Unilateral renal agenesis may be clinically silent throughout life and has minimal increased morbidity if the contralateral kidney is normal, although deterioration in renal function may occur with age. Reflux and contralateral kidney abnormalities occur in 30–50% of patients with unilateral dysplasia.

RENAL FANCONI SYNDROME

INCIDENCE

The renal Fanconi syndrome consists of generalized proximal tubular dysfunction (aminoaciduria, glycosuria, bicarbonaturia, phosphaturia) and rickets or osteomalacia. Most cases occur as part of a metabolic disorder or are secondary to drugs/toxins, renal or other diseases (**Table 10.5**).

DIAGNOSIS

Children present with both symptoms of the underlying cause and features of proximal tubular dysfunction: polyuria, polydipsia, recurrent dehydration, poor growth, vomiting and rickets. Children with cystinosis (the commonest inherited cause of the Fanconi syndrome) often have a characteristic appearance with sparse, blond hair and a pale complexion, but the condition can occur in any racial group and non-Caucasian patients have a complexion appropriate to their racial group.

INVESTIGATIONS

Urinalysis may reveal glycosuria and proteinuria but this is not invariable. Plasma biochemistry usually shows hypokalaemia, hypophosphataemia, a hyperchloraemic metabolic acidosis (e.g. normal anion gap) and sometimes hyponatraemia and hypocalcaemia. The urine is usually alkaline but will acidify in the presence of severe acidosis (bicarbonate <15 mmol/l) since it is a proximal RTA. Generalized aminoaciduria together with a low tubular reabsorption of phosphate confirm a Fanconi syndrome. Radiographs may demonstrate rickets. Specific investigations to determine the cause are listed in Table 10.5.

TREATMENT

In the acute situation, patients need rehydration with 0.9% saline usually with added potassium. Supplements of bicarbonate, potassium and phosphate are required. Vitamin D is used to treat the rickets. Specific treatments are required for the causative metabolic conditions.

PROGNOSIS

The outlook depends on the cause of the Fanconi syndrome. In addition, several of the causes lead to chronic renal failure (especially cystinosis, Lowe syndrome, tyrosinaemia and 'idiopathic' cases) although this occurs at a variable rate.

Table 10.5 Causes of renal Fanconi syndrome

Inherited (specific investigation)	Acquired
Cystinosis (leukocyte cystine concentration)	Drugs: ifosfamide, aminoglycosides, valproate, cisplatin, azathioprine
Tyrosinaemia (plasma amino acids, urine organic acids)	Heavy metals: lead, cadmium, mercury
Galactosaemia (galactose 1-phosphate uridyl transferase)	Nephrotic syndrome (rare)
Fructosaemia (fructose-1-phosphate aldolase B)	Renal transplant
Lowe's syndrome (X-linked, cataracts, hypotonia)	Tubulo-interstitial nephritis
Mitochondrial disorders (lactate, pyruvate)	Amyloidosis
Wilson's disease (copper, caeruloplasmin)	Myeloma
Glycogen storage disease (hepatomegaly, hypoglycaemia)	
Dent's disease (X-linked, hypercalciuria, nephrocalcinosis)	
Idiopathic: autosomal dominant/recessive/X-linked	

CHILDHOOD HYPERTENSION DUE TO RENO-VASCULAR DISEASE

PREVALENCE
Approximately 1 in 10,000 children.

INCIDENCE
Renovascular disease accounts for 10% of children with hypertension and is often due to fibromuscular dysplasia. In some patients, this may be associated with neurofibromatosis, William's syndrome, mid-aortic syndrome, Marfan's syndrome, thyrotoxicosis, Klippel-Trenaunay-Weber and Feuerstein-Mims syndrome.

DIAGNOSIS
A quarter of patients are diagnosed on routine blood pressure screening. Many have symptoms such as headache (50%), lethargy (39%), cardiac failure, failure to thrive, and weight loss at presentation. A significant number (10–15 %) present with neurological features alone, such as facial palsy, hemiplegia and convulsions.

INVESTIGATIONS
Most useful diagnostic tests include peripheral plasma renin activity, captopril primed isotope renal scanning, renal vein renins and arteriography. However, the vascular disease may involve intra-renal vessels and other organs (particularly the brain). Therefore, investigations should also be directed to identify these, especially if there are cerebral symptoms. Possible target organ damage due to hypertension should be assessed (e.g. formal ophthalmoscopy, echocardiography, chest x-ray and renal function studies).

TREATMENT
Children in hypertensive crisis should be treated with an intravenous antihypertensive such as labetalol or sodium nitroprusside initially, with very careful and slow reduction of blood pressure over 48–72 hours. Calcium channel blockers and beta blockers are the most useful oral pharmacological agents in the treatment of renovascular disease associated hypertension. ACE inhibitors are normally contraindicated; however they may be necessary in the management of patients with difficult to control blood pressure or in subjects with severe intra-renal vascular disease.

Renal angioplasty (**10.13**) is the treatment of choice for cases with unilateral, main or branch artery stenoses. Some patients may need vascular reconstructive procedures. Approximately one third of these achieve complete cure and most of the others a reduction in drug therapy requirement after surgery.

PROGNOSIS
Good.

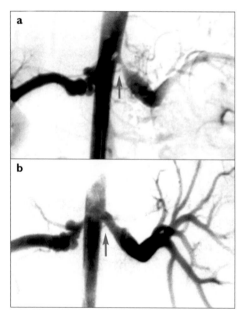

10.13 Renal artery angiogram (**a**) pre- and (**b**) post-angioplasty.

RENAL BONE DISEASE IN CHILDREN WITH CHRONIC RENAL FAILURE

PATHOGENESIS

Renal osteodystrophy is the term used to describe the disturbance of bone formation in chronic renal failure, secondary to abnormalities of vitamin D metabolism and secondary hyperparathyroidism. Reduced activity of the renal 1-α hydroxylase enzyme, with progressive renal failure, causes decreased production of the active hormone 1,25-dihydroxyvitamin D_3. This results in increased bone resorption (i.e. osteitis fibrosa due to secondary hyperparathyroidism) and impaired mineralization of osteoid (i.e. rickets). Parathyroid hormone secretion is stimulated by a fall in ionized calcium due to reduced calcium absorption mediated by 1,25-dihydroxyvitamin D_3 and hyperphosphataemia secondary to phosphate retention.

DIAGNOSIS

Children with early changes of renal osteodystrophy are usually asymptomatic but if untreated they may develop bone pain with or without fractures or slipped epiphyses, skeletal deformities and weakness secondary to proximal myopathy (**10.14, 10.15**).

A raised level of intact parathyroid hormone (PTH) is indicative of active bone disease. Measurements of intact PTH can be used to monitor treatment in conjunction with measurement of plasma phosphate, total calcium and ionized calcium. Indirect assessments of PTH activity (i.e. alkaline phosphatase, bone macrographs and tubular resorption of phosphate) are less reliable.

TREATMENT

The principles of management of renal osteodystrophy are:

- Correction of acidosis using sodium bicarbonate.
- Phosphate restriction by control of dietary intake and the use of a phosphate binder (e.g. calcium carbonate to maintain plasma phosphate within the normal range for age).
- Supplements of oral 1-α hydroxycholecalciferol or 1,25 dihydroxycholecalciferol to maintain the PTH within normal range, if not achieved by control of plasma phosphate. This may require the total calcium to be maintained at the upper end of the normal range. Total calcium is a measurement of bound, ionized and complexed calcium. The proportion may increase in chronic renal failure, reflected by total hypercalcaemia. However, if ionized calcium is within the normal range, treatment with vitamin D analogues may continue.

PROGNOSIS

Can be controlled and linear growth maintained, but progression may occur with deteriorating renal function.

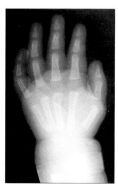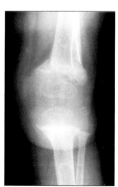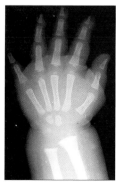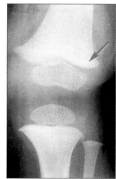

10.14 & 10.15 Bone radiographs of wrist and knee in a boy who presented aged 10 months with severe chronic renal failure secondary to posterior urethral valves and bilateral renal dysplasia.
10.14 Pre-treatment. Coarse trabecular pattern with wide irregular metaphyseal plates and subperiosteal bone resorption, with periosteal reaction in the lower femur.
10.15 Post-treatment. Resolution of bone changes with the appearance of a dense white line indicating normal bone formation at the zone of provisional calcification (arrow).

ACUTE RENAL FAILURE

INCIDENCE
Acute renal failure(ARF) is a sudden decline in glomerular filtration rate (GFR) with urine output less than 0.5 ml/kg/hour, resulting in salt and water retention, together with metabolic abnormalities.

AETIOLOGY
Pre-renal ARF has a history or signs of circulatory collapse (**Table 10.6**). There is peripheral vasoconstriction, a low blood pressure and CVP and a fractional excretion of sodium of less than 1%. If ARF is due to renal causes, there is salt and water retention with blood, protein and casts in the urine, and symptoms specific to an accompanying disease (e.g. HSP). Acute on chronic renal failure(CRF) is suggested by a poorly grown child with long-standing symptoms typical of CRF.

INVESTIGATIONS
An ultrasound is the most important investigation, in order to identify obstruction of the renal tract which may require surgery, small kidneys of CRF, or large bright kidneys with loss of cortico-medullary differentiation, typical of an acute process (**Table 10.7**). Renal biopsy is indicated if the diagnosis is unclear, in order to exclude a crescentic nephritis that would require treatment with immunosuppression (**10.16**).

TREATMENT
Conservative management is by diet (low protein, high calorie, low phosphate and potassium) and attention to fluid balance. Hypovolaemia should be corrected with normal saline or plasma. Fluid overload may respond to frusemide and fluid restriction to insensible losses. Indications for dialysis in **Table 10.8**.

Table 10.6 Causes of acute renal failure

Pre-renal
Hypovolaemia
Hypotension

Renal
Arterial (HUS, arteritis, embolic)
Venous (renal venous thrombosis)
Glomerular (glomerulonephritis)
Interstitial (interstitial nephritis, pyelonephritis)
Tubular (ATN, ischaemic, toxic, obstructive)
Acute on chronic renal failure

Post-renal
Congenital obstruction
Acquired obstruction

Table 10.7 Investigation of acute renal failure

- Ultrasound
- Full blood count, blood film and clotting
- Blood and stool culture
- Urea, Na, K, creatinine, Ca, PO4, Mg, alkaline phosphatase, albumin, HCO3, urate
- Urine, microscopy, culture, dipstick (blood and protein)
- Urine Na, urea and creatinine
- Throat swab and ASO titre
- Complement and anti-dsDNA
- Anti-GBM antibody and ANCA
- Renal biopsy if cause of ARF unclear
- X-ray hand and wrist, chest x-ray, ECG and PTH if acute on chronic renal failure

---

Table 10.8 Indications for dialysis

- Failure of conservative management
- Hyperkalaemia
- Severe hypo- or hypernatraemia
- Pulmonary oedema or hypertension
- Severe acidosis
- Multisystem failure

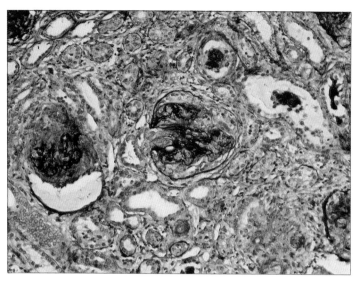

10.16 Renal biopsy showing a crescentic nephritis causing acute renal failure.

REFERENCES

General
Pediatric Nephrology (5edn) Lippincott, Williams and Wilkins, 2003

Haemolytic uraemic syndrome (HUS)
Elliott EJ, Robins-Browne RM, O'Loughlin EV et al. Australian Paediatric Surveillance Unit. Nationwide study of haemolytic uraemic syndrome: clinical, microbiological, and epidemiological features. *Arch Dis Child* 2001; **85**: 125–131.
Kaplan BS, Meyers KE, Schulman SL. The pathogenesis and treatment of hemolytic uremic syndrome. *J Am Soc Nephrol* 1998; **9(6)**: 1126–1133.
Taylor CM. Hemolytic-uremic syndrome and complement factor H deficiency: clinical aspects. *Semin Thromb Hemost* 2001; **27(3)**: 185–190.
Taylor CM, Monnens LA. Advances in haemolytic uraemic syndrome. *Arch Dis Child* 1998; **78(2)**: 190–193.
Zipfel PF, Neumann HP, Jozsi M. Genetic screening in haemolytic uraemic syndrome. *Curr Opin Nephrol Hypertens* 2003; **12(6)**: 653–657.

Nephrotic syndrome
Eddy, AA, Symons JM , Nephrotic syndrome in childhood, *Lancet* 2003; 362(**9384**): 629–639.

Polycystic kidney diseases
Igarashi P, Somlo S. Genetics and pathogenesis of polycystic kidney disease, *J Am Soc Nephrol* 2002; **13(9)**: 2384–2398.
Ong AC, Wheatley DN. Polycystic kidney disease – the ciliary connection, *Lancet* 2003; **361(9359)**: 774–776.
Woolf AS, Feather SA, Bingham C. Recent insights into kidney diseases associated with glomerular cysts. *Pediatr Nephrol* 2002; **17(4)**: 229–235.

Vesico-ureteric reflux
Dillon M J, Goonasekera CD. Reflux nephropathy. *J Am Soc Nephrol* 1998; **12**: 2377–2383.
Feather S A, Malcolm S, Woolf AS et al. Primary, nonsyndromic vesicoureteric reflux and its nephropathy is genetically heterogeneous, with a locus on chromosome 1. *Am J Hum Genet* 2000; **66(4)**: 1420–1425.

Renal agenesis and dysplasia
Winyard PJD, Chitty L. Dysplastic and polycystic kidneys: diagnosis, associations and management. *Prenat Diagn* 2001; **21(11)**: 924–935.
Woolf AS, Winyard PJD. Molecular mechanisms of human embryogenesis: developmental pathogenesis of renal tract malformations. *Pediatr Dev Pathol* 2002; **5(2)**: 108–129.
Woolf AS, Price KL, Scambler PJ, Winyard PJD. Evolving concepts in human renal dysplasia. *J Am Soc Nephrol* 2004: **15(4)**: 998–1007

Henoch Schönlein purpura
Robson WL, Leung AK. Henoch-Schonlein purpura. *Adv Pediatr* 1994; **41**: 163–194.
Saulsbury FT. , Henoch-Schonlein purpura. *Curr Opin Rheumatol* 2001; **13(1)**: 35–40.

Childhood hypertension
Dillon MJ. Renovascular hypertension. *J Hum Hypertens* 1994; **8(5)**: 367–369.

Renal bone disease in children with chronic renal failure
Ledermann SE, Johnson K, Dillon MJ, Trompeter RS, Barratt TM. Serum intact parathyroid hormone and ionised calcium concentration in children with renal insufficiency. *Pediatr Nephrol* 1994; **8(5)**: 561–565.

Blood Diseases

Owen Smith
Ian Hann

HODGKIN'S LYMPHOMA

PRESENTATION
This form of lymphoma most often develops in the 15–25-year-old age group. As with non-Hodgkin's lymphoma ('NHL'), boys are more often affected than girls.

Whereas non-Hodgkin's lymphoma usually presents at extra-nodal sites, Hodgkin's lymphoma is predominantly nodal. Presentation is usually with enlarged cervical or mediastinal lymph nodes (**11.1**), which can be massive, especially in the chest. Involvement of other node groups (axillary, inguinal, epitrochlear) is much less common. Splenic involvement (20–30% in children) is also regarded as 'nodal' disease, because the spleen is part of the so-called 'reticuloendothelial system', but liver, lung, skin, bone, bone marrow and other organ or tissue involvement is considered to be 'extra-nodal'. Around 30% of patients have systemic symptoms (so-called 'B' symptoms). These are:

- Weight loss of >10% in previous 6 months.
- Soaking night sweats (wet pillow – not just a bit of sweating if the central heating is turned up).
- Unexplained fever of >37.8°C on at least one occasion.

DIAGNOSIS AND STAGING
Diagnosis is by lymph node biopsy; lymph node aspiration (for cytology) is not recommended as it can be misleading. Hodgkin's disease can never confidently be diagnosed in the absence of Reed-Sternberg cells, which are 'transformed' B cells. In rare cases, 'atypical' Reed-Sternberg cells (often mononuclear rather than bi-nuclear) are accepted for diagnosis but, in these cases, viral infection – especially EBV infection – must be rigorously excluded. The well-known histological subtypes of Hodgkin's disease are prognostically less important these days because treatment has improved, except that nodular lymphocyte-predominant Hodgkin's disease is not, despite its name, really Hodgkin's disease at all, but a form of B-cell NHL. With diagnosis established, staging is the next step, using chest x-ray and CT or MRI scan of neck, chest and abdomen, with selected extra-nodal sites imaged if there are 'B' symptoms or clinical suspicion of disease in other organs. Up to 25% of children from 'high risk' countries will have coincident tuberculosis (TB) because of the acquired cellular immune deficiency associated with Hodgkin's lymphoma. PET (positron emission tomography) scanning is a very promising, though still 'experimental', form of scanning for Hodgkin's disease, with the capacity to image patients with metabolically 'active' residual sites of disease.

There are four stages of Hodgkin's disease, depending on the number of lymph node sites involved and the presence or absence of extra-nodal disease (see table, overleaf).

Necessary blood tests include FBC, ESR, LFTs, creatinine, serum protein and VZV/measles antibody levels.

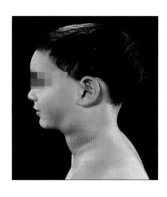

11.1 Hodgkin's lymphoma. Cervical lymphadenopathy.

TREATMENT AND PROGNOSIS

Over 85% of children with Hodgkin's can now be cured. The emphasis in recent treatment schedules has been 'cure at less cost'. What 'cost'? Both radiotherapy and chemotherapy can cause 'late-effects' (see also 'Solid Tumours and Histiocytosis' chapter), as follows:

- **From radiotherapy:** bony and soft tissue hypoplasia (any irradiated site), hypothyroidism, carotid artery narrowing (neck irradiation), myocardial disease (mediastinal irradiation) and second tumours (any site).
- **From chemotherapy:** infertility (from alkylating agents and procarbazine) and predisposition to acute non-lymphoblastic leukaemia (ANLL).

These days only around one third of patients (those with residual disease after chemotherapy) receive irradiation and usually the radiation field and doses are smaller than they were in the 1970s and 1980s. Chemotherapy regimes have also been modified, reducing the total dose of alkylating agents and procarbazine to try to preserve fertility, especially in boys – who are more susceptible to gonadotoxicity than girls – and reduce the risk of secondary leukaemia. Another important factor in higher survival is the centralization of clinical decision-making, pioneered by the German/Austrian Paediatric Oncology Group (GPOG). In future, other countries will set up similar kinds of electronically delivered central review processes, so that consistent decision-making is made by one team, rather than by each individual centre.

B-CELL NON-HODGKIN'S LYMPHOMA

PRESENTATION

In Africa, the commonest presentation would be with a jaw mass (**11.2**), commonly called Burkitt's lymphoma. In other countries, the most common presentation is an abdominal tumour which can produce an intussusception or, more often, is widely metastatic throughout the abdomen. In addition, ascites and pleural effusions are frequently found.

DIAGNOSIS

Clinical. Exclude other tumours (e.g. jaw osteosarcoma and other abdominal tumours). Ultrasound scan and CT/MRI scan of the abdomen show the presence of multiple masses. Chest x-ray may show pleural effusions. In a small proportion of cases, the bone marrow may be involved, with lymphoblasts which have the characteristics of mature B cells in that they express surface membrane immunoglobulin. These cells are large and have abundant basophilic cytoplasm; several prominent nucleoli are usually seen and cytoplasmic vacuolization is also prominent (**11.4**).

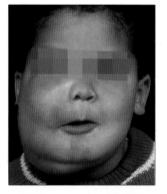

11.2 B-cell non-Hodgkin's lymphoma. Jaw mass.

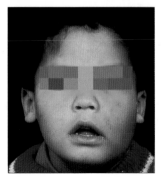

11.3 B-cell non-Hodgkin's lymphoma. Response to combination therapy.

TREATMENT

Combination anti-lymphoma chemotherapy is required. The tumours often respond dramatically (**11.3**) but there is a high risk of tumour lysis syndrome, and careful monitoring for hyperphosphataemia, hypocalcaemia, hyperkalaemia and ECG abnormalities is warranted. All patients should receive hyperhydration and allopurinol or uricozyme, although some patients may require haemodialysis.

PROGNOSIS

This depends upon the presence or absence of central nervous system disease. With localized disease, most patients will be cured and, even in the more common disseminated abdominal stage III cases, there is at least an 80% chance of five-year survival. Central nervous disease carries a worse prognosis.

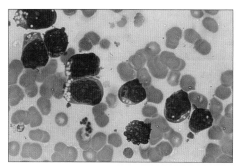

11.4 B-cell non-Hodgkin's lymphoma. Morphological characteristics.

T-CELL NON-HODGKIN'S LYMPHOMA (NHL) / LEUKAEMIA

PRESENTATION

The majority of patients present with a mediastinal mass and possibly superior mediastinal obstruction. The difference between T-NHL and T-cell acute leukaemia is largely semantic and is merely differentiated by the presence of 25% or more T-cell leukaemia cells in the bone marrow of the latter. This type of leukaemia has a relatively higher incidence of central nervous system disease and the CT scan (**11.5**) shows multiple leukaemic mass lesions within the brain substance. This type of localized 'lumpy' disease is rare. **11.6** shows meningeal infiltration over the cerebellum in a case of T-cell ALL with CNS involvement.

DIAGNOSIS

Bone marrow examination is the standard approach in diagnosing leukaemia; **11.7** shows CSF involvement with leukaemic lymphoblasts which, upon testing with T-cell specific monoclonal antibodies, was confirmed as being T-cell ALL. There is no evidence that T-cell disease responds to treatment any differently from other types of ALL in childhood and management is with standard leukaemia regimens. There is an approximately 80% chance of five-year survival with this type of treatment.

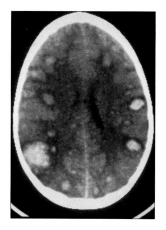

11.5 T-cell NHL/leukaemia. CT scan.

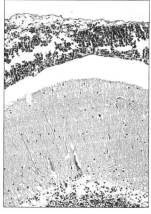

11.6 T-cell NHL/leukaemia. Involvement with leukaemic lymphoblasts.

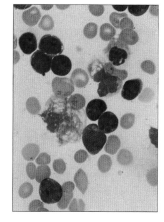

11.7 T-cell NHL/leukaemia. Meningeal infiltration.

MONOCYTIC AND MYELOMONOCYTIC LEUKAEMIA

PRESENTATION

Rarely, leukaemia can present in the newborn period and, if so, it usually presents as a mono-cytic variety of leukaemia with leukaemia cutis, the so-called 'blueberry muffin' appearance (**11.8**). Occasionally, it can also present with skin lesions in older children (**11.9**). There is also a predisposition to gum hypertrophy and for involvement of other extra-medullary sites, such as the pericardium (**11.10**) and testes.

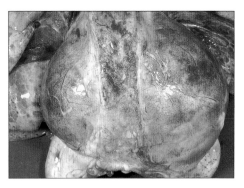

11.10 Pericardial involvement.

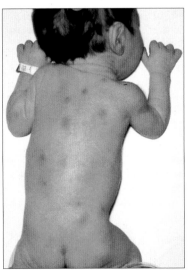

11.8 'Blueberry muffin' appearance.

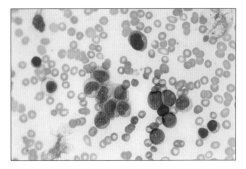

11.11 Bone marrow in monocytic and myelomonocytic leukaemia.

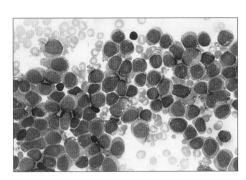

11.12 Monomorphic population of monoblasts in monocytic and myelomonocytic leukaemia.

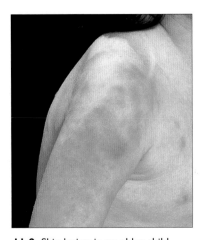

11.9 Skin lesion in an older child.

DIAGNOSIS

The bone marrow in myelomonocytic leukaemia (**11.11**) shows a mixture of myeloblasts and monocytes (AML-M4 subtype). Figure **11.12** shows the features of monocytic leukaemia (AML-M5) (monomorphic population of monoblasts). Treatment of all types of acute myeloid leukaemia includes intensive combination chemotherapy, with or without an allogeneic bone marrow transplant. Patients with a high white cell count at diagnosis and leukaemic chromosomal abnormalities involving chromosome 5 and 7 tend to have a worse prognosis. The chromosomal translocations t15:17 and t8:21, together with abnormalities involving chromosomal 16 (e.g. inv16), are associated with a better prognosis. Overall there is an approximately 60% chance of five-year survival. These patients are particularly prone to problems with bleeding and leukostasis, especially if they have high white cell counts at diagnosis.

EXTRAMEDULLARY ACUTE LYMPHOBLASTIC LEUKAEMIA

PRESENTATION

Acute lymphoblastic leukaemia can present or relapse in various sites, including the skin, ovary, eye (**11.13**) and testis (**11.14**), as well as the more conventional bone marrow and cerebrospinal fluid sites.

DIAGNOSIS

A classical hypopyon is shown in **11.13**. This is usually not associated with any pain or irritation. In a similar way, testicular relapse or testicular disease, at presentation of acute lymphoblastic leukaemia, is usually painless and obvious on routine examination. In view of the fact that most of these relapses occur in extramedullary sites following the cessation of therapy, it is essential that children are routinely examined for these abnormalities.

PROGNOSIS

Central nervous system disease relapse of lymphoblastic leukaemia can in some cases be successfully treated with cranial irradiation and continuing intrathecal methotrexate, along with intensive chemotherapy. Similarly, testicular disease, at presentation, can often be successfully managed with testicular radiotherapy, in addition to other conventional therapy. Relapse in any site has a poor prognosis, except patients who relapse in the testes following cessation of therapy. There is an approximately two-thirds chance of five-year survival in these cases.

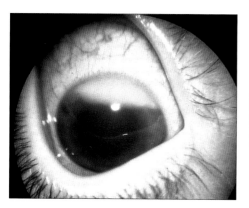

11.13 Extramedullary acute lymphoblastic leukaemia. Appearance of affected eye.

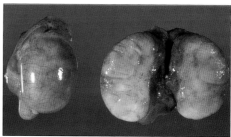

11.14 Extramedullary acute lymphoblastic leukaemia. Appearance of affected testes.

JUVENILE MYELOMONOCYTIC LEUKAEMIA

PRESENTATION
The most dramatic finding in patients with this disorder is a huge enlargement of the spleen (**11.15**). More infrequently, there is a rash (**11.16**), which can be quite subtle and may be present on the face and upper trunk.

DIAGNOSIS
The bone marrow morphology is consistent with a chronic myelomonocytic leukaemia, in that there is dysplasia in all myeloid lineages, often in association with a reduced platelet count and high fetal haemoglobin (HbF) (**11.17**). It is commoner in boys under the age of four years, with a higher incidence than expected in neurofibromatosis type 1. Bone marrow cytogenetics do not usually show any gross abnormalities. This is clearly different from the adult type of chronic myeloid leukaemia, which is a totally different disease and is associated with the t9:22 (Philadelphia) translocation.

PROGNOSIS
Adverse prognostic factors in juvenile myelomonocytic leukaemia include HbF level >20% and platelet count <50 x 10^9/l and older age. The only effective treatment at the present time is allogeneic bone marrow transplantation. Although some patients may respond to cis-retinoic acid, this is usually short lived.

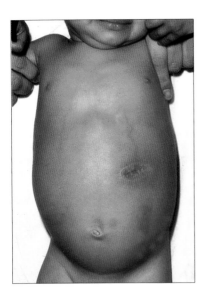

11.15 Juvenile chronic myeloid leukaemia. Enlargement of the spleen.

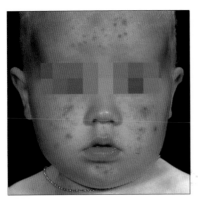

11.16 Juvenile chronic myeloid leukaemia. Rash on the face.

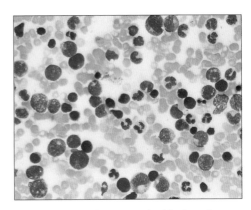

11.17 Juvenile chronic myeloid leukaemia. Bone marrow morphology showing dysplasia in myeloid lineages.

EOSINOPHILIC MYELOPROLIFERATIVE DISORDER WITH CHROMOSOMAL 5;12 TRANSLOCATION (T5;12)

PRESENTATION
This patient (**11.18**) presented with a dramatic urticarial rash and a very high eosinophilia (>5 × 10⁹/l). He also had evidence of bronchoconstriction.

DIAGNOSIS
Hypereosinophilic syndrome (HES) usually manifests as a problem with lung infiltration and right-sided heart failure, with valvular incompetence related to local infiltration with eosinophils (Loeffler's syndrome). This may be rarely associated with leukaemia and possibly more frequently with T-cell ALL. In this particular case there was a prominent skin rash only.

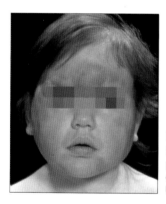

11.18 Eosinophilic myelo-proliferative disorder. Urticarial rash.

DIFFERENTIAL DIAGNOSIS
The vast majority of cases of eosinophilia in childhood are related to atopy, parasitic infestation and drugs and, less frequently, Loeffler's syndrome. The diagnosis is based on examination of the blood film (**11.19**) or bone marrow. This will show a proliferation of eosinophils which may demonstrate degranulation (not seen in this particular case) (**11.20**). The gene for the interleukin-5 ligand (eosinophil growth factor) is on chromosome 5 and it may be that the chromosomal translocation (t5:12) in this case is resulting in aberrant expression of this 'eosinopoietin'.

TREATMENT
Therapy is basically symptomatic although the interferons which are anti-proliferative have been reported to be of some value in occasional cases. Some cases have responded dramatically to the tyrosine kinase inhibitor imatinib. Bone marrow transplantation should be considered as a way of eradicating the abnormal clone. Anti-IL5 (IL5 receptor) is not available for clinical use at the present time.

PROGNOSIS
Cases of HES associated with leukaemia do not appear to confer a worse prognosis upon the primary disease. Hypereosinophilic myleoproliferative disorder is a chronic disease of uncertain prognosis.

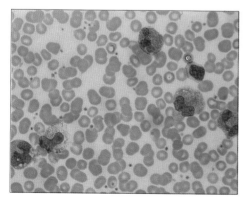

11.19 Eosinophilic myeloproliferative disorder. Blood film showing proliferation of eosinophils.

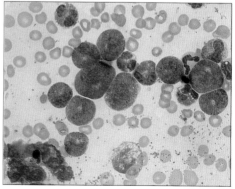

11.20 Eosinophilic myeloproliferative disorder. Bone marrow film.

SEVERE HAEMOPHILIA A AND B (CLASSIC HAEMOPHILIA AND CHRISTMAS DISEASE)

PRESENTATION

These disorders are related to severe deficiency of factor VIII and IX coagulant activity. Presentation is usually in early infancy with bleeding phenomena (from the umbilical cord, or recurrent bruising or haemarthrosis, (**11.21**). Classically, patients were described as bleeding following circumcision. Males are affected and girls are carriers, but approximately one third of new cases are through new mutations.

DIAGNOSIS

The diagnosis depends upon determination of levels of factor VIII or factor IX in coagulant assays. Treatment nowadays is with regular prophylactic therapy with high purity factor concentrates, preferably those produced by recombinant DNA technology. In the past, severe arthropathy (**11.21**, **11.22**) was common but is rarely seen with current therapy, which aims to keep the factor level above 1% at all times. The x-ray (**11.22**) shows severe joint damage with loss of joint space and cystic changes around the joint.

PROGNOSIS

An excellent prognosis is expected, providing recombinant factor concentrates are used. Patients must be regularly monitored for evidence of viral infection, especially with hepatitis viruses and for the development of inhibitors to the coagulant protein, which is a severe development leading to a refractory state of treatment.

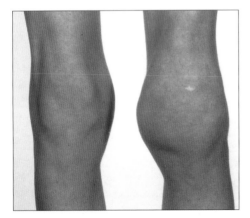

11.21 Severe haemophilia A and B. Haemarthrosis.

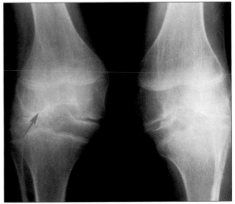

11.22 Severe haemophilia A and B. X-ray showing severe joint damage.

KASABACH–MERRITT SYNDROME

PRESENTATION
The child usually presents in the neonatal period with a massive haemangioma (**11.23**) which may be clinically obvious, as in this case, or may be occult (e.g. primary splenic haemangioma or gut haemangioma). Breathing can be compromised. Consumptive coagulopathy occurs due to production of fibrin, platelet activation and coagulation protein usage within the lesion.

The blood film usually (but not always) shows evidence of a micro-angiopathic haemolytic anaemia, with red cell fragmentation and a low platelet count, as in this case (**11.24**).

TREATMENT
In most cases, the lesion is not susceptible to surgery. Various therapies have been tried (e.g. radiotherapy, steroids, interferon and embolization of the feeding blood vessels).

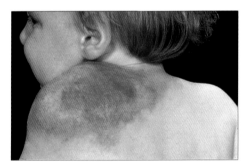

11.23 Kasabach-Merritt syndrome. Haemangioma.

VON WILLEBRAND'S DISEASE (vWD)

PRESENTATION
Patients usually present with cutaneous purpura, epistaxis and mucosal bleeding, so called 'wet purpura'. Its incidence may be as high as 1% of the population. Both autosomal recessive and dominant forms are seen. There are no specific clinical features apart from bleeding.

DIAGNOSIS
Estimation of von Willebrand factor protein (vWF) along with factor VIII coagulant activity (VIII:C) are essential in making the diagnosis. vWD is a heterogenous bleeding disorder with at least 20 distinct clinical subtypes. There are two main categories based on whether there is a quantitative (type I or type III) or qualitative (type II with its several variants) defect in vWF. Type I is the commonest (70%), has an autosomal dominant inheritance and the bleeding diathesis can be mild to severe. The bleeding seen in type III is usually severe (**11.25**) because of very low levels of VIII:C and vWF. This has a recessive mode of inheritance.

Within the type II classification, type IIB needs to be distinguished from the rest, in that DDAVP treatment exacerbates the bleeding tendency due to a worsening of the thrombocytopenia and is, therefore, contraindicated. There is increased platelet aggregation with low levels of the agonist ristocetin and intermittently low platelet counts.

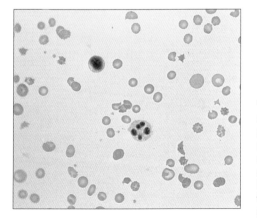

11.24 Kasabach-Merritt syndrome. Blood film.

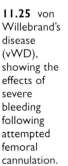

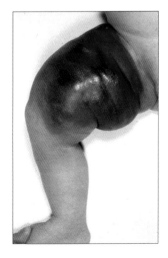

11.25 von Willebrand's disease (vWD), showing the effects of severe bleeding following attempted femoral cannulation.

TREATMENT

The majority are treated with DDAVP, which releases endogenous vWF from endothelium and megakaryocytes. Severe (type III) patients are treated with a combination of von Willebrand factor protein and factor VIII. The prognosis is excellent and the same infective risks of blood products apply to patients with von Willebrand's disease as with other bleeding disorders.

THROMBOCYTOPENIA WITH ABSENT RADIUS (TAR)

PRESENTATION

The diagnosis is usually made at birth because of the characteristic physical appearance combined with thrombocytopenia. The pathognomonic physical finding is bilateral absence of the radii with thumbs present (**11.26**) which can distinguish TAR from Fanconi anaemia (see page 324) in which thumbs may be absent and the radii are present (**11.27**).

DIAGNOSIS

Clinical observation and blood count showing severe thrombocytopenia. There may be other associated findings, including hand anomalies and abnormalities of the shoulder, neck and lower limbs. Skin haemangiomas also occasionally occur. Females are more often affected than boys, as opposed to Fanconi anaemia where there is a male predominance. The diagnosis must be distinguished from ITP and from megakaryocytic thrombocytopenia (other than ITP) because this latter condition has a propensity to the development of marrow aplasia and myelodysplasia.

TREATMENT

Most patients bleed in infancy and then improve after the first year. In the past, mortality was approximately 25%, the majority of deaths occurring in the first year. Platelet transfusions should be used during bleeding episodes or operations, including those to correct the deformities. Occasional transient responses to splenectomy have occurred and tranexamic acid may be useful for mucosal bleeding but must not be used when haematuria (macroscopic or microscopic) occurs. There are also anecdotal reports of responses to immunoglobulin therapy

PROGNOSIS

If the patient survives the first year the prognosis is excellent.

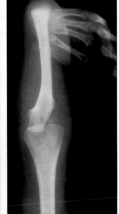

11.26 Thrombocytopenia with absent radius (TAR). X-ray showing that radii are absent.

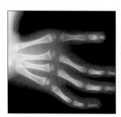
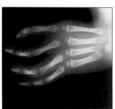

11.27 X-ray showing that thumbs are absent in Fanconi anaemia.

BERNARD–SOULIER SYNDROME

PRESENTATION
Usually with epistaxis and mucocutaneous bleeding within the first year of life. Bleeding into joints or muscles does not occur.

DIAGNOSIS
Like the other thrombocytopenias of infancy, the predominant clinical feature is bleeding (see above). The gene has been mapped to the short arm of chromosome 17 (in the region 17pter-17p12). Platelets from these patients have a reduced number of platelet membrane glycoproteins.

Bernard-Soulier syndrome is caused by mutations in GPIb-α, GPIb-β or GPIX. These proteins act as receptors for von Willebrand's factor and, when absent, platelets fail to adhere to the subendothelial matrix. The proteins are usually quantified on the platelet surface via fluorescence-activated cell-sorting (FACS) analysis, using specific monoclonal antibodies. The other main diagnostic pointer is the presence of a reduced number of platelets ($40–80 \times 10^9/l$) which are usually large in size.

Differential diagnosis for thrombocytopenia would include Wiskott-Aldrich syndrome which, unlike the Bernard-Soulier defect (**11.28, 11.29**), is associated with very small platelets, TAR, amegakaryocytic thrombocytopenia, and artefactual thrombocytopenia (**11.30**). This artefact is usually caused by an EDTA-induced antibody and the effect can be abrogated by the use of an alternative anticoagulant such as citric acid.

TREATMENT
The only available therapy is transfusion with platelet concentrates. Affected patients usually receive this therapy only for persistent and significant haemorrhage, since the transfused patient may develop antibodies against the missing blood protein, making them permanently refractory to therapy. Tranexamic acid may be used for mucosal bleeds but not for patients with haematuria.

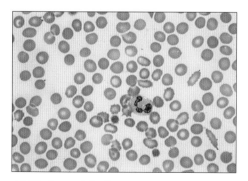

11.28 Bernard-Soulier syndrome. Blood film.

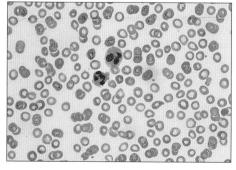

11.29 Bernard-Soulier syndrome. Blood film.

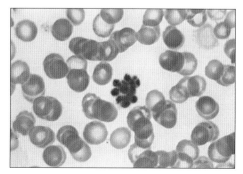

11.30 Artefactual thrombocytopenia.

TRANSCOBALAMIN II DEFICIENCY

PRESENTATION

Patients usually present at three to five weeks of age with failure to thrive, weakness, hypotonia (**11.31**) and diarrhoea, in addition to pallor due to severe progressive anaemia. Some patients present with pancytopenia. Transcobalamin II is the principal transporter for B_{12} entry into cells, and the serum vitamin B_{12} level is normal because it is transported in the plasma by transcobalamin I. The bone marrow is severely megaloblastic (**11.32**) and the blood film shows macrocytosis and other features of megaloblastic anaemia. Homocystinuria and methylmalonic aciduria have also been found in some cases. There is some evidence of autosomal inheritance associated with an abnormality in chromosome 22.

DIAGNOSIS

Absence of the protein capable of binding radio-labelled cobalamin and migrating with TCII, on chromotography or gel electrophoresis.

TREATMENT

Vitamin B_{12} must be kept high with systemic injections of hydroxycobalamin (IM) approximately 500–1,000 mg twice-weekly. The prognosis for neurological abnormalities depends upon whether or not treatment is instituted early and patients must be closely monitored for any deterioration in neurological status at which stage the vitamin B_{12} injections should be increased in dosage.

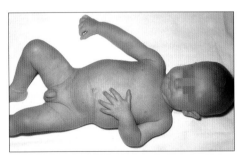

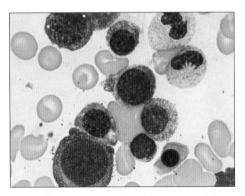

11.31 Transcobalamin II deficiency.

FANCONI ANAEMIA

PRESENTATION

Usually at around six years of age, with hyper- and hypo-pigmentation (**11.33**), short stature, abnormalities of the thumbs and radii (**11.34**), hypogonadism, microcephaly and microphthalmia (**11.35**). Renal abnormalities are also common and, being a bone marrow failure syndrome, the patients may present with bleeding and infection.

DIAGNOSIS

Laboratory: investigations include blood count showing a single cytopenia (usually thrombocytopenia but pancytopenia may also be the presenting haematological feature). Confirmation is by increased spontaneous chromosomal breakage induced with clastogenic agents (e.g. diepoxybutane [DEB]).

TREATMENT

Chromosome fragility syndromes are associated with a high risk of developing acute leukaemia. The progressive bone marrow failure may be temporarily managed with oxymetholone but the only curative procedure is bone marrow transplantation. Gene therapy may be a future possible treatment.

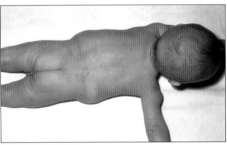

11.32 Transcobalamin II deficiency. Blood film showing megaloblastic bone marrow.

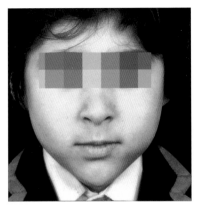

11.33 Fanconi anaemia. Facial appearance.

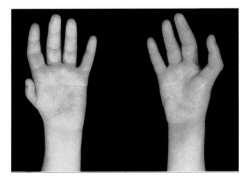

11.34 Fanconi anaemia. Thumb abnormalities.

DYSKERATOSIS CONGENITA

PRESENTATION

This is a rare form of ectodermal dysplasia. Skin and nail changes are usually seen in the first decade of life, with leukoplakia in the second. All features become more extreme with age. There is a reticulated type of pigmentation of the face, neck and shoulders, dystrophic nails (**11.36**) and mucous membrane leukoplakia. Aplastic anaemia occurs in 50% of patients, usually during the second decade and cancer in 10% by the 3rd and 4th decade.

DIAGNOSIS

Most patients present with thrombocytopenia or anaemia and then develop pancytopenia. Macrocytosis and elevated haemoglobin F are common. Chromosomal breakage studies are usually normal. The Xq28 restriction fragment length polymorphism (RFLP) might be used for prenatal diagnosis. There is an association with failure of cerebellar development (the H-H syndrome).

TREATMENT

Some patients respond to androgens, but supportive care has been the only effective holding measure, with bone marrow transplantation the only possible chance of cure.

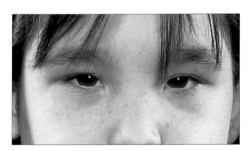

11.35 Fanconi anaemia. Microphthalmia.

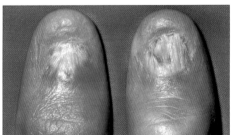

11.36 Dyskeratosis congenita. Dystrophic nails.

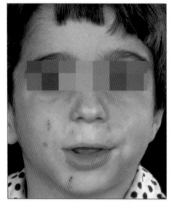

11.37 Congenital erythropoietic porphyria. Skin erosions as a result of photosensitivity.

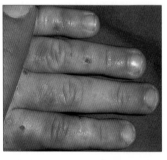

11.38 Congenital erythropoietic porphyria. Phototoxic damage to hands.

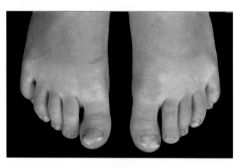

11.39 Congenital erythropoietic porphyria.

CONGENITAL ERYTHROPOIETIC PORPHYRIA (CEP)

PRESENTATION

A rare form of porphyria; this diagnosis may be suspected when pink to dark brown stains are noted in the nappy (due to large amounts of porphyrins in the urine). At an early stage, cutaneous photosensitivity is obvious and is exacerbated by any exposure to sunlight. Initial subepidermal bullous lesions progress to crusted erosions (**11.37–11.40**) which heal with scarring and (usually) increased pigmentation. Hypertrichosis and alopecia are frequent and erythrodontia (red fluorescence under ultraviolet light) (**11.41**) are virtually pathognomonic of the disease. The patients may also display symptoms of haemolytic anaemia with splenomegaly and gall stones.

DIAGNOSIS

Urinary porphyrins are greatly elevated due to decreased activity of uroporphyrinogen III cosynthase activity. The bone marrow shows porphyrin fluorescence in the red cells when exposed to UV light. The definitive diagnosis is a demonstration of a deficiency of uroporphyrinogen III cosynthase activity.

TREATMENT

Avoid sunlight and trauma to the skin. Topical sun screens may be of help, as may oral treatment with beta-carotine. The haemolysis may be mild or more severe and should be treated with blood transfusion and sometimes splenectomy. Bone marrow transplantation may be curative.

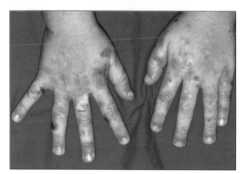

11.40 Congenital erythropoietic porphyria. Blistering on hands.

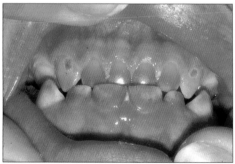

11.41 Congenital erythropoietic porphyria. Discolouration of the teeth..

IDIOPATHIC PULMONARY HAEMOSIDEROSIS

PRESENTATION

The disease may present at any time in childhood and as early as the neonatal period. It is characterized by recurrent intrapulmonary haemorrhage. The patient may have haemoptysis and dyspnoea, with a subsequent iron deficiency anaemia. The sputum is characteristically 'rusty'. There may be associated fever, tachycardia, tachypnoea, leukocytosis and occasionally abdominal pain.

DIAGNOSIS

The direct Coombs' test may be positive. The blood count shows microcytic hypochromic anaemia. Chest x-rays vary from minimal infiltrates (**11.42**) to massive ones with parenchymal involvement, atelectasis, emphysema and hilar adenopathy (**11.43**). Siderophages are found in the gastric aspirate and they stain positive with Prussian blue.

Lung biopsy shows alveolar epithelial hyperplasia, degeneration with excessive shedding of cells, large numbers of siderocytes, varying amounts of interstitial fibrosis and mast cell accumulation, elastic fibre degeneration and sclerotic vascular changes.

TREATMENT

Steroid therapy sometimes produces a remission, and there have been alleged responses to withdrawal of milk from the diet in a few cases.

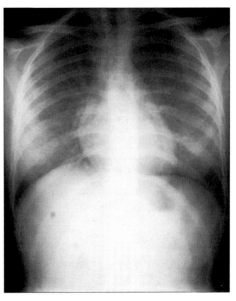

11.42 Idiopathic pulmonary haemosiderosis. Chest x-ray showing minimum infiltrates.

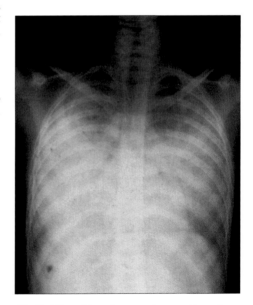

11.43 Idiopathic pulmonary haemosiderosis. Chest x-ray showing hilar adenopathy.

BETA THALASSAEMIA MAJOR

PRESENTATION

Severe anaemia, very often exacerbated by folic acid deficiency, which may lead to pancytopenia. At a later stage, patients who are severely affected develop overgrowth of the bones due to marrow expansion. A good example is shown in **11.44**, where the patient on the right was not transfusion-dependent and developed marrow overgrowth because of failure of marrow suppression. The patient on the left also had beta thalassaemia major and developed hyperpigmentation of the skin due to iron overload from blood transfusion, but the marrow was adequately suppressed and thus maxillary and other bony overgrowth did not occur.

If patients are not transfused they develop massive hepatosplenomegaly and wasting (**11.45**). The x-rays opposite (**11.46–11.48**) show expansion of the marrow cavity leading to a 'hair on end' appearance in the skull and expansion and thinning of the bones elsewhere.

DIAGNOSIS

The diagnosis depends on showing the presence of beta thalassaemia trait in the parents, along with either a raised haemoglobin A2 level or the existence of a coexisting haemoglobinopathy such as haemoglobin E. The blood film (**11.49**) shows hypochromia and microcytosis, and haemoglobin electrophoresis of the patient shows mainly HbF with some haemoglobin A2. Confirmation is either with demonstration of the lack of globin chain synthesis or by molecular methods.

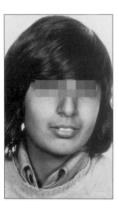 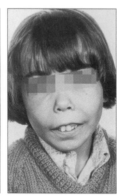

11.44 Beta thalassaemia major. The patient on the right has developed marrow overgrowth in the facial bones.

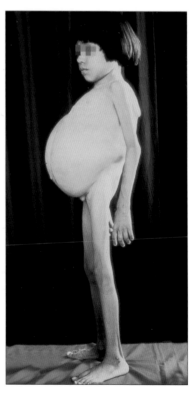

11.45 Beta thalassaemia major. Hepatosplenomegaly.

TREATMENT

The only curative treatment at present is with bone marrow transplantation, the outcome of which is excellent if a matched sibling donor is available and the transplant is carried out in the first few years of life. Otherwise, unrelated donor transplant could be considered, but the standard treatment at present is with regular blood transfusion, splenectomy following vaccination against *Pneumococcus*, *Haemophilus* and *Meningococcus C*, and supplementation with vitamin C, folic acid and penicillin prophylaxis (post splenectomy).

At a later stage, iron overload becomes a major problem and regular chelation with at least five times per week subcutaneous desferrioxamine is required. If iron overload ensues, multiple endocrinopathies including diabetes mellitus occur, with eventual cardiac failure.

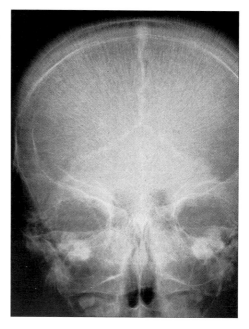

11.48 Beta thalassaemia major.

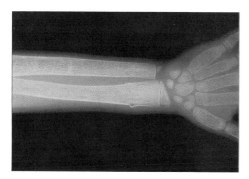

11.46 Beta thalassaemia major.

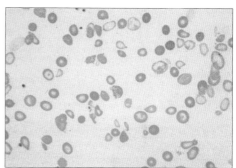

11.49 Beta thalassaemia major. Blood film.

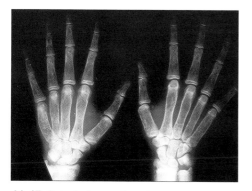

11.47 Beta thalassaemia major.

PYRUVATE KINASE DEFICIENCY

PRESENTATION
The child has a congenital non-spherocytic haemolytic anaemia which may present with hyperbilirubinaemia. Autosomal recessive inheritance is usually observed. Splenomegaly is usually present. Found predominantly in people of Northern European descent. Erythroblastopenic crisis from parvovirus B19 infection is not uncommon.

DIAGNOSIS
Blood film shows macrocytosis and occasional shrunken, spiculated erythrocytes (Echinocytes, **11.50**). Direct measurement of the pyruvate kinase (PK) enzyme shows a reduced level and there should be a concomitant high level of 2,3-Diphosphoglycerate (2,3DPG). Red cell intermediates of metabolism may be helpful in those patients with a marginally low PK level, or with a dysfunctional enzyme or very high reticulocyte count.

A severe anaemia is usually present and this may be well tolerated due to a shift to the right of the oxygen dissociation curve, secondary to a raised 2,3DPG. Hyperbilirubinaemia, low haptoglobins and raised reticulocyte levels are usually found. The enzyme level may be spuriously elevated due to relatively high PK levels in the reticulocytes and the assay must be corrected for this.

TREATMENT
The patients often tolerate a low haemoglobin of around 6g/dL very well because of the compensatory raised 2,3DPG level. Eventually the patients require splenectomy and, contrary to some previous reports, the results are usually very good. Folic acid supplementation is indicated.

SICKLE CELL DISEASE

PRESENTATION
These patients are nowadays picked up on haemoglobinopathy screening and by neonatal screening programmes. The most common problem is a painful crisis, which may involve the hand and produce dactylitis (**11.51**), possibly leading to osteomyelitis (**11.52**, **11.53**,).

Sickle chest syndrome involves sequestration in the lungs (**11.54**). The patient may also present at an early age with an aplastic crisis in which red cell production is impaired by parvovirus B19 infection. Also, an early and life threatening problem is sickle cell sequestration in the spleen and a rapid drop in haemoglobin due to pooling of blood.

DIAGNOSIS
Diagnosis is by haemoglobin electrophoresis and family studies. The electrophoretic pattern will show haemoglobin S. In haemoglobin SC

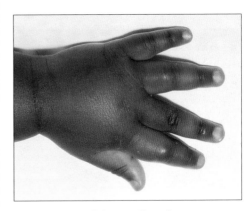

11.51 Sickle cell disease. Dactylitis.

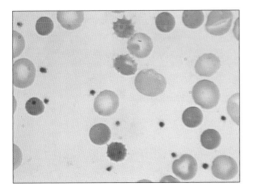

11.50 Pyruvate kinase deficiency. Blood film showing macrocytosis and spiculated erythrocytes.

disease, there is an extra band on electrophoresis and in haemoglobin S beta thalassaemia one parent will have sickle cell trait and one parent will have beta thalassaemia trait. Blood films shows the presence of sickle and target cells; the latter being more common in haemoglobin SC disease (11.55, 11.56).

MANAGEMENT
Early diagnosis is essential and may be picked up on neonatal screening. Early institution of penicillin prophylaxis is essential and treatment of painful crisis is with plentiful fluids and patient-controlled analgesia. For serious complications, such as chest syndrome and stroke, exchange transfusion is essential at a very early stage. Patients with recurrent severe problems may be considered for bone marrow transplantation.

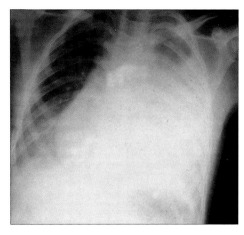

11.54 Sickle cell disease. Pulmonary sequestration.

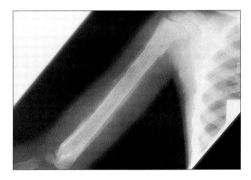

11.52 Sickle cell disease. Periosteal elevation due to osteomyelitis.

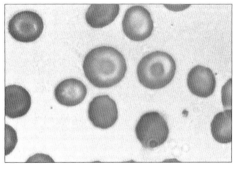

11.55 Sickle cell disease. Blood film showing sickled cells and target cells.

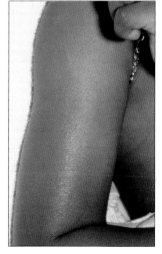

11.53 Sickle cell disease. Osteomyelitis.

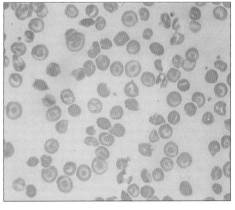

11.56 Sickle cell disease. Blood film showing sickled cells and target cells.

HEREDITARY ELLIPTOCYTOSIS

PRESENTATION
Often asymptomatic. When there is recessive inheritance, the patient may present with a severe haemolytic anaemia if homozygous.

DIAGNOSIS
This disorder is associated with classic blood film appearances (**11.57**) of many ovalocytes. In patients with the severe form of hereditary homozygous elliptocytosis, red cell fragmentation is often present.

TREATMENT
Most patients with hereditary elliptocytosis need no therapy at all. Patients with the severe homozygous form may require splenectomy.

IRON DEFICIENCY ANAEMIA

PRESENTATION
May often be asymptomatic. Can be associated with pica and is often associated with a poor diet with regard to iron content. In severe cases, cardiac failure, failure to thrive or developmental delay may be the presenting clinical features. The patient may look very pale but the ability to pick this up clinically is limited (**11.58**).

DIAGNOSIS
This is a controversial area because none of the tests are very satisfactory. A low haemoglobin with low mean red cell volume and low red cell count in the blood, associated with a low ferritin, low iron and raised total iron binding capacity (TIBC), is the classical presentation. Serum transferrin receptor level estimation may add additional information.

TREATMENT
The patient must be treated with iron until the haemoglobin rises to a normal level and then for a further three months to replete the iron stores. This must be associated with extensive dietary advice otherwise the problem will recur. If the problem is a recurrent one then causes of blood loss such as intestinal parasites, or a malabsorptive disorder such as coeliac disease should be considered. See also 'Gastroenterology' chapter.

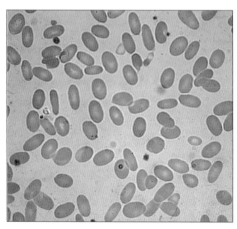

11.57 Hereditary elliptocytosis. Blood film showing ovalocytes.

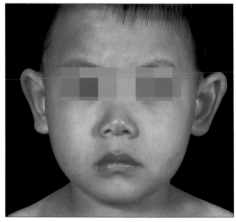

11.58 Iron deficiency anaemia. Facial appearance.

SIDEROBLASTIC ANAEMIA

PRESENTATION
The sideroblastic anaemias (SA) are a heterogeneous group of anaemias and thus can present with mild to severe anaemia at any stage during childhood. Characteristically they have a hypochromic/microcytic or normochromic/microcytic anaemia, refractory to iron therapy, and hepatosplenomegaly is not an uncommon finding at presentation.

Of the congenital types, X-linked inheritance is the commonest. When the anaemia is macrocytic and refractory to pyridoxine within the first six months of life, Pearson's syndrome should be considered. This is a multi-system disorder, characterized by deletion rearrangements of mitochondrial DNA (mt DNA), that leads to defects in respiratory chain function. Vacuolization of marrow precursors and the presence of sideroblasts, along with exocrine pancreatic insufficiency, suggest the diagnosis. Acquired sideroblastic anaemia has been associated with drugs, autoimmune disease, neoplasia and endocrinopathies.

DIAGNOSIS
Bone marrow aspirate with iron staining showing ringed sideroblasts (11.59), plus quantitative measurement of haemoglobin A2 and HbF, are necessary as a screening test for this disorder. Southern blotting analysis of mtDNA is required to make the diagnosis of Pearson's syndrome.

TREATMENT
Transfusion and iron chelation is the mainstay of treatment for SA. A trial of pyridoxine therapy is worthwhile. Allogeneic bone marrow transplantation has been used successfully in severe forms. Treatment of the underlying cause in the acquired forms usually alleviates the SA.

GLUCOSE-6-PHOSPHATE DEFICIENCY

PRESENTATION
Most patients are asymptomatic and are picked up on screening prior to surgery or drug therapy such as anti-malarial treatment. Some patients present with intravascular haemolysis and haemoglobinuria ('Coca-Cola urine'). This haemolysis is usually precipitated by the use of a drug or the ingestion of broad beans (favism). Occasional patients can present with chronic haemolysis and the consequent production of gallstones.

DIAGNOSIS
The diagnosis is based on a screening test for glucose 6 phosphate dehydrogenase (G6PD). Patients with massive intravascular haemolysis often have bucket-handle forms of the red blood cells (11.60). This is due to retraction of haemoglobin away from the red cell membrane.

TREATMENT
Specific treatment is not required except in the vary rare case of chronic haemolysis, which may respond to splenectomy. The majority of patients should be issued with a list of drugs and foods to be avoided.

Drugs and chemicals that may cause haemolysis in G6PD deficiency	
• Acetanilide	• Nitrofurantoin
• Chloramphenicol	• Pamaquine
• Daunorubicin	• Pentaquine
• Dapsone	• Phenylhydrazine
• Methylene blue	• Sulphonamides
• Nalidixic acid	

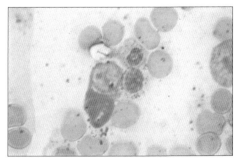

11.59 Sideroblastic anaemia. Bone marrow aspirate showing ringed sideroblasts.

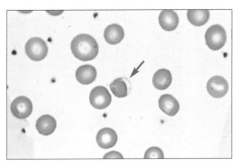

11.60 G6PD deficiency. Blood film showing 'bucket-handle' forms of red blood cells.

LEISHMANIASIS

PRESENTATION
Visceral leishmaniasis (Kala-azar) is a chronic debilitating infection that is endemic in the Mediterranean basin, East Africa, Northern East India, China and South America. The causative organism is *Leishmania donovanii* (LD), which is transmitted by the sandfly (*Phlebotomus*). The type seen in the Mediterranean usually affects younger children (*Leishmania infantum*). The protozoan infects the macrophage compartment of the reticuloendothelial system resulting in massive splenomegaly, hepatomegaly, pancytopenia and swinging fevers.

DIAGNOSIS
Usually made following analysis of the bone marrow, in which macrophages are glutted with LD bodies (amastigotes, **11.61**). Splenic aspiration and serological markers are alternative diagnostic modalities.

TREATMENT
Worldwide, antimonials are the most frequently used agents in kala-azar. These are not without serious side-effects (kidney/liver/heart) and, more recently, amphotericin B and the more effective liposomal amphotericin B have been used with impressive results.

GAUCHER DISEASE

See also 'Metabolic Diseases' chapter.

PRESENTATION
This is the commonest type of inherited lipidosis. There is great inter-individual variation in the degree of clinical involvement. Most patients have hepatosplenomegaly (**11.62**), Gaucher cells in the bone marrow and accumulation of glucosylceramide. The presentation depends on the disease type:
- **Type 1.** Chronic, non-neuronopathic adult-type Gaucher disease.
- **Type 2.** Acute, neuronopathic (infantile type) Gaucher disease.
- **Type 3.** Sub-acute, neuronopathic-type juvenile Gaucher disease.

Diagnosis is thus based on the measurement of the enzyme and detection of Gaucher cells in the marrow aspirate (**11.63**) and trephine (**11.64**).

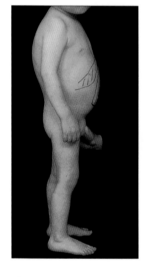

11.62 Gaucher disease. Hepatosplenomegaly.

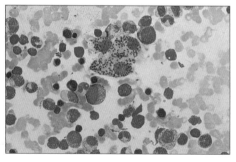

11.61 Leishmaniasis. Amastigotes in the bone marrow.

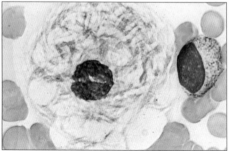

11.63 Gaucher cells in marrow aspirate.

TREATMENT

Patients with type 1, adult, chronic, neurono-pathic Gaucher disease may be treated with ceridase, which is a commercial form of the missing enzyme, or with bone marrow transplantation.

The patients with the acute, neuronopathic, type 2, infantile Gaucher disease have an early onset and fatal outcome and thus prenatal diagnosis is the most feasible alternative management course.

Patients with type 3, subacute, neurono-pathic, juvenile Gaucher disease have a relentlessly progressive neurological deterioration and are prime candidates for enzyme replacement and bone marrow replacement.

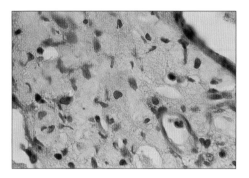

11.64 Gaucher cells in trephine.

OSTEOPETROSIS

PRESENTATION

There are two main forms, which are approximately equal in incidence – the benign autosomal-dominant form, and the severe autosomal-recessive form. Rarely, abnormalities of macrophage-colony stimulating factor (M-CSF) and carbonic anhydrase have been detected. Consanguinity is frequent and the gender ratio is equal.

The milder dominant variety is diagnosed in late childhood and is characterized by dense bones that fracture easily. These patients have no specific haematological problems.

The more severe recessive disorder presents in early infancy with fractures, because of a defect in bone resorption by osteoclasts. These patients have large heads, sclerotic bones and hepatosplenomegaly (**11.65**). They rapidly develop blindness, deafness, cranial nerve palsies and pancytopenia.

DIAGNOSIS

Based on the presence of abnormally sclerotic bones on x-ray and, in the recessive form, by the presence of a leukoerythroblastic blood film.

TREATMENT

Patients with osteopetrosis must be assessed at a very early stage for bone marrow transplantation, either from a matched sibling donor or from a haploidentical family donor and unrelated donor, before they develop problems such as blindness. Symptomatic anaemia and thrombocytopenia are treated with transfusion of red cells and platelets. The development of hypersplenism decreases the efficacy of such treatment and splenectomy is required.

Some patients with the dominant form of the disease have responded transiently to steroid therapy, an effect that is due to reticulo-endothelial suppression. Ultrasonography can be used to detect increased bone density, fractures, macrocephaly and hydrocephalus prenatally.

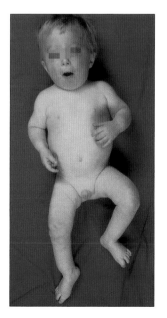

11.65 Osteopetrosis.

REFERENCES

Hodgkin's lymphoma
Donaldson SS. A discourse: The 2002 Wataru W. Sutow lecture, Hodgkin Disease in Children – perspectives and progress. *Med Pediatr Oncol* 2003; **40**: 73–81.

B-cell non-Hodgkin's lymphoma
Magrath I. Malignant Non-Hodgkins Lymphoma in Children. In: Pizzo PA, Poplach DG (eds). *Principles and Practice of Pediatric Oncology* (2nd edn). Philadelphia: Lippincott, 1993.

T-Cell non-Hodgkin's lymphoma (NHL)/Leukaemia
Hirsch-Ginsberg C, Huh Y, Kagan J *et al*. Advances in the diagnosis of acute leukaemia. *Hematol Oncol Clin N Am* 1993; **7**: 1.

Monocytic and myelomonocytic leukaemia
Odom LF. Acute Myeloid Leukaemia in Children. In: Hoffman R, Benz Jr EJ, Shattil SJ *et al* (eds). *Hematology Basic Principles and Practice* (2nd edn). Edinburgh: Churchill Livingstone, 1995.

Extramedullary and acute lymphoblastic leukaemia
Tubergen DG, Gilchrist GS, O'Brian R *et al*. Prevention of CNS disease in intermediate-risk acute lymphoblastic leukaemia: comparison of cranial irradiation and intrathecal methofrexate and the importance of systemic therapy: A Children's Cancer Group Report. *J Clin Oncol* 1993; **11**: 520–526.

Juvenile chronic myeloid leukaemia
Freedman MH, Cohen A, Grunberger T *et al*. Central role of tumour necrosis factor, GM-CSF, and interleukin 1 in the pathogenesis of juvenile chronic myelogenous leukaemia. *Br J Haem* 1992; **80**: 40–48.

Eosinophilic myeloproliferative disorder with chromosomal 5;12 translocation (t5;12)
Curnutte JT. Disorders of Granulocyte Function and Granulopoieses. In: Nathan DG, Oski FA (eds). *Hematology of Infancy and Childhood* (4th edn). Philadelphia: Saunders, 1993.

Severe haemophilia A and B (classic haemophilia and Christmas disease)
Hathway WE, Goodnight Jr SJ (eds). *Disorders of Hemostasis and Thrombosis – a Clinical Guide*. New York: McGraw Hill, 1993.

von Willebrand's disease (vWD)
Lusher JM, Kessler CM (eds). *Hemophilia and von Willebrand's Disease in the 1990s*. New York: Excerpta Medica, 1991.

Thrombocytopaenia with absent radius (TAR)
Beardsley DS. Platelet Abnormalities in Infancy and Childhood. In: Nathan PG, Oski FA (eds). *Hematology of Infancy and Childhood* (4th edn). Philadelphia: Saunders, 1993.

Bernard-Soulier syndrome
Blanchette VS, Sparling C, Turner C. Inherited Bleeding Disorders. In: Hann IM Gibson BES (eds). *Baillière's Clinical Haematology* (vol 4). Philadelphia: Baillière Tindall, 1991.

Kasabach-Merritt syndrome
Bick RL (ed). Perplexing Thrombotic and Hemorrhagic Disorders. *Hematology/Oncology Clinics of North America* (vol 6). Philadelphia: Saunders, 1992.

Fanconi anaemia
Young NS, Alter BP. Clinical Fractures of Fanconi's Anaemia. In: Young NS, Alter BP (eds). *Aplastic Anaemia Acquired and Inherited*. Philadelphia: Saunders, 1994.

Dyskeratosis congenita
Young NS, Alter BP. Dyskeratosis Congenita. In: Young NS, Alter BP (eds). *Aplastic Anaemia Acquired and Inherited*. Philadelphia: Saunders, 1994.

Transcobalamin II deficiency
Chanarin L. *The Megaloblastic Anaemias* (3rd edn). Oxford: Blackwell, 1990.

Congenital erythropoietic porphyria
Sassa S, Kappas A. The Porphyrias. In: Nathan DG, Oski FA (eds). *Hematology of Infancy and Childhood* (4th edn). Philadelphia: Saunders, 1993.

Idiopathic pulmonary hemosiderosis
Cutz E. Idiopathic pulmonaiy hemosiderosis and related disorders in infancy and childhood. *Perspect Pediatr Pathol* 1987; **11**: 47–81

Pyruvate kinase deficiency
Mentzer WC, Jr. Pyruvate Kinase Deficiency and Disorders of Glycolysis. In: Nathan DG, Oski FA (eds). *Hematology of Infancy and Childhood*. Philadelphia: Saunders, 1993.

Beta thalassaemia major
McDonagh T, Nienhuis AW. The Thalassaemia. In: Nathan DG, Oski FA (eds). *Hematology of Infancy and Childhood*. Philadelphia: Saunders, 1993.

Sickle cell disease
Davies SC, Wonke B. The Management of Haemoglobinopathies. In: Hann IM, Gibson BES (eds). *Baillière's Clinical Hematology* (vol 4). Philadelphia: Baillière Tindall, 1991.

Hereditary elliptocytosis
Becker PS, Lux SE. Disorders of the Red Cell Membrane. In: Nathan DG, Oski FA (Eds). *Hematology of Infancy and Childhood*. Philadelphia: Saunders, 1993.

Sideroblastic anaemia
Will AM. Sideroblastic Anaemias. In:Lilleyman J, Hann I, Blanchette V (eds). *Pediatric Hermatology* (2nd edn). Edinburgh: Churchill Livingstone, 1999: 112–115.

G6PD deficiency
Luzzatto L. G6PD defiency and Haemolytic Anaemia. In: Nathan DG, Oski FA, (eds). *Hematology of Infancy and Childhood*. Philadelphia: Saunders, 1993.

Leishmaniasis
Smith OP, Hann IM, Novelli V *et al*. Visceral leishmanias: rapid response to AmBisome. *Arch Dis Child* 1995; **73**: 157–159.

Gaucher's disease
Barton NW, Brady RD, Dambrosia JM *et al*. Replacement therapy for inherited enzyme defiency-macrophage-targeted glusocerebrosidase for Gaucher's disease. *N Eng J Med* 1991; **324**: 1464–1470.
Cox T, Lachmann R, Hollak C *et al*. Novel oral treatment of Gaucher's disease with N-butyldeoxynojirimycin (OGT 918) to decrease substrate biosynthesis. *Lancet* 2000; **355**: 1481–1485.

Osteopetrosis
Lenarsky C, Kohn DB, Weinberg KI *et al*. Bone marrow transplantation for genetic diseases. *Hematol Oncol Clin N Am* 1990; **4**: 589–602.

Solid Tumours and Histiocytosis

Jon Pritchard • Richard Grundy
Antony Michalski • Mark N Gaze
Gill A Levitt

INTRODUCTION

Cancer affects about 1 in 600 children worldwide. Leukaemia (bone marrow cancer) is the commonest form (30–35% of all cancer in childhood), followed by brain tumours (20–25%), lymphomas including Hodgkin's disease (10%), soft tissue sarcomas, particularly rhabdomyosarcoma (8%), neuroblastoma and Wilms' tumour (6–7%). Leukaemia and lymphoma are covered in the 'Blood Diseases' chapter. Other rarer forms of cancer also occur (see **Table 12.1**).

Fortunately, well over half of all children with cancer and leukaemia can now be completely cured. Unlike some other diseases (e.g. diabetes), patients cured of childhood cancer do not need to continue treatment for life; their treatment usually stops after three to 36 months. Today, around one in 1,000 young people in their twenties have already been cured of childhood cancer.

Table 12.1 Types of childhood cancers and cure rates

Type of Cancer	Percentage of children's cancer	Current average cure rate
Acute lymphocytic leukaemia (ALL)*	25–30%	60–70%
Brain tumour	20–25%	See**
Lymphomas – Hodgkin's disease	4%	80–90%
Non-Hodgkin's lymphomas	6%	60–90%
Sarcomas of soft tissue	8–9%	60%
Acute myeloid leukaemia (AML)	7–8%	50–60%
Neuroblastoma	7–8%	50%
Wilms' tumour (nephroblastoma)	6–7%	85%
Osteosarcoma	3–4%	60%
Ewing's sarcoma (PNET)***	3–4%	60%
Malignant germ cell tumour	2–3%	80–90%
Retinoblastoma	3%	95%
Rare tumours****	2–3%	Variable

* Chances of cure in individual children are dependent on the sub-type and stage of the cancer or leukaemia in the child and on the treatment the child receives. These figures are 'averages' – i.e. only a guide to the chance of cure for a particular patient.

** There are several types of brain tumour and the average chance of cure varies with each type.

*** PNET = Primitive neuro-ectodermal tumour outside the central nervous system.

**** e.g. hepatoblastoma, carcinomas, adrenal tumours.

WILMS' TUMOUR AND OTHER RENAL TUMOURS

See also 'Urology' chapter.

Wilms' tumour (nephroblastoma) is by far the commonest type of renal tumour in childhood, but other varieties do occur (Table 12.2). Around 80–90 cases of Wilms' tumour occur in the UK each year, representing around 6–7% of all childhood cancers.

EPIDEMIOLOGY / AETIOLOGY

With the exception of clear cell sarcoma of the kidney (CCSK), which is commoner in boys, the genders are almost equally affected. No clear environmental risk factor has emerged but Wilms' tumour is 1.5 times more common in Afro-Caribbeans than in Caucasians and least common in Asian populations.

Familial Wilms' tumour (dominant inheritance) is occasionally seen but there are other, commoner Wilms' 'predisposition syndromes', including:

- Wiedemann-Beckwith syndrome.
- Denys-Drash syndrome.
- Perlman syndrome (very rare).
- The 'WAGR' (**W**ilms' tumour, **A**niridia, abnormal **G**enitalia and growth **R**etardation) syndrome.

About 5% of tumours are bilateral. 'Sporadic' Wilms' tumours typically present in the fourth year of life, but children with bilateral disease or a predisposing syndrome usually present earlier. These observations all suggest a genetic origin for Wilms' tumour.

GENETICS

The molecular pathology of Wilms' tumour is complex, with the involvement of several genes in initiation and progression, as well as disruption of normal genomic imprinting on the short arm of chromosome 11(11p). WAGR patients have a heterozygous constitutional deletion of 11p, usually visible via standard lymphocyte karyotyping (**12.1**). To date, only one gene, WT1, has been precisely located – at 11p13. The WT1 gene is essential for kidney development. Constitutional point mutations within this gene are found consistently in Denys-Drash syndrome but fewer than 10% of sporadic tumours have any detectable abnormality of 11p.

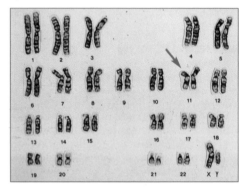

12.1 Lymphocyte karyotype from a patient with WAGR syndrome. There is a readily visible deletion from the short arm of 1 copy of chromosome 11 (arrow), designated 11p-.

Table 12.2 Types of renal tumour in childhood

Benign	Comments
Mesoblastic nephroma (*mesonephric hamartoma*)	Commonest in small infants. There are 'typical' and 'cellular' subtypes which are managed differently.
Angiomyolipoma	Occurs in association with tuberous sclerosis.
Cystic nephroma	Probably part of the Wilms' tumour 'spectrum'.
Haemangioma and lymphangioma	

Malignant	Comments
Wilms' tumour	Variable histology (see text).
Clear cell sarcoma (CCSK)	Can metastasise to bone and/or brain.
Rhabdoid tumour (RTK)	Associated with PNET of brain.
Carcinoma	May be familial.
Neuroblastoma	Can be 'intra-renal'.
Non-Hodgkin lymphoma (NHL)	Usually bilateral, diffuse involvement.

PRESENTATION

Most Wilms' tumours are discovered 'incidentally' or because parents or grandparents notice abdominal enlargement (**12.2** and **12.3**). They are often very large at diagnosis. Pain is uncommon and usually attributed to intra-tumoral bleeding, whilst haematuria occurs in only 10–15%. Presentation with tumour rupture, varicoele, hypertension or symptoms of metastatic spread is rare.

INVESTIGATIONS

Imaging: Initial screening of abdominal masses is with ultrasound, to exclude cystic lesions, which may show the blood 'lakes' characteristic of intra-tumoral bleeding in Wilms' tumour but not other types of renal tumour. CT and MRI scanning are equally effective in demonstrating the renal origin of the primary tumours, the anatomy of the 'opposite' kidney – to exclude bilateral disease (**12.4**) – and determining whether or not the IVC is involved (**12.5**). These days, because of the considerable radiation dose from CT, MRI is preferred.

Children with Wilms' tumours should have chest x-rays and chest computerized tomography (CT) to investigate for lung metastases. Those with CCSK and RTK should have, in addition, an istotope bone scan and a CT or MRI brain scan, if clinically indicated.

Other investigations: Some patients have a low haemoglobin because of intra-tumoral bleeding. The partial thromboplastin time (PTT) may be prolonged because some Wilms' tumours make an anti-von Willebrand factor. If proteinuria is present, Denys-Drash syndrome should be suspected. Constitutional karyotype studies should be carried out if the patient is dysmorphic.

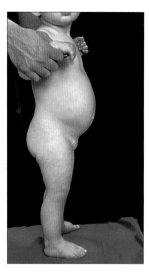

12.2 Two-year old girl on day of diagnosis of L-sided Wilms'. The tumour weighed 1 kg but was histopathologically stage I and of 'favourable' histology (FH).

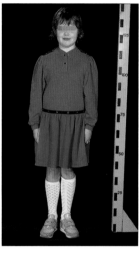

12.3 The same girl, 6.5 years later, cured by surgery and vincristine chemotherapy only. Apart from nephrectomy, there are no discernible 'late effects'.

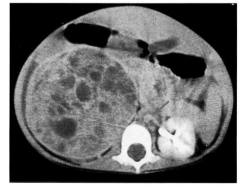

12.4 CT scan of abdomen showing huge L Wilms' tumour and a normal R kidney IVC (arrow).

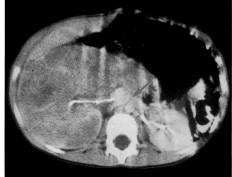

12.5 CT scan showing renal vein and IVC involvement (arrow) by direct tumour extension. Pre-operative chemotherapy is indicated.

Histopathology: Malignant tumours are stratified into those with a relatively favourable prognosis: FH ('favourable histology') and those with a lesser likelihood of cure – UH ('unfavourable histology'). **12.6** shows a standard 'triphasic', FH Wilms' tumour and **12.7** shows an area of 'anaplasia' in a UH tumour. Clear cell sarcoma of the kidney (CCSK) and rhabdoid tumour of the kidney (RTK), previously categorized as UH, are not Wilms' tumours at all.

Nephroblastomatosis, a curious tumour-like condition, is associated with Wilms' and is often assumed to be a precursor lesion.

Staging: Two staging systems are in common use. The National Wilms' Tumour System (NWTS) is most appropriate when patients have surgery first, but the International Society of Paediatric Oncology (SIOP) system is preferred for patients having preoperative chemotherapy. The NWTS system is shown in **Table 12.3**.

TREATMENT

There has been a divergence of opinion between Europe and the USA as to the merits of preoperative chemotherapy versus immediate nephrectomy. In Britain, the UKWT3 trial randomized between the two: no difference in survival was evident but less operative morbidity in the preoperative group was reported. Importantly, there was 'stage migration', with more children having lower-stage disease and less treatment. Treatment within Europe, including Britain, uses 4–6 weeks of preoperative chemotherapy with vincristine and actinomycin D. Postoperative treatment depends on the stage and histological sub-type.

PROGNOSIS

Survival for FH patients is: Stage I, >95%; Stage II, >90%; Stage III, 80–85%; Stage IV, 60–80% (overall FH survival is 85%). For UH patients (all stages) survival is: anaplastic tumours, 60%; CCSK, 80% (doxorubicin is the crucial drug for CCSK) and RTK, 20%. Cure is possible for up to half of relapsing patients, especially those who have received only one or two chemotherapy drugs and no radiotherapy 'first time around'.

LATE EFFECTS

Rather than 'cure at any cost', the objective in treating Wilms' tumour is 'cure at least cost'. Therapists try to avoid some of the 'late effects' by omitting that treatment whenever it can be shown, by clinical trial, to be unnecessary. Aside from the usual reasons for referral to a tertiary paediatric oncology centre, avoidance of unnecessary therapy is crucial for these patients.

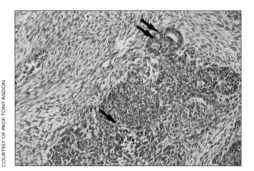

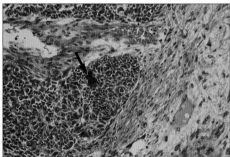

12.6 'Typical' triphasic Wilms' tumour ('FH') showing blastema (single arrow), epithelial structures (double arrow) and stroma.

12.7 'UH' tumour because of focal anaplasia. Atypical nuclei are arrowed.

COURTESY OF PROF TONY RISDON

Table 12.3 National Wilms' tumour staging system

Stage I	Single tumour confined to kidney and completely excised, pathologically.
Stage II	Single tumour invading through pseudo-capsule but completely excised, pathologically: tumour rupture into flank only.
Stage III	Single tumour either invading into adjacent tissues and incompletely excised or tumour inoperable, usually because of IVC invasion (**Figure 12.5**) any abdominal lymph nodes positive: tumour rupture with diffuse peritoneal contamination.
Stage IV	Metastatic disease, excepting abdominal lymph nodes.
Bilateral	Primary tumours in both kidneys.

LIVER TUMOURS

In sharp contrast to adults, primary liver tumours in children are more common than secondary tumours. Both benign and malignant types occur (**Table 12.4**). Overall, they represent 1–2% of all children's tumours and about 1% of all children's cancers. Males are more commonly affected than females.

AETIOLOGY

Hepatoblastoma is associated with familial adenomatous polyposis (FAP) and with Beckwith-Wiedemann syndrome. Hepatocellular carcinoma often arises in a liver previously damaged by hepatitis B virus, and is therefore commoner in epidemic areas (e.g., Taiwan), or by metabolic liver disease, especially glycogen storage disease (GSD) type I and tyrosinosis.

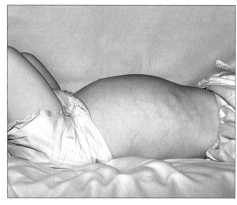

12.8 Distended upper abdomen in a child with hepatoblastoma. Note that there is no jaundice.

PRESENTATION

Liver tumours usually present with upper abdominal distension (**12.8**). Pain is unusual and jaundice only occurs in some children with biliary rhabdomyosarcoma. Besides increased levels of alpha-fetoprotein (α-FP), which must be interpreted according to the patient's age, thrombocytosis (due to release of a thrombopoietin) is characteristic of hepatoblastoma and hepatocellular carcinoma. Rarely, hepatoblastomas secrete ACTH or sex hormones and the corresponding endocrine syndrome develops. **Imaging**: The lungs are by far the most frequent site for metastatic hepatoblastoma and hepatocellular carcinoma, so chest x-ray and computerized tomographic (CT) scan of the lungs are mandatory. Magnetic resonance imaging (MRI) is probably better than CT at displaying the anatomy and focality of the primary tumour, and vividly reflects treatment response.

Table 12.4 Types of liver tumour and relationship to level* of serum α-fetoprotein (α-FP) at diagnosis

	Undetectable	Slight elevation	Very high
Benign			
Adenoma	50%	50%	–
Haemangioma	All	–	–
Haemangioendothelioma	All	–	–
Mesenchymal hamartoma	50%	50%	–
Malignant			
Hepatoblastoma	<5%	<5%	>95%
Hepatocellular carcinoma**	25%	25%	50%
Sarcoma	All	–	–
Malignant germ cell tumour***	<5%	<5%	>95%*
Non-Hodgkin's lymphoma (NHL)****	All	–	–

*Account must be taken of the child's age in interpreting values.
** Fibrolamellar variant associated with normal serum α-FP but elevated serum Vit B12 and TCII (transcobalamin II) levels.
*** Can also have elevated serum β-HCG.
****In NHL, liver enlargement is usually diffuse.

TREATMENT AND MONITORING

Benign tumours are usually treated by surgery. Exceptions are some haemangiomas, if surgery is potentially hazardous, when careful observation with serial imaging or embolization are options, and multiple adenomas (**12.9**).

Malignant tumours are treated with chemotherapy to destroy metastases and shrink the primary tumour, then with delayed surgical resection. Chemotherapy is 'PLADO' (cisplatin/ doxorubicin) for hepatoblastoma and hepatocellular carcinoma (**12.10**, **12.11**), 'JEB' (carboplatin, etoposide, bleomycin) for malignant germ cell tumours (MGCT) and 'VAC' or 'IVA' (vincristine, actinomycin D and either cyclophosphamide or ifosfamide) for sarcomas. Treatment is usually dictated by international studies.

Monitoring is by serial imaging with MRI or CT scan of tumour (see **12.9**) and chest x-rays in the case of hepatoblastoma/hepatocellular carcinoma and it is essential to monitor serum AFP 1–2 weekly during the treatment and monthly for 2 years off treatment.

PROGNOSIS

The prognosis has much improved in recent years. Overall, the cure of hepatoblastoma is now 70–80%, sarcoma >50% (biliary tumours are still difficult) and MGCT >80%. For hepatocellular carcinoma, prognosis is still relatively poor because tumours are often multifocal and/or metastatic at diagnosis; however, unifocal tumours are curable in at least 50% of cases.

Liver transplant is a realistic option for 'unresectable' tumours responding to chemotherapy, without evidence of extra-hepatic spread.

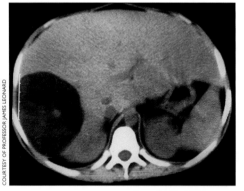

COURTESY OF PROFESSOR JAMES LEONARD

12.9 CT scan showing multiple adenomas in the liver of a boy with GSD type I. With adequate dietary control, tumour growth usually slows down and tumours may regress, as occurred in this case.

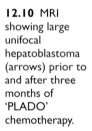

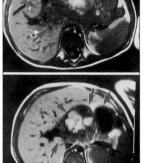

12.10 MRI showing large unifocal hepatoblastoma (arrows) prior to and after three months of 'PLADO' chemotherapy.

12.11 Serum α-FP response to courses of 'PLADO' chemotherapy (solid arrows – see text) in a 1.5-year-old child with hepatoblastoma. The $t^{1/2}$ is 4–5 days, indicating a major tumour response. Complete surgical resection was achieved (open lozenge). The MRI scans of this patient, who is a long-term survivor, are shown in 12.9.

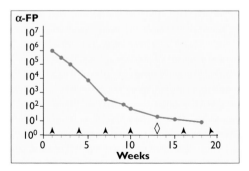

HISTIOCYTOSIS

There are two main types of histiocytes, both derived from pluri-potential stem cells of the bone marrow. The principal function of one type is antigen-processing, chiefly by phago-cytosis: members of the family of cells include the circulating blood monocyte, the pulmonary alveolar macrophage, the hepatic Kupffer cell and the so-called 'microglia' of the central nervous system (CNS). The other type of histiocyte is chiefly concerned with antigen presentation and the Langerhans cell, which forms a 'network' at the dermo–epidermal junction, over the entire body surface, is the most notable member of this cell family.

Pathologically and clinically, distinct types of histiocytosis arise from these two cell types. Haemophagocytic lymphohistiocytosis (HLH) and Rosai Dorfman disease seem to be disorders of phagocytes (Type I histiocytosis) while Langerhans cell histiocytosis (LCH) is a disease of Langerhans cells (Type II histiocytosis). Although sometimes progressive and (especially in the case of HLH) fatal, none of these disorders is currently regarded as 'malignant'. True malignant histiocytosis (Type III) is exceptionally rare in children and will not be discussed here.

LANGERHANS CELL HISTIOCYTOSIS
Aetiology/epidemiology
Langerhans cell histiocytosis (LCH) is caused by a clonal proliferation of pathological Langer-hans cells (LCH cells) which invade a range of organs in which their normal counterparts are never found and attract several types of 'inflam-matory' cells, forming an infiltrate. LCH is commoner in boys than in girls, and also occurs in adults.

Inheritance
The cause of LCH has not been identified. Epidemiological studies reveal a uniform racial and geographical distribution, with no 'clus-tering' of cases in time or space and, to date, no specific cytogenetic or molecular lesion has been identified in LCH cells. On the other hand, familial clustering, including identical twins, have been reported.

Clinical presentation
Histiocytosis can affect many organ systems. Lytic bone lesions often heal slowly but com-pletely, although deformity and disability can occur. The skull bones are commonly affected (**12.12**, **12.13**) resulting in sequelae including deafness and proptosis. Skin involvement can resemble seborrhoeic dematitis involving the

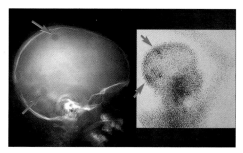

12.12 High resolution CT scan of skull, showing soft tissue mass in middle ear with adjacent destruction of the petrous temporal bone and invasion of the structures of the middle and inner ear. The patient, a five-year-old girl, presented with an aural polyp and deafness. Only the skeleton was involved in this patient ('single-system disease').

12.13 Skull radiograph showing 'punched-out' lytic deposits in the skull table of a five-year old boy with 'multi-system' LCH. The inset shows the corresponding radionuclide scan after injection of an ^{111}In radiolabelled mouse anti-CD1a antibody. There is increased uptake in the skull lesions and in Waldeyer's ring.

flexural creases (**12.14**) and purpura can appear if platelets are low (**12.15**).

Restrictive lung defects with cysts and bullae formation may result in pneumothoraces; pulmonary fibrosis is a chronic sequela (**12.16**, **12.17**). Liver disease may progress to biliary cirrhosis. Lymph node and splenic enlargement can be massive and lymph nodes may erode to create sinuses. Small and large gut involvement is often underdiagnosed. Selective invasion of the pituitary/hypothalamus region (**12.18**) causes diabetes insipidus and growth hormone deficiency in 40% and 10% of cases respectively. Other CNS complications include cerebellar white matter involvement, resulting in ataxia (**12.19**) and cerebral mass lesions.

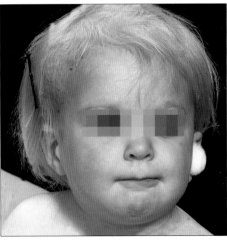

12.14 Seborrhoea-like rash involving the scalp and external ear of a two-year-old girl with multi-system LCH. The condition had previously been diagnosed as 'seborrhoeic eczema'; the cotton-wool plug provides the diagnostic clue! Eighteen years later, she is alive and disease-free.

Classification

LCH is classified according to whether one ('single-system disease') or more ('multi-system disease') organs is/are affected. The commonest form of LCH (around 50%) is single-system bony disease, with one or more lytic lesions in almost any bone. These lesions are also known as 'eosinophilic granuloma'. Skin involvement (**12.14**) is also common, in a characteristic distribution (see also 'Dermatology' chapter). Some 5–10% of patients have severe multi-system disease, with organ failure ('Letterer-Siwe disease') and the remaining 40–45% suffer disease with intermediate severity. Diabetes insipidus, in up to 40% of patients, is the commonest chronic sequel of LCH.

Diagnosis

The picture is similar in all forms of LCH. The infiltrating lesion is heterogeneous but LCH cells, characterized by CD1a positivity are present in every case, together with 'ordinary' histiocytes, neutrophils, eosinophils, giant cells and T lymphocytes. In chronic disease, CD1a-positive cells disappear and fibrosis or, in the brain, gliosis are the dominant features.

Full blood count, liver function tests with plasma albumin and coagulation studies, chest x-ray, radiographic skeletal survey (preferred to isotope bone scanning) and early morning urine osmolarity are needed in each patient. This initial screening may indicate the need for other investigations including bone marrow, liver or gut biopsy, CT scan of lungs and/or respiratory function tests, dental or aural radiographs, MRI scan of pituitary and brain.

Using these results, patients are categorized into those with single-system disease and those with multi-system LCH with/without organ dysfunction.

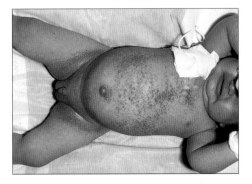

12.15 Widespread, confluent central truncal rash and petechiae in an infant with multi-system LCH and thrombocytopenia due to 'haemopoietic failure' despite treatment. This 14-month-old boy died six months later, from progressive LCH.

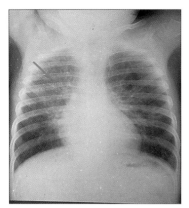

12.16 LCH pulmonary disease. X-ray showing a four-year old boy at diagnosis, with interstitial infiltrate and bilateral pneumo-thorax. The same patient aged 18 years had a much-reduced chest volume secondary to lung fibrosis with secondary cyst formation.

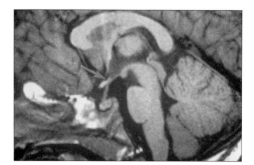

12.18 Pituitary stalk thickening (increased from 1 to 2–3 mm) and absence of the posterior pituitary 'bright signal' in this T1-weighted MRI scan of a two-year-old boy with proven diabetes insipidus (DI) but normal growth. The DI was well-controlled with oral DDAVP tablets. Anterior pituitary function was normal.

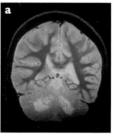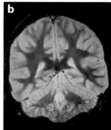

12.19 MRI scans (T2 weighted) of 10-year-old patient with multi-system LCH since birth and cerebellar ataxia, evolving over the previous four years. The symmetrical changes in the white matter of both cerebellar hemispheres (**a**) are characteristic of 'burnt-out' LCH. Scan in a normal 9–10 year old (**b**).

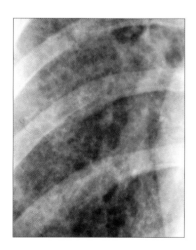

12.17 A high magnification view of the lung of another patient, who was a smoker, showing intense interstitial shadowing; biopsy confirmed 'active' LCH.

Treatment/prognosis

Patients with single-system disease usually have an excellent prognosis. Systemic treatment is rarely needed and spontaneous regression is common. Helpful 'local' therapies include topical anti-inflammatory lotions and tar-based shampoos, intra-lesional steroids and/or oral indomethacin for bone pain and surgical debridement of aural/oral lesions.

Patients with multi-system LCH require systemic therapy with steroids and cytotoxic drugs; however, 'local' therapies can be a helpful 'adjuvant' to management. Diabetes insipidus is managed by replacement DDAVP and GH deficiency by GH supplementation. Hepatic failure may be treated with transplantation.

Adverse prognostic factors for multi-system LCH include age <2 years; involvement of many organs; low serum albumin, prolonged clotting times or pancytopenia ('organ failure'); and poor response to initial chemotherapy.

The outcome for single-system disease is excellent, with virtually no deaths and few sequelae. Patients with multi-system disease have a more guarded prognosis: 10–20% (mostly young children with 'organ failure' and a poor initial response to chemotherapy) die of LCH, despite intensive support. Of the survivors, at least 50% will have one or more chronic, debilitating sequelae.

HAEMOPHAGOCYTIC LYMPHOHISTIOCYTOSIS (HLH) (12.20)

The disease is characterized by activated T cells and hypercytokinaemia, especially increased circulating levels of TNF and soluble IL2 receptor. Linked genetic loci have been identified on chromosomes 9q and 10q but the exact pathogenetic mechanism has not yet been clarified.

There are two varieties of HLH, as summarized in Table 7.5. Clinical features are similar, except that the genetic form (autosomal recessive) is common in societies where intermarriage is prevalent and tends to present at an earlier age – almost always within the first year of life – than sporadic HLH. The sporadic form seems to be commoner in the Far East. Viral infections may precipitate 'sporadic' HLH and exacerbate the genetic form. The genders are equally affected.

Clinical presentation

HLH can present in a variety of ways. Characteristic features include hepatosplenomegaly, coagulopathy and bi- or pan-cytopenia. Signs of CNS involvement, varying from minor irritability to seizures and 'meningism', are common in the genetic form (see **Table 12.5**). However, in some patients, involvement of one system (hepatic, neurological) can predominate and delay diagnosis. Lymphadenopathy and skin rash (except purpura) are uncommon.

Diagnosis

Any or all of the following may be present: anaemia, neutropenia, thrombocytopenia, raised liver transaminases, low plasma albumin, raised low-density lipoproteins, and prolonged coagulation times (PT, PTT and thrombin time) with low plasma fibrinogen levels. Bone marrow aspirates and CSF cytofuge preparations may show haemophagocytosis but repeated sampling is sometimes necessary.

Some centres advocate splenic aspiration instead. Liver biopsy shows a periportal infiltrate, similar to that of chronic active hepatitis, and haemophagocytosis. However, none of these tests is diagnostic; the differential diagnosis includes leukaemia, myelodysplasia, aplastic anaemia, primary immune deficiency and vasculitis.

Treatment/prognosis

Mild cases of 'sporadic' HLH may resolve spontaneously or with blood product support and antimicrobials. Genetic and severe sporadic HLH are usually life-threatening and often progress at an alarming speed. Initial treatment is with etoposide (VPI6) and high-dose cortico-steroids: CNS-directed treatment (intrathecal methotrexate-MTX) is only used if there are CNS symptoms because MTX may contribute to brain damage; if the systemic component of the disease is controlled, CSF pleocytosis resolves spontaneously. As soon as clinical remission is achieved, patients with genetic HLH should proceed to marrow ablation and bone marrow transplantation, otherwise the condition recurs and ultimately proves fatal. Siblings may develop the disease up to the age of 5–6 years so older siblings or 'MUDs' (matched unrelated donors) are preferred. If no donor is available, remission may be maintained with cyclosporin A (CyA), for months or even years.

Follow-up and counselling

Recurrences of HLH are generally heralded by re-enlargement of the spleen and liver but regular blood counts may be indicated, especially in patients who have not been treated by BMT, for 1–2 years. CSF monitoring is not needed, unless there are worrying symptoms.

'Curative' BMT for HLH has only been in use since the early 1990s, so long-term prognostication is difficult, but patients who survive >5 years after their transplant, disease-free, are regarded as cured.

If patients with 'sporadic' HLH survive the first episode, they usually do well, though vigilance is needed, especially in younger patients, in case this is the first episode of 'genetic' HLH.

Families of children with definite (positive family history or consanguinity) or probable (presentation under 1 year of age) genetic HLH should consult a clinical geneticist, especially in 'borderline' cases, especially now that definitive 'HLH genes' have been identified.

This is a very rare form of Type I histiocytosis.

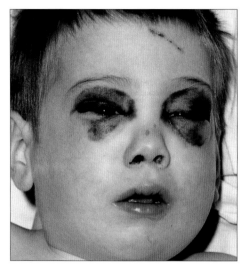

12.20 Petechiae and ecchymosis in a sick seven-year-old with pancytopenia due to haemophagocytic lymphohistiocytosis (HLH) of the sporadic variety. In this case, the illness was precipitated by Epstein-Barr virus (EBV) infection.

Table 12.5. Sporadic and genetic Haemophagocytic Lymphohistiocytosis

	Genetic form	Sporadic form
Age at onset	3–12 months	Any age
Inheritance	Autosomal recessive	Not inherited
Precipitated by infection	Sometimes	Often
Skin rash	None	May be present if precipitated by virus.
CNS involvement	Common	Less common
Clinical course and prognosis	Recurrent episodes and ultimately poor prognosis unless BMT* performed.	Relatively good but can be very severe and fatal. Recurrences unusual.

* BMT = Bone marrow ablation and transplant

RHABDOMYOSARCOMA, OTHER SOFT TISSUE SARCOMAS AND FIBROMATOSIS

INCIDENCE

Soft tissue sarcomas (STS) occur in all age groups but rhabdomyosarcoma (RMS) is the commonest type (60–70% of all STS), in children. Conversely, 'adult' types of sarcomas occur, albeit rarely, in children. In aggregate, STS represent 8–10% of all children's cancers. Apart from haemangioma and lymphangioma, benign mesenchymal tumours are very rare indeed: probably the best documented example is cardiac rhabdomyoma, in children with tuberous sclerosis.

RHABDOMYOSARCOMAS (RMS)
Inheritance

More than 90% of RMS are 'sporadic' but 5–10% can be explained by inheritance of a 'cancer predisposition gene', most often a constitutional mutation of the TP53 gene on chromosome 17p, causing the Li-Fraumeni syndrome. TP53 is classified as an 'anti-oncogene' because 'loss of function' mutations cause cells to lose regulatory control. Cell production and apoptosis become uncoupled and, if other mutations occur, clonal expansion leads to development of tumours. Brain tumours, adrenal tumours and early-developing breast cancer are also characteristic of the Li-Fraumeni syndrome and a meticulous three- or four-generation family history is essential when RMS is diagnosed and annually thereafter. Genetic and oncological counselling is available for family members with TP53 mutations.

Clinical presentation

Around 40% of RMS arise in the head or neck, 20–25% in the pelvis and 25–30% in the trunk and limbs. The orbit is the commonest head and neck site. Painless proptosis (**12.21**, **12.22**) is usual but inflammation can occur and the differential diagnosis includes orbital cellulitis or pseudotumour, Langerhans cell histiocytosis (LCH) and other cancers, especially acute leukaemia, secondary neuroblastoma and optic nerve glioma. Middle ear tumours may present with aural pain or chronic discharge and delay in diagnosis is common because the problem is often first regarded as 'inflammatory'. At this and other head and neck sites, the primary tumour is often regarded as 'parameningeal' with the potential to invade directly through the meninges into the central nervous system (CNS). Genitourinary and pelvic primary tumours present either as a visible mass with or without bleeding and discharge, for example at the vaginal introitus (**12.23**) or by causing symptoms of pelvic outlet obstruction, most often retention of urine. Tumours arising under mucosa often have a tell-tale 'botryoid' appearance (**12.23**).

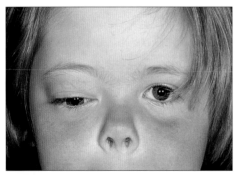

12.21 Orbital rhabdomyosarcoma of L eye showing downward and outward displacement of globe. Occasionally, the swelling looks 'inflammatory' (see text).

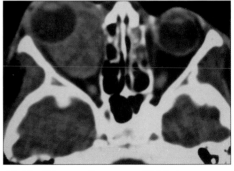

12.22 CT scan of patient in 12.21 showing tumour mass, probably arising from one of the intrinsic muscles, on the medial and posterior walls of the orbit.

Limb and trunk primaries arise as painless swellings, if they grow 'outwards' (centrifugally) or with one or more of a variety of symptoms (spinal stiffness or pain, pleural effusion, intestinal obstruction) if they grow internally. Some 'primaries' can be tiny, and hard to identify, while others reach 15–20 cm or more in diameter. Presentation with symptoms of metastasis (bone pain, marrow failure) is virtually limited to tumours with 'alveolar' histology (see below).

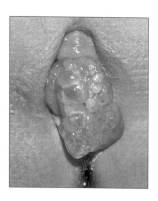

12.23 Vaginal sub-mucosal embryonal rhabdomyo-sarcoma with characteristic 'botryoid' appearance.

Diagnosis

As well as anatomical location, the histology of RMS varies, with three main sub-types (**Table 12.6**).

Risk factors for relapse therefore include: trunk or limb primary; alveolar histology; the t(2;13) translocation; age >10 years; and presence of metastases.

Biopsy, with cytogenetic studies, can be performed percutaneously or endoscopically. Bone marrow tests can be carried out at the same time. Special stains for actin, myoglobin and the microfilament desmin (**12.24**) are especially useful.

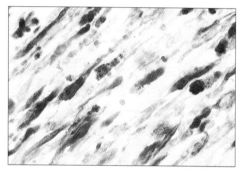

12.24 High-power microphotograph of embryonal rhabdomyosarcoma showing positive (brown) immunohistochemical stain for desmin in tumour cells.

Table 12.6 Subtypes of rhabdomyosarcoma

Histological sub-type	Age group and usual location of primary	Tumour cell cytogenetics	Clinical behaviour	Prognosis
*Embryonal ** (70–80%)	Usually <5 yrs; Head and neck, pelvis	Non-specific abnormalities of chromosome 11p15	i Often arises under mucosa causing 'botryoid' appearance ii Associated with Li-Fraumeni syndrome iii Low risk of metastasis	Good (70+% cure)
***Alveolar **(15–25%)	Often >10 yrs; Trunk and limb primaries	Specific translocation t(2;13)(q35;q14) or variant	i Primary tumour may be very small ii Risk of metastasis high	Poor (<30% cure)
Pleomorphic **(5–10%)	Varies	None identified to date	i Intermediate risk of metastasis	Moderate****

*so-called because of resemblance of tumour cells to normal embryonal myocytes
**% of all rhabdomyosarcomas
***so-called because 'spaces' within clusters of tumour cells are reminiscent of lung alveoli
****Also depends on stage/group of tumour

The primary tumour is best imaged by MRI (**12.25**), because it delineates soft tissue planes better than CT. Lung CT and isotope bone scan are also needed with bone marrow aspirates and trephines. CSF cytofuge examination is indicated if the tumour is 'parameningeal'. There is no 'tumour marker', measurable in serum or plasma, for RMS.

There is no consensus as regards 'staging'. In Europe, tumours are usually categorized according to their clinical and imaging characteristics, using the so-called TNM (tumour-node-metastasis) system, while in the USA, RMS are 'grouped' according to their resectability. In either case, the higher the stage or group, the worse the prognosis.

Treatment/prognosis

Multimodality treatment is often required. Patients receive primary chemotherapy, either the 'VAC' (vincristine, actinomycin D, cyclophosphamide) or 'IVA' (ifosfamide, vincristine and actinomycin D) combinations. Other drugs, such as carbo-platin/cisplatin, etoposide and doxorubicin arealso used in high risk patients. Local control may involve radiotherapy (RT) and/or surgery. RT is effective in RMS and well tolerated by young patients but affects bony and soft tissue growth, sometimes with disastrous cosmetic results. These days, primary surgery is only used for easily-resected 'peripheral' tumours, such as paratesticular primaries, to reduce morbidity, but less extensive surgery may be used after chemotherapy.

Response is best monitored with MRI andis usually good, initially, though shrinkage is relatively slow in most cases. If the mass disappears, surgery and RT can be deferred as long as the primary site is monitored carefully by scanning and, if appropriate, by serial endoscopy. If a mass remains, it can be removed surgically, or RT can be used, or both. Many children still need surgery and RT for cure, but around 50% can be spared the 'late effects' of these treatments (**12.26–12.29**).

Embryonal tumours have the best prognosis (see **Table 12.6**) and alveolar tumours the worst, with pleomorphic tumours intermediate. 'Local' regrowth of tumour, or non-response, may be treated with 'second-line' chemotherapy, surgery and/or RT if indicated, but the prognosis is guarded.

Follow-up should include annual enquiry about any 'new' tumour in the family (see the section at the beginning of this chapter).

OTHER SOFT TISSUE SARCOMAS

Other STS sub-types are individually so rare as to merit little space here but, in general, 'local' control of the primary tumour is the main problem and metastases are unusual. Some centres therefore advocate 'aggressive' surgery and RT for these patients while others prefer to use primary chemotherapy, as for RMS.

FIBROMATOSIS

Two types of fibromatosis occur in children. 'Aggressive' fibromatosis, sometimes misleadingly called 'infantile fibrosarcoma', usually occurs in young children and affects the limbs, especially the legs. Histologically, the tumours look 'aggressive', with many mitoses, but they do not metastasize. Treatment is conservative and 'gentle' chemotherapy (usually vincristine and actinomycin D) often initiates sustained regression (**12.30, 12.31**).

'Adult' type fibromatosis (desmoid tumour), by contrast, is histologically bland. Tumours can occur at almost any site. Intra-abdominal desmoids are often a feature of mutations in the 'FAP' (familial adenomatous polyposis) gene and FAP should also be ruled out when desmoids are multiple and/or arise in young

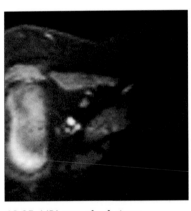

12.25 MRI scan of soft tissue rhabdomyosarcoma involving the hamstrings and subcutaneous fat, demonstrated on axial image, inversion recovery sequence; note the tumour is high signal. It is separate from the neurovascular bundle, behind the femur.

children. Besides intestinal polyposis, which develops during the teenage years, other manifestations of FAP include sebaceous cysts, osteomas and congenital hypertrophy of the retinal pigment epithelium ('CHRPE'). Desmoids are difficult to manage successfully.

Complete surgical excision is usually impossible and incomplete resection often provokes regrowth at a more rapid rate than that of the original tumour. Anti-oestrogens (tamoxifen or toremifene), multi-agent 'aggressive' chemotherapy and radiotherapy may be helpful.

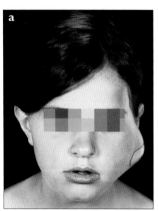
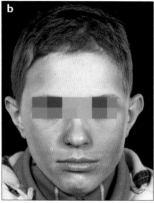
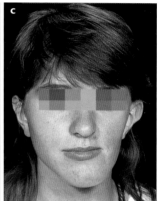

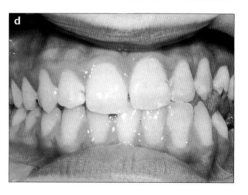

12.26–12.29 Facial appearance of girl with facial, non-parameningeal primary rhabdomyosarcoma: at diagnosis, aged 7 years (**a**); at the end of treatment with chemotherapy ('VAC' combination) and external beam radiotherapy (RT) to area of primary tumour, aged 8.5 years (**b**); and aged 15 years (**c**), showing marked facial hemiatrophy due to RT. She also had severe dental caries on the side of the RT (**d**). Multiple plastic surgical and orthodontic procedures were needed but she is now married with two normal sons, despite a high cumulative dose of cyclophosphamide.

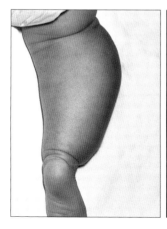
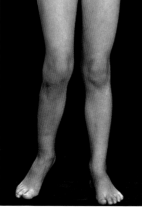

12.30 & 12.31 Aggressive fibromatosis ('infantile fibrosarcoma') of R calf: (**left**) at diagnosis (posterior view) in an infant girl. She received six months 'gentle' chemotherapy (vincristine and actinomycin D), which initiated tumour regression. Spontaneous shrinkage continued and (**right**) shows her legs, aged 5.5 years. The patient's only handicap, at that time, was a short Achilles tendon, later successfully corrected by surgery.

NEUROBLASTOMA

Neuroblastoma is thought to arise from neural crest cells that go on to form the sympathetic nervous system; primary tumours are located in the adrenal glands or sympathetic ganglia. It is the commonest extracranial solid tumour, accounting for 8% of all childhood malignancy. The clinical behaviour of neuroblastoma is very variable, with some tumours undergoing spontaneous regression and others progressing rapidly with a poor prognosis, in spite of aggressive multimodality therapy. Patients can be stratified into 'risk groups' using criteria such as age, clinical stage, and characteristic abnormalities in the molecular biology of the tumours.

STANDARD-RISK NEUROBLASTOMA
Incidence
The true incidence of low-stage disease is unknown. Screening all infants for urinary catecholamine metabolites detects those with good-risk disease, but it is unlikely that these tumours would have progressed if left un-diagnosed.

Presentation
Infants with stage 4S disease present with rapidly increasing hepatomegaly and may have skin deposits (**12.32, 12.33**). Stage 1 and 2 tumours may be detected as incidental findings on x-rays performed for other reasons.

Genetics
Good-risk tumours express Trk A protein but do not have amplification of MYCN, deletions of chromosome 1 or diploid DNA index.

Essential investigations
An MIBG scan is essential to exclude distant disease and CT or MRI imaging should rule out lymph node involvement. Bone marrow aspirates and trephines will be free of disease in stage 1 and 2 tumours though stage 4S disease may show <10% of nucleated cells in the bone marrow to be tumour.

Treatment
Resection of the primary tumour is performed in stage 1 and 2 disease. Stage 4S disease usually regresses spontaneously but, in infants with rapid liver enlargement, chemotherapy and occasionally radiotherapy may be needed.

Prognosis
Over 95% of patients with stage 1 and 2 disease survive. Seventy percent of stage 4S patients survive, with uncontrolled hepatic growth accounting for the majority of the mortality.

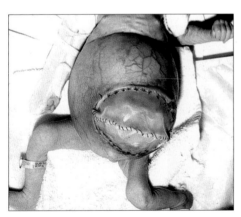

12.32 Massive hepatomegaly in stage 4S neuro-blastoma. A 'silo' procedure was attempted.

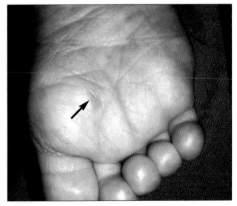

12.33 Skin nodules in stage 4S neuroblastoma.

HIGH-RISK NEUROBLASTOMA

Incidence

Forty percent of neuroblastoma cases are diagnosed in infants of less than 1 year, 35% are aged 1–2 years and 25% are older than 2 years, with the disease becoming rare after the age of 10. Of the cases that present clinically, up to 80% are stage 3 or 4 disease.

Presentation

Metastatic 'high-risk' disease would exhibit signs of the mass, catecholamine excess and bone or bone marrow involvement. The 'classic' presentation is with a hard abdominal mass in a sweaty, hypertensive, irritable child with black eyes (orbital metastases) and a limp. Tumours arising in paraspinal ganglia can present with spinal cord compression.

Genetics

Although no characteristic chromosomal translocations have been identified, a number of genetic changes occur in tumour cells. The following are associated with a poor prognosis: amplification of the MYCN oncogene, deletion of genetic material from 1p or 11q, gain of genetic material on 17q, reduced expression of the high affinity nerve growth factor receptor (TrKA) and diploid DNA index. Of these, MYCN amplification is used to stratify therapy.

Diagnosis and staging

Elevation of urinary catecholamine metabolites is helpful in establishing the diagnosis. Abdominal masses are adrenal or paraspinal in origin and may be calcified. Bone marrow aspirates and trephine biopsies are essential and a radionuclide bone scan is the optimal method of establishing the presence of bony disease. A radio-iodine labelled MIBG (metaiodobenzyl-guanidine) scan delineates soft tissue disease (**12.34**). CT or MRI scans of the primary site will allow identification of disease which crosses the midline as well as the presence of nodal enlargement (**12.35**). A biopsy of the primary tumour is mandatory in the absence of identifiable bone marrow involvement and histological criteria for the predication of outcome have been developed. Measurement of neurone-specific enolase, ferritin and lactate dehydrogenase may provide further prognostic information. Staging should be performed using the criteria developed by the International Neuroblastoma Staging Study group (INSS) and young children (<1 year of age) fare better than older patients.

Treatment

High-risk neuroblastoma is sensitive to both chemotherapy and radiation. Dose-intense chemotherapy aims to reduce the size of the primary tumour and clear metastatic disease. Further therapy involves resection of the primary tumour and high dose chemotherapy with autologous rescue (either marrow or peripheral stem cells). Oral 13-cis-retinoic acid may 'differentiate' residual tumour and improve outcome.

Prognosis

The 5-year survival for patients with extensive local but non-metastatic disease is 70%, whereas only 20–40% of patients greater than 1 year of age with metastatic disease live 5 years or more.

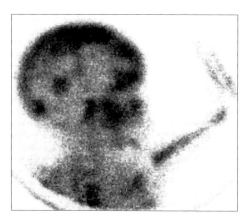

12.34 An mIBG scan showing multifocal abnormal uptake.

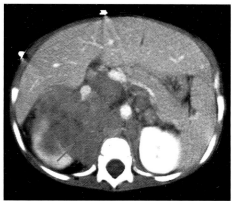

12.35 CT showing a right-sided mass crossing midline and undermining great vessels.

RETINOBLASTOMA

INCIDENCE

Retinoblastoma affects 1 in 20,000 children. More than 90% of cases are diagnosed before five years of age (see also 'Ophthalmology' chapter). Children with a family history of retinoblastoma present earlier and have a higher incidence of bilateral or multifocal disease.

CLINICAL PRESENTATION

Presenting signs are leukocoria (**12.36**), strabismus, glaucoma or poor vision. Disease is bilateral in 30% of cases. Five percent of patients are dysmorphic with microcephaly, hypertelorism, dental and digital abnormalities characteristic of constitutional deletions of 13q14.

GENETICS

Tumours arise due to the loss of function of both copies of the RB tumour suppressor gene. In sporadic cases, both copies of the gene are mutated by random genetic events, whereas in familial cases there is a constitutional mutation of one copy of the gene and only a single somatic event is necessary for tumorigenesis (Knudson hypothesis). Patients with familial retinoblastoma are predisposed to a variety of tumours in later life of which osteosarcoma is the most prevalent.

INVESTIGATIONS

Skilled ocular examination is mandatory to define the extent of intra-ocular disease. Ultrasound examination of the globe may be helpful. CT or MRI scanning of the head will define extra-orbital local disease and exclude trilateral retinoblastoma. In the very rare cases with spread outside the orbits abnormalities of CSF cytology, bone scans or MIBG scans may be seen.

TREATMENT

Treatment of intra-ocular tumours is complex and involves the use of local therapy such as laser therapy, cryotherapy, chemotherapy, localized radioactive plaques, external beam radiation and surgery. Chemotherapy now has a proven role in the treatment of RB, in particular to reduce the use of radiotherapy in bilateral disease and hence second malignant neoplasms. Screening of the relatives of the index case is recommended and in young children involves full ocular examination under anaesthetic. In families with more than one affected member, polymorphic DNA probes can be used to identify carriers of the defective gene and antenatal diagnosis is feasible. In families with a single affected member, direct identification of the mutation can be performed and relatives can then be screened for this mutation.

PROGNOSIS

Localized retinoblastoma has an excellent prognosis; disseminated disease can be cured with high-dose chemotherapy, but CNS dissemination is almost universally fatal.

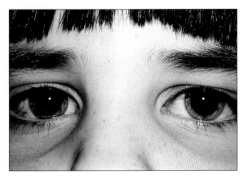

12.36 Leukocoria in the right eye of a child with retinoblastoma.

EWING'S SARCOMA AND PERIPHERAL PRIMITIVE NEUROECTODERMAL TUMOUR (pPNET)

INCIDENCE
Ewing's sarcoma classically occurs in the second decade of life, affecting fewer than three in every 1 million children under 15 years of age. Ewing's sarcoma is very rare in black children and those of Chinese origin. The true incidence of peripheral primitive neuroectodermal tumours is unclear, as their distinction from other small round blue cell tumours of childhood is difficult.

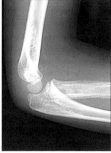

12.37 Plain radiograph of humerus showing periostial reaction, bone loss and sclerosis.

CLINICAL PRESENTATION
Ewing's sarcoma of bone presents as pain and swelling with the pelvis, femur, tibia and fibula being most commonly affected. The soft tissue Ewing's tumours or peripheral primitive neuroectodermal tumours present with intra-thoracic disease (Askin's tumour), or as para-vertebral or retroperitoneal masses.

GENETICS
Both Ewing's sarcoma and PNET share the same characteristic chromosome translocation, t(11;22), though variant translocations have been described.

DIAGNOSIS
Plain radiographs may reveal 'moth-eaten' bone with periosteal elevation (**12.37**). MRI scans define the extent of soft tissue involvement (**12.38**). Metastatic disease should be sought in the lungs (CT chest, **12.39**), bones (bone scan) and bone marrow (aspirate). Samples of the tumour should be analyzed histopathologically (characteristically MIC2 is positive on immuno-histochemistry) and in the case of diagnostic doubt the presence of the t(11;22) translocation in tumour material can be helpful.

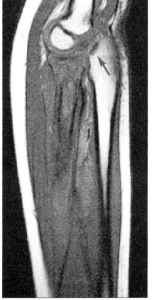

12.38 MRI showing expansion of the bone with destruction of the cortex, but without joint involvement.

TREATMENT
Chemotherapy with alkylating agents and anthracyclines reduces disease bulk and treats micrometastatic disease. Good local control with surgery or radiotherapy is essential but difficult to achieve in pelvic sites.

PROGNOSIS
The size of the mass (>100 cm^3) and the presence of metastatic disease are both poor prognostic factors. With aggressive therapy, around 65% of patients can be cured.

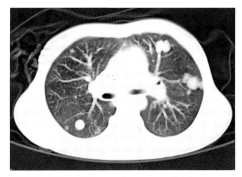

12.39 Chest CT scan showing multiple metastasis.

OSTEOSARCOMA

INCIDENCE
Osteosarcoma occurs in both children and adults. There are age peaks in adolescence and in the elderly. Peak incidence in adolescent females is 11–14 years. Peak incidence in adolescent males is 15–18 years. Male: female ratio is 2:1.

AETIOLOGY
Genetic predisposition: Li-Fraumeni syndrome (TP53); retinoblastoma (chromosome 13).
Radiation exposure: Radium dial workers (historical).
Rapid bone growth: Paget's disease of bone; adolescence.

PRESENTATION
Bone pain. Swelling.

SITES
In order of frequency:
- Distal femur.
- Proximal tibia.
- Proximal humerus.
Axial tumours constitute 10%.

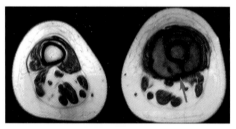

12.40 T$_1$-weighted axial MRI of the distal femora, showing swelling of the left thigh caused by a tumour of the femur, which both involves the intramedullary region and extends into the soft tissues around the cortex.

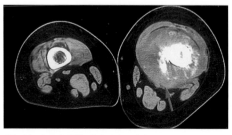

12.41 Axial CT of the distal femora, showing partly calcified extension of tumour into the soft tissues of the thigh around the left femur.

DIAGNOSIS
Plain radiographs classically show a partly lytic, partly sclerotic lesion affecting the metaphysis of a long bone, eroding the cortex, elevating the periosteum to cause a Codman's triangle, with 'sunburst' calcification extending into soft tissues.
Magnetic resonance imaging of the primary site will show the extent of intramedullary tumour, and spread into surrounding soft tissues including neurovascular bundles (**12.40, 12.41**).
Computed tomography of the primary site may show calcification in extraosseous tumour. CT of the lungs is mandatory to identify pulmonary metastases in 10–15% at presentation (**12.42**).
Skeletal scintigraphy will show the primary tumour and any bone metastases. Pulmonary or other soft tissue metastases may also be demonstrated.
Histologically, there is usually osteoid with osteoblastic, chondroblastic and fibroblastic areas. Intracytoplasmic alkaline phosphatase can be demonstrated in the malignant cells.

TREATMENT
Surgery has improved dramatically in recent years. Amputation is now only rarely necessary as the initial surgical procedure in limb osteosarcoma. In most cases, limb conserving surgery, usually with a customized endoprosthesis (**12.43**), is undertaken to replace part of the affected bone, and sometimes the neighbouring joint. For growing children, expandable endoprostheses can be used. Occasionally, a bone allograft is used. In some parts of the world, amputation of the knee region, with re-union

---

Table 12.7 Classification of osteosarcoma

1 High grade central osteosarcoma
    Osteoblastic
    Chondroblastic
    Fibroblastic
    Osteoclast-rich
    Telangiectatic
    Small cell
2 Periosteal osteosarcoma
3 Parosteal osteosarcoma
4 Low-grade central osteosarcoma
5 Osteoblastoma-like osteosarcoma
6 Paget's osteosarcoma
7 Post-irradiation osteosarcoma

of the rotated distal limb is undertaken. Occasionally, thoracotomy and resection of pulmonary metastases is undertaken.

Chemotherapy has improved the prognosis of operable osteosarcoma from approximately 20% to about 60%. It is usually given both prior to and after definitive surgery. The standard chemotherapy regimen includes doxorubicin, cisplatin and methotrexate. Chemotherapy is also used for inoperable and metastatic osteosarcoma, but survival rates are poor.

Radiotherapy has a very limited role in osteosarcoma, but it may be a useful means of achieving local control of inoperable tumours.

EXTRACRANIAL MALIGNANT GERM CELL TUMOURS

INCIDENCE
Malignant germ cell tumours, derived from primordial germ cells, occur in gonadal and extragonadal sites and affect 4 children per million of the population per annum, with a childhood female to male ratio of around 3:1.

CLINICAL PRESENTATION
Sites affected include sacrococcygeal (**12.44**), gonadal, mediastinal, vagina and uterus and abdominal. Malignant tumours may develop in patients who have had previously 'benign' tumours resected.

DIAGNOSIS
The measurement of tumour markers α-FP and β-HCG helps in diagnosis and follow-up. Teratomas and germinomas secrete neither α-FP nor β-HCG. Yolk-sac tumours and endodermal sinus tumours secrete α-FP, choriocarcinomas secrete β-HCG, and embryonal carcinomas secrete both markers. Individual tumours may have a mixture of histopathological types within them. Accurate imaging of the primary site and evaluation for metastatic disease with a CT scan of the chest and a bone scan are important.

TREATMENT / PROGNOSIS
Initial surgery should not be 'mutilating' as chemotherapy results in rapid shrinkage of disease. Chemotherapy with platinum compounds, bleomycin and etoposide has vastly improved the prognosis for children.

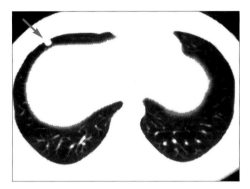

12.42 Thoracic CT scan showing small solitary pulmonary metastasis at the right lung base anteriorly.

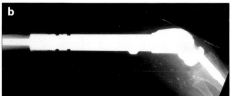

12.43 Anteroposterior (**a**) and lateral (**b**) radiographs after resection of the distal femur with endoprosthetic replacement.

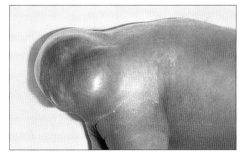

12.44 Sacrococcygeal teratoma in an infant.

TUMOURS OF THE CENTRAL NERVOUS SYSTEM

Primary malignancies of the central nervous system account for 25% of all cancers in childhood. Although there are over 120 distinct histological sub-types, the commonest tumours are low-grade gliomas, primitive neuro-ectodermal tumours, ependymomas, high-grade gliomas and intracranial germ cell tumours. The clinical behaviour of these tumours differs from that of their adult counterparts.

EPENDYMOMA
Incidence
Ependymomas comprise 10% of all CNS tumours of childhood; Seventy percent arise in the posterior fossa and 30% supratentorially. The mean age at diagnosis is 5 years but the peak age of incidence is 2 years. Ependymomas account for 25% of primary spinal cord tumours but present later.

Presentation
Posterior fossa tumours present with raised intracranial pressure and ataxia. Cranial nerve palsies and vomiting are more common than in medulloblastoma due to adherence of the tumour to the floor of the fourth ventricle. Patients with supratentorial tumours present with seizures, focal neurological deficits or raised intracranial pressure.

Diagnosis
MRI or CT scanning will reveal the primary tumour (**12.45**). Metastases within the CNS can occur but are infrequent at diagnosis (10%). The prognostic value of histological grading is unclear.

Treatment/prognosis
Complete surgical resection is prognostically important but sometimes difficult to achieve due to adherence of tumour to vital structures. Involved field radiotherapy, rather than cranio-spinal radiation, is recommended, as the vast majority of relapses are at the site of the primary tumour. Second-look surgery should always be considered for residual disease. Chemotherapy is used in children under 3 and its role in older children is being investigated. Current 5-year survival is 45%.

MEDULLOBLASTOMA / PNET
Incidence
Medulloblastoma arises in the cerebellar vermis but, as other histopathologically similar tumours arise elsewhere in the brain, the term primitive neuroectodermal tumour (PNET) has been used for the whole group irrespective of the site of origin (see also 'Neurology' chapter). Classical cerebellar medulloblastoma affects 6.6 children per million per year with a median age at diagnosis of 5 years.

Presentation
Cerebellar tumours present with ataxia and signs of raised intracranial pressure. Patients with tumours in the pineal region may have Parinaud syndrome (failure of upward gaze, dilated pupils that react to convergence but not light, nystagmus and lid retraction).

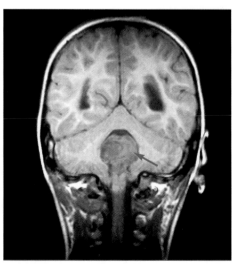

12.46 MRI scan of posterior fossa mass which proved to be medulloblastoma.

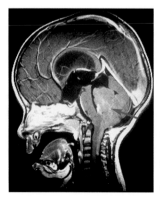

12.45 T$_1$-weighted MRI scan showing a mass in posterior fossa.

Diagnosis

MRI or CT scanning will reveal the presence of the tumour (**12.46**). Spinal imaging (with MRI) is mandatory to exclude spinal metastases (**12.47**) and CSF should be checked for the presence of malignant cells. Abnormalities of chromosome 17 may predict a bad outcome.

Treatment/prognosis

Complete surgical resection correlates with improved survival, and surgery combined with radiotherapy to the craniospinal axis is curative in around 60–70% of children. The role of chemotherapy in patients with metastatic disease has been established and is now also used in children without disease spread. For children younger than 3 years, chemotherapy is used to try to delay radiotherapy, thereby decreasing the neuropsychological and endocrine sequelae. Relapses are local or disseminated through the craniospinal axis.

HIGH-GRADE SUPRATENTORIAL GLIOMA

Incidence

Malignant supratentorial gliomas comprise around 10% of childhood brain tumours and have a bimodal incidence with a peak at around 2 years of age and another in early adolescence. Forty percent occur in the cerebral hemispheres and the remainder in the thalami, hypothalamic regions or basal ganglia.

Presentation

Over half the patients present with signs of raised intracranial pressure. Weakness, visual disturbances, cranial nerve palsies and hemiplegia are found in around 50% of cases.

Diagnosis

MRI or CT scanning (**12.48**). Spread within the neuraxis is uncommon. Patients with glioblastoma multiforme fare worse than those with anaplastic astrocytoma.

Treatment/prognosis

The completeness of surgical resection is of vital prognostic significance. Radiotherapy certainly delays regrowth but may not actually improve long-term survival, especially in children under 3. The use of chemotherapy is contentious, with only a small randomized study supporting its use. Prognosis for all high-grade tumours is 20% event-free 5-year survival.

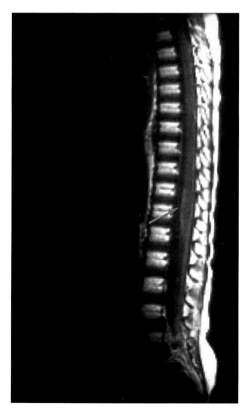

12.47 Saggital MRI scan of spine showing enhancing spinal deposits.

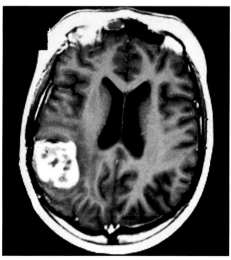

12.48 MRI scan showing huge high-grade astrocytoma, arising in the left parietal lobe.

BRAIN STEM GLIOMA

Incidence
Brain stem gliomas account for 10–20% of childhood CNS tumours, with a peak incidence at 5–8 years of age.

Presentation
May present with mood changes, cranial nerve dysfunction, hemiparesis, cerebellar signs, sensory disturbances, raised intracranial pressure.

Diagnosis
MRI scan. Biopsy not generally indicated as may cause neurological damage and does not change therapy or accurately predict prognosis.

Treatment/prognosis
Dorsally exophytic tumours or tumours of the cervico-medullary junction benefit from aggressive surgical management. Diffuse intrinsic pontine tumours (**12.49**) are not amenable to surgery. Radiotherapy is useful in controlling symptoms and extends survival. Chemotherapy has currently not been shown to be of benefit. Prognosis is poor with a median survival of 9–13 months in patients with diffuse instrinsic pontine tumours. The prognosis for localized tumours is better.

LOW-GRADE ASTROCYTOMA

Incidence
Cerebellar astrocytoma accounts for 10–20% of all childhood CNS tumours and has a peak incidence in the first decade of life. Low grade gliomas of the optic pathways comprise about 5% of CNS tumours, but patients with neurofibromatosis type I are predisposed to developing these tumours.

Presentation
Cerebellar astrocytomas present with raised intracranial pressure and ataxia. Optic pathway tumours (**12.50**) lead to squint, proptosis or visual loss. Hypothalamic involvement can produce growth disturbance, diabetes insipidus and changes in mood.

Diagnosis
MRI or CT scan (**12.51**), no routine spinal imaging. Ophthalmological assessment mandatory in optic pathway tumours.

Treatment
Over 90% of children with cerebellar astrocytoma are cured by surgery alone. Surgery has a role in unilateral optic nerve tumours with total visual loss, but the majority of optic pathway tumours can be managed with chemotherapy or radiotherapy treatment being instituted for tumour growth or an increase in symptoms.

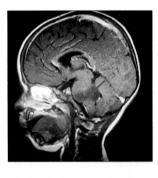

12.49 MRI scan showing diffuse intrinsic pontine glioma.

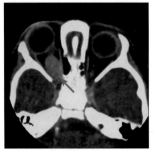

12.50 MRI scan showing optic nerve tumour in a child with neurofibromatosis type I.

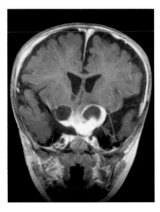

12.51 Coronal MRI scan showing chiasmatic glioma with cyst formation.

Table 12.8 Conditions predisposing to carcinoma

Predisposing syndromes	Cancer	Molecular abnormality	
		Gene symbol	Chromosomal location
Li-Fraumeni syndrome	Adrenocortical	TP53	17p13
Beckwith-Wiedemann syndrome	carcinoma	WBS	11p15
Multiple endocrine neoplasia type 1		MEN1	11q13
Familial adenomatous polyposis	Colon carcinoma	APC	5q21
Juvenile polyposis coli			
Familial melanoma	Melanoma	MLM	9p21
Von Hippel-Lindau syndrome	Renal cell carcinoma	VHL	3p25

RARE TUMOURS AND RARE MANIFESTATIONS OF COMMON TUMOURS

Although more than 95% of childhood tumours are 'common' types of leukaemia or solid tumours, rare types also occur. These tumours may pose particular problems for clinicians because there is often no standard approach to their treatment. The formation of a rare tumour group within the United Kingdom Children's Cancer study group may ease this problem. Once the diagnosis is confirmed, however, a careful family history is mandatory, as rare tumours often provide clues to a underlying genetic predisposition (**Table 12.8**).

Table 12.9 Sites of five most common carcinomas in children, in order of frequency

- Thyroid
- Nasopharyngeal
- Adrenocortical
- Salivary gland
- Hepatocellular

CARCINOMAS

Carcinomas are cancers that arise from the epithelium.

INCIDENCE

Only 2–3% of childhood cancers are carcinomas, compared with 85–90% of all cancers in adults. Therefore, in one year, only 20–40 children with carcinomas will be diagnosed in the entire UK. The sites of carcinomas in children differ from those in adults (**Table 12.9**).

AETIOLOGY

The cause of most carcinomas in childhood is unknown, but there are notable exceptions. Carcinomas may arise as 'second primaries' in those previously treated for cancer. Viruses seem to be critical in the pathogenesis of certain tumours, notably Epstein-Barr virus (EBV) in nasopharyngeal carcinoma, and hepatitis B virus in hepatocellular carcinoma. In others, carcinoma may reflect genetic predisposition (**Table 12.8**). The molecular basis of some of these genetic associations is now being unravelled; in the case of the Li-Fraumeni syndrome, the inheritance of a defective TP53 gene (whose product acts as a checkpoint control in cell cycle progression) has been identified in numerous families.

TREATMENT / PROGNOSIS

Due to their rarity in children, carcinomas are usually treated on protocols designed for adults. However, carcinomas in children are often more responsive to treatment than carcinomas of similar histology in adults.

THYROID CARCINOMA

Only 5–7% of all thyroid cancers occur in children, more frequently in girls than boys, with a peak incidence in adolescence. Exposure to ionising radiation is a known risk factor

Papillary carcinoma accounts for 80–90% of thyroid cancer with follicular, medullary and anaplastic occurring less commonly in sequential order.

Presentation

A painless thyroid nodule and enlargement of a lateral cervical lymph nodes is the commonest presenting complaint (**12.52**). A solitary thyroid nodule in a child should always be investigated, as up to 50% may be malignant. Metastatic disease, usually to the lungs, is uncommon.

Diagnosis

The avid uptake of radioactive ^{123}I or ^{131}I by thyroid tumours makes radionucleotide scanning the investigation of choice. Chest x-rays (PA + lateral) are also indicated. Serum calcitonin is a useful 'marker' in the management of medullary carcinoma and thyroglobulin in differentiated thyroid carcinoma.

Treatment/prognosis

Papillary thyroid carcinomas run a more indolent course in children than adults and concerns over late effects of treatment influence management decisions. Intra-thyroidal disease can usually be safely resected leaving sufficient residual thyroid tissue for normal function. In more extensive disease the choice is between radical surgery and radioiodine, balancing the risks of damage to the recurrent laryngeal nerve against concern over the potential oncogenicity of ^{131}I in later life. Medullary and anaplastic carcinoma are usually treated by radical resection. Lifelong surveillance is advised.

NASOPHARYNGEAL CARCINOMA (NPC)

Incidence

Nasopharyngeal carcinoma arises from the epithelial lining of the nasopharynx and is therefore a squamous cell carcinoma. It represents around 1% of all malignant disease in children. Boys are more commonly affected than girls.

Presentation

Presentation is usually with either lymphadenopathy, signs of nasopharyngeal obstruction or both. Nasal bleeding or discharge, deafness, tinnitus or trismus may be found. Direct extension of the primary tumour into the cavernous sinus may cause multiple cranial nerve palsies. Lymph node spread is very common but metastases to other sites (bone marrow, bone, lung and CSF) occur in only 5–10% of patients. The TNM system is used for staging disease.

Treatment/prognosis

Chemotherapy is effective in inducing remission, but radiotherapy is usually used to consolidate treatment. Thyroid irradiation leads to hypothyroidism in over 50% of children, and all children are at risk of subsequent thyroid tumours. Growth hormone deficiency is common because the pituitary gland is often within the radiotherapy field.

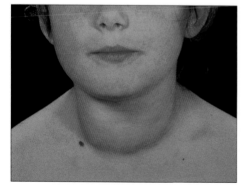

12.52 A discrete, painless thyroid nodule in a young girl.

ADRENOCORTICAL CARCINOMA (ACC)

Incidence
ACC is rare (only around 0.2% of childhood malignancies) and occurs more commonly in girls than boys.

Presentation
This is usually with signs of virilization or Cushingoid features (**12.53**). There is an increased incidence of ACC in patients with isolated hemihypertrophy and the Beckwith-Wiedemann syndrome and it may be the first manifestation of the Li-Fraumeni syndrome within a family.

Diagnosis
There is no reliable histopathological distinction between adrenal adenomas and carcinomas so diagnosis is difficult.

Treatment/prognosis
Tumour size is the best available predictor of biological behaviour, and tumours greater than 200 cm^3 are associated with a worse prognosis. Other adverse prognostic factors include older age at presentation, increased urinary steroid levels and delay in diagnosis. Complete surgical resection, especially of small tumours, may be curative. In patients with incomplete resection or metastatic spread, treatment options include chemotherapy (cisplatin/carboplatin, etoposide, vincristine and cyclophosphamide). Control of endocrine systems (with possibly some cytotoxicity) may be achieved by the use of mitotane.

SALIVARY GLAND TUMOURS

Incidence
Two to four percent of all salivary gland tumours occur in patients under 16 years of age. In children, tumours occur more commonly in the parotid gland (e.g. haemangioma, lymphangioma and pleomorphic adenoma) than in the sub-mandibular glands or orolingual salivary tissues and are usually benign. Mucoepidermoid carcinoma, the most common salivary gland carcinoma, usually presents as a painless mass in children aged 5–15 (**12.54**). The incidence in boys and girls is about equal.

Diagnosis
The pathological distinction between high-grade and low-grade tumours is not always helpful in predicting recurrence, although distant metastases are commonly found in children with high-grade tumours.

Treatment/prognosis
Wide surgical excision is recommended, as local recurrence rate is high after more conservative operations; 'shelling out' procedures are contra-indicated. Most children are cured by surgery alone. These tumours are not particularly radiosensitive, but postoperative RT decreases the local relapse rate in 'high risk' patients. Chemotherapy is sometimes effective. Treatment of the very rare actinic cell and adenoid cystic carcinomas is the same as for this carcinoma.

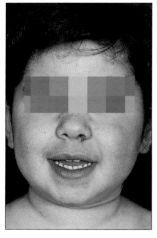

12.53 Virilization in a 5-year-old girl due to a functioning adrenal tumour.

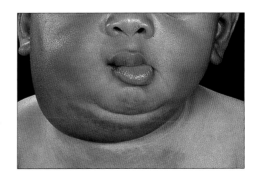

12.54 Salivary gland tumour.

RENAL-CELL CARCINOMA (RCC)
Incidence
Also known as Grawitz tumour or hyper-nephroma, this tumour is occasionally reported in children, particularly older children and adolescents. RCC arise from the proximal tubular cells and are, therefore, ultimately derived from metanephric blastema. The incidence of this tumour is estimated at between 0.3 and 3 % of all renal tumours in children.

Presentation
Clinical presentation is usually with an abdominal mass and often with haematuria. Metastasis is to liver, lungs, bone and abdominal lymph nodes. RCC is associated with Von-Hippel-Lindau (VHL) syndrome (hereditary angiomatosis of the retina and cerebellum).

Inheritance
The VHL gene is a tumour suppressor gene and is located on the short arm of chromosome 2. Familial renal cell carcinoma may be assoc-iated with a constitutional translocation involv-ing chromosome 3p t(3;8) (p14;q24).

Treatment/prognosis
Radical nephrectomy is the treatment of choice and, since prognosis is stage-related, may be sufficient in well-encapsulated tumours. Chemo-therapy and radiotherapy are used, without consistent success, for unresectable tumours. Immunotherapy is of interest for patients with metastatic disease.

SKIN CANCERS

INCIDENCE
Melanoma is the commonest skin cancer in children, but basal cell and squamous cell carci-nomas may occur.

AETIOLOGY
Exposure to ultraviolet light provides the most important stimulus for skin cancers, followed by ionizing radiation and immunodeficiency/immunosuppression. Hereditary cutaneous melanoma is well recognized (see **Table 12.8**) as is the link between melanoma and the dysplastic naevus syndrome.

TREATMENT / PROGNOSIS
Metastatic spread is via satellite lesions to regional lymph nodes before widespread dis-semination. Surgery is usually sufficient for small basal cell and squamous cell carcinomas, though radiotherapy may be required. Treatment of melanomas is more complex, due to the propen-sity for these tumours to metastasize. Staging depends on the depth of invasion of the tumour and the involvement and size of local lymph nodes. Melanomas are sometimes responsive to multiagent chemotherapy, cyclophosphamide, actinomycin-D and vincristine, DTIC and cisplatin. Because melanomas are 'immuno-genic', interleukin 2 and vaccine therapy also have a role.

Table 12.10 Very rare carcinomas in children

Cancer	Comments
Gastric	Patients with immune deficiency are at increased risk.
Colorectal	Less than 1% of cases occur in patients under 30 years of age. Prognosis may be worse in children than in adults. Predisposing factors include APC and juvenile polyposis coli.
Bladder	Usually transitional cell carcinoma. May occur years after treatment with cyclophosphamide/iphosphamide.
Laryngeal	Usually squamous cell. Present with hoarseness and upper airways obstruction. Manage on adult protocols.
Ovarian	Extremely rare before menarche. Critical distinction from germ cell tumour.
Vaginal	Clear cell adenocarcinoma linked to maternal stilboestrol ingestion. Now very rare.
Pancreatic	As in adults, the prognosis is poor for adenocarcinomas.
Breast	Female breast development may be asynchronous and mimic a breast lump. Breast lumps in childhood should always be investigated, especially in boys.
Lung	Bronchogenic carcinoma has been reported, mostly in adolescents. Treat on adult protocols.
Oesophageal	Usually squamous cell carcinomas. More common in boys. Present with dysphagia, regurgitation, vomiting, weight loss. Multimodal therapy is indicated.
Sweat gland	Extremely rare. Histologically usually a clear cell acrospiroma. Wide surgical excision is the treatment of choice.

LATE EFFECTS OF CANCER TREATMENT

Present-day multimodality cancer treatment has improved overall survival in children, so that more than 70% can expect to live to adulthood. Unfortunately, the cytotoxic effects of surgery, chemotherapy and radiotherapy are not specific to tumour cells and therefore damage to normal tissue can occur. The functional damage can remain static, progress or improve over time, depending upon the organ characteristics (cell turnover, treatment sensitivity), age and development of the patient, gender and the synergistic effects of the treatments. Furthermore, psychological problems can occur in both patients and their families following the effects of cancer and its treatment.

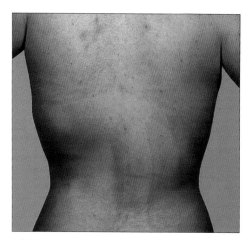

12.55 Right flank hypoplasia after radiation for treatment of Stage III Wilms' tumour.

Two frequently discussed issues are 'fertility' and 'second tumours'. Fertility is impaired after gonadal radiation, often permanently and also after certain forms of chemotherapy, especially procarbazine, alkylating agents and nitrosureas, particularly in boys. Pre-treatment storage is offered to boys capable of producing a semen specimen. Second tumours – solid tumours in radiation fields and leukaemia after etoposide, doxorubicin and alkylating agents – occur in a small number of patients, diminishing as oncogenic drugs are substituted by alternative agents via clinical trials.

SURGERY

Definitive surgical treatment usually occurs after chemotherapy, and involves the removal of the tumour with wide excision margins which may also include the organ of origin. This can cause functional impairment and, if extensive surgery is required, may affect the patient's body image perception, particularly during adolescence. Morbidity from surgery is becoming less severe as improved chemotherapy regimes result in shrinkage of tumour, allowing conservative surgery.

RADIOTHERAPY

Conventionally-planned radiotherapy will include a margin of normal tissue. Hypoplasia of the surrounding musculoskeletal tissue will occur, the degree being dependent on the growth potential of the child; the younger the child, the worse the effect. Other manifestations of radiation will depend on the organs within the radiation field, the type of radiation, dose and fractionation. (**12.55**)

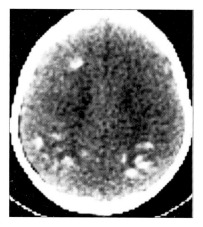

12.56 Head CT scan showing calcification after intramuscular methotrexate.

CHEMOTHERAPY

The different chemotherapy agents have various modes of action and their own spectrum of toxicities. Risk factors include cumulative dose, dose intensity and method of administration. (**12.56**)

Long-term follow-up is an important part of the total care of cancer patients. Surveillance identifies late effects that require treatment, provides psychosocial support and information to survivors of possible late effects. Research is vital to identify toxicities, study risk factors and so influence future protocols.

REFERENCES

Pinkerton CR, Michalski AJ, Veys PA (eds). *Clinical challenges in paediatric oncology.* Oxford: Isis Medical Media Ltd, 1999.

Renal tumours
Pritchard Jones K. Controversies and advances in the management of Wilms' tumour. *Arch Dis Child* 2002; 87: 241–242.

Liver tumours
Pritchard J, Brown J, Shafford E et al. Cisplatin, doxorubin, and delayed surgery for childhood hepatoblastoma: a successful approach – results of the first prospective study of the International Society of Pediatric Oncology. *J Clin Oncol* 2000; 18(22): 3819–3828.

Soft Tissue sarcoma
Stevens MC. Treatment of childhood rhabdomyosarcoma: the cost of cure. *Lancet Oncol* 2005; 2: 77–84.

Neuroblastoma (standard risk)
Woods WG, Lemieux B, Tuchman M. Neuroblastoma represents distinct clinical-biologic entities: a review and perspective from the Quebec neuroblastoma screening project. *Pediatrics* 1992; 89: 114–118.

Silber JH, Evans AF, Friedman M. Models to predict outcome from childhood neuroblastoma: the role of serum ferritin and tumor histology. *Cancer Res* 1991; 51: 142–1433.

Neuroblastoma (high risk)
Brodeur GM, Pritchard J, Berthold F et al. Revisions of the International Criteria for Neuroblastoma diagnosis, staging and response to treatment. *J Clin Oncol* 1993; 11: 1466–1477.

Pinkerton CR. Where next with therapy in advanced neuroblastoma? *Br J Cancer* 1990; 61: 351–353.

Ewing's sarcoma and peripheral primitive neuroectodermal tumour (PNET)
Jurgens H, Exner U, Gadner H et al. Multidisciplinary treatment of Ewing's sarcoma of bone. A six year experience of a European Cooperative Trial. *Cancer* 1988; 61: 23–32.

Marina NM, Etcubanas E, Parham DM et al. Peripheral primitive neuroectodermal tumour (peripheral neuroepithelioma) in children. *Cancer* 1989; 64: 1952–1960.

Osteosarcoma
Souhami RL, Craft AW, Van Der Eijken JW et al. Randomised trial of two regimens of chemotherapy in operable osteosarcoma: a study of the European Osteosarcoma Intergroup. *Lancet* 1997; 350: 911–917.

Extracranial malignant germ cell tumours
Kramarova E, Mann JR, Magnani C, Corraziari I, Berrino F. Eurocare Working Group. Survival of children with malignant germ cell, trophoblastic and other gonadal tumours in Europe. *Eur J Cancer* 2001; 37(6): 750–759.

Ependymoma
Bouffet E, Perilongo G, Canete A, Massimino M. Intracranial ependymomas in children: a critical review of prognostic factors and a plea fro cooperation. *Med Ped Oncology* 1998; 30(6): 319–329.

Goldwein JW, Leahy J, Packer RJ et al. Intracranial ependymomas in children. *Int J Radiat Oncol Biol Phys* 1990; 19: 1497–1502.

Medulloblastoma/PNET
Gajjar A, Kühl J, Epelman S, Bailey C, Allen J. Chemotherapy of medulloblastoma. *Child's Nerv Syst* 1999; 15: 554–562.

High grade supratentorial glioma
Finlay JL, Wisoff JH. The impact of extent of resection in the management of malignant gliomas of childhood. *Child's Nerv Syst* 1999; 15: 786–788.

Brain stem glioma
Packer RJ, Nicholson HS, Johnson DL, Vezina LG. Dilemmas in the management of childhood brain tumours: Brainstem Gliomas. *Ped Neurosurg* 1991; 17: 37–43.

Low-grade astrocytoma
Janss AJ, Grundy R, Cnaan A et al. Optic pathway and hypothalamic/chiasmatic gliomas in children younger than age 5 years with a 6-year follow-up. *Cancer* 1995; 75: 1051–1059.

Late effects of cancer treatment
Green D and Wallace H (eds). *Late effects of childhood cancer.* London: Arnold, 2004.

Skinner R, Levitt G, Wallace WHB. Therapy based long term follow up: Practice Statement. UKCCSG 2005. www.UKCCSG.org

Endocrinology

Mehul Dattani • David Grant*
Harry Baumer • Katie Mallam
Charles Brook

*Dr David Grant sadly died before the publication of this chapter

AMBIGUOUS GENITALIA

See also 'Urology' chapter.

INCIDENCE / GENETICS

Congenital adrenal hyperplasia and 5α-reductase deficiency (**13.1, 13.2**) are inherited as auto-somal recessive disorders. Mutations of the genes encoding 5α-reductase, 21-hydroxylase, steroidogenic factor (SF), Wilms' tumour (WT) and the androgen receptor have been described. The incidence of CAH is 1 in 15,000, while 5α-reductase deficiency and androgen insensitivity are much rarer (**Table 13.1**).

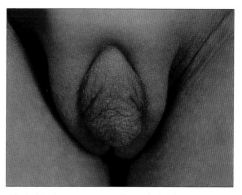

13.1 Virilization in newborn baby (karyotype 46XX) due to 21-hydroxylase deficiency.

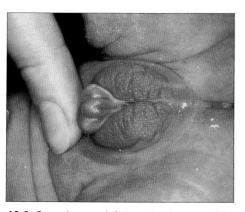

13.2 5α-reductase deficiency in nine-year-old boy.

Table 13.1 Aetiology of ambiguous genitalia

Inadequate masculinization
Leydig cell hypoplasia
Inborn errors of testosterone biosynthesis in adrenals, testes or both
5a-reductase deficiency (**13.2**)
Defect in target tissues, e.g. androgen insensitivity
Associated with dysmorphic syndromes – e.g. Smith-Lemli-Opitz, Dubowitz, Aniridia-Wilms, etc.

Virilized female
Virilization by androgens of fetal origin – e.g. congenital adrenal hyperplasia (**13.1**)
Virilization by androgens of maternal origin – e.g. anabolic steroids, danazol, virilizing maternal tumour
Dysmorphic syndromes – e.g. Seckel, Zellweger
Presence of testicular tissue – e.g. ovotestis

DIAGNOSIS

Usually present at birth. Presence of bilaterally palpable gonads suggest an inadequately virilized male; a unilateral palpable gonad may suggest a diagnosis of XO/XY mosaicism or a hermaphrodite. May be associated with salt loss (salt-losing congenital adrenal hyperplasia – see page 392). There may be associated dysmorphic features.

INVESTIGATIONS

Pelvic ultrasound scan, karyotype, plasma electrolytes, serum 17-hydroxy progesterone, urinary steroid profile, plasma ACTH, testosterone, dihydro-testosterone, adrenal androgens, LH, FSH, plasma renin activity, aldosterone, HCG test and DNA analysis. Urethrography may delineate the anatomy more clearly.

TREATMENT

Gender assignment: aim to achieve unambiguous and functionally normal external genitalia through surgery and appropriate hormonal therapy. The decision is usually based upon the anatomy of the internal and external genitalia, and future potential for fertility is a much less important consideration. Medical treatment (e.g. hormone replacement in congenital adrenal hyperplasia, androgens for micropenis treatment). Surgery (e.g. clitoral reduction, vaginoplasty, hypospadias repair, correction of chordee). Gonadectomy: patients with dysgenetic or non-functional gonads, especially those with Y-bearing cell lines, have an increased risk of malignant change in the gonad. Psychological support is essential.

PROGNOSIS

Dependent on underlying condition and appropriateness of gender assignment.

THE SHORT CHILD

This is the commonest reason for referral of a child to an endocrinologist, and the algorithm (on opposite page) gives an approach to the management of this condition. See following pages for a description of some of these conditions in more detail.

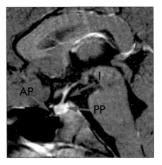

13.3a MR scan showing a normal anterior pituitary (AP) with the posterior pituitary (PP) located normally in the sella turcica. Note the infundibulum (I) connecting the pituitary to the hypothalamus.

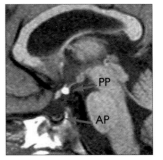

13.3b MR scan of a child with congenital growth hormone deficiency (GHD) showing severe hypoplasia of the anterior pituitary (AP) with an undescended posterior pituitary (PP) at the level of the tuber cinereum. Note the absence of the infundibulum. This appearance reflects a developmental abnormality and is commonly observed in patients with isolated GHD and combined pituitary hormone deficiency.

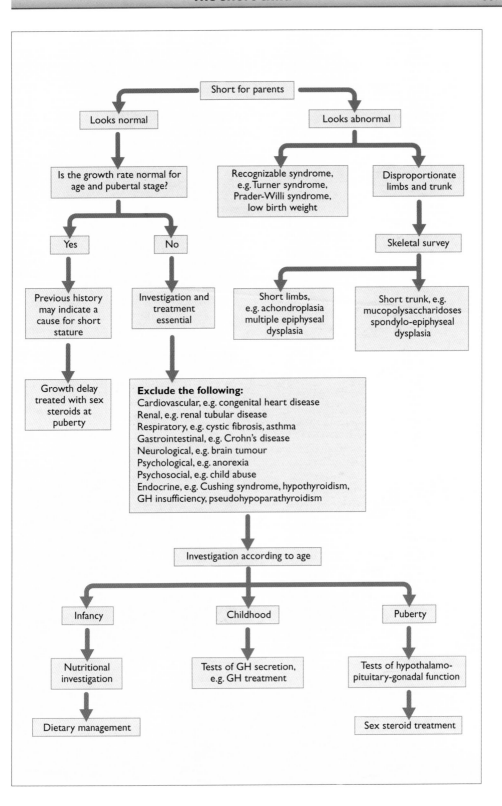

TURNER SYNDROME

See also 'Genetics' chapter.

INCIDENCE / GENETICS

This is the commonest abnormality of the sex chromosomes, affecting an estimated 3% of all females conceived. However, the incidence is 1 in 1,500–2,500 live female births. Approximately 50% of cases have a 45XO karyotype, 50% demonstrating mosaicism with one 45XO cell line and another cell line often containing an abnormal X chromosome (or Y chromosome). If more than one tissue is studied, the incidence of mosaicism rises to 70% for two tissues and 90% for three tissues.

PATHOGENESIS / AETIOLOGY

Loss of one of the sex chromosomes after formation of the zygote. In 70–80% of cases, the retained X chromosome is maternal. More than 50% of all patients with Turner syndrome have a mosaic chromosomal complement.

DIAGNOSIS

May present in the neonatal period with lymphoedema of the hands and feet (**13.4**) or co-arctation of the aorta. Birth weight may be low (~1 Standard Deviation Score [SDS] below the mean). The short stature of females with Turner syndrome is a combination of several factors:

- Turner girls often have feeding difficulties in the first year of life, with loss of growth in the critical nutrition phase of growth.
- They grow at a 25th centile height velocity during childhood, which leads to a further gradual loss of stature.
- They have a skeletal dysplasia, with a coarse trabecular pattern in the long bones and tall vertebrae and, similar to skeletal dysplasias, growth during the pubertal years is extremely poor.

Ovarian failure with streak gonads is observed in the vast majority of patients. Other clinical features include widely-spaced nipples, anomalous auricles, epicanthic folds, micrognathia, low posterior hairline, webbed neck, cubitus valgus, osteoporosis, narrow hyperconvex nails (**13.5**), excessive pigmented naevi, renal anomalies, idiopathic hypertension, aortic stenosis, recurrent middle ear infections, sensorineural deafness, specific learning abnormalities, diabetes mellitus, autoimmune hypothyroidism and Crohn's disease. Essential investigations are karyotype, echocardiogram, renal and pelvic ultrasound scans and thyroid function.

TREATMENT

Appropriate treatment of cardiac abnormalities, if present. Monitor blood pressure. Growth promotion may be achieved with the use of low-dose anabolic steroids (oxandrolone), growth hormone and oestrogen, although the timing of these interventions remains a source of much debate. Pubertal induction with ethinyloestradiol and the later addition of progestogens is required in the majority of cases at the appropriate age. Twenty percent of girls with Turner syndrome have a spontaneous onset of puberty but very few go on to achieve menarche (5–10%) and fertility (1%). Complications such as hypothyroidism are treated as they arise. If a Y chromosomal cell line has been demonstrated, the dysgenetic gonads should be removed because of the possibility of malignant change.

PROGNOSIS

The prognosis for final height is determined to a large extent by the parental heights. In the Western world, the mean final height of women with Turner syndrome is in the region of 143–146 cm, which is approximately 20 cm less than the average final height for normal adult females. The use of *in vitro* fertilization and embryo implantation techniques have improved the prospects for childbearing.

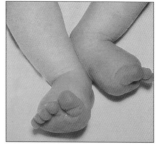

13.4 Turner syndrome. Lymphoedema of feet in a child.

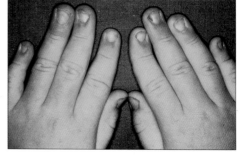

13.5 Turner syndrome. Dysplastic nails (child).

LOW BIRTH WEIGHT SYNDROME

INCIDENCE
Common. The inheritance pattern is dependent on the underlying cause (see below). The majority are sporadic. Children with familial Russell-Silver syndrome have been described.

PATHOGENESIS / AETIOLOGY
Chromosomal disorders, recognized environmental insult *in utero* (e.g. rubella, cytomegalovirus, alcohol, maternal smoking, anticonvulsants, placental dysfunction). The aetiology of Russell-Silver syndrome remains unknown, although genetic factors may play a role.

DIAGNOSIS
May present with hypoglycaemia in the neonatal period. The majority have short stature and are usually very slim. Feeding problems in the first year of life are very common in this group of children. Birth weight which is inappropriately low for gestation and in relation to the birth weights of other siblings. The Russell-Silver syndrome shares many of these features. Additionally, clinical features include asymmetry of the face (**13.6**) and limbs (**13.7**), clinodactyly (**13.8**), a small triangular facies, café-au-lait spots, excessive sweating. If hypoglycaemia is proven, investigations should be performed to exclude other pathology (e.g. hyperinsulinism, β-oxidation defect). If a reduced growth velocity is documented, investigations should be carried out to exclude coincident pathology (e.g. GH insufficiency). A karyotype may be indicated if a genetic syndrome is suspected.

TREATMENT
Growth hormone treatment has recently been approved for children who are born small for gestational age and fail to catch up. Additionally, treatment may be required for complications such as hypoglycaemia (frequent feeds)..

PROGNOSIS
The prognosis for height is highly variable, and a significant proportion (~40%) will have final heights that fall considerably short of their midparental target height. Growth hormone treatment has been demonstrated to improve height in the short term, but effects on final height remain unknown.

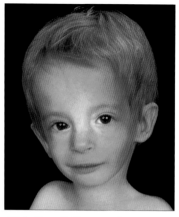

13.6 Russell-Silver syndrome in a child, showing facial asymmetry.

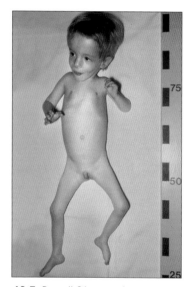

13.7 Russell-Silver syndrome. Full view of child in 13.6.

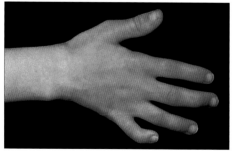

13.8 Russell-Silver syndrome in a child showing clinodactyly.

PRADER–WILLI SYNDROME

GENETICS

Chromosomal analysis reveals a deletion in the long arm of the paternally-derived chromosome 15 (deletion of 15q11-13) in approximately 50% of cases Recently, it has been demonstrated that Prader-Willi syndrome can be an example of uniparental disomy, whereby both sections of chromosome 15 are derived from the mother.

DIAGNOSIS

Usually presents in the neonatal period with hypotonia and feeding difficulties. Birth weight may be low or normal. Characteristic facial features include a narrow forehead, almond-shaped eyes, strabismus and micrognathia. Small hands and feet are a feature of the condition, with tapering fingers and clinodactyly. Scoliosis, congenital dislocation of the hips, neurodevelopmental delay and hypogonadism with a micropenis, hypoplastic scrotum and bilateral cryptorchidism are other features of the condition.

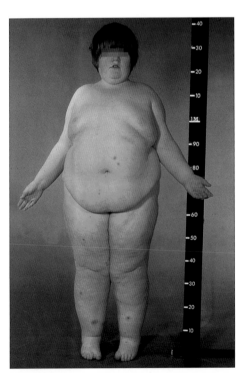

13.9 Prader-Willi syndrome. Gross obesity in a child. Note the small hands and feet.

Insatiable appetite from the age of one to two years leads to gross obesity (**13.9**) with the ensuing complications of genu valgum, cellulitis, intertrigo, and the Pickwickian syndrome. Endocrine features include poor secondary sexual development, delayed menarche and insulin-resistant diabetes mellitus. Short stature is a feature in a significant proportion of cases, with a poor pubertal growth spurt. Investigation often reveals a diagnosis of growth hormone deficiency/insufficiency.

Essential investigations: detailed genetic analysis of chromosome 15; exclusion of other causes of obesity and hypotonia; investigation of gonadal function (luteinizing hormone releasing hormone [LHRH] and human chorionic gonadotrophin [HCG] tests); investigation of hypothalamo-pituitary axis in children with a low growth velocity.

TREATMENT

The mainstay of treatment is severe dietary restriction. Energy requirements for growth are low, and these should be calculated and calorie intake appropriately restricted. Neurodevelopmental delay compounds the difficulties inherent in dietary restriction. In boys, bilateral orchidopexies may be required. Testosterone in the form of depot preparations has a role in the treatment of hypogonadism.

In girls, menarche may be delayed and oestrogen treatment may be required. Growth hormone treatment is indicated if dietary restriction is successful and the height velocity poor, with documented GH insufficiency on provocative testing. More recently, growth hormone treatment has been used in an attempt to improve the hypotonia associated with this condition.

PROGNOSIS

Poor. Attempts at dietary restriction are often doomed to failure, particularly in view of the neurodevelopmental delay which is a feature of the condition, with the consequence of gross obesity. Premature death due to bronchopneumonia or cardiorespiratory failure and Pickwickian syndrome with hypoventilation is usual. Additionally, the stress on the family is considerable.

SKELETAL DYSPLASIAS

Several of these exist but only the commoner forms are described here – namely, achondroplasia, hypochondroplasia, spondylo-epiphyseal dysplasia and multiple epiphyseal dysplasia.

INCIDENCE / GENETICS

- Achondroplasia. 1 in 10,000 to 15,000. Inherited as an autosomal dominant condition with a fresh mutation rate of 90%. Recent work has suggested that a mutation in the fibroblast growth factor receptor-3 (*FGFR3*) accounts for most cases.
- Hypochondroplasia. This condition is much more common than was previously thought. Inherited as an autosomal dominant trait with mutations in *FGFR3* being implicated.
- Spondylo-epiphyseal dysplasia/mutiple epiphyseal dysplasia. Rare. Inherited as autosomal dominant conditions.

DIAGNOSIS

Achondroplasia (**13.10**) presents in the neo-natal period with short-limbs and characteristic craniofacial features. These include a large head with marked frontal bossing, a low nasal bridge and mild mid-facial hypoplasia. Skeletal abnormalities include small cuboid vertebral bodies with short pedicles and progressive narrowing of lumbar interpedicular distance. Lumbar lordosis, mild thoraco-lumbar kyphosis, small iliac wings, short tubular bones and a short trident hand are other features of the condition. There is sometimes mild hypotonia with some early motor delay. Hydrocephalus secondary to a narrow foramen magnum is an associated feature. Spinal cord and/or root compression can occur as a consequence of kyphosis, spinal canal stenosis or disc lesions. Associated features include upper airways obstruction and recurrent otitis media. Pseudoachondroplasia resembles achondroplasia clinically.

Hypochondroplasia patients usually present with short stature in relation to mid-parental target height centile. The growth rate is initially normal, with a compromised pubertal growth spurt (**13.11**). Skeletal abnormalities

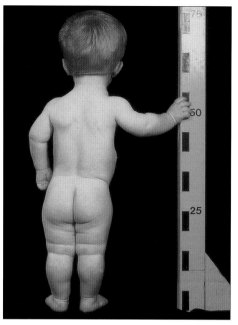

13.10 Achondroplasia. Typical childhood appearance.

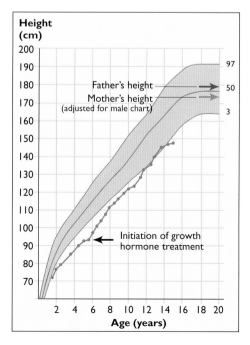

13.11 Growth chart of a boy with hypochondroplasia, who was treated with recombinant hGH from the age of 5.4 years (arrow). The final height is well below the target height.

are characteristic. Disproportion may only be apparent in puberty, although more severe cases may present earlier with disproportion (**13.1**). Family history often reveals disproportionate short stature in one or both parents.

Spondylo-epiphyseal dysplasia is characterized by prenatal onset growth deficiency, malar hypoplasia, cleft palate, short spine, lumbar lordosis, kyphoscoliosis, decreased arm span, weakness, talipes varus and developmental dysplasia of the hip.

Multiple epiphyseal dysplasia is characterized by short stature, with short metacarpals and phalanges, ovoid, flattened vertebral bodies, waddling gait, slow growth and early osteoarthritis. These features are by no means invariable.

Essential investigations include a skeletal survey, especially an antero-posterior view of the spine to show diagnostic radiological features. In hypochondroplasia, there is loss of the normal widening of the interpedicular distance proceeding down the lumbar spine. In achondroplasia, neuroradiological imaging may be indicated if hydrocephalus is suspected.

TREATMENT

Correction of hydrocephalus and orthopaedic abnormalities. The use of growth hormone (GH) to treat these conditions is the subject of clinical trials. Final height data are not as yet available, although the early response to GH in achondroplastic children is often encouraging. In hypochondroplasia, GH treatment may enhance the pubertal growth spurt, although the effects of recombinant human growth hormone (rhGH) are variable and uncertain. GH treatment is of little use in pseudo-achondroplasia, multiple epiphyseal dysplasia and spondylo-epiphyseal dysplasia. Limb lengthening may be an option in achondroplasia and severe cases of hypochondroplasia. The gain in height needs to be balanced against the time and discomfort involved in these procedures.

PROGNOSIS

Without intervention, the height prognosis can be poor in achondroplasia, and variable in hypochondroplasia. The effect of growth hormone treatment on final height is, as yet, unknown.

GROWTH HORMONE DEFICIENCY / INSUFFICIENCY

INCIDENCE / GENETICS

The incidence of GH deficiency/insufficiency (GHD/GHI) in its classical form is 1 in 3,000. Hereditary forms of GH deficiency arising as a result of, e.g. a GH gene deletion, are rare, accounting for 5–10% of cases. (**Table 13.2**).

DIAGNOSIS

GH deficiency may rarely present with neonatal hypoglycaemia. Later presentation is usually with short stature (**13.13**). The child classically looks chubby with a round immature face (**13.14**). Micropenis may be a feature (**13.15**). The birth weight is usually normal. However, the height velocity is slow from around the end of the first year of life. Breech delivery with obstetric trauma may be associated.

GH insufficiency may be associated with other pituitary hormone deficiencies as part of an evolving endocrinopathy. There may be evidence of associated disorders (e.g. midline cleft palate, optic nerve hypoplasia, agenesis of the corpus callosum, absence of the septum pellucidum and Fanconi's anaemia). The bone age is usually delayed, as is the dentition. Investigations should initially be performed to exclude non-endocrine pathology (e.g. renal and coeliac disease). The level of insulin-like growth factor (IGF-1) and its binding protein (IGF-BP3) may be low in GHD/GHI, but the sensitivities and specificities of these tests are poor. A skeletal age may be delayed.

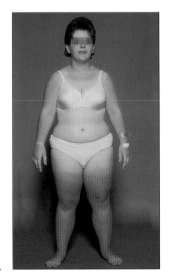

13.12 Hypochondroplasia. The clinical appearance shows obvious skeletal disproportion.

**Table 13.2 GH deficiency/insufficiency –
pathogenesis and aetiology**

Congenital
- Hereditary – gene deletion/mutation
- Idiopathic GHRH deficiency
- Developmental abnormalities –
  pituitary aplasia, hypoplasia, midline brain
  and facial defects, many of which are associated
  with mutations in transcription factors such as
  HESX1, LHX3, LHX4, PROP1 and PIT1.

Acquired
- Perinatal trauma
- Hypothalamic/pituitary tumours

Secondary to
- Cranial irradiation
- Head injury
- Infection
- Sarcoidosis
- Histiocytosis

Transient due to
- Low sex hormone concentration
- Psychosocial deprivation
- Hypothyroidism

If the diagnosis of GHD or GHI is suspected, pharmacological or physiological tests of GH secretion may be indicated. Although physiological tests of GH secretion may be of greater relevance, they entail sampling of blood for GH concentrations at 20 minute intervals over a 12–24 hour period and are therefore expensive and time-consuming. Pharmacological testing in the form of provocative tests of GH secretion (e.g. insulin-induced hypoglycaemia, glucagon provocation, arginine provocation, clonidine stimulation and growth hormone-releasing hormone) should only be performed in children in whom a low growth velocity has been documented. Of these biochemical tests, insulin-induced hypoglycaemia and glucagon provocation are the most widely used. The results are dependent on the assay in use, and so the test results for any one centre need to be carefully evaluated. It should be noted that these tests can be dangerous if performed by inexperienced operators in units which are not tertiary referral centres.

TREATMENT

Replacement with rhGH (15–20 units/m^2/week or 0.02–0.05 mg/kg/day). Restores normal growth velocity after a period of catch-up growth. The smallest, most slowly growing and most severely GH-insufficient children will respond best. GH is given as a daily subcutaneous dose and is associated with minimal side-effects in replacement doses.

PROGNOSIS

The prognosis for final height in GHD/GHI is excellent, provided that treatment is begun at an early stage. If treatment is commenced late, a loss of height will ensue.

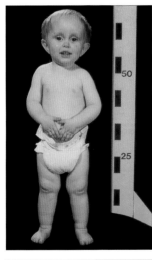

13.13
GHD. Child
presenting
with short
stature and
classic
appearances.

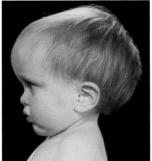

13.14
GHD. Typical
immature,
chubby facies
of a child.

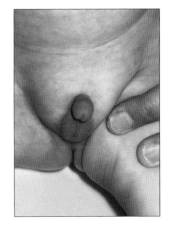

13.15 GHD.
Micropenis in
a child.

LARON-TYPE DWARFISM

INCIDENCE / GENETICS
Classic Laron-type dwarfism is extremely rare. It is commoner in consanguinous unions as it is inherited as an autosomal recessive condition. Clusters of patients have been identified in Mediterranean countries, the Middle East and Ecuador. At least 19 molecular defects in the GH receptor gene have been described, including gene deletions, nonsense and frame-shift mutations and missense mutations. Recently, mutations in the GH receptor gene have been described in children with what has been previously been described as idiopathic short stature, who are thought to have a partial form of GH insensitivity.

PATHOGENESIS / AETIOLOGY
The genetic lesion leads to an abnormal GH receptor. GH fails to interact appropriately with this abnormal receptor, with an inability to generate IGF-1 and ensuing growth failure.

DIAGNOSIS
It may present with hypoglycaemia in the neonatal period and, later on, with extreme short stature (**13.16**) and an extremely poor growth rate. The birth weight may be low. Clinically, they resemble GH deficient children, but with extreme short stature. Bone age is delayed with respect to chronological age, but advanced with respect to height age. Other features include micropenis, small hands and feet, craniofacial anomalies such as a saddle nose (**13.17**), excess subcutaneous fat, sparse hair growth, delayed closure of anterior fontanelles, and a prominent forehead. Hip dysplasia and a chubby appearance are other associated features. Pubertal delay may be a feature. More recently, partial insensitivity to GH has been described in children who present with idio-pathic short stature.

Essential investigations are as for GHD/GHI (see previous pages). Unlike GHD/GHI, the basal concentration of GH in serum is elevated, with an exaggerated peak GH in response to provocation and low basal IGF-1 and IGF-BP3 levels. Additionally, an IGF-1 generation test should be performed, and this fails to demon-strate an increase in the IGF-1 level following the administration of rhGH. GH-binding protein may be present or absent, depending on the underlying molecular lesion. In children with short stature secondary to partial GH resistance, GH-binding protein levels are low. GH levels are high, with low IGF-1 levels.

TREATMENT
Trials are currently under way in children with Laron-type dwarfism using recombinant IGF-1 treatment. Initial results are promising, with an initial increase in the height velocity, but close monitoring of patients is essential as the treatment is not without its side-effects (hypo-glycaemia, hypokalaemia and papilloedema). In children with partial GH resistance, it would theoretically be possible to treat with high doses of GH, which might then improve the height velocity. However, at present, this remains purely speculative.

PROGNOSIS
The height prognosis is extremely poor. The role of recombinant IGF-1 treatment with respect to an increase in final height remains to be established.

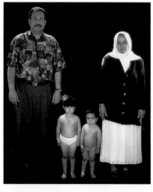

13.16 Laron-type dwarfism. Extreme short stature in two siblings, shown here with their parents.

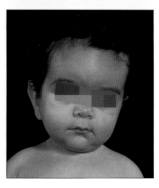

13.17 Laron-type dwarfism. Facial features of a child.

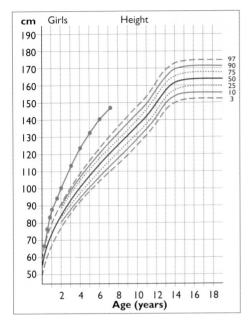

TALL STATURE

Tall children become tall adults by growing continuously at a rate greater than their smaller peers. A growth rate which is constantly around the 90th centile, a height attained which is greater than one might expect for the family, and an increasing height prediction are all reasons to investigate the tall child. The flow chart below suggests a plan of management for children with tall stature.

Some of the conditions leading to tall stature will be further discussed in the next sections.

13.18 Cerebral gigantism. Typical growth chart of a child with an extremely rapid rate of growth.

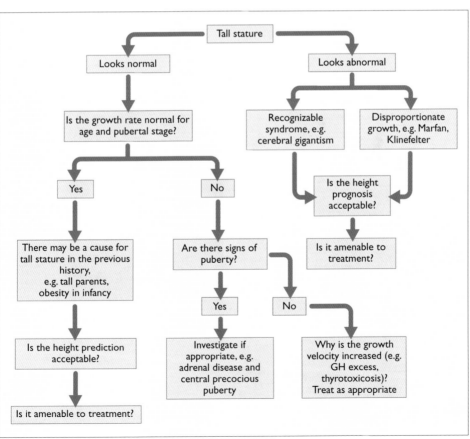

MARFAN SYNDROME

See also 'Genetics' chapter.

INCIDENCE / GENETICS

Autosomal dominant, with a high *de novo* mutation rate.

PATHOGENESIS / AETIOLOGY

The mutation in the fibrillin gene on chromosome 15 leads to widespread connective tissue abnormalities, and the characteristic lesions of Marfan syndrome.

DIAGNOSIS

Patients present with tall stature. Other features include arachnodactyly (**13.19, 13.20**), wide arm span, joint laxity, kyphoscoliosis, narrow face, high-arched palate, bluish sclerae, upward lenticular dislocation, aortic incompetence, dissecting aneurysm of aorta, mitral valve prolapse and inguinal or femoral herniae. The diagnosis is clinical. Investigations should include an echocardiogram, chromosomal analysis, and measurement of urinary homocystine to exclude homocystinuria, the main differential diagnosis.

TREATMENT

Tall stature may be limited by early induction of puberty. Cardiac lesions may need surgical intervention.

PROGNOSIS

This is dictated by the cardiac anomalies.

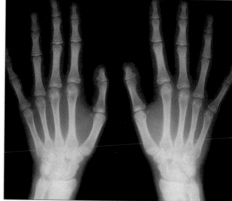

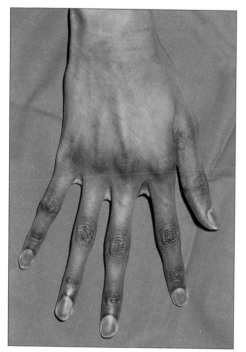

13.19 & 13 .20 Marfan syndrome in a child demonstrating arachnodactyly (clinical and radiological appearances).

PITUITARY GIGANTISM

INCIDENCE / GENETICS
Extremely rare. Recent research has suggested that an activating Gs mutation in signal-transducing G-proteins may account for some adult cases of acromegaly and hence, by extrapolation, for some cases of pituitary gigantism.

PATHOGENESIS / AETIOLOGY
The underlying lesion is usually a somatotroph adenoma. These lesions are commoner in the McCune-Albright syndrome (see page 383).

DIAGNOSIS
Usually presents with tall stature, irrespective of the mid-parental target centile (**13.21, 13.22**). The height velocity is generally greater than the 75th–97th centiles. Precocious puberty should be excluded by clinical examination. Visual fields may reveal a deficit, although it is unlikely that a GH-secreting adenoma will be large enough to lead to such a deficit. A 24-hour GH secretory profile may be diagnostic. This entails measurement of serum GH concentrations at 20-minute intervals. The profile is often difficult to distinguish from that of a child with constitutional tall stature. However, in gigantism, it is characterized by an inability of GH concentrations to achieve undetectable levels (ie. there are no troughs of GH secretion). The IGF-1 level is elevated.

Although in acromegalic adults there is a paradoxical increase in GH secretion in response to an oral glucose load or thyrotrophin-releasing hormone (TRH), in childhood, the situation is somewhat more complex. Paradoxical GH responses are often seen in both short and tall normal children during puberty. Imaging of the pituitary gland using magnetic resonance should be undertaken in all cases of suspected pituitary gigantism.

TREATMENT
In the first instance, medical treatment can be instituted using either somatostatin or bromo-criptine. Somatostatin switches off GH secretion. However, it also switches off insulin secretion and is associated with unacceptable gastrointestinal side-effects such as diarrhoea, fat intolerance and the formation of gall stones. Bromocriptine, a dopamine agonist, has the paradoxical effect of switching off GH secretion in children with pituitary gigantism. It can, however, also be associated with unacceptable side-effects, particularly nausea and vomiting. The definitive treatment entails surgical removal of the adenoma, via the trans-sphenoidal approach.

PROGNOSIS
The overall prognosis in cases of isolated pituitary adenomata is generally good, once the lesion has been removed. However, there is a possibility that the lesion will recur. In the McCune-Albright syndrome, the prognosis must be guarded, in view of the other complications associated with this condition (see page 383).

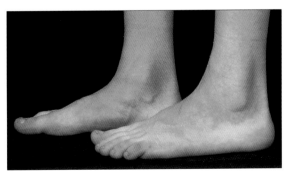

13.21 & 13.22 Pituitary gigantism in a child. Note the large feet.

EARLY PUBERTY

The algorithm on this page gives an approach to the diagnosis of early puberty. Subsequent sections will discuss some of these conditions in more detail. Of essence to the diagnosis is the clinical assessment as to whether puberty is consonant or not (i.e. whether the sequence of pubertal development is normal or not), with enlargement of testicular size in boys and breast development in girls being the first signs of gonadotrophin-dependent precocious puberty.

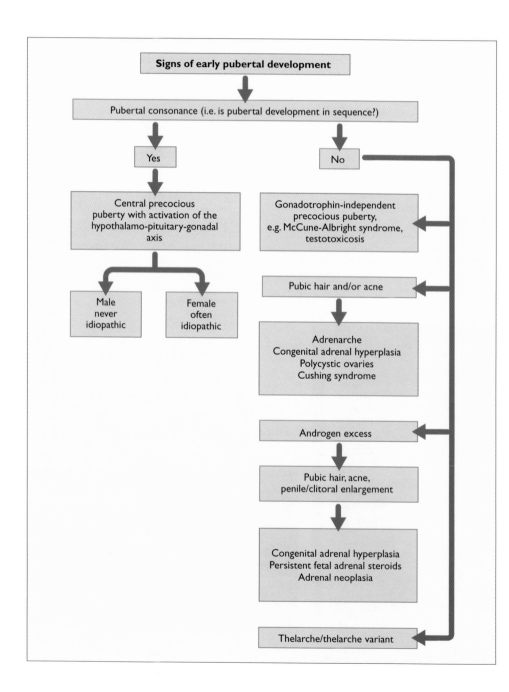

PREMATURE THELARCHE / THELARCHE VARIANT OR 'BENIGN' PRECOCIOUS PUBERTY

INCIDENCE / GENETICS
Premature thelarche is a sporadic condition which is commonly observed, particularly in neonates. Thelarche variant is also not uncommon.

PATHOGENESIS / AETIOLOGY
Ovarian cyst development due to isolated pulsatile FSH secretion results in the secretion of oestrogen and isolated breast development.

DIAGNOSIS
These girls usually present with isolated early breast development (13.23). Over 80% of girls have cyclical breast development which waxes and wanes at intervals of 4–6 weeks. The age of onset is usually below two years and frequently continues as an extension of the neonatal breast enlargement, due to placental transmission of maternal oestrogens. Such development is usually associated with isolated ovarian cyst development, which is due to premature but isolated pulsatile FSH secretion. The uterus is of an appropriate size and shape for age, with no endometrial echo and only exceptionally is there a vaginal bleed.

Growth is at a normal rate, and the bone age is not advanced. There are no other signs of puberty. In thelarche variant, increased stature, advanced bone age, a small uterus and an ovarian morphology which is between that for premature thelarche and precocious puberty, are characteristically associated with isolated breast development. Investigations should include a bone age in children over the age of three years (advanced in thelarche variant, but not in premature thelarche) and a pelvic ultrasound scan (13.24). FSH levels are raised, with a pulsatile secretory pattern, and the response of FSH to GnRH (gonadotrophin-releasing hormone) is brisk. Thyroid function should be tested, since in primary hypothyroidism, isolated breast development may occur due to elevated FSH concentrations.

TREATMENT
No treatment is required for these conditions.

PROGNOSIS
Both conditions are benign with no effect on the growth prognosis. The conditions may continue largely unchanged with waxing and waning of breast size in parallel to ovarian cyst size until puberty.

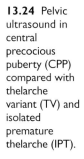

13.23 Thelarche in a five-year-old girl.

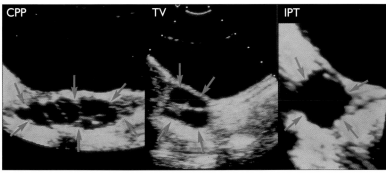

13.24 Pelvic ultrasound in central precocious puberty (CPP) compared with thelarche variant (TV) and isolated premature thelarche (IPT).

GONADOTROPHIN-DEPENDENT (CENTRAL) PRECOCIOUS PUBERTY

INCIDENCE / GENETICS
The condition is relatively common in girls (M:F ratio of 1:10). Most cases are sporadic. However, familial forms are now recognized, and may be due to an activating mutation in G-proteins associated with the gonadotrophin-releasing hormone receptor.

PATHOGENESIS / AETIOLOGY
In girls, often no underlying cause can be demonstrated. In boys, pineal and other intra-cranial tumours and hamartomata may be present. Other causes include hydrocephalus and neurofibromatosis. Previous cranial irra-diation frequently leads to precocious sexual development in both sexes.

DIAGNOSIS
Usually presents with early signs of puberty. The sequence of sexual maturation is identical to that of normal puberty (i.e. in boys, testicular enlargement is the first sign while in girls, breast development is the first sign) (**13.25**). In boys, the aetiology is rarely idio-pathic (**13.26**), and signs of an underlying condition may be present (e.g. neurological abnormalities secondary to a brain tumour, hydrocephalus, neurofibromatosis).

Tall stature with an increased height velocity is a feature of central precocious puberty in both boys and girls. Behavioural disturbances may also be evident, with an inappropriate degree of sexualization. A pelvic ultrasound scan in girls will reveal a multicystic ovarian morphology in response to pulsatile gonado-trophin secretion. The demonstration of a physiological pulsatile pattern of gonadotrophin secretion over a 24-hour period is the investi-gation of choice, but can be expensive and time-consuming. An LHRH test shows a brisk pubertal LH and FSH response to LHRH (luteinizing hormone-releasing hormone).

A bone age will be advanced. The sex inci-dence of intracranial lesions is equal. However, since girls outnumber boys with precocious puberty, the majority of girls do not have an underlying lesion accounting for the precocious puberty. Neuroradiological imaging of the brain is indicated in all boys with precocious puberty, and in all girls with neurological signs and symptoms.

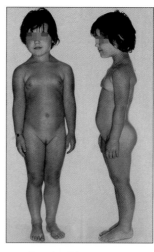

13.25 Idiopathic gonadotrophin-dependent precocious puberty in a six-year-old girl.

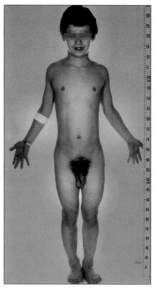

13.26 Gonadotrophin-dependent precocious puberty in a seven-year-old boy with a sub-arachnoid cyst. Note the body disproportion with the short limbs in relation to the spine.

TREATMENT
Treatment is indicated if puberty occurs at an early age with consequent psychological dis-turbance. Masturbation and other forms of inappropriate sexual behaviour can lead to major problems for the family, particularly in boys. Additionally, the onset of menarche at primary school is a cause of much distress and is also an indication for treatment. Treatment can alter the final height prognosis in only the youngest children, and the use of growth hormone has not been shown to improve the height prognosis.

Agents such as progestogens (e.g. medroxy-progesterone and cyproterone acetate or the gonadotrophin-releasing hormone analogues) are used in the treatment of this complex condition. Although pubertal development is arrested, growth also slows down considerably and this may necessitate the use of growth hormone in conjunction with the above agents. This is not without its own problems, the chief drawback being the development of polycystic ovaries (see page 384). The use of cyproterone is not without hazard, since it can lead to adrenal suppression and hepatotoxicity.

PROGNOSIS

Although pubertal development can be arrested, the final height of these children may be unaffected by treatment. Early sexual maturation is associated with the early growth acceleration of puberty. In addition, rapid epiphyseal maturation occurs in response to increased sex steroid secretion, which ultimately limits growth. Although children with early puberty tend to be tall when they are young, their final height prognosis is compromised. The earlier the onset of puberty and the shorter the parental heights, the shorter the child's final height will be. Polycystic ovarian syndrome can be a late problem.

McCUNE–ALBRIGHT SYNDROME

INCIDENCE / GENETICS

McCune-Albright syndrome is a rare condition. An activating missense mutation in the gene for the α-subunit of Gs, the G-protein that stimulates cAMP formation, has recently been discovered in these patients. The mutation is found to a variable extent in different affected endocrine and non-endocrine tissues, consistent with the mosaic distribution of abnormal cells generated by a somatic cell mutation early in embryogenesis. Substitution of Arg201 with either Cys or His inhibits the GTPase activity of Gs and leads to inappropriate stimulation of adenylyl cyclase.

DIAGNOSIS

Patients with this condition can present at any age. Clinical features include the presence of large irregular pigmented lesions (50% unilateral) (**13.27**), polyostotic fibrous dysplasia, sexual precocity (**13.28**) and other endocrinopathies (e.g. Cushing syndrome, excessive GH secretion by pituitary somatotroph adenomata, and thyrotoxicosis). Non-endocrine abnormalities include chronic hepatic disease, thymic hyperplasia, and cardiopulmonary disease.

A skeletal survey and a bone scan show the characteristic bony abnormalities of polyostotic fibrous dysplasia (**13.29**). GnRH stimulation

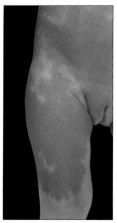
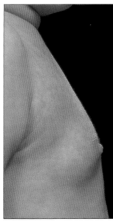
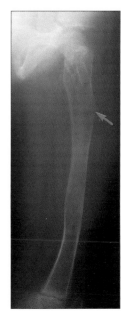

13.27 McCune-Albright syndrome. Typical large *café-au-lait* pigmented area with an irregular margin in a child.

13.28 McCune-Albright syndrome. Precocious puberty (gonadotrophin-independent) in a two-year-old girl.

13.29 McCune-Albright syndrome showing polyostotic fibrous dysplasia in a child.

fails to increase gonadotrophin levels, since the precocious puberty is gonadotrophin-independent. Appropriate investigations for Cushing syndrome, thyrotoxicosis and pituitary adenomata leading to GH excess are performed as and when necessary. Other investigations should include liver function tests and an echocardiogram.

TREATMENT

The precocious puberty can be difficult to control. Agents used include cyproterone acetate, testolactone and medroxyprogesterone. Abnormalities of other endocrine glands are treated as and when the problems arise (e.g. bilateral adrenalectomy for Cushing syndrome, carbimazole for thyrotoxicosis).

PROGNOSIS

This is variable. The prognosis is much poorer for early-onset McCune-Albright syndrome with multi-organ involvement. Sudden death can occur due to cardiopulmonary involvement.

POLYCYSTIC OVARIAN DISEASE

INCIDENCE / GENETICS

The incidence shows a familial predisposition, although the gene has not been identified to date. Polycystic ovaries can be found in 6% of six-year-old girls and this increases to 25% of the female adult population on pelvic ultra-sound scanning.

PATHOGENESIS / AETIOLOGY

Predisposing factors include hyperandrogenism (e.g. congenital adrenal hyperplasia), hyper-insulinism, tall stature and obesity. Treatment with growth hormone is also associated with PCO, as is diabetes mellitus.

DIAGNOSIS

This condition usually presents with late menarche and menstrual irregularities, and accounts for 87% of irregular menstrual cycles in unselected adult females. The polycystic ovarian syndrome (PCOS; Stein-Leventhal syndrome) presents with oligomenorrhoea, acne, hirsutism and obesity. Acanthosis nigricans and insulin-resistance are other associations. In several patients, symptoms referrable to the polycystic ovaries are not present, and the diagnosis is only made by pelvic ultrasound scan examination.

Pelvic ultrasound scan (USS) shows the classical appearance of large ovaries with increased stroma and a characteristic arrangement of follicles around the periphery of the ovary (**13.30**). Other investigations include serum LH (usually elevated), raised levels of androgens, an elevated fasting glucose and an oral glucose tolerance test with measurement of plasma insulin levels reveals hyperinsulinism with insulin resistance. The diagnosis of late-onset congenital adrenal hyperplasia (page 392) needs to be excluded in children who present predominantly with hirsutism.

TREATMENT

Irregularities of the menstrual cycles can be controlled with the oral contraceptive pill. An anti-androgen (cyproterone acetate) can be used to alleviate the effects of hyperandrogenism. However, recent reports have linked high doses of this agent with hepatotoxicity and adrenal suppression. Metformin can be used in obese patients with PCOS.

PROGNOSIS

Fertility can be impaired in up to 25% of women. However, in the vast majority of individuals fertility is normal. The long-term outlook is also determined by the presence of obesity, hypertension and diabetes mellitus.

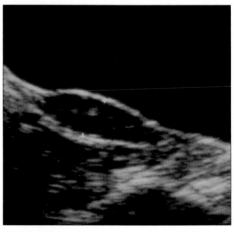

13.30 PCOS. Classic ovarian ultrasound appearance, with a 'necklace' of cysts around the periphery of the ovary.

LATE PUBERTY

The algorithm offers an approach to the diagnosis of conditions leading to late puberty.

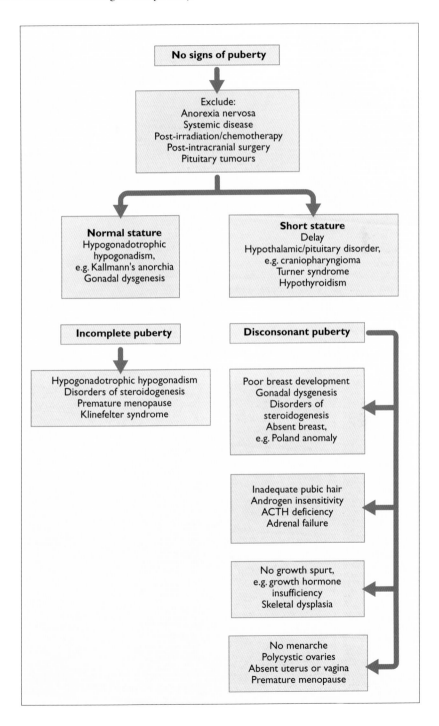

KLINEFELTER SYNDROME

INCIDENCE / GENETICS
The incidence is 1 in 500 male births. Chromosomal analysis reveals a karyotype of 47 XXY.

PATHOGENESIS / AETIOLOGY
See above. Tall stature results not only from the presence of additional chromosomal material but also from inadequate sexual development, which allows growth to continue at a normal rate far beyond its usual age of cessation.

DIAGNOSIS
This condition usually presents with tall stature and excessively long legs (**13.31**). The patients tend to be slim initially, but can be obese as adults. Other features include hypogonadism with small testes and inadequate virilization, infertility and gynaecomastia (**13.32**). Children with this condition can have a low IQ with poor school performance. Diabetes mellitus is commoner in adults with Klinefelter syndrome than in the general population. Investigations should include a karyotype and serum LH and FSH which are usually elevated (hypergonadotrophic hypogonadism). The serum testosterone is consequently low. A pelvic USS is indicated if cryptorchidism is a feature.

TREATMENT
Treatment with testosterone in the form of depot injections administered at two- to four-weekly intervals is indicated. Earlier treatment with testosterone can prevent the onset of gynaecomastia and can limit the tall stature associated with this condition. Other forms of therapy for growth-limitation include the possible use of somatostatin. However, its mode of administration (as a subcutaneous infusion) and unacceptable gastrointestinal side-effects limit its use.

PROGNOSIS
With the addition of testosterone therapy, pubertal development ensues. However, patients are generally infertile.

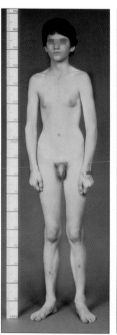 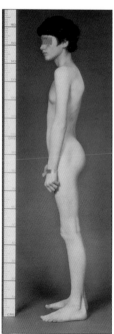

13.31 & 13.32 Klinefelter syndrome. Tall stature and slim build with eunuchoid appearances in a boy.

CONGENITAL HYPOTHYROIDISM

INCIDENCE / GENETICS

The incidence is 1 in 4,000 newborn infants. Those cases due to an inborn error of hormonogenesis are inherited in an autosomal recessive fashion, while those due to a dysgenetic gland have a low recurrence rate (1 in 100). Mutations in the transcription factors PAX8, TTF1 and TTF2 are associated with the latter.

PATHOGENESIS / AETIOLOGY

The primary form of the disease is due to agenesis of the thyroid gland, a dysgenetic gland or dyshormonogenesis. The much rarer secondary form of the disease is due to TSH deficiency, either isolated or due to pituitary hypoplasia, when it may be associated with other pituitary hormone deficiencies.

DIAGNOSIS

This condition is usually detected on neonatal screening. Few infants now manifest clinical evidence of thyroxine deficiency. Clinical features, when present, include an umbilical hernia, macroglossia, constipation, feeding problems, lethargy, respiratory distress, prolonged jaundice, hoarse cry, hypotonia, coarse facies (**13.33**), growth failure, abundant hair, delayed closure of fontanelles, hypothermia and a dry, mottled skin. Retarded bone maturation with delayed epiphyseal ossification and epiphyseal dysgenesis are other features. These usually appear if the diagnosis has been missed for more than six weeks. Other congenital malformations are present in 7% of cases.

Investigations include a free thyroxine level (low) and serum TSH (elevated). If the hypothyroidism is secondary (due to congenital TRH or TSH deficiency), a TRH test together with assessment of GH, cortisol, prolactin and gonadotrophin secretion may be indicated. A radioisotope scan may differentiate between thyroid dysgenesis and dyshormonogenesis, locate the thyroid gland and enable a decision to be made regarding life-long therapy. Since transient hypothyroidism may occur in some children, it would be wise to recheck thyroid function in children with congenital hypothyroidism after switching to tri-iodothyronine and then stopping treatment for a week before re-testing. In view of the association between congenital hypothyroidism and deafness, audiological assessment should be performed in these children.

TREATMENT

Treatment is with thyroxine ($100\mu g/m^2/day$). Subsequent monitoring entails careful documentation of the growth rate, which is an extremely sensitive measure of thyroid function. Biochemical assessment, measuring the free thyroxine level and the TSH level, is particularly important in the first year of life.

PROGNOSIS

Before the introduction of screening, the major complications of late treated congenital hypothyroidism were impaired intelligence and a range of abnormalities of neurological function, particularly with respect to coordination. These neuro-psychological sequelae are now much less marked, following the advent of screening. Nevertheless, the intelligence quotient (IQ) of these patients is closely related to the pre-treatment thyroxine level in serum. For example, in those children with a low pre-treatment thyroxine concentration (total thyroxine below 42 nmol/L or free thyroxine <5 pmol/L), a mean deficit of approximately 10 IQ points can be observed compared with controls. Subjects with pre-treatment thyroxine concentrations over 42 nmol/L have similar IQ scores to normal children.

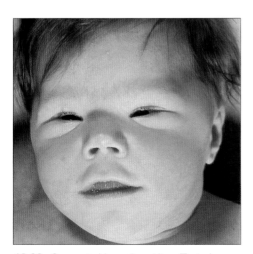

13.33 Congenital hypothyroidism. Typical coarse facies of a child.

ACQUIRED HYPOTHYROIDISM

INCIDENCE / GENETICS

Autoimmune hypothyroidism is associated with a family history in 30–40% of cases and is one of the commonest forms of acquired hypothyroidism.

PATHOGENESIS / AETIOLOGY

Worldwide, iodine deficiency is the commonest cause of hypothyroidism. Causes of acquired hypothyroidism include goitrogenic agents, thyroid dysgenesis, auto-immune thyroiditis, pituitary TSH deficiency (e.g. post-cranial irradiation and craniopharyngioma), endemic iodine deficiency and cystinosis. Chromosomal disorders (i.e. Turner, Down and Klinefelter syndromes) are associated with an increased incidence of hypothyroidism, which is probably autoimmune in origin.

DIAGNOSIS

This can present at any age, usually with a gradual onset. The most important sign in childhood is growth failure. A goitre may be present. There is a modest weight gain, with disproportion between weight and height gain (**13.34**). Isolated breast development or testicular enlargement, without other signs of puberty or an increase in height velocity, results from excessive FSH secretion. In contrast, pubertal delay or arrest can also be a feature. Other signs of classical hypothyroidism are slow to develop (e.g. mental sluggishness, cold intolerance, fatigue, constipation, bradycardia, dry skin, coarse facies, proximal myopathy). Classically, tendon reflex contraction is slow and the bone age is delayed.

These children are usually extremely well-behaved and compliant and do well at school. There may be features of other autoimmune conditions (e.g. Addison's disease, myasthenia gravis, insulin-dependent diabetes mellitus, pernicious anaemia, malabsorption and vitiligo) as thyroid disease may be a component of polyglandular autoimmune disease.

Investigations should include free thyroxine and triiodothyronine levels, serum TSH, thyroid autoantibodies (especially antimicrosomal and anti-thyroglobulin), a TRH test if the TSH level is low, and FSH and prolactin levels (may be elevated in primary hypothyroidism). Ideally, the rest of the family should be screened for hypothyroidism by performing thyroid function and a thyroid auto-antibody screen.

TREATMENT

Treatment with thyroxine should be commenced cautiously, at a dosage of $50\mu g/m^2/$ day initially, with a subsequent increase to 100 $\mu g/m^2/$day. Commencement of treatment can lead to severe behavioural changes, with considerable disruption to family life and the child's schooling. The model compliant child's return to a normal level of activity is often extremely traumatic. When treatment begins there is a catch-up phase of growth, followed by a subsequent return to a normal height velocity.

PROGNOSIS

The prognosis for final height, fertility and general health is excellent, provided treatment is commenced early and the compliance is good.

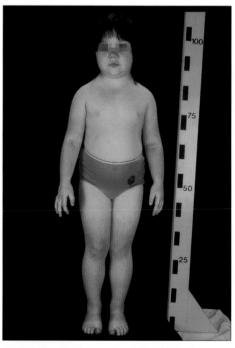

13.34 Acquired hypothyroidism. Typical appearance of a child. Note the disproportion between height and weight.

PRIMARY ADRENAL INSUFFICIENCY

INCIDENCE / GENETICS

The incidence of congenital adrenal hypoplasia has been reported as 1 in 12,500 births. Inheritance is either as an autosomal or X-linked recessive condition. Mutations in the DAX1 gene are associated with the X-linked form of the disease. Autoimmune adrenal insufficiency is associated with the two types of polyglandular autoimmune syndrome (**Table 13.3**). Type I is associated with mutations in the *AIRE* (Autoimmune Regulator) gene on chromosome 21.

PATHOGENESIS / AETIOLOGY

Causes of primary adrenal insufficiency include congenital adrenal hypoplasia, defects of adrenal steroid biosynthesis, adrenal haemorrhage, autoimmune adrenalitis, multiple endocrinopathy, infections (e.g. tuberculosis and Waterhouse-Friederichsen syndrome), adrenoleukodystrophy (see also 'Metabolic Diseases' chapter) and iatrogenic [chemical or surgical] causes.

DIAGNOSIS

Congenital adrenal hypoplasia usually presents in the neonatal period with hypoglycaemia, salt loss, apnoeic episodes, dehydration, poor feeding, failure to thrive, vomiting and hyperpigmentation. In Addison's disease, presentation is usually later and symptoms and signs include lethargy, anorexia, vomiting, weight loss, irritability, salt-losing adrenal crisis, hypoglycaemia, syncope and hyperpigmentation of the skin and mucosal surfaces (**13.35**).

In adrenoleukodystrophy, neurological symptoms and signs may develop first, with features of adrenal insufficiency developing between the ages of four and eight years. In the polyglandular autoimmune syndrome, features of other autoimmune conditions such as

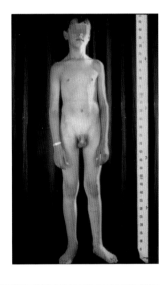

13.35 Addison's disease. Hyperpigmentation in a child.

Table 13.3 Polyglandular autoimmune syndrome

	Type 1	Type 2
Inheritance (autosomal)	Recessive (due to mutations in *AIRE*)	Dominant
Age at onset	Childhood (<12 years)	Adulthood (>30 years)
Female : male ratio	1.5:1	1.8:1
HLA association	None	B6, -Dw3, -DR3
Disease components:		
Addison disease	65%	100%
Hypoparathyroidism	80%	None
Mucocutaneous candidiasis	75%	None
Alopecia	25%	<1%
Malabsorption	22%	None
Gonadal failure	20%	20%
Pernicious anaemia	13%	<1%
Autoimmune thyroid disease	10%	70%
Chronic active hepatitis	10%	None
Diabetes mellitus	8%	5%
Vitiligo	8%	5%

hypoparathyroidism, diabetes mellitus, vitiligo, myasthenia gravis, coeliac disease and pernicious anaemia may also be present. Mucocutaneous candidiasis is a feature of Type 1 polyglandular autoimmune syndrome.

Investigations should include plasma urea and electrolytes (hyponatraemia, hyperkalaemia), a cortisol profile (low values of cortisol), a synacthen test (no cortisol response to exogenous ACTH), a plasma ACTH level (elevated), plasma renin activity and aldosterone level (renin is raised with a low aldosterone level if mineralocorticoid deficiency is associated), an auto-antibody screen, thyroid function, plasma calcium, and fasting glucose (low in Addison disease, but may be elevated if associated with diabetes mellitus). Plasma very long-chain fatty acids (VLCFA) levels are useful in excluding a diagnosis of adrenoleukodystrophy.

TREATMENT

Initially, hypovolaemia should be corrected with adequate fluid and sodium replacement, followed by maintenance treatment with replacement doses of glucocorticoids in the form of hydrocortisone, with added mineralocorticoid treatment in the form of 9α-fludrocortisone if the diagnosis of mineralocorticoid deficiency is confirmed. Indication of adequate dosage is given by general well-being, normal appetite and activity, weight gain and normal growth. When hypothyroidism is present in a child with chronic adrenal insufficiency, adequate glucocorticoid therapy should be established before commencing thyroxine therapy, otherwise an adrenal crisis would be precipitated.

PROGNOSIS

Given correct treatment and adequate parental support, patients with congenital adrenal hypoplasia and Addison disease can lead a normal life with a normal life-span. However, growth and pubertal development need careful monitoring. In congenital adrenal hypoplasia, hypogonadotrophic hypogonadism is associated with the condition, and so puberty will need to be induced. The prognosis in polyglandular autoimmune disease is poor if chronic active hepatitis is also present. The prognosis in adrenoleukodystrophy is that of the underlying neurological disorder, which progresses inexorably.

CUSHING SYNDROME

INCIDENCE / GENETICS

Iatrogenic Cushing syndrome is relatively common. Endogenous Cushing syndrome is rare. Adrenal tumours predominate in female infants under two years of age, in whom the underlying diagnosis may be that of the McCune-Albright syndrome. In older individuals, the underlying lesion is usually a pituitary adenoma. Ectopic ACTH production in children leading to Cushing syndrome is extremely rare. Cushing syndrome is sporadic, although very rare forms of familial hypercortisolism have been described.

PATHOGENESIS / AETIOLOGY

Cushing syndrome can be iatrogenic, due to a CRH- or ACTH-secreting tumour (either in the pituitary gland or due to ectopic secretion of the stimulating hormone), or due to an adrenal neoplasm or nodular adrenal hyperplasia. McCune-Albright syndrome (see page 383) can lead to primary adrenal Cushing syndrome.

DIAGNOSIS

Children with this syndrome present with excessive weight gain leading to rapidly progressing obesity which is mainly truncal in nature (**13.36**). Other features include 'moon-like' facies (**13.37**), a 'buffalo-hump', hypertension, purple striae (**13.38**), hirsutism, osteoporosis, hypogonadism, proximal myopathy, susceptibility to bruising and infection, cataracts, pubertal arrest, amenorrhoea, emotional lability and growth arrest, although, initially, androgen secretion may lead to acceleration of the height velocity.

In Cushing disease (due to a pituitary adenoma), headaches and visual disturbance may be a feature, with impaired visual fields, and even papilloedema. Diagnosis can be extremely difficult, and is based upon elevated plasma cortisol concentrations with a loss of circadian rhythm and elevated 24-hour urinary free cortisol. In pituitary-dependent Cushing disease, ACTH levels are detectable in the face of raised cortisol levels. In primary adrenal Cushing syndrome, ACTH levels will be suppressed in the face of elevated cortisol levels.

In ectopic Cushing syndrome, both cortisol and ACTH levels are extremely high. Once the diagnosis is established, the source of the excess cortisol production needs to be established. Dexamethasone suppresses cortisol production in normal individuals. In pituitary-dependent

Cushing disease, low-dose dexamethasone will not suppress cortisol secretion, but high-dose dexamethasone will suppress it in approximately 80% of cases.

Adrenal and ectopic Cushing syndrome will not suppress with any dose of dexamethasone. Administration of CRH (corticotrophin-releasing hormone) can be helpful in differentiating an adrenal and pituitary cause of the syndrome. Imaging of the pituitary and adrenals using an MRI scanner is usually indicated in order to locate the tumour. In difficult cases, inferior petrosal sinus sampling can be performed to locate a pituitary lesion.

TREATMENT

Pituitary-dependent Cushing disease is usually treated by trans-sphenoidal removal of the adenoma by an experienced neurosurgeon. Where an adrenal tumour is defined, surgical removal of the tumour is indicated. Medical treatment with metyrapone or ketoconazole is not without its own problems and can only be used as a temporary measure.

PROGNOSIS

In untreated patients, the mortality and morbidity from this condition is high, with osteoporosis, glucose intolerance and hypertension accounting for this. Following surgical treatment of Cushing disease, there is a strong possibility that the condition either does not remit, or relapses. In this case, further exploration of the pituitary with a possible total hypophysectomy may be indicated. This will mean that the child will then need replacement hydrocortisone, thyroxine, gonadotrophins or sex steroids, growth hormone and DDAVP treatment. However, the outlook is nevertheless better than that following a bilateral adrenalectomy with consequent Nelson's syndrome. If the Cushing syndrome is due to an adrenal carcinoma or an ectopic source (usually a lung carcinoid), the prognosis is much worse.

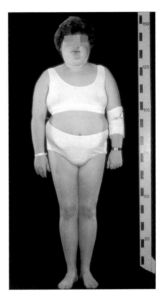

13.36 Cushing syndrome. Central obesity.

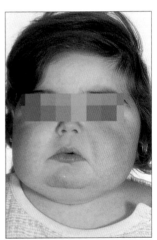

13.37 Cushing syndrome showing 'moon-like' facies in a child.

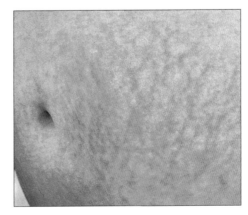

13.38 Cushing syndrome. Purple abdominal striae in a child.

CONGENITAL ADRENAL HYPERPLASIA

INCIDENCE / GENETICS

21-hydroxylase deficiency is the commonest cause of CAH, with a frequency of between 1 in 5,000 to 23,000 for the homozygous affected state, depending on the population studied. Simple virilizing or non-classical CAH is commoner in Ashkenazi Jews. The inheritance for all forms of CAH is autosomal recessive. At the molecular level, the inheritance is best understood for 21-hydroxylase deficiency, where the gene encoding the microsomal cytochrome P450 21-hydroxylase enzyme system (CYP21B) and a pseudogene (CYP21A) are located in the HLA complex. Mutations and deletions in the CYP21B gene are associated with the variable phenotype seen in this condition.

PATHOGENESIS / AETIOLOGY

These autosomal recessive conditions result in enzyme deficiencies in the adrenal glands. These glands cannot synthesize vital steroids, with a resulting accumulation of the substrate steroid which precedes the block as a result of the excessive ACTH drive consequent upon loss of feedback. Cholesterol incorporation into the adrenal cortex is promoted by the ACTH drive, giving rise to the adrenal hyperplasia. Early genotype-phenotype studies have already shown that the correlation between clinical, biochemical and molecular genetic findings in patients with classical 21-hydroxylase deficiency is not absolute.

DIAGNOSIS

Children with congenital adrenal hyperplasia may present with ambiguous genitalia at birth, a salt-losing crisis in the newborn period, hypertension, precocious puberty in males, virilization in females and 'bilateral cryptorchidism' with breast development in puberty (i.e. females raised inappropriately as males) (**13.39**). Hypoglycaemia is a rare feature of the condition.

In non-classical 21-hydroxylase deficiency, females are born with normal external genitalia. Subsequently, clinical manifestations from increased androgen production can occur at any time. Symptoms in female patients appearing later in childhood or adolescence include hirsutism, temporal baldness, acne, delayed

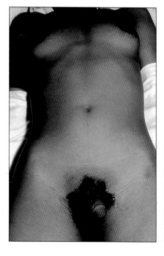

13.39 Congenital adrenal hyperplasia. Excessive virilization in a female raised as a male.

Table 13.4 Phenotypes associated with congenital adrenal hyperplasia

Enzyme defect	Ambiguous genitalia		Salt loss	Hypertension	Puberty
	Male	Female			
CYP11A/StAR (Steroidogenic Acute Regulatory Protein)	+	−	+	−	Absent
3β-hydroxy-steroid dehydrogenase	+	+	+	−	Absent
17-hydroxylase (P450c17)	+	−	−	+	Absent
21-hydroxylase (P450c21)	−	+	+	−	Precocious
11-hydroxylase (P450c11β)	−	+	−	+	Precocious

menarche, menstrual irregularities, clitoro-megaly and infertility. An accelerated linear growth velocity, a short final height and an advanced bone age may be other features of this condition.

In cases with genital ambiguity or virilization, a karyotype and pelvic ultrasound scan to identify the internal organs are mandatory. A raised plasma 17-hydroxyprogesterone level (17 OHP) indicates a diagnosis of 21-hydroxylase deficiency. The definitive diagnosis is based upon the analysis of a urine sample, with the measurement of various urinary steroids. This will define the enzyme block. In cases of simple virilizing CAH, a synacthen test (flat cortisol response, raised 17OHP levels) with the collection of appropriate plasma and urine samples will assist in the diagnosis. Urea and electrolyte measurements, plasma renin activity and plasma aldosterone levels are essential in the diagnosis of salt-losing CAH. A bone age (usually advanced) may be helpful in the management of simple virilizing CAH. Genetic analysis is useful, particularly if future pregnancies are being considered.

TREATMENT

In the first instance, a salt-losing crisis needs to be treated by adequate fluid and saline replacement, as well as glucocorticoid (hydrocortisone) and mineralocorticoid (9-α fludrocortisone given as crushed tablets) replacement. Subsequently, the child is maintained on these replacement hormones, the doses being altered according to surface area (20 mg/m^2/day of hydrocortisone, 150 μg/m^2/day of fludrocortisone). Salt supplements should be continued until an infant is switched to normal cow's milk. Girls with ambiguous genitalia may need surgical correction in the form of clitoral reduction and a genitoplasty within the first 3–12 months. Late-onset, simple-virilizing CAH is best treated with hydrocortisone in order to suppress the ACTH drive. Puberty may need to be induced in CYP11A/StAR deficiency, 3β-hydroxysteroid dehydrogenase deficiency and 17-hydroxylase deficiency.

Monitoring of the condition is by regular auxology and biochemical monitoring. Both under-treated and over-treated congenital adrenal hyperplasia result in an abnormal growth pattern, with an increased or decreased growth velocity respectively. Skeletal age is advanced in under-treated congenital adrenal hyperplasia. Measurement of plasma renin activity and 17OHP is useful in monitoring salt-losing CAH.

PROGNOSIS

In well-controlled CAH where compliance with medication is satisfactory, the prognosis for final height and pubertal development is good in males, while that for fertility is more guarded. Females with CAH invariably develop polycystic ovarian disease and the prognosis for fertility may be affected by this complication. With late diagnosis and/or poor compliance, the children grow extremely rapidly with a considerable advance in bone age and early fusion of the epiphyses leading to a compromised final height.

RICKETS

INCIDENCE / GENETICS

The incidence is dependent on the underlying cause of the condition. Nutritional rickets is generally commoner in children in Asian communities, possibly due to a combination of genetic and dietary factors, and a lack of sunlight. Vitamin-D-dependent rickets, which can be due to 1-hydroxylase deficiency (type 1) or an end-organ receptor resistance to vitamin D (type 2), is inherited as an autosomal recessive condition. Familial hypophosphataemic rickets is inherited as an X-linked dominant condition, with a frequency of 1 in 25,000.

PATHOGENESIS / AETIOLOGY

Calciopenic causes include dietary calcium and vitamin D deficiency, malabsorption, lack of sunlight, hepatic disease, anti-convulsant treatment, renal disease, 1-α hydroxylase deficiency and end-organ resistance to vitamin D. Phosphopenic causes include Fanconi syndrome, X-linked hypophosphataemic rickets, renal tubular acidosis and oculo-cerebro-renal syndrome (Lowe syndrome).

DIAGNOSIS

This condition usually presents with bone deformity exhibiting different patterns, depending on the child's age at the onset of disease and the relative growth rate of different bones. In the first year of life, the most rapidly growing bones are the skull, the upper limbs and ribs. Rickets at this time presents with craniotabes, widening of the cranial sutures, frontal bossing, enlarged swollen epiphyses, particularly of the wrists, bulging of the costochondral joints (rachitic rosary) and a Harrison's sulcus.

After the first year of life, genu varum (13.40), genu valgum, abnormal dentition with enamel hypoplasia, bone pain and proximal myopathy are the dominant clinical features. In severe cases, tetany, laryngeal stridor, paraesthesiae and convulsions result from the hypocalcaemia. Growth failure is a common feature. Alopecia is a feature of Vitamin-D-dependent rickets type 2.

X-linked hypophosphataemic rickets usually presents in the male during late infancy with hypophosphataemia. Subsequently, untreated patients present with slow growth, bowing of the legs and a waddling gait. The clinical presentation is extremely variable, ranging from biochemical abnormalities to severe bony disease. Other features include poor dental development and abscesses of the teeth.

Biochemically, hypocalcaemia and hypophosphataemia may be present. The alkaline phosphatase level is high, while the 1,25-dihydroxy vitamin D level is low. The serum parathyroid hormone level may be high. Radiologically, widening of the growth plate and fraying, cupping and widening of the metaphyses occur. Pseudofractures and signs of secondary hyperparathyroidism may also be seen (e.g. sub-periosteal erosions). Other investigations may be abnormal, depending on the underlying cause (e.g. acidosis, aminoaciduria, chronic renal failure, anaemia).

TREATMENT

Calcium, phosphate and vitamin D are used in varying combinations, in an attempt to correct the clinical, radiological and biochemical abnormalities. Underlying abnormalities (e.g. coeliac disease) need appropriate treatment. Growth needs to be carefully monitored. In hypophosphataemic rickets, large doses of vitamin D are required. In patients with 1α-hydroxylase deficiency or end-organ resistance to vitamin D, 1,25-dihydroxy-cholecalciferol is usually required in significant doses. Regular renal ultrasound scanning is important.

PROGNOSIS

The prognosis for growth and cure of radiological and biochemical abnormalities is excellent in most children with rickets, provided that the condition is adequately treated. However, in hypophosphataemic rickets, the prognosis is less certain, and severe deformities of the limbs may result, particularly if compliance is poor.

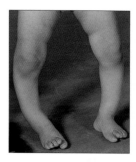

13.40 Rickets. Genu varum in a child.

GRAVES' DISEASE

INCIDENCE / GENETICS

Autoimmune thyrotoxicosis is six to eight times more common in girls. Often, a family history of autoimmune thyroid disease can be elicited.

PATHOGENESIS / AETIOLOGY

Thyroid-stimulating antibodies are present in the serum of these patients and are responsible for the clinical picture observed. Autonomous functioning thyroid nodules are rare in children, as is autonomous TSH production from the thyrotroph or pituitary tumours.

DIAGNOSIS

This can occur in preschool children, but there is a sharp increase in incidence in adolescence. The onset may be abrupt or insidious. Presenting features may include nervousness, palpitations, tremor, excessive perspiration, an increased appetite, muscle weakness, marked weight loss and behavioural abnormalities. Tachycardia, a widened pulse pressure, an overactive praecordium and heart failure may dominate the clinical picture. A goitre may be present, the size being variable (13.41). A bruit and a thrill may be features of the goitre. Eye signs of Graves' disease are variable. Severe Graves' ophthalmopathy is much less common in children than in adults. Malignant exophthalmos is virtually unknown.

Features in childhood include lid retraction, lid lag, exophthalmos proptosis (13.42), ophthalmoplegia, chemosis of the conjunctiva, pain, swelling and irritation. Graves' dermopathy, whereby there is accumulation of mucopolysaccharides in skin and subcutaneous tissues, is rare in children.

There may be evidence of other autoimmune conditions (e.g. vitiligo, Addison's disease, myasthenia, pernicious anaemia and insulin-dependent diabetes mellitus). Investigations of free thyroxine, free triiodothyronine and TSH levels (suppressed) are mandatory. A TRH test shows no TSH response to TRH, but is not necessary as newer TSH assays are highly sensitive. An auto-antibody screen may show thyroid-stimulating antibodies. Thyroid radioactive iodine uptake assessment is usually unnecessary, although an ultrasound scan may be required if a solitary nodule is suspected. The family should also be given thyroid function tests and an auto-antibody screen.

TREATMENT
Treatment entails reducing the secretory rate of thyroxine with the use of anti-thyroid medication such as carbimazole or propylthiouracil and blunting its effects using propranolol. The drugs have certain side-effects, and there may be a relapse once medication is stopped. In the long-term, definitive treatment in the form of a thyroidectomy may be indicated.

Complications of surgery include hypoparathyroidism and recurrent laryngeal nerve damage. Alternatively, radioactive iodine may be used and is easy to administer and cheap. To date, concern about radiation oncogenesis and genetic damage has limited its use to adolescents, although anxieties regarding the former have largely been alleviated in adults. Post-treatment hypothyroidism needs to be treated with thyroxine.

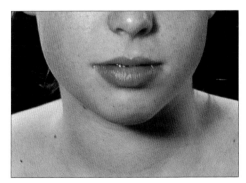

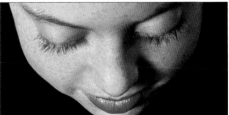

13.41 & 13.42 Graves' disease. Thyroid goitre and bilateral proptosis.

PROGNOSIS
Once definitive treatment has been performed, life-long thyroxine treatment is indicated. With this, the prognosis is good providing compliance is satisfactory. The course of the eye manifestations and the thyroid disease may differ, and exophthalmos may persist in spite of satisfactory treatment of the hyperthyroidism.

HYPOPARATHYROIDISM / PSEUDO-HYPOPARATHYROIDISM

INCIDENCE / GENETICS
When due to polyglandular autoimmune syndrome type I, hypoparathyroidism is inherited as an autosomal recessive condition. DiGeorge syndrome may be due to monosomy 22q11. In pseudohypoparathyroidism, inheritance is as an autosomal dominant, and the condition is rare.

DIAGNOSIS
Usual presentation for both conditions is with symptomatic hypocalcaemia. Children with hypoparathyroidism may present with symptoms and signs of hypocalcaemia *per se*. These include jitteriness, apnoeas in the neonatal period, convulsions, tetany, muscle cramps, laryngospasm, carpopedal spasm, positive Chvostek and Trousseau signs, neurodevelopmental delay, basal ganglia calcification and lenticular cataracts.

In DiGeorge syndrome, hypoparathyroidism is associated with thymic aplasia and consequent T-cell defects, congenital heart disease (especially truncus arteriosus) facial anomalies such as micrognathia, cleft lip and palate and ear malformations (**13.43**). (See also 'Immunology' chapter.)

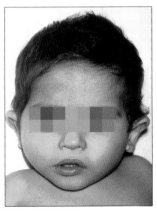

13.43 DiGeorge syndrome. Facial appearance of a child.

In pseudohypoparathyroidism, many of the children have neurodevelopmental delay and show unique somatic features, termed Albright's hereditary osteodystrophy. These include short stature, round facies (**13.44**), a short neck, obesity and subcutaneous calcification, especially near joints. A pathognomic feature of this condition is shortening of the fourth and fifth metacarpals and metatarsals (**13.45**). Symptoms of chronic hypocalcaemia may predominate, and include convulsions, cataracts and ectodermal changes such as dry, scaling skin and enamel hypoplasia.

In Albright's syndrome, hormonal resistance may be generalized and the clinical picture includes diabetes insipidus, hypogonadism and hypothyroidism. The condition is characterized biochemically by hypocalcaemia, hyperphosphataemia and reduced parathyroid hormone levels in hypoparathyroidism.

In pseudohypoparathyroidism, parathyroid hormone levels are elevated, and the diagnosis is confirmed by an inability to increase urinary cyclic AMP levels and phosphate excretion in response to an infusion of parathormone. A skeletal survey may help in the diagnosis, and reveals short metacarpals and metatarsals with ectopic subcutaneous calcification. Pseudopseudohypoparathyroidism refers to the phenotype associated with pseudohypoparathyroidism but with normal biochemistry.

PATHOGENESIS / AETIOLOGY
Hypoparathyroidism may be due to mutations in or near the PTH gene on chromosome 11, polyglandular autoimmune syndrome and post-surgery. DiGeorge syndrome is due to developmental defects of the structures which derive from the third and fourth pharyngeal pouches and branchial pouches. Pseudohypoparathyroidism is due to a mutation in the α-subunit of the G-protein coupled to the PTH receptor.

TREATMENT
Treatment is with calcium supplements and vitamin D, with close biochemical monitoring and regular renal ultrasound scans to detect nephrocalcinosis. In DiGeorge syndrome, recurrent infections need appropriate treatment as do cardiovascular abnormalities.

PROGNOSIS
In DiGeorge syndrome, the prognosis is dictated by the immunological and cardiovascular anomalies. In pseudohypoparathyroidism, mild to moderate neurodevelopmental delay is observed in 50–75% of cases. The prognosis in isolated hypoparathyroidism is very good, provided that the condition is not associated with chronic active hepatitis.

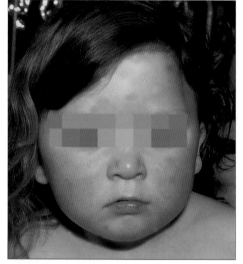

13.44 Pseudohypoparathyroidism. Characteristic facial appearance of a child.

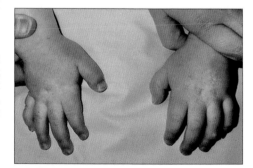

13.45 Pseudohypoparathyroidism. Clinical appearance of the hands with short fourth and fifth metacarpals.

WILLIAMS SYNDROME

See also 'Genetics' chapter.

INCIDENCE / GENETICS
The condition is due to a deletion or mutations in the elastin gene on chromosome 7q11.

PATHOGENESIS / AETIOLOGY
A genetic defect in the elastin gene is responsible for the diverse features of the condition.

DIAGNOSIS
Infantile hypercalcaemia is associated with neurodevelopmental delay, facial, cardiovascular, and other features in Williams syndrome. The facial features include a broad prominent forehead, a short and turned up nose with a flat nasal bridge, full cheeks and lips with a prominent overhanging upper lip, low- set ears, epicanthic folds and strabismus (**13.46, 13.47**). Dental anomalies are characteristic. Cardiovascular anomalies are present in 75% and include supravalvular aortic stenosis and peripheral pulmonary artery stenosis. Low birth weight, short stature, microcephaly, hoarse voice, hyperacusis and kyphoscoliosis are other features. Infantile hypercalcaemia usually resolves spontaneously.

Investigations reveal an elevated serum calcium level, a high normal phosphate level, low normal alkaline phosphatase and PTH level, and hypercalciuria. Radiographic features include increased density at the metaphyseal ends of the long bones, osteosclerosis of the base of the skull, nephrocalcinosis and soft tissue calcification. The pathogenesis of the hypercalcaemia remains unclear.

TREATMENT
The hypercalcaemia usually resolves spontaneously. A low calcium diet is indicated until the calcium level falls. If the calcium level is persistently elevated and leads to symptoms, prednisolone may be indicated. The cardiovascular abnormalities will also require treatment.

PROGNOSIS
The prognosis is determined by the cardiovascular anomalies and the neurodevelopmental delay. The outlook for the hypercalcaemia is good.

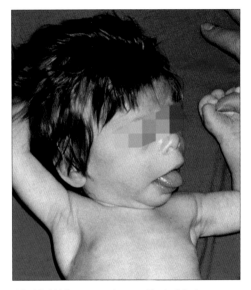

13.46 Williams syndrome. Typical facies in a child.

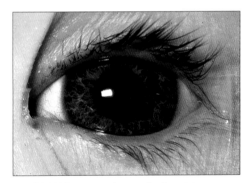

13.47 Williams syndrome. Stellate iris in a child.

HYPERINSULINISM

INCIDENCE / GENETICS

Persistent hyperinsulinaemic hypoglycaemia of infancy (PHHI) or nesidioblastosis has an incidence of approximately 1 in 50,000 births. The majority of cases are sporadic. Familial cases occur, and a genetic basis has been proposed to underlie these. Linkage analysis in these families has mapped the hyperinsulinism gene to chromosome 11p14-15.1. More recent studies have suggested that mutations in the sulphonylurea receptor gene, which has been mapped to 11p15.1, lead to inappropriate secretion of insulin in these children. Beckwith-Wiedemann syndrome is very rare. The majority of cases are sporadic, but an abnormal chromosome 11 has again been identified in this condition.

PATHOGENESIS / AETIOLOGY

A developmental abnormality in the β-cells in the Islets of Langerhans in the pancreas leads to an excessive secretion of insulin, with a consequent reduction in glycogenolysis, lipolysis and gluconeogenesis, all culminating in hypoglycaemia. Focal and diffuse forms exist.

DIAGNOSIS

The majority present within three days of birth with symptoms of neonatal hypoglycaemia. These include tremor, jitteriness, apnoea, hypotonia, feeding difficulties, convulsions and coma. Examination generally reveals macrosomia, plethora, chubby cheeks and generalized adiposity. Hepatomegaly is usually present. In the Beckwith-Wiedemann syndrome, hyperinsulinism is accompanied by other abnormal somatic features. These include exomphalos, macroglossia, visceromegaly, polycythaemia, hemi-hypertrophy and gigantism. Abnormalities of the ears are also present, and include transverse creases in the ear lobes.

The diagnostic investigation is a sample of blood drawn at the time of spontaneous or induced (by fasting) hypoglycaemia (blood glucose <2.6mmol/l). The insulin is inappropriately elevated, with decreased levels of free fatty acids, ketone bodies, glycerol and branched chain amino acids. Serum growth hormone and cortisol values are generally raised. An increased glucose requirement is also helpful in the diagnosis.

Other investigations include a urine organic acid screen taken at the time of hypoglycaemia. A glucagon provocation test leads to a large increase in blood glucose levels due to mobilization of excess glycogen stores to glucose. Infusion of somatostatin is useful as it suppresses insulin secretion and leads to an increase in blood glucose levels.

TREATMENT

The aim of treatment is to establish normoglycaemia by using infusions of glucose. Medical treatment consists of diazoxide in combination with chlorothiazide, or somatostatin. Diazoxide can lead to hypertrichosis lanuginosa (**13.48**). Surgical treatment is indicated for failure of medical treatment or unacceptable side-effects of medical treatment. The procedure of choice is 95% pancreatectomy in diffuse cases, with more conservative surgery in focal cases.

PROGNOSIS

In the past, the prognosis for neurological outcome was poor, with up to 50% of children suffering from neurodevelopmental delay. The risk for this is particularly marked because of the unavailability of ketone bodies as an alternative fuel for the brain starved of glucose. With early referral and diagnosis, there has been a considerable improvement in the outcome. Following a pancreatectomy, the patient may suffer from diabetes mellitus, characterized by an excessive sensitivity to insulin. Ketotic hyperglycaemia is very rare. Malabsorption may develop and requires treatment with exocrine pancreatic supplementation.

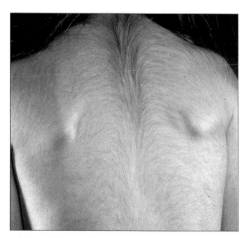

13.48 Hyperinsulinism. Diazoxide-induced hypertrichosis lanuginosa in a child.

INSULIN RESISTANCE SYNDROMES

INCIDENCE / GENETICS
There is a familial predisposition to the type A syndrome, and also in non-insulin-dependent diabetes mellitus.

PATHOGENESIS / AETIOLOGY
There is a resistance to insulin at the receptor level, although the underlying pathogenetic mechanism is unclear. In the type A syndrome, insulin receptor mutations may cause defects in receptor expression on the cell surface, or in the signalling capacity of the receptor. Similar mutations have been described in patients with leprechaunism and lipodystrophy.

DIAGNOSIS
The common form of the condition presents with obesity, but can occur in lean adolescent girls (type A syndrome). It is associated with acanthosis nigricans (**13.49, 13.50**), which is characterized by the presence of hyperkeratotic epidermal papillomatosis with increased melano-cytes, leading to hyperpigmented, velvety areas of skin predominantly in apposed and flexural regions (**13.49, 13.50**). In girls, the condition is associated with polycystic ovarian disease, where it is associated with hyperandrogenism leading to hirsutism. Patients may go on to develop glucose intolerance and hypertension.

Leprechaunism is an extreme form of the syndrome which is characterized by intrauterine growth retardation, dysmorphic facies, lipo-atrophy, acanthosis nigricans, and extreme insulin resistance (**13.51**). Affected newborn girls have cystic ovaries, hirsutism and clitoro-megaly. Lipoatrophy or lipodystrophy is also associated with insulin resistance and hyper-triglyceridaemia, as are obesity and non-insulin-dependent diabetes mellitus.

Fasting plasma glucose and lipid levels may be abnormal. A glucose tolerance test may reveal extremely high insulin levels with or without elevated glucose levels. In girls, a pelvic ultrasound scan may reveal polycystic ovaries.

TREATMENT
At present, the main form of treatment is dietary restriction with weight loss. Oral hypoglycaemic agents such as metformin may have a role to play. Severe insulin resistance, such as that observed in leprechaunism, may be extremely difficult to treat.

PROGNOSIS
There is an increased incidence of diabetes mellitus, hypertension and coronary heart disease with this condition.

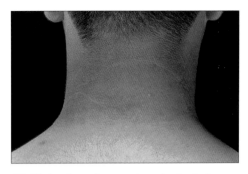

13.49 Insulin resistance. Acanthosis nigricans in the nuchal folds of a child.

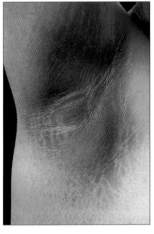

13.50 Insulin resistance. Acanthosis nigricans in the axillary folds of a child.

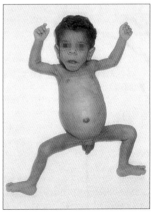

13.51 Leprechaunism in a child presenting with hyper-insulinism.

DIABETES MELLITUS

TYPE 1 DIABETES

Pathogenesis/aetiology

Absolute insulin deficiency results from auto-immune destruction of the beta cells in the pancreas. HLA-DR and -DQ alleles are associated with varying degrees of predisposition to, and protection against, the development of type 1 diabetes. However, 50% concordance rates for type 1 diabetes in monozygotic twins and a rapid increase in the incidence of type 1 diabetes over recent decades, suggest that as yet unidentified environmental factors moderate genetic risk.

Epidemiology

Type 1 diabetes is by far the commonest form of diabetes in childhood. Between 1990 and 1994, Sardinia, Finland, Sweden, Norway, Portugal, the United Kingdom, Canada and New Zealand were the countries in the world with the highest incidence of type 1 diabetes in childhood (>20/100,000 per year). The lowest incidence (<1/100,000 per year) was in populations from China and South America. An annual increase in incidence of 3.2% was reported in Europe between 1989 and 1998. The rate of increase is highest in young children. It has been suggested that this is attributable to earlier clinical manifestation rather than a global increase in disease incidence.

Presentation

The vast majority of children with type 1 diabetes will present with the classic triad of polydipsia, polyuria and weight loss. Diabetes may also present with secondary enuresis and recurrent infections. Children may present in diabetic keto-acidosis with vomiting, dehydration, abdominal pain, hyperventilation (Kussmaul's breathing), hypovolaemia and altered consciousness.

Necrobiosis lipoidica is a rare skin condition associated with diabetes, but not the level of glycaemic control. It is most commonly found on the shins and is characterized by yellow plaques with a violaceous border, which often scale, crust or ulcerate.

Rarely, a child may be found to have a high plasma glucose without having symptoms of diabetes, e.g. following the use of a family member's home blood-glucose monitoring kit. In this case diabetes should be confirmed by the presence of a fasting plasma glucose ≥ 7.0 mmol/l, or a 2-hour plasma glucose >11.0 mmol/l during a standard oral glucose tolerance test (OGTT). When performing these tests, results may be obtained that are outside normal limits, but which don't meet the requirements for diagnosis of diabetes. In this case, the diagnosis might be impaired fasting glycaemia, or impaired glucose tolerance.

Presymptomatic screening of at risk children, such as siblings, should not be undertaken, as it confers no benefit to the child and has the potential for psychological harm.

Essential investigations

The diagnosis can be confirmed by a random plasma glucose of >11.0 mmol/l. A urine dipstick test for ketonuria should also be undertaken as the absence of ketonuria might indicate type 2 diabetes or maturity onset diabetes of the young (MODY).

Glycated haemoglobin (HbA1c) reflects medium-term glycaemic control and predicts the risk of long-term complications. It should be checked 3 – 4 times a year. The target is less than 7.5%.

Home blood-glucose monitoring is used to guide insulin dose, using meters with a memory.

There is an increased risk of other auto-immune disorders, particularly coeliac disease and hypothyroidism. Screening for both of these conditions is recommended, as they can be asymptomatic with a significant morbidity if left untreated.

Management outline

The aim is to decrease the risk of microvascular complications without severe hypoglycaemia. Intensified treatment improves glycaemic control and delays the onset and slows the progression of microvascular complications, and also increases hypoglycaemia.

Many newly diagnosed children not in diabetic ketoacidosis may be managed initially at home, with support from the diabetes team, depending on age and absence of psychosocial difficulties. A vital part of initial management is education. This should include the aims of diabetes management in preventing complications, the basic physiology of glucose and insulin, the likely honeymoon phase, practical issues surrounding glucose monitoring and insulin injections, recognition and management of hypoglycaemia, management of intercurrent illness – including advice never to omit insulin, dietetic advice, advice on exercise including benefits and effects, psychological issues, Medicalert identification, available support services and emergency contact numbers. Adolescents need to be given information on smoking, alcohol and substance misuse. This education should continue after diagnosis, be adapted to a child's age, stage of diabetes, maturity, lifestyle and beliefs, as well as to the needs of individual parents. It should empower and motivate children and their families to make informed choices relating to diabetes management.

A multidisciplinary team, including a specialist paediatric diabetes nurse, consultant paediatrician and a paediatric dietitian, should provide the care of children with diabetes in designated diabetes clinics. There should also be easy access to psychology, podiatry and ophthalmology. Transfer to adult services should be planned with the young person and occur at a time of relative stability.

Home blood-glucose monitoring and a diary improve glycaemic control and reduce hypoglycaemia. New systems for continuous and non-invasive blood-glucose monitoring are being investigated and may improve the detection of asymptomatic hypoglycaemia.

Dietary advice should encourage 'healthy eating' with a reduction in highly refined foods, adequate carbohydrate intake and avoiding saturated fat. Carbohydrate counting is no longer advised. A number of other dietary approaches, such as the use of the glycaemic index, are untested in children. Knowledge of the glycaemic index of foods (rate of rise in blood glucose following carbohydrate ingestion) and the use of a low glycaemic index diet might reduce blood glucose variability, but has not yet been adequately researched in children. An active lifestyle is encouraged.

Children with diabetes have an increased risk of psychological problems, such as depression, eating and behavioural disorders, which are likely to have a significant impact on diabetes control. Psychological interventions in adolescents improve metabolic control. Social work support is sometimes needed.

Choice of insulin

Currently, only subcutaneous insulin is available, although inhaled and intranasal insulin are being developed. The injection technique should avoid intramuscular injection (with its risk of exercise-induced hypoglycaemia) or leakage of insulin from the skin. Injections should be rotated to avoid lipohypertrophy (**13.52**), which results in variable absorption. Lipoatrophy (**13.53**) is now rare with the available insulins.

Short-acting human insulin, or the recently available insulin analogues insulin aspart and lispro, with a faster action, are combined with intermediate-acting isophane insulin or long-acting insulin analogues, insulin glargine and detemir. Insulin is delivered either via needle and syringe, or via a pen device for which pre-mixed short- and intermediate-acting insulins are available. Two to four injections a day are used. In the former, a mixture of short and intermediate insulins are given before breakfast and tea. In the latter, a short-acting insulin is given before each main meal, with long-acting insulin before bed. In a three-injection regime, the lunchtime insulin is omitted and a mixture of short and intermediate insulin given before breakfast. Continuous subcutaneous short-acting insulin can be administered via a pump, which provides a fixed or variable basal dose and which delivers a bolus at mealtimes.

Guidelines for the management of diabetes have been produced by the Scottish Intercollegiate Guidelines Network and by the National Institute for Clinical Excellence.

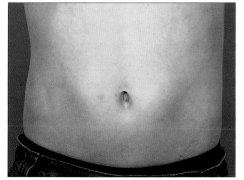

13.52 Lipohypertrophy in a boy who injected subcutaneously into his abdomen.

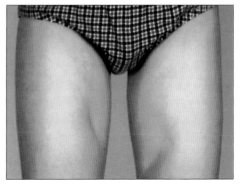

13.53 Lipoatrophy.

Short-term prognosis
Acute complications
The symptoms and signs of hypoglycaemia relate to autonomic activation (tremor, sweating) and neuroglycopaenia (irritability, headache, confusion, convulsions, coma). Although death is an extremely rare consequence of hypoglycaemia, severe hypoglycaemia may cause long-term neuropsychological impairment. The risks of hypoglycaemia need to be balanced against the benefits of good glycaemic control. Hypoglycaemia is treated with oral glucose followed by carbohydrate containing food or, if severe, with intramuscular glucagon or intravenous glucose.

Death from diabetes in childhood is rare (standardized mortality ratio 2.3 in the UK). Diabetic ketoacidosis is the commonest cause of death (implicated in over 80% of such cases), usually as a result of cerebral oedema, which has a mortality rate of 25% and a risk of developing severe neurological sequelae in over a third of survivors. Treatment of diabetic ketoacidosis includes rehydration with intravenous fluids, insulin and careful monitoring of fluid, electrolytes, blood glucose and neurological status.

Longer-term prognosis
Diabetes is the commonest cause of end-stage renal failure and of blindness in people of working age. Retinopathy and nephropathy surveillance (the former using a retinal camera with pupils dilated, the latter by testing for microalbuminuria) should be performed annually from 12 years of age. Both can be modified if identified early. Microalbuminuria precedes hypertension in nephropathy, but blood pressure should also be monitored regularly. Although the macrovascular complication of coronary heart disease is common in middle age, routine screening for elevated blood lipids is not recommended in childhood and adolescence. Regular podiatry reviews are important, to emphasize preventative foot care but are not likely to identify early manifestations of diabetic foot pathology. Cataracts can occur early, unrelated to the degree of glycaemic control. Other clinical manifestations of poor diabetes control include limited finger-joint mobility (**13.54**).

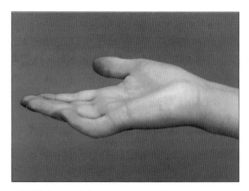

13.54 Limited finger-joint mobility.

Table 13.5 Comparisons between actions required for hypoglycaemia and hyperglycaemia

	Clinical state	Management principles
Hypoglycaemia	Conscious	Simple carbohydrate orally e.g. sugary drink. Then, complex carbohydrate orally e.g. biscuits. Unlikely to need hospital admission.
	Unconscious, fitting, or vomiting	Glucagon IM, or Hypostop PO, or, if IV access immediately available, 10% dextrose IV (5 mls/kg). May require hospital admission.
Hyperglycaemia	No vomiting and no ketonuria	'Sick day rules': frequent blood glucose monitoring, possible increase (or decrease in young children) in short-acting insulin dose. Usually can avoid hospital admission.
	Unwell, drowsy, vomiting or ketonuria	Admit to hospital. A, B, C assessment and resuscitation. Check blood gas and electrolytes. IV fluids to correct dehydration over 48hrs. IV insulin infusion. BEWARE: cerebral oedema; hypokalaemia

TYPE 2 DIABETES

Aetiology

This results from insulin resistance and a relative insulin deficiency when insulin secretion is insufficient to compensate for insulin resistance. Previously known as 'adult-onset' diabetes, type 2 diabetes is now occurring in childhood, particularly in some ethnic groups. These include American Indian, Canadian Indian, African American, Hispanic, Japanese, Pacific Island and Australian Aboriginal children. In the United Kingdom, type 2 diabetes is more common in children from Asian backgrounds, but has recently been reported in Caucasian children. Attempts have been made to calculate the prevalence of type 2 diabetes, but these studies have mainly been in clinic populations and are therefore likely to have underestimated the prevalence, as type 2 diabetes is often asymptomatic. Children are usually obese, are more likely to come from ethnic minority backgrounds, and usually have a stronger family history of diabetes than children with type 1 diabetes.

Presentation

Children may have acanthosis nigricans, a velvety thickening of the skin in the neck or axillae (**13.49, 13.50**) and symptoms or signs of polycystic ovarian disease (oligomenorrhoea, hirsutism), both of which are associated with insulin resistance.

Type 2 diabetes should be considered if the child is obese and particularly:
- is of Asian, American Indian, Canadian Indian, African American, Hispanic, Japanese, Pacific Island or Australian Aboriginal ethnic origin
- has a strong family history of type 2 diabetes
- has acanthosis nigricans
- has symptoms/signs of polycystic ovarian disease
- has no ketones in their urine at presentation or when hyperglycaemic
- has a prolonged honeymoon phase or no insulin requirement.

Some children with type 2 diabetes can present with ketonuria.

Essential Investigations
- Auto-antibodies (islet cell, insulin and GAD)
- insulin and c-peptide levels – fasting and during OGTT
- fasting lipid levels.

MATURITY ONSET DIABETES OF THE YOUNG (MODY)

Aetiology

A group of disorders characterised by autosomal dominant inheritance of a single gene defect resulting in pancreatic β-cell dysfunction. Diabetes often develops before the age of 25. Currently, six genes have been identified, which account for nearly 90% of MODY in the UK.

- HNF1α mutations account for 70%. The amount of insulin produced is normal in childhood but reduces with age. Diabetes usually develops during adolescence or the early twenties. Glycosuria may be present before diabetes due to a low renal threshold for glucose. Complications develop if the blood glucose is not controlled, and patients often need treatment with sulphonylureas and may go on to need insulin.
- Glucokinase acts as the body's 'glucose sensor' and controls insulin secretion. Mutations in the glucokinase gene account for nearly 15% and result in a higher set-point for glucose. It is very rare for people with glucokinase mutations to develop complications or require treatment other than dietary modulation. Although the resulting blood glucose abnormality is present from birth, it may not manifest for many years.
- HNF4α mutations account for only 3% and are similar in presentation and course to HNF1α.
- HNF1β mutations result in a syndrome known as Renal Cysts and Diabetes (RCAD), which accounts for 3%. Features include renal cysts that might be detected antenatally, genital tract malformation, early-onset non-insulin-dependent diabetes and hyperuricaemia with early-onset gout.
- Mutations in IPF1 and NeuroD1 each account for less than 1%.

Presentation

MODY should be considered if:
- the child has no ketones in their urine at presentation or when hyperglycaemic,
- or the child has a prolonged honeymoon phase, or no insulin requirement,
- and there is diabetes (insulin or non-insulin dependent) in one parent,
- or the child and one parent has persistent, stable, mild hyperglycaemia (fasting blood glucose 5.5–8 mmol/l), which might indicate a glucokinase mutation,

- or there is glycosuria in the presence of relatively normal blood glucose levels, suggesting an HNF1α mutation.

Essential investigations
Molecular genetic testing.

OTHER FORMS OF DIABETES
Diabetes may also be caused by genetic defects in insulin action (leprechaunism), diseases of the exocrine pancreas (cystic fibrosis), endocrinopathies (Cushing syndrome), drugs or chemicals (glucocorticoids) and infections (congenital rubella), and may also be associated with other genetic syndromes (Wolfram syndrome).

REFERENCES

Ambiguous genitalia
Warne GL, Zajac JD. Disorders of sexual differentiation. *Endocrinol Metab Clin N Am* 1998 27(4): 945–967.

The short child
Tanner JM, Lejarraga H, Cameron N. The natural history of the Silver-Russell syndrome: a longitudinal study of thirty-nine cases. *Ped Res* 1975; **9**: 611–623.

Turner syndrome
Saenger P. Turner syndrome. *N Engl J Med* 1996; **335**(23): 1749–1754.
Lippe B. Turner Syndrome. *Endocrinol Metab Clin N Am* 1991; **20**: 121–152.

Prader-Willi syndrome
Donaldson MDC, Chu CE, Cooke A *et al*. The Prader-Willi syndrome. *Arch Dis Childhood* 1994; **70**: 58–63.
Wharton RH, Loechner KJ. Genetic and clinical advances in Prader-Willi syndrome. *Curr Opin Paed* 1996; **8**(6): 618–624.

Skeletal dysplasias
Horton WA, Hecht JT, Hood OI *et al*. Growth hormone therapy in achondroplasia. *Am J Med Genet* 1992; **42**: 667–670.
Shiang R, Thompson LM, Zhu Y-Z et al. Mutations in the transmembrane domain of FGFR3 cause the most common genetic form of dwarfism, achondroplasia. *Cell* 1994; **78**: 335–342.
Rousseau F, Bonaventure J, Legcai-Mallet L *et al*. Mutations in the gene encoding fibroblast growth factor receptor-3 in achondroplasia. *Nature* 1994; **371**: 252–254.
Bellus GA, McIntosh I, Smith EA *et al*. A recurrent mutation in the tyrosine kinase domain of fibroblast growth factor receptor-3 causes hypochondroplasia. *Nature Genet* 1995; **10**: 357–359.

Growth hormone deficiency insufficiency
Rosenfeld RG, Albertsson-Wikland K, Cassorla F *et al*. Diagnostic controversy: the diagnosis of childhood growth hormone deficiency revisited. *J Clin Endocrinol Med* 1995; **80**: 1532–1540.
Hindmarsh PC, Brook CGD. Short stature and growth hormone deficiency. *Clin Endocrinol* 1995; **43**: 133–142.

Laron-type dwarfism
Rosenbloom AL, Guevara-Aguirre J. Lessons from the genetics of Laron syndrome. *Trends Endocrinol Metab* 1998 52(9/7): 276–283.
Rosenfeld RG, Rosenbloom AL, Guevara-Aguirre J. Growth hormone insensitivity due to primary GH receptor deficiency. *Endoc Rev* 1994; **15**: 369–390.

Tall stature
Dietz HC, Cutting GR, Pyeritz RE *et al*. Marfan syndrome caused by a recurrent *de novo* missense mutation in the fibrillin gene. *Nature* 1991; **352**: 337–339.
Tsipouras P, Del-Mastro R, Sarfarazi M *et al*. Genetic linkage of the Marfan syndrome, ectopia lentis, and congenital contractual arachnodactyly to the fibrillin genes on chromosomes 15 and 5. The International Marfan Syndrome Collaborative Study. *N Engl J Med* 1992; **326**: 905–909.

Pituitary gigantism
Hindmarsh PC, Brook CGD. Tall stature. In: Brook CGD (ed). *Clinical Paediatric Endocrinology* (3rd edn). Oxford: Blackwell Science, 1995: 195–209.

Early puberty
Bridges NA, Christopher JA, Hindmarsh PC, Brook CGD. Sexual precocity: sex incidence and aetiology. *Arch Dis Childhood* 1994; **70**: 116–118.

Premature thelarche/thelarche variant or 'benign' precocious puberty
Stanhope RG, Brook CGD. Thelarche variant: a new syndrome of precocious sexual development? *Acta Endocrinol* 1990; **123**: 481–486.
Salardi S, Cacciari E, Mainetti B, Mazzanti L, Pirazzoli P. Outcome of premature thelarche: relation to puberty and final height. *Arch Dis Childhood* 1998; **79**(2): 173–174.

Polycystic ovarian disease

Goudas VT, Dumesic DA. Polycystic ovary syndrome. *Endocrinol Metab Clin N Am* 1997; **26**(4): 893–912.

Bridges NA, Cooke A, Healy MJR, Hindmarsh PC, Brook CGD. Ovaries in sexual precocity. Clin Endocrinol 1995; 42: 135–140.

McCune-Albright syndrome

Weinstein LS, Shenker A, Gejman PV et al. Activating mutations of the stimulatory G-protein in the McCune-Albright syndrome. *N Engl J Med* 1991; **325**: 1688–1695.

Late puberty

Schibler D, Brook CGD, Kind HP, Zachmann M, Prader A. Growth and body proportions in 54 boys and men with Klinefelter syndrome. *Helv Paed Acta* 1974; **29**: 325–333.

Congenital hypothyroidism

Grant DB. Congenital hypothyroidism: optimal management in the light of 15 years' experience of screening. *Arch Dis Childhood* 1995; **72**: 85–90.

Tillotson SL, Fuggle PW, Smith I, Ades AE, Grant DB. Relation between biochemical severity and intelligence in early treated congenital hypothyroidism: a threshold effect. *BMJ* 1994; **309**: 440–445.

Acquired hypothyroidism

Delange F, Fisher DA. The Thyroid Gland. In: Brook CGD (ed). *Clinical Paediatric Endocrinology* (3rd edn). Oxford: Blackwell Science, 1995: 397–433.

Graves disease

Rivkees SA, Sklar C, Freemark M. The management of Graves' disease in children, with special emphasis on radioiodine treatment. *J Clin Endocrinol Metab* 1998; **83**(11): 3767–3775.

Primary adrenal insufficiency

Grant DB, Barnes ND, Moncrieff MW, Savage MO. Clinical presentation, growth and pubertal development in Addison's disease. *Arch Dis Childhood* 1985; **60**: 925–928.

Forest M. Adrenal Steroid Deficiency States. In: Brook CGD (ed). *Clinical Paediatric Endocrinology* (3rd edn). Oxford: Blackwell Science, 1995: 453–498.

Cushing syndrome

Newell-Price J, Trainer P, Besser M, Grossman A. The diagnosis and differential diagnosis of Cushing's syndrome and Pseudo-Cushing's states. *Endoc Rev* 1998; **19**(5): 647–672.

Congenital adrenal hyperplasia

New MI. Diagnosis and management of congenital adrenal hyperplasia. *Ann Rev Med* 1998; **49**: 311–328.

Rickets

Thacher TD, Fischer PR, Pettifor JM et al. A comparison of calcium, vitamin D, or both for nutritional rickets in Nigerian children. *N Engl J Med* 1999; **341**(8): 563–568.

Kruse K. Disorders of Calcium and Bone Metabolism. In: Brook CGD (ed). *Clinical Paediatric Endocrinology* (3rd edn). Oxford: Blackwell Science, 1995: 735–778.

Hypoparathyroidism/pseudohypoparathyroidism

Patten JL, Johns DK, Valle D et al. Mutation in the gene encoding the stimulatory G protein of adenylate cyclase in Albright's hereditary osteodystrophy. *N Engl J Med* 1990; **322**: 1412–1419.

Williams' syndrome

Ewart AK, Morris CA, Atkinson D et al. Hemizygosity at the elastin locus in a developmental disorder, Williams syndrome. *Nature Genet* 1993; **5**(1): 11–16.

Hyperinsulinism

Thomas PM, Cote GJ, Wohlik N et al. Mutations in the sulfonylurea receptor gene in familial persistent hyperinsulinaemic hypoglycaemia of infancy. *Science* 1995; **268**: 426–429.

Aynsley-Green A. The management of islet cell dysregulation syndromes in infancy and childhood. *Zeitschr Kinderchir* 1988; **43**: 267–272.

Insulin resistance syndromes

Tritos NA, Mantzoros CS. Syndromes of severe insulin resistance. *J Clin Endocrinol Metab* 1998; **83**(9): 3025–3030.

Diabetes mellitus

Karvonen M, Viik-Kajander M, Moltchanova E, Libman I, LaPorte R, Tuomilehto J. Incidence of childhood type 1 diabetes worldwide. Diabetes Mondiale (DiaMond)Project Group. *Diabetes Care* 2000 Oct; **23**(10):1516–1526.

Green A, Patterson CC; EURODIAB TIGER Study Group. Europe and Diabetes; Trends in the incidence of childhood-onset diabetes in Europe 1989–1998. *Diabetologia* 2001 Oct; 44 Suppl 3: B3–8.

Weets I, De Leeuw IH, Du Caju MV, Rooman R, Keymeulen B, Mathieu C, Rottiers R, Daubresse JC, Rocour-Brumioul D, Pipeleers DG, Gorus FK; Belgian Diabetes Registry. The incidence of type 1 diabetes in the age group 0-39 years has not increased in Antwerp (Belgium) between 1989 and 2000: evidence for earlier disease manifestation; *Diabetes Care* 2002 May; 25(5): 840–6.

www.sign.ac.uk. Management of diabetes. SIGN publication number 55.

www.nice.org. Type 1 diabetes; diagnosis and management of type 1 diabetes in children and young people. Publication reference CG15.

Edge JA, Ford-Adams ME, Dunger DB. Causes of death in children with insulin dependent diabetes 1990–96. *Arch Dis Child* 1999; 81: 318–323.

www.bsped.org.uk. Julie Edge. Guidelines for the Management of Diabetic Ketoacidosis. British Society for Paediatric Endocrinology and Diabetes.

Rosenbloom AL, Joe JR, Young RS, Winter WE. Emerging epidemic of type 2 diabetes in youth. *Diabetes Care* 1999 Feb; **22**(2): 345–354.

Ehtisham S, Barrett TG, Shaw NJ. Type 2 diabetes mellitus in UK children – an emerging problem. *Diabet Med* 2000 Dec; **17**(12): 867–71.

Ehtisham S, Hattersley AT, Dunger DB, Barrett TG. British Society for Paediatric Endocrinology and Diabetes Clinical Trials Group; First UK survey of paediatric type 2 diabetes and MODY. *Arch Dis Child* 2004 Jun; **89**(6):526–529.

Metabolic Diseases
Callum Wilson

ADRENOLEUKODYSTROPHY

CLINICAL PRESENTATION

Adrenoleukodystrophy (ALD) is a peroxisomal disorder with a variable phenotype. The most severe form is childhood onset cerebral ALD (COCALD) (approximately 50% of those affected). They typically present between the ages of 6 and 8 years with progressive neurological impairment. This may manifest as behavioural problems or deterioration in school performance. Alternatively they may present with an adrenal crisis. Approximately 25% of patients present in early adult life with evidence of spinal cord and peripheral nerve involvement; this form is known as adrenomyeloneuropathy or AMN. About 8–10% may have only Addison's disease; the child is abnormally tanned and a Synacthen® test reveals the adrenal insufficiency. A smaller number may remain entirely asymptomatic.

INVESTIGATIONS

The finding of elevated plasma very-long-chain fatty acids (VLCFAs) and in particular the C26:22 and C24:22 ratios, in the presence of suggestive clinical features, is diagnostic. Once the diagnosis has been confirmed, the extent of the illness must be assessed. Neuropsychometric testing, nerve conduction studies, MRI brain (14.1), visual and hearing assessment and a Synacthen® test are all required.

BIOCHEMISTRY / GENETICS

ALD is an X-linked disorder caused by a defect in a peroxisomal transmembrane transporter protein. This leads to defective oxidation of VLCFAs, that is, fatty acids with carbon chains lengths of 24 and 26. The exact pathogenesis of this condition is unclear. The condition is not fully recessive and women are at risk of symptoms in adulthood.

TREATMENT

Cortisol and fludrocortisone are used to manage the adrenal insufficiency. Lorenzo's Oil, which is a mixture of mono-unsaturated fatty acids, normalizes the plasma VLCFA level in many patients and may, in some, improve the neurological outcome. A number of alternative medical therapies, which also appear to improve the biochemistry, are currently undergoing trial.

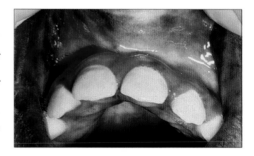

14.2 Pigmentation of the buccal mucosa in a ALD patient with Addison's disease.

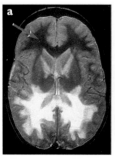
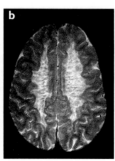

14.1 MRI scan showing moderately advanced leukodystrophy in a boy with COCALD (**a**). This pattern of severe temporal and parieto-occipital involvement is typical for ALD. In contrast, (**b**) shows the more diffuse white matter involvement seen in metachromatic leukodystrophy.

Bone marrow transplantation (BMT) is currently the only successful treatment. If performed early, it can reverse the neuropathology. However, it needs to be performed before there is significant neurological impairment, due to the risks involved in this procedure it is only indicated in early COCALD.

PROGNOSIS

The prognosis of COCALD without BMT is very poor. Once neurological regression has commenced there is rapid progression to a decorticate state over a period of months to years. Death usually occurs after a few years. With BMT the prognosis is much improved although long term follow-up studies are not available. The prognosis for AMN is less clear

See also 'Endocrinology' chapter.

GAUCHER DISEASE

CLINICAL PRESENTATION

Gaucher disease is a heterogeneous disorder which can present at any time from birth (with hydrops fetalis) to adulthood. The severe form of the disease, the acute neuronopathic infantile (type 2) disorder, presents with a rapidly progressive neurodegeneration in the first year of life. They have marked hepatosplenomegaly and go on to develop the classical signs of trismus, strabismus and opisthotonos.

The most common form of the disease, the non-neuronopathic or type 1 form, can present at any age with a range of symptoms. These include asymptomatic hepatosplenomegaly, and in children, growth failure or failure to thrive. The type 3 or subacute neuronopathic form has similar features to type 1, but affected patients initially also have a subtle oculomotor apraxia and slowly progressive neurological disease.

INVESTIGATIONS / DIAGNOSIS

The diagnosis is often made by the finding of the classical foamy 'wrinkled tissue-paper' Gaucher cell in a bone marrow aspirate (**14.3**). The enzyme chitotriosidase, which is markedly elevated in blood in Gaucher disease, can be used as a screening test and to monitor treatment. Confirmation of the disease is by enzyme analysis in leukocytes or fibroblasts. All patients need to be monitored. Baseline bloods, abdominal ultrasound, MRI brain, chest x-ray, skeletal survey (**14.4**), visual and neurological assessment may all be needed in varying combinations.

BIOCHEMISTRY / GENETICS

The disease is caused by deficiency of the lysosomal enzyme glucocerebrosidase, leading to an accumulation of glucosylceramide. Prenatal diagnosis can be offered. Mutation analysis is available. However, with a few exceptions, there is no genotype/phenotype correlation.

TREATMENT

Enzyme replacement therapy (fortnightly intravenous infusion) is the treatment of choice in type 1 and 3 disease. Bone marrow transplantation is also effective but carries significant morbidity. The bone disease may be treated with bisphosphonates. Supportive therapy is all that is available for the acute neuronopathic form of the disease.

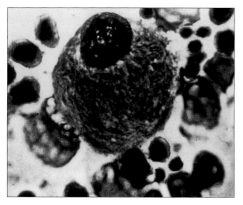

14.3 Typical appearance of a Gaucher cell in bone marrow.

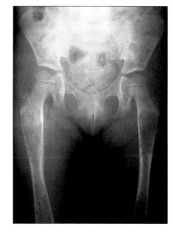

14.4
Severe bony involvement of the proximal femurs in a patient with Gaucher disease.

PROGNOSIS

The prognosis for the non-neuronopathic form of the disease is generally favourable. The long term prognosis for the subacute neurological disease in type 3 disease is still unclear.

See also 'Blood Diseases' chapter.

HURLER'S DISEASE

CLINICAL PRESENTATION

Hurler's disease is the prototype of a group of disorders collectively known as the mucopolysaccharidoses (MPS). Children with Hurler's disease usually present in infancy with failure to attain normal developmental milestones. Affected children have hepatomegaly, thickened skin, macrocephaly and the classical 'coarse' facial features of mucopolysaccharidoses (MPS). A bone dysplasia known as 'dysostosis multiplex' is evident radiologically and later becomes obvious clinically with short stature, 'claw-like' hands (14.5), a lumbar gibbus and joint contractures. Children often have corneal clouding at presentation (14.6) although other well described features such as deafness, cardiac valvular disease and carpal tunnel disease are typically seen later. A mild variant of the disorder, Scheie's disease, presents in late childhood with similar physical problems but without cognitive impairment.

INVESTIGATIONS/DIAGNOSIS

Measurement of urine glycosaminoglycans (GAGs) is the screening test of choice for suspected MPS disease. Children with Hurler's disease have an increased secretion of dermatan sulphate and heparan sulphate. The diagnosis can then be confirmed by measurement of enzyme activity in leukocytes. There is useful genotype phenotype correlation, which aids selection of patients for BMT.

The extent and severity of disease needs to be established in all children with MPS. A skeletal survey including neck views, MRI brain, neurological, visual and audiological assessment and cardiac echo are all required.

BIOCHEMISTRY/GENETICS

Hurler's disease is caused by a defect in the gene coding for α-L-iduronidase, a lysosomal enzyme essential for the degradation of GAGs (glycosaminoglycans). They are important structurally in the extracellular matrix.

TREATMENT

Until recently, treatment focused on identifying and treating the various complications of the disease. This included the obstructive respiratory disease, instability of the cervical vertebrae, cardiac disease, carpal tunnel syndrome, sleep disturbances and visual and hearing impairment.

Bone marrow transplantation (BMT) significantly slows the progression of the disease although it does not reverse bone or neurological disease. Recent trials suggest enzyme replacement therapy will become an important adjunct to treatment in the future.

PROGNOSIS

The prognosis for classic Hurler's is poor, with progressive and severe neurodevelopmental regression. Death usually occurs before the age of 10 years from cardiac, respiratory or neurological causes. Following BMT, disease progression is slowed down and some features are reversed, though not completely.

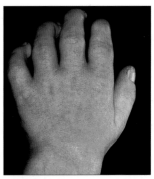

14.5 Typical 'claw' hand of MPS disease

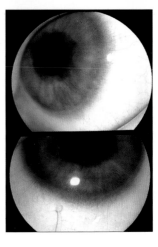

14.6 Corneal clouding in a patient with Hurler's disease.

UREA CYCLE DISORDERS

CLINICAL PRESENTATION

The disorders often present with lethargy, poor feeding, apnoea and encephalopathy in the neonatal period. These symptoms are usually initially mistaken for sepsis. Ammonia is a respiratory stimulant and a respiratory alkalosis may be found early in the illness.

Older children with milder disease present with variable symptoms. These can range from episodic nausea, vomiting and behavioural changes to encephalopathy. There may be a history of protein intolerance. On examination there may be hepatomegaly but few other diagnostic clues. In the most common condition, ornithine transcarbamylase deficiency (OTC) there is frequently a family history of neonatal male deaths.

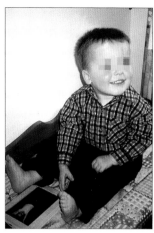

14.7 Three-year-old boy with the urea-cycle disorder citrullinaemia. He has short stature and failure to thrive secondary to his restrictive diet and recurrent episodes of illness. He is of normal intelligence.

DIAGNOSIS / INVESTIGATIONS

The key investigation is the plasma ammonia. Ammonia is often falsely elevated but a concentration greater than 200 µmol/l in neonates and 100 µmol/l in older children is highly suspicious of a metabolic condition. Plasma amino acids and urine organic acids are urgent to establish the diagnosis. Further tests to confirm this are essential.

BIOCHEMISTRY / GENETICS

The urea cycle converts toxic ammonia to urea. Deficiencies in the enzymes of this cycle result in hyperammonemia. OTC is an X-linked condition that is frequently fatal in boys. All other disorders, for instance citrullinaemia and arginosuccinic aciduria (ASA), are autosomal recessive.

TREATMENT

Seek expert advice and transfer to a metabolic centre. Ammonia is neurotoxic and lowering the plasma concentration is essential. In general, stopping the normal feeds and commencing intravenous 10% dextrose is recommended. The sick neonate will frequently require haemofiltration. Sodium benzoate and sodium phenylbutyrate lower the ammonia by conjugating with amino acids and reducing the nitrogen load. Likewise arginine is used in ASA. Once the situation has stabilized, protein is gradually reintroduced. The long-term management of these patients includes a high calorie, low protein diet and the use of the nitrogen removing medications. Metabolic control is monitored with plasma amino acids.

PROGNOSIS

The outcome often depends on the severity of the initial presentation. Children who presented in the neonatal period with severe encephalopathy will frequently die and those that survive will invariably have some degree of neurodevelopmental delay. Once treated, children will have further episodes of metabolic decompensation, especially during periods of intercurrent illness. Children who present later may do remarkably well (**14.7**) but the outcome is often dependent on the speed of diagnosis. Prenatal testing is available.

GALACTOSAEMIA

CLINICAL PRESENTATION

Classically, these children present in the early neonatal period with jaundice, vomiting, and lethargy. They are often initially thought to have sepsis. If the lactose (galactose) containing feeds are stopped and antibiotics started, the children improve. The frequent finding of an E coli-positive blood culture may confuse the diagnosis. When milk feeds are reintroduced the child becomes unwell again. Children may present in infancy with failure to thrive (**14.8**) and vomiting. Hepatomegaly and jaundice are present on examination and there is usually biochemical evidence of liver dysfunction. Cataracts are characteristically present (**14.9**).

DIAGNOSIS / INVESTIGATIONS

Positive urine reducing substances can suggest the diagnosis although this is a poor test as 'sick' neonates will often have a positive test and galactosaemia patients will have a negative test if not receiving galactose. Direct measurement of the enzyme galactose-1-phosphate uridyl-transferase (Gal-1-PUT) in red blood cells is diagnostic. The parents of affected children will have Gal-1-PUT levels in the heterozygotes range and this is useful in diagnosing the infant who has received a recent blood transfusion. All affected children should have their eyes examined and their renal tubular and liver function assessed. Prenatal testing is available.

BIOCHEMISTRY / GENETICS

The disease is autosomal recessive and is caused by a deficiency in the enzyme galactose-1-phosphate uridyl transferase. Lactose, the disaccharide in breast, formula and cows' milk is made up of galactose and glucose, and it is the metabolites of galactose which are toxic.

TREATMENT

Eliminate galactose (i.e. lactose) in the diet. Essentially this means switching to a soya-based formula and later a dairy-products-free and 'minimal galactose foods' diet. Galactose is present in many processed foods; these should also be avoided. Calcium supplements are usually needed.

PROGNOSIS

Death from liver failure or sepsis is seen if the patient remains on a lactose diet. With treatment, however, the immediate prognosis is generally good, although early feeding problems and speech delay due to an oral-motor dyspraxia are common. Older children and adults have problems with verbal planning and 'concepts' in mathematics and science. Motor function, co-ordination and balance may also be affected. Women usually have hypergonadotrophic hypogonadism and are infertile. The cataracts are reversible if treatment is started early.

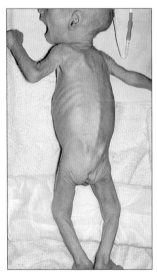

14.8 Severe failure to thrive seen in a late-diagnosed patient with galactosaemia.

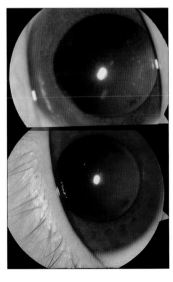

14.9 'Oil-drop' cataracts seen in the condition.

FATTY ACID OXIDATION DEFECTS

CLINICAL PRESENTATION

Children with fatty acid oxidation defects (FAOD's) frequently present with encephalopathy. They are often hypoglycaemic and there may be evidence of hepatic dysfunction. Usually there is a history of a preceding viral-like illness and a period of catabolic stress such as a missed meal. There is often little to find on examination apart from some hepatomegaly. 'Found dead in bed' during an intercurrent illness is unfortunately also a relatively common presentation. Muscle preferentially oxidizes fat as an energy source, so alternative presentations are with cardio-myopathy, especially in infancy, or with myopathy as an adult.

DIAGNOSIS / INVESTIGATIONS

The finding of hypoglycaemia with inappropriately low ketones (urine or blood) is suggestive of a FAOD.

There may be acidosis, transaminaemia, an elevated CK and/or hyperammonaemia. The specific disorder can usually be diagnosed on the acylcarnitine profile (**14.10**). This is a simple test using a blood spot on a Guthrie card. Confirmation of the diagnosis is by fatty acid oxidation studies of fibroblasts (skin biopsy and culture) or in MCAD and LCHAD by looking for the common mutations.

BIOCHEMISTRY / GENETICS

There are a series of enzymes necessary for the oxidation of fat to ketones and energy. The most common condition is medium-chain acyl-co-A dehydrogenase (MCAD) deficiency. The FAODs are inherited in an autosomal recessive fashion and a molecular diagnosis is usually possible.

TREATMENT

Avoid catabolism. The patient, parents and doctor need to understand that that the child must not be subjected to significant catabolic stress, especially during periods of intercurrent illness. If the child is unwell, they should take a high calorie carbohydrate drink 2–4 hourly until well (the 'emergency regime'). If they are not tolerating this, or if there are any other concerns, then they should be admitted to their local hospital. Carnitine supplements may be useful in some of the conditions, while avoidance of long-chain fats and regular feeds are necessary in the long-chain disorders.

PROGNOSIS

Once diagnosed and treated, the prognosis is generally favourable. Many children, however, die or suffer significant morbidity, prior to diagnosis.

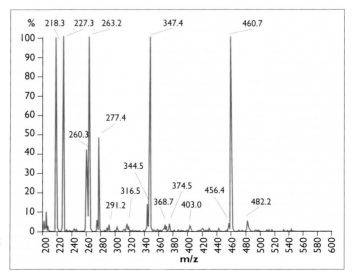

14.10 Acylcarnitine profile of a patient with MCAD deficiency showing the characteristic peak of octanylcarnitine at 344.5.

TYROSINAEMIA

CLINICAL PRESENTATION

Tyrosinaemia, or more correctly tyrosinaemia type 1, often presents as 'acute' neonatal liver failure with jaundice, a coagulopathy, failure to thrive and often sepsis. These children are often very sick and prior to NTBC the mortality was high. Alternatively, the 'chronic' presentation is in later infancy with failure to thrive, rickets (**14.11**) (due to renal tubular dysfunction) and liver dysfunction (**14.12, 14.13**). Other problems include neurological crises with porphyria-like pain and paraesthesia, renal failure and hepatocarcinoma.

DIAGNOSIS / INVESTIGATIONS

The presence of elevated levels of succinyl-acetone in the urine organic acids is diagnostic.

BIOCHEMISTRY/GENETICS

The defect is in the enzyme fumarylaceto-acetase, the last enzyme in the breakdown of the amino acids phenylalanine and tyrosine. The 'upstream' metabolites are alkylating agents and are thought to be responsible for the hepatorenal damage. Decreased activity of fumarylacetoacetase in fibroblasts or lympho-cytes, in the presence of the classical bio-chemical and clinical features, confirms the diagnosis. The disorder is recessive.

TREATMENT

Normal feeds should be stopped and the hepatorenal dysfunction and rickets treated as indicated. Prior to 1991, the only successful long-term treatment of tyrosinaemia type I was liver transplantation but, with the advent of NTBC (2-(2-nitro-4-trifluoromethylbenzoyl)-1,3-cyclohexanedione) – a potent inhibitor of the up-stream enzyme 4-hydroxyphenyl-pyruvate dioxygenase, effective treatment is now available. NTBC prevents the 'toxic' metabolites forming and is effective in both the acute and chronic forms of the disease. A dose of 1 mg/kg/day is recommended. Because the children still have a 'metabolic block', they require a low phenylalanine and tyrosine diet with a supplementary phenylalanine/tyrosine free amino acid formula. Growth, tyrosine levels and residual liver damage all need to be monitored, including liver imaging for hepatoma.

PROGNOSIS

Provided there is no substantial liver damage or malignant transformation, the long-term prognosis is likely to be excellent.

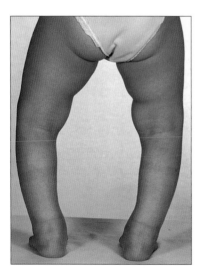

14.11 Tyrosinaemia: involvement of the bones (rickets) is seen in untreated tyrosinaemia.

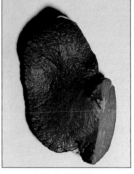

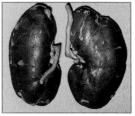

14.12 & 14.13 Tyrosinaemia: involvement of the liver (left) and kidneys (below).

GLYCOGEN STORAGE DISEASE TYPE 1

CLINICAL PRESENTATION

Children with glycogen storage disease type 1 (GSD1) usually present in infancy with failure to thrive, abdominal distention and/or signs and symptoms of hypoglycaemia. The later can occur after a short fast, yet the child, especially in early infancy, may surprisingly be asymptomatic. On examination there is often massive hepatomegaly (**14.14**), truncal obesity, short stature, mild hypotonia and a 'doll-like' face.

DIAGNOSIS / INVESTIGATIONS

There is often a significant lactic acidosis that decreases with feeding. Hypertriglyceridaemia and hyperuricaemia are also characteristically present. These findings, along with the typical clinical appearance, are highly suggestive of GSD1 and the diagnostic investigation is now molecular analysis rather than a liver biopsy for enzymology.

BIOCHEMISTRY / GENETICS

GSD1a is caused by a deficiency of glucose-6-phosphatase. A transport protein, responsible for the transport of glucose-6-phosphate, is defective in GSD1b. This disorder is associated with neutropenia and immune deficiency. Molecular analysis has recently become available for both GSD 1a and 1b.

TREATMENT

Maintaining normal glucose homeostasis is the key and is likely to greatly reduce the long-term complications. This is achieved by the use of frequents daytime oral feeds and a continuous overnight feed via a nasogastric tube or gastrostomy. Specialist dietary input is essential. After the age of 2 years, uncooked cornstarch may be used. Allopurinol lowers uric acid levels while GCSF can improve the neutropenia seen in GSD1b. Long term management also includes the regular monitoring of the biochemistry (lactate, triglycerides and glucose profiles), growth, renal function, liver (ultrasound for adenomas) and bone mineralization status.

PROGNOSIS

Adults who have had relatively poorly controlled disease frequently have the complications of short stature, renal disease, osteoporosis and liver adenomas. The latter may become malignant. It is hoped the current treatment guidelines will greatly reduce the frequency and severity of these complications. It is likely that there is a good correlation between metabolic control (i.e. normoglycaemia) and outcome.

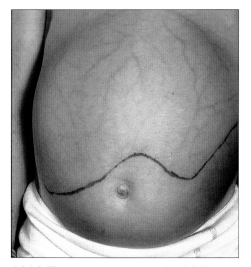

14.14 The massive hepatomegaly of GSD 1.

PEROXISOMAL BIOGENESIS DISORDERS

CLINICAL PRESENTATION

Peroxisomal biogenesis disorders (PBD) are a group of disorders which include the phenotypes Zellweger's, neonatal adrenoleukodystrophy and infantile Refsum's disease. The most severe form, Zellweger's, presents at birth with severe hypotonia, hepatomegaly and the characteristic features of a prominent forehead, huge anterior fontanelle and stippled epiphiseal calcification (**14.15**). The much milder infantile Refsum's disease presents with subtle facial features and developmental delay in early childhood. They may have autistic features and/or seizures.

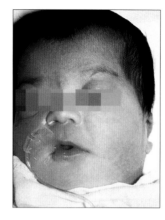

14.15
Typical facial appearances of Zellweger syndrome.

INVESTIGATIONS / DIAGNOSIS

Elevation of the very-long-chain fatty acids (VLCFA's) is the key diagnostic investigation. This finding establishes the broad diagnosis although measurement of plasma bile acids, red cell plasmalogens and fibroblast enzyme analysis is needed to further elucidate the aetiology.

Liver and renal function are often impaired in these patients and need to be assessed.

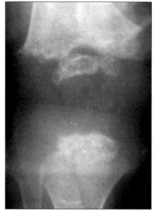

14.16
Radiograph showing the punctate calcification seen in peroxisomal disorders.

BIOCHEMISTRY / GENETICS

Peroxisomal biogenesis disorders are caused by a failure of protein (enzyme) import into the peroxisome. A variety of gene defects can result in the same phenotype (locus heterogeneity) and yet the various phenotypes can also be allelic. In addition there are single enzyme peroxisomal disorders which can give rise to an infantile Refsum's-like phenotype. All the conditions are inherited in an autosomal recessive manner, and mutation analysis is currently available on a research basis.

TREATMENT

There is no specific treatment for these disorders.

PROGNOSIS

The prognosis for the severe Zellweger's form of the disease is very poor, with death usually in the first year of life. Children with infantile Refsum's can live much longer with very little disease progression.

LEIGH SYNDROME

CLINICAL PRESENTATION
Leigh syndrome (LS) is a neurodegenerative disease characterized clinically by neurological regression and basal ganglia and brainstem dysfunction. The course of the illness is unpredictable although the onset is frequently in infancy and may coincide with an intercurrent illness. The child may present acutely with encephalopathy or a stroke-like illness. Alternatively, there may be no clear onset of symptoms or there are non-specific symptoms such as failure to thrive and developmental delay.

The children usually have evidence of basal ganglia dysfunction on examination, with variable combinations of abnormal eye movements, dysarthria, dystonia, ataxia and cognitive delay present. They are not dysmorphic and there is normally no significant hepatomegaly.

INVESTIGATIONS / DIAGNOSIS
While LS remains a neuropathological diagnosis, the characteristic clinical features, typical radiological findings of basal ganglia and brainstem lesions and the frequent finding of an elevated blood and/or CSF lactate, allow a diagnosis to be made *ante mortem* in most patients (**14.17**). A muscle biopsy for histology, histochemistry and respiratory chain enzymology will often help to confirm the diagnosis.

Other causes of neurodegenerative disease should also be considered.

BIOCHEMISTRY / GENETICS
Recent studies have demonstrated a molecular or biochemical defect of the pyruvate dehydrogenase complex (PDHC) or of the mitochondrial respiratory chain complexes in up to 75% of patients with definitive LS. The genetics of the condition are complex. While the majority of defects are likely to be inherited in an autosomal recessive manner, some forms of LS are caused by mutations in the mitochondrial genome and thus genetic counselling is difficult. Many of the nuclear genes for mitochondrial disease are now being identified and, depending on the exact enzyme defect (i.e. which complex of the respiratory chain), mutational analysis may be possible.

TREATMENT
There is no curative therapy so treatment is generally supportive. Episodes of decompensation during intercurrent illness should be prevented as far as possible.

This may require early admission to hospital and the administration of intravenous dextrose to prevent catabolic stress. A variety of vitamins and other medications are used in mitochondrial disease with anecdotal reports of their benefit.

PROGNOSIS
The long-term prognosis is generally poor although there may be long periods (i.e. many years) of stability. Children who present in early infancy can be expected to have a very poor prognosis.

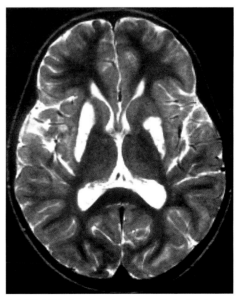

14.17 MRI showing changes typical of Leigh syndrome, with involvement of the lentiform nuclei bilaterally.

MENKE'S DISEASE

CLINICAL PRESENTATION
Menke's disease is a disorder of copper transport which, in the classic form, causes severe neurological disease. Apart from neonatal jaundice, children are usually relatively normal during early infancy but develop symptoms of poor feeding. vomiting and failure to thrive at 2–4 months (**14.18**). Seizures and developmental delay are often the presenting features. Neurological regression is rapid, with a wide range of symptoms reported. Seizures are often difficult to control. Death is usually within the first 2 years of life.

The facial appearance is highly characteristic, with a pale complexion, sagging jowls, wide nasal bridge and abnormal hair. The hair is striking; it is lustreless, brittle and has an unkempt appearance (**14.19**). Microscopically it shows pili torti. Menke's patients, because of the role of copper in elastin and collagen synthesis, can also have problems with joint laxity, bladder diverticulum and rupture, arterial bleeds and bony abnormalities. These features are also seen in the milder forms of the disease such as the occipital horn syndrome (Ehlers-Danlos IX).

INVESTIGATIONS / DIAGNOSIS
The clinical features are usually highly suggestive, and the subsequent finding of low serum copper and caeruloplasmin establishes the diagnosis. Copper uptake and release studies in fibroblasts are usually performed to confirm this. Blood for DNA should also be obtained, as mutational analysis is also available and is important for future prenatal testing.

BIOCHEMISTRY / GENETICS
Menke's disease is caused by a defect in copper transmembrane transporter that results in enhanced uptake but decreased efflux in intestinal and renal tubular cells. This results in an increased concentration of copper in these areas but a deficiency elsewhere. This deficiency affects copper-containing enzymes such as cytochrome oxidase and lysyl oxidase, essential in cellular energy production and collagen/elastin synthesis respectively. The disease is inherited as an X-linked recessive trait.

TREATMENT / PROGNOSIS
Treatment is palliative, as with any child with seizures and a rapidly progressive neurological condition. Intravenous or subcutaneous copper histidinate therapy may be partially successful if started very early (less than one month old) although these children still have a significant morbidity, with a severe connective tissue disorder and mild developmental delay.

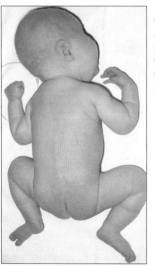

14.18 Infant with Menke's disease who presented with failure to thrive and seizures.

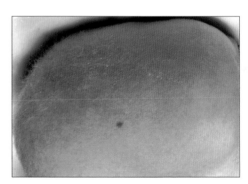

14.19 The short, brittle hair of Menke's disease.

WILSON'S DISEASE

See also 'Gastroenterology' chapter.

CLINICAL PRESENTATION

The presentation of Wilson's disease is variable, with two main phenotypes described. Sometimes patients will present with features of both. The hepatic presentation rarely occurs before mid-childhood and ranges from asymptomatic hepatomegaly to acute severe liver failure. An acute or chronic hepatitis is probably the most common liver problem. Wilson's disease therefore must be ruled out in any child with liver disease. A coexisting haemolytic anaemia can occasionally be the presenting feature.

The neurological presentation is unusual in childhood. The neurological disease in teenagers affects motor function, with symptoms of dysarthria, poor coordination, involuntary movements and dystonia. They may also present with poor school performance, behavioural and psychiatric problems.

Clinically, patients may have features of liver disease such as jaundice, spider naevi (**14.20**), palmar erythema and hepatosplenomegaly. Neurological signs include increased tone, basal ganglia signs and an abnormal gait.

The classic sign of Kayser-Fleischer rings should also be looked for. They are seen in the outer margin of the cornea as a reddish-brown ring and represent deposition of copper in the Descemet membrane. While apparent on slit-lamp examination in all patients with neurological disease and in most patients with hepatic disease, they are not easy to distinguish with the naked eye.

INVESTIGATIONS / DIAGNOSIS

The diagnosis of Wilson's disease can be difficult, especially in established hepatic disease. Simple tests such as plasma caeruloplasmin (low in Wilson's disease), serum copper (marginally low) and an elevated 24-hour urinary copper after penicillamine are helpful but are neither sensitive nor specific. A liver biopsy for copper content is required if the diagnosis is likely. A normal value rules out Wilson's disease while a high level, in the absence of significant liver disease, confirms the diagnosis. 'Non-Wilson's' liver disease can also lead to elevated hepatic copper and this makes the diagnosis difficult in the child with established liver disease. A copper isotope study may be useful in these patients. Molecular methods may make the diagnosis easier in the future. All patients with Wilson's disease require a full assessment of liver and renal function including a GFR and tubular markers, and an MRI of the brain if indicated.

BIOCHEMISTRY / GENETICS

Wilson's disease is caused by a defect in a autosomal recessive gene important for copper transport. There is a failure to incorporate copper into caeruloplasmin and an accumulation of copper in the liver and brain.

TREATMENT

There are a number of effective copper chelators available. D-penicillamine is usually the first line of treatment. Clinical improvement, especially neurological, may take some months, and the drug frequently causes sensitivity reactions and, less commonly, marrow or renal damage. Alternatively zinc has been used in the long tern management. The management of the acutely unwell patient with liver disease is best carried out in specialist centres and may require haemofiltration or the powerful chelator ammonium tetrathiomolybdate. Occasionally liver transplant is necessary.

PROGNOSIS

The prognosis is generally favourable in early diagnosed, well-treated patients. Patients with severe brain or liver disease at presentation often have some degree of damage that is irreversible.

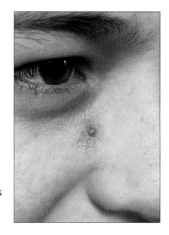

14.20
Teenage boy with Wilson's disease. He has a spider naevus secondary to liver disease. The Kayser-Fleischer rings can be just seen.

PHENYLKETONURIA

CLINICAL PRESENTATION

The classical childhood features of phenylketonuria (PKU) are now rarely seen, as a result of the highly effective neonatal screening programmes of Western countries. This is based on the detection of elevated phenylalanine concentrations in the neonatal Guthrie card blood spot, taken when the child is 2–10 days old.

Untreated, PKU leads to progressive mental retardation over the first few years of life. Patients may also have mild spasticity and an abnormal gait, while a minority have focal neurological signs and seizures. The severe neurodevelopmental delay may be partially reversible if treatment is started in early childhood. If treatment is not started until late childhood, an improvement in behaviour is the best one can expect. Children with untreated PKU tend to have blond hair, blue eyes and fair skin due to metabolic defect restricting melanin production.

INVESTIGATIONS / DIAGNOSIS

PKU is easily diagnosed by measuring the concentration of phenylalanine in blood (Guthrie card blood spot or plasma). In classical PKU, the levels are well above 1000 µmol/l (normal 40–100 µmol/l). Some children have transient hyperphenylalaninaemia, which usually resolves over the first year of life. Enzymology is not necessary and molecular analysis is available but not essential. A rare but important group of disorders, the pterin defects, also presents with elevated levels of phenylalanine on the neonatal blood spot. Tests for defects in the 'pterin' pathway must be done in all patients with raised blood phenylalanine, as the treatment and prognosis are different from that for PKU.

BIOCHEMISTRY / GENETICS

PKU is caused by a defect in the gene for phenylalanine hydroxylase, the enzyme responsible for the conversion of phenylalanine to tyrosine. It is the high concentrations of phenylalanine that cause the cognitive damage. The disease is inherited in an autosomal recessive manner.

TREATMENT

The aim of treatment is to maintain the phenylalanine concentrations in the range 100–350 µmol/l in the first five years of life and less than 600 µmol/l throughout childhood. The immature brain is much more susceptible to hyperphenylalaninaemia and thus good control is essential in early childhood. The diet can be relaxed in adulthood, except for women contemplating pregnancy (see below), although the long-term consequences of this are unknown.

Treatment consists of a very restricted natural protein (phenylalanine) intake and a supplementary formula which contains various concentrations of fat, carbohydrates, vitamins, minerals and amino acids, depending on the age of the child. This diet can be difficult and compliance is often a problem.

PROGNOSIS

With early treatment, the prognosis is excellent (**14.21**) although there is probably a mild deficit in IQ. Women with PKU are at risk of having children with severe complications due to intrauterine exposure of high concentrations of phenylalanine and thus must be on a very strict diet prior to and throughout the pregnancy.

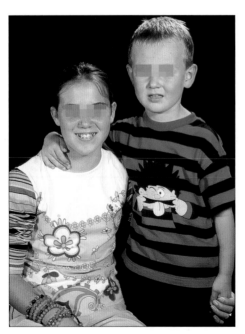

14.21 Brother and sister with early diagnosed and treated PKU. They are healthy and of normal intelligence.

BIOTIN DISORDERS

CLINICAL PRESENTATION

There are two main forms of biotin disorders: Holocarboxylase synthetase deficiency and biotinidase deficiency. The former tends to present in the neonatal period while the latter usually presents in infancy. The presentation is variable and ranges from acute metabolic decompensation with ketosis, lactic acidosis and a 'septic'-like picture, to failure to thrive and developmental delay. Frequently, children present with neurological complaints such as ataxia, hypotonia and especially seizures. There may be a characteristic erythematous rash, which may be generalized or confined to the perioral regions (**14.22, 14.23**). There may be a blepharoconjunctivitis and a glossitis.

INVESTIGATIONS / DIAGNOSIS

Acutely unwell children have lactic acidaemia with the typical urinary organic acid picture of 3-methylcrotonylglycine and methylcitrate – highly suggestive of a biotin pathway defect. The child with the chronic form of the conditions may not always have the typical organic acids, although lactic acidemia is often present. Biotinidase activity can be directly measured in blood, while holocarboxylase synthetase enzymology requires fibroblasts.

BIOCHEMISTRY / GENETICS

The carboxylase enzymes require the attachment of biotin to their apocarboxylase precursors to be active. Biotinidase recycles biocytin to supply biotin while holocarboxylase synthetase is involved in catalyzing the attachment of biotin to the apoenzyme. Both conditions are autosomal recessive.

TREATMENT / PROGNOSIS

Treatment is with 5–40 mg of biotin daily. This dramatically improves the biochemical abnormality, the skin rash and general wellbeing. Seizures tend to improve but significant neurological impairments to hearing, vision and cognition may remain.

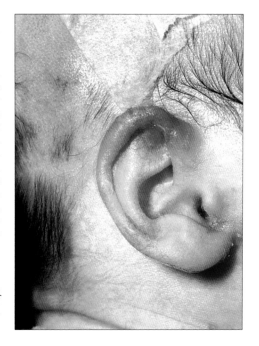

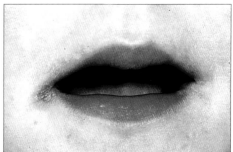

14.22 & 14.23 Typical skin manifestations of biotinidase deficiency.

ALPHA-1-ANTITRYPSIN DEFICIENCY (AT)

Alpha-1-antitrypsin deficiency (AT) is a heterogeneous condition that mainly affects the liver and the lungs. Around 10% of affected children have neonatal cholestasis with nearly half having transient sub-clinical transaminaemia in early childhood. While the majority make a full recovery, some, especially those with the more severe genetic variants of the condition, can have progressive hepatic symptoms with jaundice, vomiting, failure to thrive and liver dysfunction. AT can also cause associated hepatitis. Liver histology may reveal signs of hepatitis, fibrosis and cirrhosis, with hepatocytes classically showing globular membrane-bound inclusions of α-1-antitrypsin (**14.24**).

The lung pathology is that of emphysema, with destruction of the alveolar and small airways.

BIOCHEMISTRY/GENETICS

The diagnosis of AT is easily made by measuring the α-1-antitrypsin activity and PI phenotype in blood. AT is inherited in a co-dominant autosomal manner with the normal phenotype known as PIMM and the classically deficient patient having the PIZZ form. People with PIZZ have α-1-antitrypsin levels around 15% of normal. There are numerous other phenotypes, with most having normal α-1-antitrypsin levels.

The abnormal Z alleles self-aggregate in the hepatocyte and, through a process that is not entirely clear, cause variable liver damage. A deficiency of α-1-antitrypsin protein itself results in uninhibited protease induced destruction of the alveolar wall and thus the pulmonary pathology.

TREATMENT

The avoidance of smoking is the most effective preventative therapy for lung disease. Recombinant α-1-antitrypsin, either by infusion or by aerosol, has recently been shown to be effective at increasing protease inhibition and improving pulmonary function tests in many patients. Medium to long-term data on these therapies are not available.

Liver transplantation is well established for those with end-stage liver disease, while lung transplantation has also proved very successful in some patients.

PROGNOSIS

The long-term prognosis in patients with established disease is traditionally poor, although recent advances in management have improved this.

14.24 Liver biospy taken at the time of liver transplantation for α-1-antitypsin deficiency. The liver shows cirrhosis with fatty change and the characteristic PAS-stained red globules within many hepatocytes, that represent accumulations of α-1-antitypsin.

REFERENCES

Scriver CR, Beaudet A, Valle D (eds). *The Metabolic and Molecular Basis of Inherited Disease* (8th edn). New York: McGraw Hill, 2001.

Fernandes J, Suadubray JM, Van den Berghe G (eds).- Inborn Errors of Metabolism (3rd edn). Berlin: Springer Verlag, 2000.

Genetics
Robin Winter*
Michael Baraitser

*Professor Robin Winter sadly died before the publication of this chapter

DOWN SYNDROME (TRISOMY 21)

PRESENTATION

There is hypotonia and a recognizable 'gestalt' at birth due to the upslanting palpebral fissures, prominent epicanthus, small mouth, relatively large tongue, short nose with flat bridge, and brachycephaly (**15.1**). Thirty to forty percent will have congenital heart disease, most commonly an endocardial cushion defect. Minor features include a third fontanelle, bilateral single palmar creases, fifth finger clinodactyly (**15.2**), a sandal-gap between toes 1 and 2 and Brushfield spots of the iris.

INVESTIGATIONS

Chromosome analysis. If regular trisomy 21 is found, then parental chromosomes analysis is not necessary. If the child has a translocation, then both parents should be tested.

PROGNOSIS

In the absence of cardiac involvement, the main problem is mild to moderate neurodevelopmental delay. Patients may develop features of early Alzheimer disease in adulthood.

GENETICS

Full trisomy is usually sporadic and risks increase with maternal age. Recurrence risks after a child with simple trisomy are 1% in younger mothers, with a maternal age-related risk for mothers over 40 years. Recurrence risks for translocation carrier parents depend on the sex of the parent and the nature of the translocation. Prenatal diagnosis should be offered in all cases. Either chorionic villus sampling at 11 weeks (risk of miscarriage 1–2%) or amniocentesis at 16 weeks (risk 1%). The triple test,

measuring maternal α–FP/hCG and oestriols, and ultrasound scans looking at increased nuchal thickness, are used as screening tests in low-risk parents.

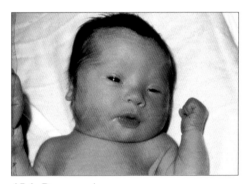

15.1 Down syndrome.

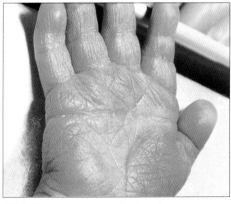

15.2 Down syndrome. Single palmar crease, fifth-finger clinodactyly.

EDWARDS SYNDROME
(TRISOMY 18)

PRESENTATION
Usually soon after birth, due to dysmorphism (**15.3**) and low birth weight. The head is long from front to back with a prominent occiput. The jaw is small, the palpebral fissures are short, the nose is short, the mouth is small and the ears are low-set. Cleft lip and palate occur in 10–20% of cases. The fingers overlap (the fist is clenched, the fifth finger overlaps the fourth and the second overlaps the third) and the nails are small. The feet have a rocker-bottom profile. Other malformations include congenital heart defects, renal anomalies, and abnormal lung segmentation.

INVESTIGATIONS
Chromosome analysis to confirm the trisomy. In the small proportion of cases with an unbalanced translocation, parental chromosomes should be examined.

PROGNOSIS
Poor. 90% die within the first year of life. Those who survive are usually profoundly delayed.

GENETICS
Recurrence risks for a baby with a chromosome defect (including other trisomies) are 1% and CVS or amniocentesis should be offered.

PATAU SYNDROME
(TRISOMY 13)

PRESENTATION
At birth, with microcephaly, a sloping forehead, aplasia cutis congenita of scalp, microphthalmia (cataracts, colobomas, retinal dysplasia and even anophthalmia can all occur). There might be facial features of underlying holoprosencephaly of the brain (i.e. agenesis of the premaxilla or single nostril). Midline facial haemangiomas are frequent (**15.4**). In the hands and feet, post-axial polydactyly is frequent and the feet might be rocker-bottom in shape. Congenital heart defects and renal anomalies are also frequent.

INVESTIGATIONS
Chromosome analysis to confirm the diagnosis.

PROGNOSIS
Most cases die within the first year of life.

GENETICS
Similar recurrence risks to those for trisomy 18 for standard trisomies.

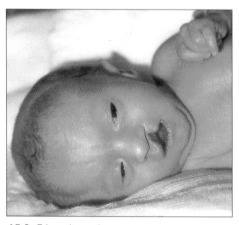

15.3 Edwards syndrome.

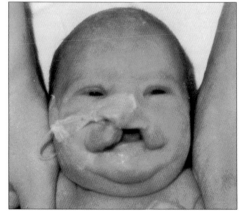

15.4 Patau syndrome.

WOLF–HIRSCHHORN SYNDROME (4P–)

PRESENTATION
This condition presents in the neonatal period with hypotonia and microcephaly. The diagnosis is suggested by the characteristic gestalt, the so-called 'Greek helmet' appearance. The eyes are widely spaced, there is a prominent glabella and parallel borders to the nose. The philtrum is short but well formed. In profile, there is an absent angle between the forehead and the nasal bridge (**15.5**). The ears are simple and low set and there may be preauricular pits. Cleft lip and palate are common, as are abnormalities of the genitalia in males.

INVESTIGATIONS
Chromosome analysis in child and parents. Some cases have an extremely small deletion and fluorescent *in situ* hybridization (FISH) studies should be asked for if there is a clinical suspicion.

PROGNOSIS
Poor in terms of development. Survival is reduced because of associated malformations and hypotonia, with poor feeding in infancy.

GENETICS
De novo deletions carry a small recurrence risk. If a parent has a balanced translocation, recurrence risks are high at 20–30% and prenatal chromosome analysis should be offered.

CRI-DU-CHAT SYNDROME (5P–)

PRESENTATION
Usually at birth because of the characteristic 'cat cry' (more like the mewing of a kitten) in an infant who is microcephalic and has a round 'moon-shaped' face. There are usually prominent epicanthic folds, hypertelorism, a broad nasal bridge and a small chin. Cleft palate and heart defects occur. The phenotype changes with age, with the face becoming elongated (**15.6**).

INVESTIGATIONS
The diagnosis must be confirmed cytogenetically and parental translocations looked for.

PROGNOSIS
Poor; those who survive have profound neurodevelopmental delay.

GENETICS
Recurrence risks are small in *de novo* cases. Prenatal diagnosis must be offered if a parent is a translocation carrier.

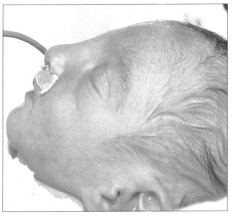

15.5 Wolf-Hirschhorn syndrome.

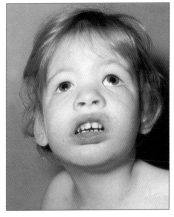

15.6 Cri-du-chat syndrome.

TURNER SYNDROME (XO)

See also 'Endocrinology' chapter.

PRESENTATION
This might be at birth, with a female with pedal oedema, a webbed neck (**15.7**), or coarctation of the aorta. The chest might be broad and the nipples wide-spaced. Later presentation might be with poor growth, or an adolescent might present with amenorrhea or infertility.

INVESTIGATIONS
Chromosome analysis will usually show a 45,X karyotype, but there are many variants of this including mosaicism, i.e. X/XX or X/XXX or X/XX/XXX, and partial deletions of the X chromosome.

PROGNOSIS
This concerns growth and fertility (in those without cardiac abnormalities). Average eventual height is between 135–150cms. Five to ten percent menstruate, but this is often late and there might be premature cessation of menstruation. Individuals with mosaic Turner syndrome are more likely to menstruate and be fertile. Intelligence is usually normal, although there might be problems with spacial orientation.

GENETICS
Mostly sporadic; recurrence risks are very small where an XO karyotype is detected.

NOONAN SYNDROME

PRESENTATION
The phenotype is variable and also changes with age. The immediate concern in the infant might be major feeding difficulties, with some puffiness of the feet. The dysmorphic features at that stage are the prominence of the eyes, which are widely spaced and downslanting, posteriorly rotated ears and extra folds of skin in the neck. The hair is often sparse and curly. As the infant gets older, ptosis replaces the prominence of the eyes (**15.8**), the neck might appear webbed and the chest wall shows a pectus excavatum.

INVESTIGATIONS
A cardiology opinion concerning a possible pulmonary stenosis or hypertrophic cardiomyopathy. Chromosome analysis to rule out Turner syndrome in a female.

PROGNOSIS
Variable. Intelligence and even stature might be normal, although there may be some learning difficulties. Severe neurodevelopmental delay is uncommon.

GENETICS
Autosomal dominant; both parents should be examined for features of the condition. The gene for one form has been found but there is more than one locus.

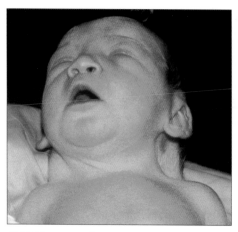

15.7 Turner syndrome.

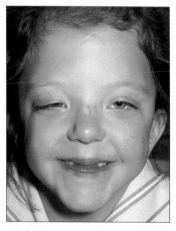

15.8 Noonan syndrome.

CHROMOSOME MOSAICISM

PRESENTATION

The features will differ depending on the chromosome involved but there are specific clinical clues. The first is hypomelanosis of Ito, where pigmented or depigmented linear skin streaks or swirls are seen (**15.9**). The second clue is body or limb asymmetry. Seizures and non-specific neurodevelopmental delay are common.

Some chromosome mosaicisms have specific clinical features. Deep grooves on the soles of the feet (**15.10**) and deep palmar creases (**15.11**), together with absent or hypoplastic patellae are indicative of mosaic trisomy 8. Mosaic tetrasomy 12p presents with neurodevelopmental delay, a rather coarse, heavy looking face (**15.12**) and poor hair growth over the temples.

INVESTIGATIONS

The abnormality might be detected in blood chromosomes but, if normal, and mosaicism is suspected, a skin biopsy should be performed.

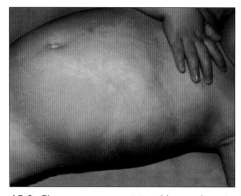

15.9 Chromosome mosaicism. Hypomelanosis of Ito.

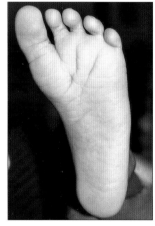

15.10 Trisomy 8 mosaicism. Grooves on soles of feet.

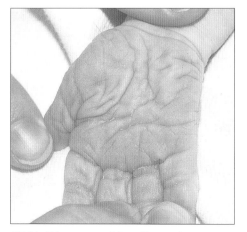

15.11 Trisomy mosaicism. Deep palmar creases.

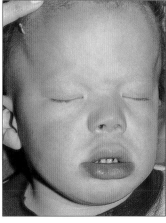

15.12 Tetrasomy 12p mosaicism. Heavy-looking face; poor hair-growth over temples.

FRAGILE X SYNDROME

PRESENTATION
Either with developmental delay, especially speech delay, or a combination of delay and hyperactive behaviour. The head might be relatively large and the joints lax. Alternatively, there may be a positive family history of males and/or females with a learning disorder. The males are not particularly dysmorphic although the ears might be big, the face long (**15.13**) and testes large after puberty.

INVESTIGATIONS
Chromosome analysis – specifically looking for fragile sites – may not be reliable. DNA analysis is now the definitive test.

PROGNOSIS
This depends on the degree of neurodevelopmental delay which is usually in the mild to moderate range.

GENETICS AND COUNSELLING
The well-documented phenomenon of phenotypically-normal transmitting males in pedigrees has been explained by the finding of an unstable $p(CCG)n$ trinucleotide repeat sequence in the gene (FMR-1). Affected individuals have greater than 200 copies of this repeat (a full mutation allele), normal individuals have ~6–60 copies and normal transmitting males ~60–200 (a premutation allele). All mothers of affected males must be assumed to be carriers of the full or pre-mutation. All daughters of normal transmitting males carry the premutation but are unaffected. About 50% of female carriers of the full mutation will have developmental delay, although not usually as severe as affected males.

WILLIAMS SYNDROME

PRESENTATION
The cheeks are sagging, the lips full and there is supra-orbital fullness (**15.14**, **15.15**). There may be a stellate iris pattern in children with blue eyes. Children have feeding difficulties, are initially floppy, are subsequently delayed and are hyperactive with a poor attention span. A supravalvular aortic stenosis should be looked for. Parents will often comment on hypersensitivity to noise and the deep, gruff voice.

INVESTIGATIONS
Serum calcium in the neonatal period might be elevated; an echocardiogram to look for the supravalvular aortic stenosis and a FISH chromosome study, looking for deletion of the elastin gene on chromosome 7, should be carried out. Most but not all clinically classic cases will have a micro-deletion. If deleted, FISH analysis of parental chromosomes should be undertaken.

PROGNOSIS
Children are often loquacious, sociable and tend to mix well. Few adults live and work totally independently, although many cope with help. Severe neurodevelopmental delay is the exception.

COUNSELLING
Sporadic, especially if the FISH studies on parental chromosomes are normal.

Occasional patients have had an affected child (50% risk).

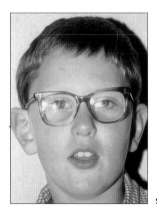

15.13 Fragile X syndrome.

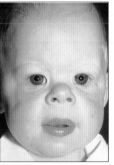

15.14 Williams syndrome.

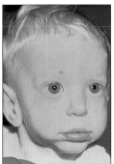

15.15 Williams syndrome.

RUBINSTEIN–TAYBI SYNDROME

PRESENTATION
Dysmorphic features are usually noted from birth and these are: a small head size, a beaked nose with a prominent columella, ptosis and downslanting palpebral fissures (**15.16, 15.17**). Broad, deviated thumbs (**15.18, 15.19**) and toes are helpful for the diagnosis. The facial dysmorphism might be difficult in the neonate, and the child might 'grow into' the diagnosis.

INVESTIGATIONS
Standard chromosome analysis will usually be normal, but the laboratory could be asked to pay attention to chromosome 16p, as 20–30% of cases have now been found to have a small (usually submicroscopic) deletion in this area using DNA probes. Mutations in the CBP gene have been found.

PROGNOSIS
Neuroevelopmental delay is the main problem, but the affected children seem happy and are good natured.

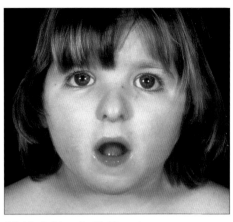

15.16 Rubinstein-Taybi syndrome.

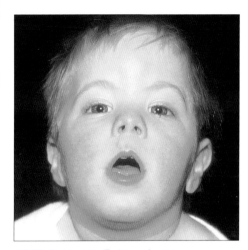

15.17 Rubinstein-Taybi syndrome.

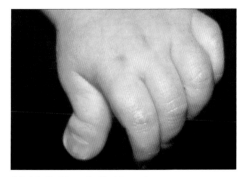

15.18 Rubinstein-Taybi syndrome. Broad deviated thumb.

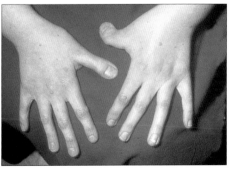

15.19 Rubinstein-Taybi syndrome. Broad deviated thumbs.

DE LANGE SYNDROME

PRESENTATION

Infants are usually small at birth and are, in addition, microcephalic. There is hypertrichosis, synophrys, a short nose with a long philtrum, and a thin upper lip (**15.20–15.22**). The hands and feet are short and the thumbs and fifth digits may be small. Oligodactyly or mono-dactyly occasionally occur (**15.23**). There is a milder variant of this condition with similar facial features, which must be diagnosed with care. Duplication of the long arm of chromosome 3 can give a somewhat similar clinical appearance.

INVESTIGATIONS

Chromosome analysis should be carried out although this is usually normal.

PROGNOSIS

Most children will have significant neuro-developmental delay. Marked short stature is to be expected in severe cases.

COUNSELLING

Nearly always sporadic, with recurrence risks of 1% or less if the parents are normal.

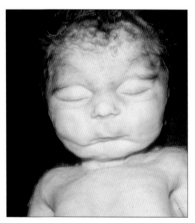

15.21 De Lange syndrome.

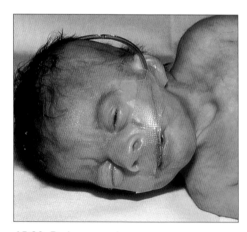

15.20 De Lange syndrome.

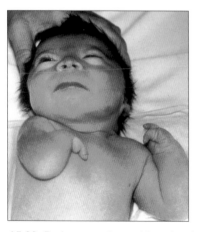

15.22 De Lange syndrome. Monodactyly.

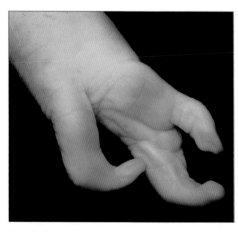

15.23 De Lange syndrome. Split hand.

ANGELMAN SYNDROME

PRESENTATION
Mostly with developmental delay, the dysmorphic features (wide mouth, small jaw) not being helpful in early stages. Likewise, the characteristic jerky movements might only become obvious when the child is trying to sit (often late in the first year of life). Seizures might be the first feature to cause concern. It is the happy disposition (**15.24**, **15.25**), the frequent laughter, often inappropriate, that will initially suggest the diagnosis.

INVESTIGATIONS
The EEG (electroencephalogram) is extremely useful as the majority of patients will have a characteristic pattern. DNA analysis is the investigation of choice. This will show a deletion of l5q in 70-80% of cases. Uniparental disomy (2 copies of the paternal gyromosome 15) occurs in a small percentage. In about 20% of cases, no DNA abnormalities are found.

GENETICS
If there is a deletion or disomy and parental chromosomes are normal, recurrence risks are small (1%). If all tests are negative, but the clinical and EEG features are highly suggestive, then recurrence risks may be as high as 50%. Some non deletion/disomy cases have been found to have mutations in the UBE3A gene and some abnormalities of DNA methylation.

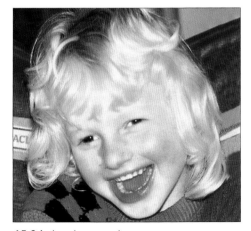

15.24 Angelman syndrome.

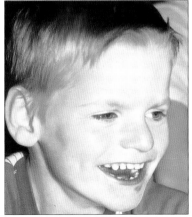

15.25 Angelman syndrome.

FRONTONASAL DYSPLASIA

PRESENTATION
Mostly at birth because of the bifid nose or grooved nasal tip (**15.26, 15.27**) and severe hypertelorism. There might be an anterior encephalocele.

INVESTIGATIONS
A brain scan is indicated as occasionally agenesis of the corpus callosum is present.

PROGNOSIS
Despite the major cosmetic problems which can require extensive plastic surgery, the outlook in terms of mental development can be good, depending on the absence of major brain malformations.

GENETICS
Recurrence risks to normal parents are small, and offspring risks might likewise be small.

VATER ASSOCIATION

PRESENTATION
The acronym stands for **V**ertebral anomalies, **A**no-rectal malformations, **T**racheo-oesophageal fistula, oesophageal atresia, **R**adial (**15.28**) (or **R**enal) anomalies. VACTERL is sometimes used – **C** for cardiac and **L** for limb defects other than radial. Occasionally there is an overlap with CHARGE association (see below).

INVESTIGATIONS
In some cases Fanconi syndrome should be ruled out by specific chromosome analysis, especially where there are CNS abnormalities.

PROGNOSIS
Intelligence is often normal, and the outlook depends on the complications encountered with the structural lesions noted above.

GENETICS
Mostly sporadic, cause is unknown and recurrence risks are small (1–2%).

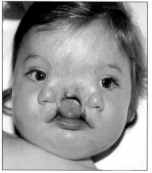

15.26 Fronto-nasal dysplasia.

15.27 Fronto-nasal dysplasia.

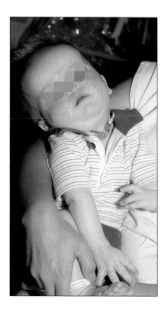

15.28 VATER association. Note absent thumb.

GOLDENHAR SYNDROME

PRESENTATION
At birth with ear malformations, pre-auricular or facial skin tags (usually asymmetrical), facial asymmetry, and a lateral extension to the corner of the mouth on the more severely affected side (**15.29, 15.30**). A subconjunctival dermoid is a frequent and, some would say, essential finding for the diagnosis (**15.31**). In its absence, the diagnosis of 'first and second branchial arch syndrome' or 'hemifacial microsomia' might be made.

INVESTIGATIONS
Radiographs to look for cervical spine anomalies; cardiac and renal scans; chromosome analysis, although this is likely to be normal.

PROGNOSIS
Deafness is frequent and cosmetic facial surgery may be necessary.

GENETICS
Mostly sporadic (1–2% recurrence) although both parents should be examined, especially for pre-auricular ear tags, as there are rare dominant families.

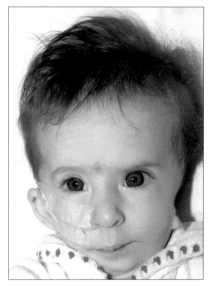

15.29 Goldenhar syndrome. Facial appearance.

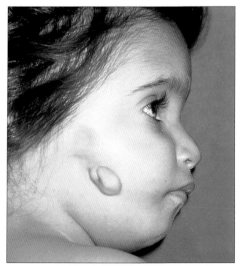

15.30 Goldenhar syndrome, showing skin tags.

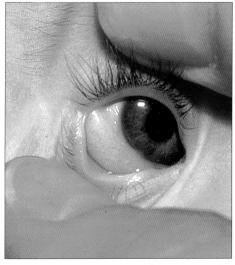

15.31 Goldenhar syndrome. Subconjunctival dermoid.

BARDET–BIEDL SYNDROME

PRESENTATION
This diagnosis might be suggested by postaxial polydactyly (**15.32**) noted at birth, but it cannot be made conclusively at this stage. Developmental delay and obesity (**15.33**) help to confirm the diagnosis later in childhood. A pigmentary retinopathy frequently develops, also renal failure due to nephronophthisis. Other renal anomalies include cysts, diverticulae and calyceal clubbing. The problem diagnostically is the variability of the condition; neuro-developmental delay might occur in only 50% of cases.

INVESTIGATIONS
An ophthalmological opinion and possibly an electroretinogram to detect early signs of a retinal dystrophy; renal imaging and urine concentration studies.

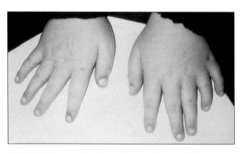

15.32 Bardet-Biedl syndrome. Postaxial polydactyly.

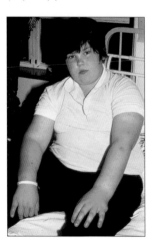

15.33 Bardet-Biedl syndrome. Obesity.

PROGNOSIS
The main problems are educational difficulties, visual problems (many will be blind by early adulthood) and progressive renal failure. Obesity and diabetes mellitus also occur.

COUNSELLING
Autosomal recessive. Eight separate loci have been identified.

CHARGE ASSOCIATION

PRESENTATION
The letters of the acronym stand for **C**oloboma (iris, retina or both) **H**eart defects, **A**tresia choanae, **R**etardation of growth and/or development, **G**enital anomalies (often hypogenitalism), and **E**ar abnormalities (a simple cup-shaped anteverted ear is the commonest) (**15.34**).

INVESTIGATIONS
Less than 5% of cases have a small deletion on the long arm of chromosome 22. The laboratory should be asked to carry out FISH analysis of chromosome 22. Growth might be slow and, if a major problem, growth hormone studies should be undertaken.

PROGNOSIS
Learning difficulties are variable, and visual and hearing problems must be taken into account.

GENETICS
Most cases are sporadic and recurrence risks for parents of a case with normal chromosomes are 1–2%. The gene has been mapped to chromosome 8q12.

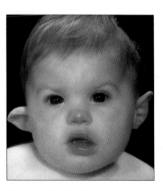

15.34 CHARGE association.

MARFAN SYNDROME

See also 'Endocrinology' chapter.

PRESENTATION
Tall stature may be the presenting feature. Further examination will reveal an aesthenic build, long fingers (**15.35**) and toes, a high arched palate (**15.36**), joint laxity, skin striae and a pectus excavatum.

INVESTIGATIONS
Formal ophthalmological examination to look for lens dislocation. Regular echocardiography to look for mitral valve prolapse and aortic root dilatation.

PROGNOSIS
The potential for aortic root dilatation with rupture lowers the average life expectancy.

GENETICS
Autosomal dominant. Mutations in the fibrillin gene at 15q have been identified.

VELOCARDIOFACIAL SYNDROME

PRESENTATION
There is a bulbous tip to the nose, but the nose itself appears pinched (**15.37, 15.38**). There are upslanting, narrow, palpebral fissures and tapering fingers. The cardiac defect is variable but is commonly a conotruncal anomaly (tetralogy of Fallot, aortic arch defects). Some patients will present to ear, nose and throat clinics with a nasal voice due to palatal incompetence or a submucous cleft palate. (See also 'Speech and Language Therapy' chapter.)

INVESTIGATIONS
A chromosome analysis asking the laboratory to carry out FISH analysis on chromosome 22. The majority of cases will have a submicroscopic deletion of 22q11. Calcium levels and immune function (T cells) should be checked because of the overlap with Di George syndrome (see also 'Immunology' chapter).

PROGNOSIS
The degree of neurodevelopmental delay is variable and can be mild. Features of psychosis in later life have been reported in some cases.

GENETICS
If both parental sets of chromosomes are normal, using FISH, then recurrence risks are small.

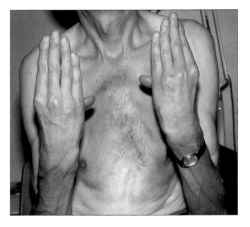

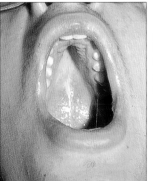
15.35 & 15.36 Marfan syndrome. Note arachnodactyly and high-arched palate.

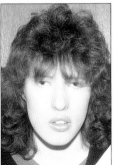 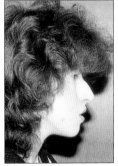
15.37 & 15.38 Velocardiofacial syndrome.

TUBEROUS SCLEROSIS

PRESENTATION

May be in infancy, with infantile spasms and, on closer inspection, depigmented macules are found usually over the trunk. Presentation can occur later in childhood, with generalized seizures; the characteristic adenoma sebaceum might be the first sign in adolescence (**15.39**). Periungual fibromas (around or under the nail bed) (**15.40**), shagreen patches (**15.41**) (often on the back), and retinal phakomata (**15.42**) should be looked for.

INVESTIGATIONS

Examination of the skin under Wood's lamp for depigmented macules. Periventricular calcification should be sought by a CT brain scan and cardiac rhabdomyomas by echocardiography. This latter lesion might occur in 90% of gene carriers under the age of two years, after which they regress. Retinal phakomata and renal lesions (cysts, angiolipomas) should also be looked for.

PROGNOSIS

Seizures occur in 60% of gene carriers and neurodevelopmental delay in 40%.

COUNSELLING

Autosomal dominant. If parents have no skin lesions, normal eyes and a normal renal scan, recurrence risks are 3% (this covers the risk of gonadal mosaicism). The condition is genetically heterogeneous; the disorder has been mapped to both 16p and 9q and the genes have been isolated.

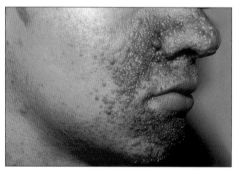

15.39 Tuberous sclerosis. Adenoma sebaceum.

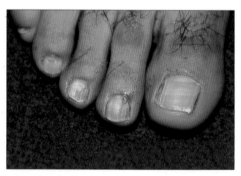

15.40 Tuberous sclerosis. Periungal fibromas.

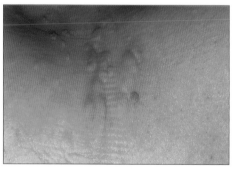

15.41 Tuberous sclerosis. Shagreen patches.

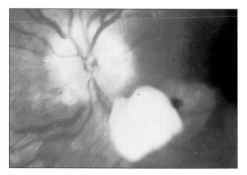

15.42 Tuberous sclerosis. Retinal phakomata.

NEUROFIBROMATOSIS TYPE 1

PRESENTATION

In childhood, with an increasing number of café-au-lait patches (15.43). If more than 5 develop, measuring more than 1.5cm in diameter, the diagnosis is highly probable. Axillary freckling is also a significant finding (15.44). Occasionally, children present with a plexiform neuroma (15.45), with pseudo-arthrosis of the tibia, or with scoliosis. Some children (about 10%) present with learning difficulties. Subcutaneous neurofibromas develop later in childhood and increase in number into adulthood (15.46).

INVESTIGATIONS

Once the diagnosis has been made, an annual follow-up should be arranged to check for hypertension secondary to renal artery stenosis or (more rarely) phaeochromocytomas, for optic nerve gliomas, for scoliosis, for deafness and for plexiform neuromas.

PROGNOSIS

One-third never come to medical attention, one-third have remediable problems not requiring major intervention and one third have serious complications.

GENETICS

Autosomal dominant. A half of cases are fresh mutations, but careful examination of the parents should be carried out. The gene maps to 17q11 and has been isolated.

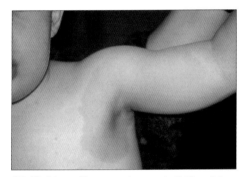

15.43 Neurofibromatosis type 1. Café au lait spot.

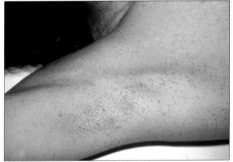

15.44 Neurofibromatosis type 1. Axillary freckles.

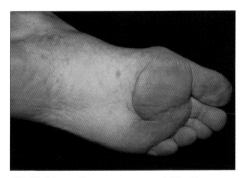

15.45 Neurofibromatosis type 1. Plexiform neuroma.

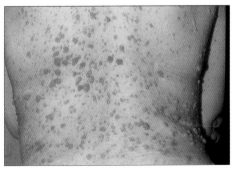

15.46 Neurofibromatosis type 1. Subcutaneous neurofibromas.

MOEBIUS SYNDROME

PRESENTATION
There are bilateral VIIth and VIth nerve palsies causing facial weakness and inability to abduct the eyes (**15.47**). Moebius syndrome can involve bulbar muscles and infants can have major swallowing problems. Some have, in addition, a small tongue and transverse limb defects (the Hanhart or hypoglossia–hypodactylia syndrome). A hand malformation (symbrachydactyly – a small hand, with short fingers partially joined together) is a frequent finding in classic Moebius syndrome (**15.48**). A small proportion of children will also have the Poland anomaly.

INVESTIGATIONS
If there are serious brain-stem problems then an MRI might show some atrophy in this region and posterior fossa calcification is occasionally noted.

PROGNOSIS
Mostly good, although the inability to show expression facially can disturb interpersonal relationships. Neurodevelopmental delay can complicate the more severe cases but should be diagnosed with caution.

GENETICS
Mostly sporadic when the full spectrum including hand abnormalities is present. Recurrence risks are 2%.

STICKLER SYNDROME

PRESENTATION
This condition may present at birth with features of the Pierre Robin association (micrognathia, cleft palate, glossoptosis). Later there is also a flat midface and nasal bridge (**15.49, 15.50**). The eyes are often prominent and a high myopia is common.

INVESTIGATIONS
Regular ophthalmological opinion to look for severe myopia, vitreous changes, cataracts, and retinal detachment, and an audiological opinion to check hearing (a mixed hearing loss is frequent). Epiphyseal changes are common, involving the hips, knees and the vertebral end-plates. In infancy, the bony changes can be marked with a dumb-bell shape to the long bones, but this improves with age.

PROGNOSIS
Good in terms of growth and development, but serious eye disease, deafness and premature arthritis are the main problems.

GENETICS
Autosomal dominant with variable expression. Gene carriers can be difficult to detect and early pictures should be looked at. There are two loci known to be responsible for the condition, one is the COL2A1 gene on chromosome 12q and the other the COL11A2 gene at 6p. These code for the alpha 1 chain of type 2 collagen and the alpha 2 chain of type 11 collagen.

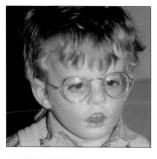

15.47 Moebius syndrome.

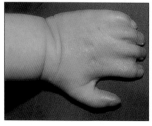

15.48 Moebius syndrome.

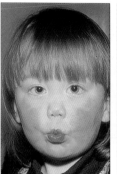 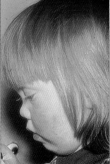

15.49 & 15.50 Stickler syndrome.

RUSSELL–SILVER SYNDROME

PRESENTATION
There is a 'pseudohydrocephalic' appearance, suggested by a relatively large head, a broad forehead, a small triangular face (**15.51**), in a child who is of low birthweight. Body asymmetry and clinodactyly should be looked for, but are not essential for the diagnosis. See also 'Endocrinology' chapter.

INVESTIGATIONS
This is almost a diagnosis of exclusion and other causes of failure to grow should be excluded. A skeletal survey might be necessary to exclude bone dysplasias such as slender bone nanism (3M syndrome)

PROGNOSIS
Good in terms of development. Initial long-term results of growth hormone treatment, despite initial promise, have been disappointing.

GENETICS
Most cases are sporadic and the sib risk is small. Offspring risks are not yet known with certainty but there have been possible parent to offspring recurrences. Some possible cases have been shown to have uniparental disomy for maternal chromosome 7.

ACHONDROPLASIA

PRESENTATION
There is rhizomelic short stature (proximal segments more involved than distal), a disproportionately large head, lumbar lordosis (**15.52**) and a trident configuration of the hands (**15.53**).

INVESTIGATIONS
A skeletal survey is needed to confirm diagnosis. The long bones are short and, in infancy, the proximal end of the femur has a round translucent area. The iliac wings are hypoplastic. The greater sacrosciatic notch is narrow and, in the lumbar spine, the interpedicular spaces narrow instead of widening as one progresses down the spine. See also 'Endocrinology' chapter.

PROGNOSIS
Eventual height is 131 +/- 5.6 cm in males and 124 +/- 5.9 cm in females. Leg lengthening might be suitable in some cases. Neurological problems might arise because of abnormalities in the region of the foramen magnum causing an obstructive hydrocephalus, and spasticity of the lower limbs can result from spinal cord stenosis.

GENETICS
Autosomal dominant, most cases being fresh mutations. There is a 1% recurrence risk to normal parents to cover gonadal mosaicism. Mutations have been found in the fibroblast growth factor receptor 3 gene at 4p16.

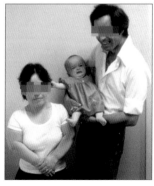

15.52
Achondroplasia.

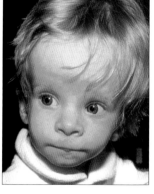

15.51
Russell-Silver syndrome.

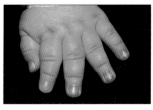

15.53
Achondroplasia, showing trident configuration of the hand.

HYPOCHONDROPLASIA

PRESENTATION
The condition rarely presents at birth, but short stature is noticed in childhood. The children look as if they have mild achondroplasia, in that limb shortening is rhizomelic (**15.54**) and there might be a pronounced lumbar lordosis. The head might be disproportionately large, but this is not always the case.

INVESTIGATIONS
A skeletal survey will confirm the rhizomelic shortening, the interpedicular narrowing in the lower spine, short femoral necks and relatively long fibulae. Radiographs might be normal or inconclusive in early childhood and may need to be repeated to confirm the diagnosis.

PROGNOSIS
The average height is 126–145 cm.

GENETICS
Autosomal dominant. Mutations have been found in the fibroblast growth factor receptor 3 gene at 4p16 in some cases.

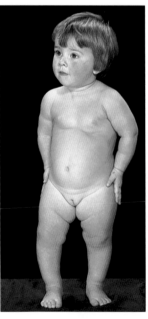

15.54
Hypochondro-
plasia.

OSTEOGENESIS IMPERFECTA

PRESENTATION
Clinically there are four types. In type I presentation might be with fractures at any time during childhood, but seldom at birth. The ocular sclerae are blue (**15.55**) and dentition may show poorly formed, discoloured enamel (dentogenesis imperfecta) in some. Type II presents with multiple fractures at birth and is mostly lethal. In type III, there are often fractures at birth and the bones become progressively deformed (**15.56**). Type IV is similar to type I but the sclerae are white and there might be mild limb-bowing.

INVESTIGATIONS
Skeletal radiographs to confirm the diagnosis and to classify the patient into one of the four types, especially when fractures are from birth. Multiple wormian bones (on a Townes skull view) and osteoporosis are additional features.

GENETICS
- **Type 1.** Autosomal dominant
- **Type II.** Mostly new dominant mutations. Five percent recurrence risk for sibs of isolated cases.
- **Type III.** Seven percent recurrence risk for sibs of isolated cases.
- **Type IV.** Seven percent recurrence risk for sibs of isolated cases.

Mutations in the COL1A1 and COL1A2 genes have been found.

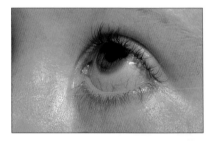

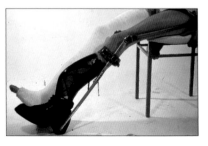

15.55 Osteogenesis imperfecta – type I.

15.56 Osteogenesis imperfecta – type III.

EHLERS–DANLOS SYNDROME

PRESENTATION

There are at least nine types, but the commonest are types I, II, and III, in which joint hypermobility (**15.57**), causing motor problems, is a frequent mode of presentation. On examination, the skin is soft and hyperelastic (**15.58**), the joints hypermobile and even dislocatable. Patients bruise easily and scars are often paper thin (**15.59**).

INVESTIGATIONS

Collagen biochemistry may help to diagnose some types. However, the diagnosis is still mainly clinical.

PROGNOSIS

There may be multiple dislocations, especially of the hips. Complications present in certain forms include bowel and bladder diverticulae, arterial and bowel rupture and rupture of the globe of the eye.

GENETICS

The three common types are autosomal dominant but rarer forms can be autosomal recessive.

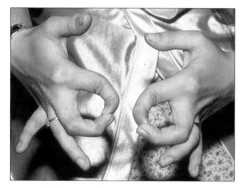

15.57 Ehlers-Danlos syndrome. Joint hypermobility.

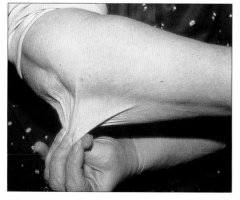

15.58 Ehlers-Danlos syndrome. Hyperelastic skin.

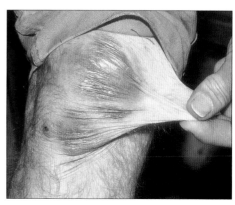

15.59 Ehlers-Danlos syndrome. Paper-thin scars.

BECKWITH–WIEDEMANN SYNDROME

PRESENTATION

The diagnosis is often made at birth in an infant of high birthweight with a prominent tongue (**15.60**) and exomphalos (EMG is the other name – **E**xomphalos, **M**acroglossia, **G**igantism). The face is often coarse and characteristic grooves or pits are found either on the front of the lobe, the helix, or behind the ear. Profound hypoglycaemia can occur and hemihypertrophy of limbs is a feature.

INVESTIGATIONS

Ultrasound of the abdomen, looking for enlarged organs, especially kidneys, liver and spleen. Chromosome analysis is usually normal but 11p duplications should be looked for.

PROGNOSIS

Good, if the neonatal hypoglycaemia is swiftly dealt with. The risk of a Wilms' tumour is 7.5% if there is hemihypertrophy and 1% if there is not. Screening for this tumour, either by the parents by means of palpation or by ultrasound scanning, is recommended (three-monthly). After five years, the frequency can be reduced until growth stops.

GENETICS

This is complicated. Recurrence risk if there is no family history is 5%. Occasional dominant pedigrees are seen. Deletions and gene mutations at 11p15 have been reported and these must be looked for. About 17% of cases are due to uniparental disomy (patem-1) for 11p15 markers.

SOTOS SYNDROME

PRESENTATION

This is an overgrowth syndrome, first coming to attention because of a large birth weight in 75% of cases. Thereafter, growth remains accelerated and measurements for weight, length and head circumference are above the 98th centile. This can sometimes go unnoticed and young children might present with global developmental delay and are then found to be dysmorphic. There is mild hypertelorism with downslanting palpebral fissures. The forehead is broad and the chin is pointed (**15.61**, **15.62**). Hair may be sparse in the temporal regions.

INVESTIGATIONS

An advanced bone age is necessary to confirm the diagnosis, but this normalizes after the age of eight years. CT brain scan sometimes shows mildly dilated ventricles. Some cases have developed hypothyroidism.

PROGNOSIS

The main problems are clumsiness and learning difficulties, although these might be mild, and increased growth velocity. Although a minority of patients are tall as adults, the majority show a spontaneous reduction of growth velocity and final height may be average.

GENETICS

Possibly autosomal dominant but most cases seen will be sporadic, with small recurrence risks if parents are normal. The condition maps to 5q35 and mutations have been found on the NSD1 gene.

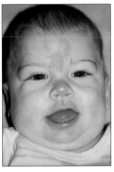

15.60 Beckwith-Wiedemann syndrome.

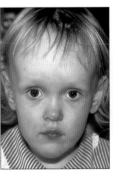

15.61 Sotos syndrome.

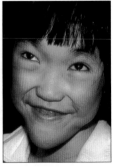

15.62 Sotos syndrome.

ROBINOW SYNDROME

PRESENTATION

Also called the fetal face syndrome, it is often the face that first suggests the diagnosis. The eyes are widely spaced, the mouth is wide, the upper lip is especially long (this might be obscured by a cleft lip and palate) and the corners of the mouth are downturned (**15.63**). The gums are hypertrophied (**15.64**), the limbs are short (either mesomelic or rhizomelic) and, in males, the penis is very small or embedded in the scrotum (**15.65**).

INVESTIGATIONS

Radiographs of the spine, as vertebral anomalies are frequent.

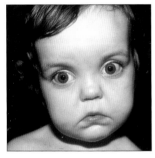

15.63 Robinow syndrome. Facial appearance.

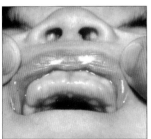

15.64 Robinow syndrome. Broad gums.

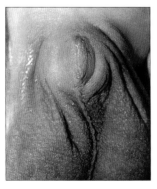

15.65 Robinow syndrome. Micropenis.

PROGNOSIS

Reasonably good in terms of intelligence as the majority are normal

GENETICS

Both autosomal recessive and autosomal dominant families have been reported. Those with severe mesomelic limb shortening and multiple vertebral anomalies are perhaps more likely to be autosomal recessive, but caution is necessary in counselling. The recessive type has been mapped to 9q22 and mutations found.

EEC SYNDROME

PRESENTATION

The acronym EEC stands for **E**ctrodactyly (**15.66**), **E**ctodermal dysplasia and **C**lefting (**15.67**). The condition is variable and often only two of the three cardinal features are present. The degree of ectrodactyly (split hand or foot) is also variable and careful examination should be made for minor clefting. The ectodermal dysplasia usually takes the form of poor hair growth and poor dentition, with some nail dysplasia.

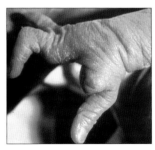

15.66 EEC syndrome. Note cleft hand.

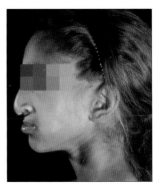

15.67 EEC syndrome.

INVESTIGATIONS

This remains a clinical diagnosis, although there is an increased incidence of renal anomalies, including ureteric obstruction and vesicouretero reflux, and these should be looked for.

PROGNOSIS

Intelligence is usually normal. There may be psychological problems because of the hand malformation and the cosmetic sequelae of clefting and poor hair growth.

GENETICS

Autosomal dominant with variable penetrance and expression. There might be a small recurrence risk even where parents seem unaffected. Some cases are associated with chromosomal abnormalities of 7q. Other families map to 3q and 19q. Mutations in the p63 gene have been found.

COCKAYNE SYNDROME

PRESENTATION

The classic presentation is with developmental delay, regression, light sensitivity involving skin but especially eyes (photophobia) and deafness. The facial appearance, with loss of subcutaneous fat around the orbits giving the eyes a sunken appearance, is characteristic (**15.68**). There is an early onset form, which presents because of failure to thrive, cataracts, joint contractures (**15.69**) and rocker-bottom feet.

INVESTIGATIONS

An ophthalmological opinion to look for either cataracts or a retinal dystrophy, peripheral electrophysiology (if ankle jerks are unobtainable) to look for a demyelinating neuropathy and an MRI brain scan to look for basal ganglia calcification and evidence of a leukodystrophy. The diagnosis can be confirmed by looking for increased sensitivity to UV irradiation in cultured skin fibroblasts.

PROGNOSIS

There is increasing cachexia and neurological impairment, with death in late teens or early adulthood in the classic form.

GENETICS

Autosomal recessive. Mutations in DNA repair genes have been found.

APERT SYNDROME

PRESENTATION

The facial manifestations of this craniosynostosis syndrome are usually severe, in that the forehead is markedly broad, there is midfacial underdevelopment, the nose is conspicuously beaked and the jaw small (**15.70**). The head shape is characteristically tall (acrocephaly) (**15.71**) but flat at the back. The fingers are joined together (syndactyly) and the thumb might be involved in the web. The toes are similarly affected (**15.72**).

INVESTIGATIONS

Combined neurosurgical, craniofacial and hand surgery opinions should be sought at an early stage (preferably from a unit specializing in this).

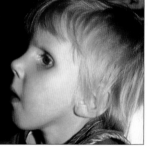

15.68 Cockayne syndrome.

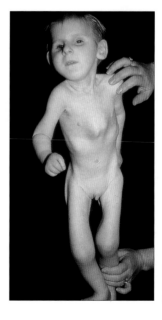

15.69 Cockayne syndrome.

PROGNOSIS

Postoperatively the degree of neurodevelopmental delay has not been found to be as great as previously suggested but this complication does occur.

GENETICS

Autosomal dominant. Small recurrence risks (1%) should be quoted if parents are normal. Mutations in the fibroblast growth factor receptor 2 (FGFR2) gene have been found.

PFEIFFER SYNDROME

PRESENTATION

At birth, because of the unusual brachycephalic head shape. Some neonates with this condition have a pronounced phenotype with severe proptosis and the skull shape is in the form of a clover leaf (**15.73**). The forehead is broad, there is hypertelorism, downslanting palpebral fissures and the nasal bridge is flat. The most important diagnostic signs are in the feet, where the big toe is broad and medially deviated (**15.74**). There might be significant syndactyly between the second and third toes (**15.75**). The thumbs are variably involved and may be broad and deviated.

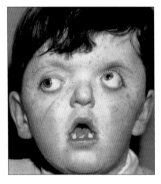

15.70 Apert syndrome. Craniosynostosis.

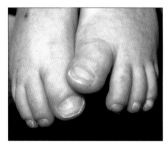

15.73 Pfeiffer syndrome.

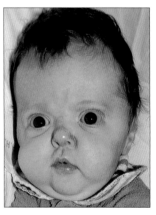

15.71 Apert syndrome. Acrocephaly

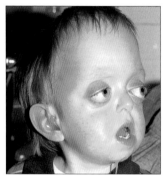

15.74 Pfeiffer syndrome. Note broad big toes.

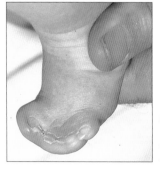

15.72 Apert syndrome. Note complete syndactyly.

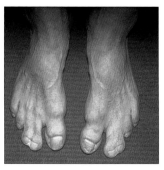

15.75 Pfeiffer syndrome. Broad big toes and 2–3 toe syndactyly.

INVESTIGATIONS

Skull radiograph to confirm craniosynostosis. All sutures might be fused if the skull is clover-leaf shaped and a CT brain scan might be necessary to look for hydrocephalus.

GENETICS

Autosomal dominant with variable expression. Mutations in both the fibroblast growth factor receptor 1 and 2 genes have been found.

CROUZON SYNDROME

PRESENTATION

At birth, because of the brachycephalic head shape, prominent eyes, beaked nose and small chin (15.76). The fingers and toes are normal.

INVESTIGATIONS

A skull radiograph to confirm the bi-coronal synostosis; intracranial pressure monitoring.

PROGNOSIS

It is the cosmetic sequelae which are most troublesome. Intelligence is usually normal.

GENETICS

Autosomal dominant. Most gene carriers will manifest some of the facial features. Mutations in the fibroblast growth factor receptor 2 gene have been identified.

HOLOPROSENCEPHALY

PRESENTATION

At birth, with hypotelorism and an absent premaxilla resembling a severe bilateral cleft lip and palate (15.77, 15.78) but on closer inspection quite different (the central tissue is missing). More severe cases may have a single nostril or cyclopia.

INVESTIGATIONS

A karyotype, because trisomy 13 and deletions of chromosomes 2, 3, 7, 13, 18 can result in this phenotype. A brain scan will be necessary to confirm the undivided frontal lobes.

PROGNOSIS

Poor, especially in those with alobar holoprosencephaly. Those with minor degrees of fusion (hypotelorism with an intact upper lip might be the only sign) might survive and have neurodevelopmental delay.

GENETICS

If the karyotype is normal, recurrence risks are 5%. There are some dominant pedigrees, and gene carriers might only have a single central upper incisor. This should be looked for in both parents. Mutations in the sonic hedgehog and other genes have been found.

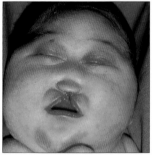

15.77 Holo-prosencephaly.

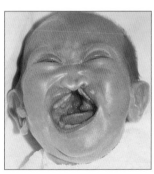

15.78 Holo-prosencephaly.

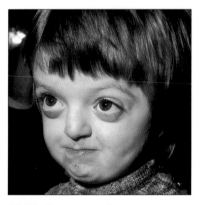

15.76 Crouzon syndrome.

COFFIN–LOWRY SYNDROME

PRESENTATION
Most males present with severe developmental delay. They are then noted to be dysmorphic and, in particular, the eyes are widely spaced, downslanting and the lips are prominent, giving the face a heavy look (**15.79**). The fingers are fleshy and tapered (**15.80**). Later in life a scoliosis develops. Female carriers might have similar hands and mild facial features.

INVESTIGATIONS
Tufting of the distal segments of the phalanges is a useful sign, but might not always be present. Vertebral anomalies may also be present.

GENETICS
X-linked recessive but females should be examined for minor features. The gene has been cloned and is at Xp22.

BLEPHAROPHIMOSIS, PTOSIS EPICANTHUS INVERSUS SYNDROME (BPES)

PRESENTATION
As the name implies it is with bilateral ptosis, small eye openings (blepharophimosis) and an epicanthus inversus, which consists of a fold of skin covering the lower medial portion of the eye (**15.81**). At birth, the configuration of the eye openings gives the impression that the eyes slant upwards and an erroneous diagnosis of Down syndrome might be made. The other dysmorphic facial feature is overfolding of the helix (the rim) of the ear.

INVESTIGATIONS
Chromosome analysis, especially to look for rearrangements of 3q. Note that there are many causes of blepharophimosis, but most do not have the epicanthus inversus.

PROGNOSIS
Usually good, although mild neuro-developmental delay has been observed. It should be noted that the children are often floppy during the first year of life and the motor delay can be exacerbated by the tendency of the infant to throw its head backwards in order to see under the eyelids. There is good evidence that there are two types of BPES, distinguished from each other by the presence of female infertility in type 1.

GENETICS
Autosomal dominant. The gene maps to 3q in some families and mutations have been found in FOXL2, a transcription factor.

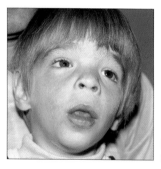

15.79 Coffin-Lowry syndrome.

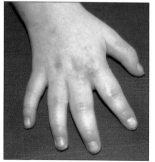

15.80 Coffin-Lowry syndrome. Note tapering fingers.

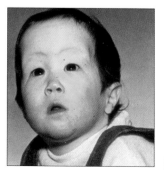

15.81 BPES.

MECKEL–GRUBER SYNDROME

PRESENTATION

This condition often results in a stillbirth but it is important to diagnose because of its genetic implications. The full clinical picture is that of an infant with a posterior encephalocele, a distended abdomen due to polycystic kidney disease (**15.82**), and a post-axial polydactyly (**15.83**).

INVESTIGATIONS

Renal investigation to confirm the cystic renal disease, as this is the most constant feature. At death, a detailed postmortem examination should be arranged to look for associated features such as hepatic fibrosis.

PROGNOSIS

Poor, with those surviving infancy having severe neurodevelopmental delay.

GENETICS

Autosomal recessive, with a 25% recurrence risk. Prenatal diagnosis by detailed anomaly scans should be possible, looking for the encephalocele, renal cysts and postaxial polydactyly. At least two genetic loci have been mapped.

GREIG SYNDROME

PRESENTATION

There is a broad forehead and nasal bridge, and pre- and postaxial polydactyly of the hands and feet with syndactyly (**15.84**).

INVESTIGATIONS

Nothing further if the diagnosis is secure. There has been the occasional child where there has been a communicating hydrocephalus and a CT brain scan might be necessary.

PROGNOSIS

In general, good. The hand and foot anomalies might need surgery

GENETICS

Autosomal dominant. The gene (GLI3) maps to 7p13.

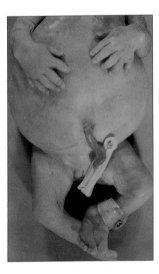

15.82 Meckel-Gruber syndrome. Polydactyly and large cystic kidneys.

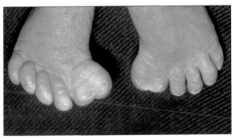

15.84 Greig syndrome. Pre-axial polysyndactyly.

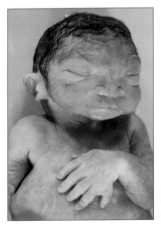

15.83 Meckel-Gruber syndrome.

HOLT–ORAM SYNDROME

PRESENTATION
The limb abnormality (classically, a radial ray defect) will be noted from birth but this can be variable. For example, there may be an absent thumb, a triphalangeal thumb (15.85) or a more extensive defect manifesting as a transverse limb deficiency. The cardiac lesion is classically an ASD, but there are families in which obligate gene carriers are without a heart lesion.

INVESTIGATIONS
Limb radiographs and cardiac investigations in both patient and parents.

PROGNOSIS
Good for mental development.

GENETICS
Autosomal dominant. Because of the variability of the condition, care should be taken in examining family members and advice should include risk of severe limb defects. The gene (TBX5) maps to 12q in some families but not others.

ROBERTS SYNDROME

PRESENTATION
Limb shortening is severe and the upper limbs are usually more severely affected than the lower (15.86). The upper limb deficiencies might be radial or phocomelic. The face is dysmorphic, with hypertelorism, clefting, a prominent pre-maxilla and a mid-facial capillary haemangioma. The ears might be small and dysplastic.

INVESTIGATIONS
Chromosome analysis asking specifically about 'chromosome puffing'. This occurs because of premature centromere separation and is diagnostic of the condition.

PROGNOSIS
Many die in the neonatal period and those who survive may have moderate to severe neuro-developmental delay.

GENETICS
Autosomal recessive.

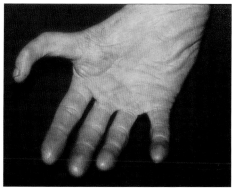

15.85 Holt-Oram syndrome. Triphalangeal thumb.

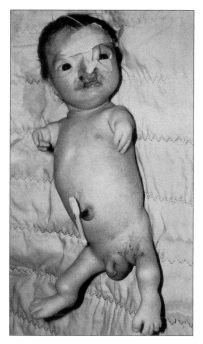

15.86 Roberts syndrome.

MICROCEPHALY – 'TRUE', AUTOSOMAL RECESSIVE

PRESENTATION
At birth, with a small head. In 'true' recessive microcephaly, early development is usually normal and delay might only become apparent after the first year of life, when the child falls behind in speech and more complex understanding. Other dysmorphic facial features are slight but might include relatively big ears and a small chin (**15.87**). Note that there are other types of recessive microcephaly with serious neurological problems, including severe delay, seizures and spasticity.

INVESTIGATIONS
If no normal sibs, exclude maternal phenylketonuria by testing the mother. A CT brain scan, chromosome, urinary aminoacid and organic acid analysis are basic requirements in those with minimal neurological signs, and a more extensive neurological work-up is needed in those with more serious manifestations. Intrauterine infections should be excluded.

PROGNOSIS
The degree of neurodevelopmental delay is variable, but is usually mild to moderate.

GENETICS
Autosomal recessive. At least six loci are involved (8p, 9q, 19q, 15q, 13q).

FANCONI ANAEMIA
See also 'Blood Diseases' chapter.

PRESENTATION
Although the hallmark of this condition is the pancytopenia, this might not be present in the first years of life (mean age of onset is eight years). The only clue at birth might be radial aplasia or thumb anomalies (hypoplasia) (**15.88**). Microcephaly, growth delay and café-au-lait patches are seen. Renal anomalies (hypoplasia, horseshoe kidneys or double ureters) occur in a third of cases.

INVESTIGATIONS
Haematological investigations, to check for pancytopenia, and bone marrow examination when indicated. The diagnosis is confirmed cytogenetically by challenging the cells with mitomycin C, to look for increased chromosome breakage.

GENETICS
Autosomal recessive. There are several complementation groups with at least five loci.

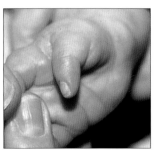

15.88 Fanconi anaemia.

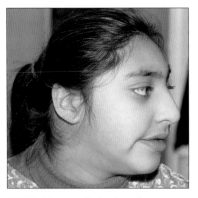

15.87 Microcephaly – 'true', autosomal recessive.

REFERENCES

Rimoin DL, Connor JM, Pyeritz RE. *Emery and Rimoin's Principles and Practice of Medical Genetics* (4th edn). Edinburgh: Churchill Livingstone, 2002.

Harper PS. *Practical Genetic Counselling* (5th edn). Oxford: Butterworth-Heinemann, 1998.

Winter RM, Baraitser M. *The London Dysmorphology Database: a Computerised Database for the Diagnosis of Rare Dysmorphic Syndromes.* Bushey: London Medical Databases, 2003.

Donnai D, Winter RM (eds). *Congenital Malformation Syndromes.* London: Chapman and Hall, 1995.

Baraitser M, Winter RM. *Colour Atlas of Congenital Malformation Syndromes.* London: Mosby-Wolfe, 1996.

Immunology
Alison Jones • Bert Gerritson
David Goldblatt • Stephan Strobel

COMMON VARIABLE IMMUNODEFICIENCY (CVID)

INCIDENCE
The commonest immunodeficiency encountered in later childhood and adult life. Minor immunoglobulin abnormalities in infancy or early childhood may evolve to become CVID. Probably approximately 1 in 20,000 live births.

AETIOLOGY
Unknown – almost certainly more than one underlying defect.

PRESENTATION
Recurrent bacterial and viral infections (16.1–16.3). Unusually severe episodes of common infections. Non-specific symptoms – fatigue, general malaise. Poor growth. Chronic diarrhoea. Autoimmune manifestations – e.g. arthritis, autoimmune haemolytic anaemia.

INHERITANCE
No clear pattern, but definite increased familial incidence. Suggestion of autosomal dominant pattern with variable penetrance in some families. Co-inheritance with certain HLA haplotypes (HLA-A1, HLA-B8, HLA-DR3 and HLA-DQB1*0201). Other family members may have selective IgA deficiency.

DIAGNOSIS
Demonstration of hypogammaglobulinaemia – variable patterns. May be abnormal lymphocyte subpopulations – low T cells and/or low B cells. May be poor specific antibody production and/or low isohaemagglutinins. May be autoantibody production. Exclusion of other defined genetic defects, e.g. X-linked agammaglobulinaemia (BTK deficiency) or hyper IgM syndrome (CD40 ligand deficiency)

TREATMENT
Depends on severity. Antibiotic prophylaxis/early recourse to antibiotics for infections.

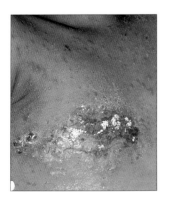

16.1 Herpes zoster becoming generalized in a child with common variable immunodeficiency.

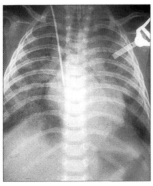

16.2 Varicella pneumonitis in common variable immunodeficiency.

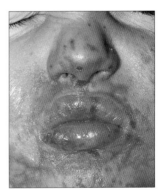

16.3 Scarring impetigo in a boy with IgA and IgG subclass I deficiency.

Immunoglobulin replacement – probably life-long once commenced. Symptomatic treatment for complications.

COMPLICATIONS

End-organ damage, particularly lungs and ears. 'Immune enteropathy'. Lymphoid hyperplasia of liver, gut. Enteroviral meningo-encephalitis. Increased incidence of lymphoma.

PROGNOSIS

Reasonably good with adequate treatment/ prevention of infection. Depends on early recognition before onset of end-organ damage.

HYPOGAMMAGLOBULIN-AEMIA WITH HYPER-IGM (CD40 LIGAND DEFICIENCY)

INCIDENCE

A rare immunodeficiency which is most usually X-linked, and manifests as functional defects of both humoral and cell-mediated immunity, with a particular susceptibility to liver disease. Probably approximately 1 in 50,000 to 100,000 live births.

AETIOLOGY

X-linked: mutations in the CD40 ligand gene, located at Xq26, causing defective expression of CD40 ligand on activated T cells. Autosomal recessive: some cases have mutations in the 'AID' (activation-induced cytidine deaminase) gene.

PRESENTATION

Recurrent bacterial infections. Susceptibility to *Pneumocystis carinii* pneumonia (PCP) (**16.4**). Usually after six months of age, when maternal IgG has declined. Oral ulceration and gingival hypertrophy secondary to neutropenia.

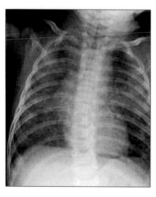

16.4
Interstitial pneumonitis caused by *Pneumocystis carinii* as the presentation of CD40 ligand deficiency.

INHERITANCE

X-linked. Autosomal recessive. Similar syndrome may also be triggered by congenital rubella infection, drugs (e.g. phenytoin), pulmonary disease, tumours and haemolytic anaemia.

DIAGNOSIS

May be positive family history with a typical 'X-linked pedigree', but approximately 30% are new mutations in X-linked type.
- Normal lymphocyte subpopulations and T cell proliferative responses to mitogens.
- Abnormal antigen-induced T-cell proliferation.
- Low IgG and IgA, normal or high IgM.
- May be absence of isohaemagglutinins.
- X-linked:
  – Absence of CD40 ligand expression on activated T cells (**16.5**).
  – Diagnosed by demonstration of disease-causing mutation in the CD40 ligand gene.

TREATMENT

Lifelong regular immunoglobulin replacement (maintain trough IgG levels into age-related normal range). Prophylaxis against *Pneumocystis carinii* with co-trimoxazole, cryptosporium with paromomycin. Boil drinking water. Bone marrow transplantation may be indicated before onset of irreversible liver disease.

COMPLICATIONS

End-organ damage, particularly lungs, ears. Autoimmune manifestations: haemolytic anaemia, thrombocytopenia, neutropenia, arthritis, etc. Chronic cryptosporidial infection. Liver disease, particularly sclerosing cholangitis (autoimmune or infection related – e.g. cryptosporidial cholangitis). High incidence of liver tumours.

PROGNOSIS

High incidence of liver disease by age 20, but phenotype very variable.

GENETICS

X-linked form: CD40 ligand mutation screening available - allows accurate carrier assessment and prenatal diagnosis. Several autosomal recessive subtypes also described.

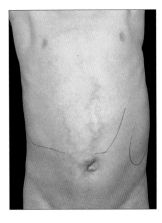

16.5 Caput medusae and hepatospleno-megaly (outlined) in a boy with CD40 ligand deficiency complicated by sclerosing cholangitis.

WISKOTT–ALDRICH SYNDROME

INCIDENCE
A rare X-linked disorder which results in thrombocytopenia, atypical eczema and immunological abnormalities, with a high risk of autoimmune disease and lymphoma. Probably approximately 1 in 50,000 to 100,000 live births.

AETIOLOGY
Mutations in the 'WASP' (Wiskott-Aldrich Syndrome Protein) gene, located at Xp11.

PRESENTATION
Bruising, bleeding, bloody diarrhoea in infancy. Recurrent infections: upper and lower respiratory tract infections, otitis media, atypical eczema (**16.6**). Clinical variant = 'X-linked thrombocytopenia' (a mild form of WAS rather than a distinct disorder).

INHERITANCE
X-linked recessive.

DIAGNOSIS
Suggested by clinical features combined with compatible immunological investigations. May be a positive family history with a typical 'X-linked pedigree' but 30% new mutations. Confirmation of diagnosis by demonstration of lack of expression of 'WASP' protein and/or disease-causing mutation in the 'WASP' gene.

INVESTIGATION
- Platelets – low numbers and small size.
- Immunoglobulin levels: typically normal IgG, low IgM, high IgA.
- Isohaemagglutinin levels may be low.

- Specific antibody production to poly-saccharide antigens may be defective.
- Lymphocyte subpopulations and T-cell function usually normal in the first few years of life, but later progressive reduction in T-cell numbers and function.

TREATMENT
- Immunoglobulin replacement. Even in the absence of *in vitro* immunological abnormalities, affected boys usually suffer from recurrent infections. Early immunoglobulin replacement is indicated, and may also be beneficial in thrombocytopenia.
- Prophylaxis against *Pneumocystis carinii*: even without demonstrable T-cell abnormalities there is a risk of PCP and prophylaxis with co-trimoxazole (dapsone or pentamidine if co-trimoxazole is not tolerated) should be given.
- Thrombocytopenia: Severe thrombo-cytopenia may respond to high dose immunoglobulin therapy. If there is evidence of autoimmune thrombo-ctyopenia, immunosuppression may be effective (e.g. steroids, azathioprine, vincristine). Resistant thrombocytopenia may require splenectomy, which usually results in normal platelet numbers. Splenectomy should be avoided if bone marrow transplantation is planned.
- Bone marrow transplantation (BMT): The long-term outlook for boys with WAS is poor, with a risk of malignancy and autoimmune complications. Early BMT is recommended, as results are significantly better if performed before 5 years of age.
- Complications: Autoimmune vasculitis. End-organ damage as a result of repeated infections. Risk of lymphoma.

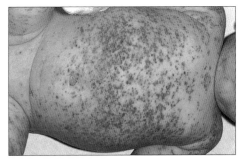

16.6 Wiskott-Aldrich syndrome. Extensive eczema and purpuric skin rash.

PROGNOSIS

Variable. The phenotype can vary even within families. Some boys survive to adulthood with few complications. The overall outlook is poor because of the above risks. Successful BMT cures the underlying WAS, but the effect of BMT on the risk of malignancy is unknown.

GENETICS

Female carriers show 'non-random' X chromosome inactivation in whole blood (which is also the case in about 5% of non-carrier females). 'WASP' mutation screening is available and allows accurate carrier testing and prenatal diagnosis where requested.

X-LINKED AGAMMAGLOBULINAEMIA (BRUTON'S DISEASE)

INCIDENCE

Accurate incidence unknown – probably approximately 1 in 50,000 to 100,000 live births.

AETIOLOGY

Mutations in the 'BTK' (Bruton tyrosine kinase) gene, located at Xq22. Precise function of BTK protein not known – involvement in B cell signalling pathway.

PRESENTATION

Recurrent bacterial infections, often severe (e.g. pneumonia, osteomyelitis, bacterial meningitis). Usually after six months of age, when maternal IgG has declined.

INHERITANCE

X-linked.

DIAGNOSIS

May be positive family history with a typical 'X-linked pedigree' but approximately 30% new mutations.

- Absent or very low circulating mature B cells.
- Absent or very low immunoglobulins of all isotypes.
- Absent specific antibody responses.
- Confirmation of diagnosis by demonstration of lack of expression of BTK protein and/or disease-causing mutation in the 'BTK' gene.

'Leaky' variants of XLA now recognized – less severe hypogammaglobulinaemia, some circulating mature B cells. These boys also have mutations in the 'BTK' gene. The severity of the clinical phenotype may vary within families.

TREATMENT

Lifelong regular immunoglobulin replacement (IgG levels maintained well into age-related normal range). Antibiotic prophylaxis, if evidence of chronic lung disease (**16.7**).

COMPLICATIONS

End-organ damage, particularly lungs and ears. Chronic enteroviral meningoencephalitis. Neutropenia, which may respond to immunoglobin therapy.

PROGNOSIS

Good with adequate immunoglobulin replacement, but risk of enteroviral infection seems to persist.

GENETICS

Female carriers show 'non-random' X chromosome inactivation in purified B cells. 'BTK' mutation screening available, and allows accurate carrier assessment and prenatal diagnosis where requested.

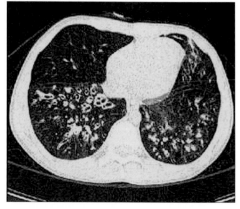

16.7 Bronchiectasis as a complication of recurrent lung infection (associated with insufficient immunoglobulin supplementation) in XLA.

CHRONIC MUCOCUTANEOUS CANDIDIASIS (CMC)

Also known as Louis-Bar syndrome and Vogt's disease.

INCIDENCE
Unknown (rare).

PRESENTATION
Children present often during infancy with persistent, occasionally treatment-resistant oral thrush and extensive rashes in the perianal and perigenital region (nappy or diaper rash). Skin superinfections with bacterial pathogens, increased mucosal spread of *Candida* infections leading also to extensive involvement of buccal mucosae and spreading to lips and finger or toe nails. Endocrinopathies are usually a feature of older infants (see Diagnosis). Some children show persistent localized severe *Candida* infections of nails and of otherwise normal skin (**16.8–16.10**).

GENETIC INFORMATION
Equal male:female ratio. Mostly sporadic, autosomal recessive inheritance (chromosome 22?) has been reported.

DIAGNOSIS
The mainstay of the diagnosis is the clinical observation of excess *Candida* colonization of the patient, with evidence of organ-specific autoantibody production affecting mainly the parathyroid, adrenal and thyroid glands. Vitiligo and alopecia may be more common in those patients with an endocrinopathy. Other autoantibodies affecting pancreatic islet cells, gastric parietal cells and others are part of the chronic mucocutaneous candidiasis and polyendocrinopathy complex. The occurrence of organ-specific auto-antibodies is not necessarily associated with organ dysfunction. Children with CMC have an increased susceptibility to infections and oral aphthous ulcerations, but these symptoms can also be associated with other disorders.

DIFFERENTIAL DIAGNOSIS
Primary and secondary (acquired) immunodeficiency syndromes where *Candida* overgrowth is part of the clinical spectrum. Systemic *Candida* infection (e.g. septicaemia) is not a feature of CMC.

IMMUNOPATHOLOGY
Consistent with the heterogeneity of the syndrome, abnormalities of T-cell function (lack of *Candida* specific responses), B-lymphocyte, phagocytic and monocytic functions have been described. *In vitro* tests show great individual variation and are at times suggestive of the diagnosis, but they are not diagnostic. Several different subgroups of patients have been classified according to their clinical presentations and immunological findings.

TREATMENT
In most cases the treatment is symptomatic, with topical and/or systemic antifungals.

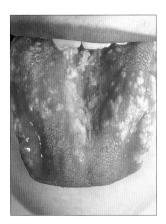

16.8 Appearance of the tongue in chronic mucocutaneous candidiasis.

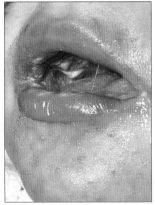

16.9 Mouth of toddler with chronic mucocutaneous candidiasis.

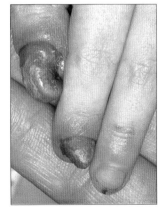

16.10 Nail infection in chronic mucocutaneous candidiasis.

Intravenous therapy is only rarely required. Hormone replacement therapy is required for restoration of endocrine function, if this is abnormal. Immunosuppressive therapies to modulate the autoantibody production are of no proven benefit and contraindicated. In extreme cases, bone-marrow transplantation can be considered.

PROGNOSIS
Probably satisfactory (no reliable data available) with adequate long term surveillance and early treatment of infections and underlying endocrinopathies.

ATAXIA-TELANGIECTASIA

See also 'Neurology' chapter.

INCIDENCE
Unknown (very rare).

PRESENTATION
This boy presented at the age of two years with recurrent sinopulmonary infections, slight but constant drooling of saliva (note slight reddening of his chin), suspicion of early developmental delay, mask-like facies and an unsteady gait with discrete ocular telangiectasias (**16.11, 16.12**).

GENETIC INFORMATION
Autosomal recessive inheritance. The defective gene is the ATM (ataxia-telangiectasia mutated) gene, located on chromosome 11q22-23. Prenatal diagnosis and carrier detection are available for affected families.

DIAGNOSIS
There is great variability in the onset of symptoms and the features mentioned above are not always recognisable at presentation. Slurred speech, strabismus, cerebellar and extrapyramidal signs, and muscle weakness usually develop during progression of the disease. Neurodevelopmental delay is present in some patients. A common feature is recurrent sinopulmonary infections with secondary bronchiectasis. Despite a progressive immunodeficiency involving T- and B-cell function, opportunistic infections are not a feature of this condition.

LABORATORY FINDINGS
Lymphopenia and eosinophilia, together with an IgA deficiency and IgG subclass deficiency, are common findings in 60–70% of patients.

T-cell subset analysis may show a reduced CD4+ population, at times with an overall increased TCRγδ expression. Mitogen responses *in vitro* and delayed hypersensitivity responses *in vivo* are often (~50–60%) reduced. There is increased radiosensitivity as an indication of a DNA repair defect (and increased chromosomal breakage) after radiation of cells *in vitro*.

IMMUNOPATHOLOGY
Ataxia-telangiectasia is characterized clinically by cerebellar ataxia, oculocutaneous telangiectasias, immunodeficiency, sensitivity to radiomimetic agents, and cancer predisposition. The ATM gene product is a member of a novel family of large proteins implicated in the regulation of the cell cycle and response to DNA damage.

TREATMENT
Supportive treatment, with prophylactic antibiotics and intravenous gammaglobulin administration usually every three weeks, follows the principle outlined for the management of X-linked agammaglobulinaemias and common variable immunodeficiency. There is no cure for the disease. Bone marrow transplantation may correct the immunodeficiency but will not halt the progressive neurological deterioration of these patients and is contraindicated because of the underlying defect in DNA repair.

PROGNOSIS
There is great variability but frequently the patient is wheelchair bound in the second decade of his/her life. Early deaths as well as survival into the twenties to forties have been reported.

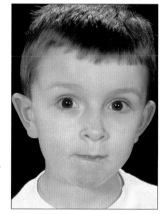

16.11 Ataxia-telangiectasia. Typical facial appearance.

X-LINKED LYMPHOPROLIFERATIVE DISEASE (XLP, DUNCAN SYNDROME)

Also known as Duncan's disease or Purtilo syndrome. Genetic inability to mount appropriate immune response to Epstein-Barr Virus (EBV) infection (infectious mononucleosis).

INCIDENCE
Rare, exact incidence is unknown, more than 80 kindreds have been described worldwide.

PRESENTATION
Severe, fulminant, sometimes fatal infectious mononucleosis, often with CNS and liver involvement (**16.13**). Survivors of initial EBV infection may develop progressive hypogamma globulinaemia, aplastic anaemia or B-cell lymphoma/lymphoproliferative disease.

GENETIC INFORMATION
X- linked, Xq26. The gene defective in XLP has been designated SH2D1A and encodes a protein called SLAM-associated protein ('SAP'). Although mutation analysis has only identified a mutation in 60% of patients with a typical clinical and family history, most cases are associated with absence of 'SAP' protein in T cells.

DIAGNOSIS
Clinical presentation with a suggestive family history (early male deaths indicating an X-linked pedigree) and evidence of EBV-infection. Patients may show raised titres of antibodies to EBV virus capsid and nuclear antigen.

Immunological abnormalities, such as a markedly reversed CD4/CD8 ratio and panhypogammaglobulinaemia. Polymorphic lymphocyte infiltration (lymphocytes, plasma cells, histiocytes) are recognized in the liver, spleen, central nervous system and lymph nodes.

Absence of 'SAP' expression in all cases. Mutations in 'SAP' genes in 60% of cases. Genetic defect in remaining cases not known.

IMMUNOPATHOLOGY
Deficient immune response to EBV with a failure to control B cell proliferation caused by the viral infection.

TREATMENT
Antiviral therapy with aciclovir and ganciclovir, and intravenous immunoglobulins with conventional supportive treatments have been tried but remain unsatisfactory. A fatal outcome is expected in about 75–80% of affected patients who present with fulminant disease. Anti-CD20 monoclonal antibodies may be useful.

Preventive therapy with high dose intravenous immunoglobulins in susceptible individuals may be indicated but not entirely successful. Bone marrow or peripheral stem cell transplantation has been attempted with some successes.

PROGNOSIS
Current overall mortality rate around 75–80 % (without transplantation).

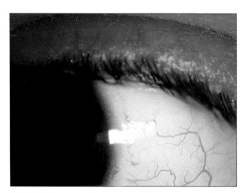

16.12 Ataxia-telangiectasia. Appearance of the eye.

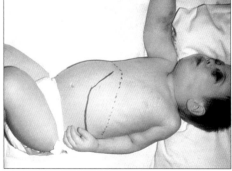

16.13 Patient with hepatosplenomegaly, bruises and oedema in ICU.

CHEDIAK–HIGASHI SYNDROME

INCIDENCE
Unknown (very rare).

PRESENTATION
This six-year-old patient, of Asian origin, with partial oculocutaneous albinism (a distinct greyish tint of his dark hair and small areas of depigmented skin) presented with recurrent pyogenic infections (**16.14**, **16.15**).

GENETIC INFORMATION
The disease occurs sporadically but can be inherited in an autosomal pattern. Prenatal diagnosis has been achieved by demonstration of large lysosomes in chorionic villus cells. The underlying defect is in the LYST gene. The precise role is unknown but is involved in lysosomal function.

DIAGNOSIS
The physical appearance of the patient together with a history of recurrent infections and the demonstration of large cytoplasmic inclusions (**16.16**, **16.17**) in neutrophils are diagnostic. Patients may also present in the 'accelerated phase' of the disease characterized by fever, hepatosplenomegaly, jaundice, lymphadeno-pathy, pancytopenia, severe bleeding disorder and evidence of diffuse mononuclear cell infiltrates. This stage of the disease carries a high mortality.

LABORATORY FINDINGS
Unlike most functional neutrophil disorders, the Chediak-Higashi Syndrome is associated with neutropenia. Functional neutrophil assays (random and directed migration, microbicidal activity) are abnormal.

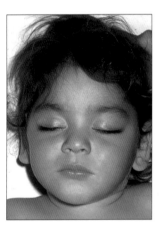

16.14 Chediak-Higashi syndrome in a boy, showing greyish appearance of hair.

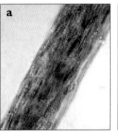

16.15 Chediak-Higashi syndrome. Appearance of hair under the microscope, **(a)** normal hair, **(b)** patient with Chediak-Higashi syndrome.

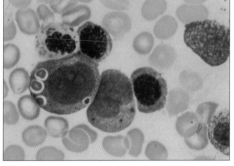

16.16 Bone marrow with giant inclusions in Chediak-Higashi syndrome.

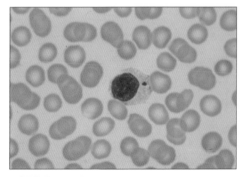

16.17 Normal marrow.

IMMUNOPATHOLOGY
The underlying pathology is not completely understood. The giant granules fail to discharge during phagocytosis and the cytoskeletal abnormalities may explain the abnormal migration properties of cells of the monocyte series (**16.16, 16.17**).

TREATMENT
Prophylaxis and early treatment of recurrent bacterial infections is essential in managing these patients. The role of ascorbic acid in partially restoring the neutrophil defect is not conclusive. Treatment of the accelerated phase includes steroids, cytotoxic and immunosuppressive agents. Bone marrow transplantation should be considered.

PROGNOSIS
The prognosis is poor once the patient presents in the accelerated phase. It is unclear when and whether all or most patients reach this phase.

LEUKOCYTE ADHESION DEFECTS

Leukocyte adhesion deficiency syndrome (LAD-syndrome) LFA-1 deficiency and delayed cord separation syndrome.

INCIDENCE
Unknown (very rare).

PRESENTATION
Patients with these defects present with recurrent necrotic soft tissue and skin infections. Severe forms of the disease can present with omphalitis, neonatal septicaemia and delayed cord separation (>3 weeks), where the umbilical cord remains 'fleshy' and often needs to be manually separated. Mucous membranes and the gastrointestinal tract may also be involved. Superficial lesions begin as small non-purulent nodules which may fail to heal and progress to large ulcers (**16.18**) and cellulitis without normal pus formation. Healing of wounds is delayed leaving dysplastic scars (**16.19**). Gingivitis and peridontitis are common features in older children (**16.20**).

GENETIC INFORMATION
Sporadic and autosomal recessive pattern of inheritance. LAD 1 is caused by mutations within the common beta subunit (CD18) gene of the lymphocyte function-associated antigen 1 (LFA-1, CD 11a) located on chromosome 21. Second-trimester prenatal diagnosis can be performed by measuring expression of the molecule on fetal lymphocytes.

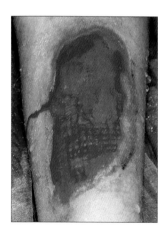

16.18 Large clean ulcer in LAD.

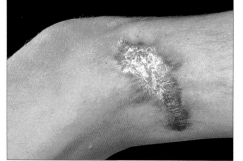

16.19 Dysplasic scar in LAD.

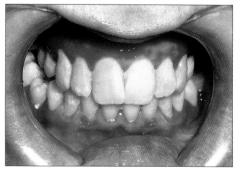

16.20 Gingivitis in LAD.

DIAGNOSIS

Recurrent infections and poorly healing wounds associated with neutrophil counts of over 15,000 granulocytes/μl under normal conditions, rising to over 40,000 granulocytes/μl during infections, are hallmarks of the disease. The absence of neutrophilia generally rules out this diagnosis.

LABORATORY FINDINGS

The diagnosis is confirmed by flow cytofluorometric analysis (FACS – **16.21**) of white blood cells, using monoclonal antibodies for CD11, CD18 and CD15s (the latter to rule out a rare LAD 2 variant – sialyl-Lewis X deficiency), demonstrating absence of the cell adhesion molecule. A subgroup of patients with less severe infections often has low grade expression of the adhesion molecules (1–10% of normal). Functional assays show severe impairment of adhesion-dependent functions such as adhesion, migration and complement receptor 3 binding. Adhesion-independent functions (microbicidal activity and the oxidative burst) are unaffected.

IMMUNOPATHOLOGY

The β2 subfamily of leukocyte integrins includes three complexes, each with a different alpha-chain, but sharing a common beta subunit (CD18). Defects in the beta subunit gene result in quantitative or qualitative reduction in these integrins, which include LFA-1(CD11a), Mac-1 (CR3, CD11b) and CR4 (p150,95 CD11c). Abnormal function or lack of these molecules leads to diminished margination and an increase in the circulating neutrophil pool in the circulation.

TREATMENT

Early and aggressive treatment of bacterial infections and prophylactic antibiotic therapy are essential for managing these patients. Viral infections are not a feature. Dental hygiene with antiseptic mouthwashes reduces the painful gingivitis in some patients. Anti-inflammatory agents and steroids may be of benefit. Bone marrow transplantation is curative in these patients.

PROGNOSIS

The prognosis is severe and dependent on the residual expression and function of the adhesion molecule. Patients with moderate phenotypes can live into the second or third decade of life (without bone marrow transplantation).

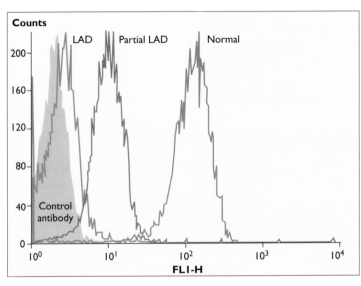

16.21 Leukocyte adhesion defects. Fluorescence-activated cell sorter profile showing severe and partial deficiencies.

DI GEORGE SYNDROME

INCIDENCE
Varies from 1 in 20,000 to 66,000, depending on population studied.

PRESENTATION
Characterized clinically by hypocalcaemic tetany, congenital heart disease, characteristic facies, neurodevelopmental delay, growth retardation and an increased susceptibility to infection. A marked variation in the phenotype exists and not all the above mentioned abnormalities may be present.

DIAGNOSIS
Characteristic facies (16.22, 16.23): Low set, posteriorly rotated ears, hypertelorism, short philtrum, small mandible. **Congenital heart disease:** A spectrum of abnormalities occur with the commonest being the interrupted aortic arch (type B). Recognized but less common associations include truncus arteriosus and tetralogy of Fallot. **Hypocalcaemic tetany:** Onset is usually within 24–48 hours of birth and persists after 14 days. It is usually associated with low levels of parathyoid hormone (PTH).

INHERITANCE
Most cases are sporadic and an autosomal dominant form is recognized. The majority will have an associated microdeletion of the long arm of chromosome 22 (22q11).

IMMUNOLOGY
The variability of the immunological findings is partly explained by the degree of thymic hypoplasia and consequent T-cell abnormalities. Clinically, frequent bacterial infection, persistent thrush, diarrhoea and failure to thrive may occur. T-cell function may improve spontaneously. Classically, patients have reduced CD4 counts and poor mitogen responses. B-cell function is usually normal.

TREATMENT
Patients may require complex cardiac surgery. HLA indentical non-T-cell-depleted bone marrow transplants have been performed successfully as have earlier and more recent attempts to reconstitute the immune system with thymic transplants. The hypoparathyroidism can be treated with calcium supplements and vitamin D administration. It may be necessary to reduce phosphorus in the diet to maintain control. Patients may require antibiotic prophylaxis. Live vaccines should be avoided if T-cell numbers are low, with live polio vaccine also being avoided by family members.

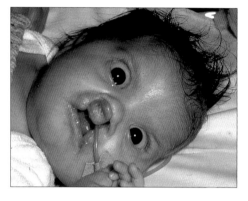

16.22 Di George Syndrome. Characteristic facies.

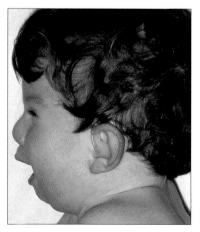

16.23 Di George Syndrome. Lateral view of face showing small jaws and low ears.

CHRONIC GRANULOMATOUS DISEASE (CGD)

CGD is a chronic disorder of neutrophil function, characterized by recurrent bacterial infection of the skin, lungs and lymph nodes and other deep sites, with formation of widespread granulomata (**16.24–16.27**).

PRESENTATION

Patients may present at any age but usually present in early childhood. Clinical characteristics are suppurative lymphadenitis, recurrent staphylococcal skin infections, perianal abscesses, hepatosplenomegaly and pneumonia. Characteristic pathogens are catalase-positive bacteria and fungi, especially *Aspergillus*.

GENETICS

Two-thirds of cases are X-linked and are due to the absence of the 91kDa phagocyte oxidase protein, part of the membrane bound NADPH

oxidase system. One third of patients inherit a mutation in the genes encoding cytosolic proteins, the most common being the 47phox and 67phox, and such mutations are inherited in an autosomal recessive fashion.

IMMUNOPATHOLOGY

The disease is due to the failure of phagocytic cells to generate superoxides secondary to defects in the NADPH oxidase.

DIAGNOSIS

The diagnosis can be established by means of the nitro-blue tetrazolium test (NBT). This test depends on the conversion of the yellow dye (NBT) to dark blue formazan by superoxides generated by normal phagocytes. In affected individuals, >90% of phagocytes fail to reduce the dye. Carriers of the X-linked form of the disease may demonstrate reduction by 10–90% of the phagocytes.

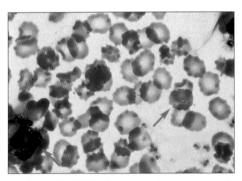

16.24 CGD. NBT of a carrier showing normal (blue-stained, left) and abnormal phagocytes.

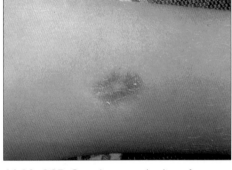

16.26 CGD. Granulomatous healing of a forearm.

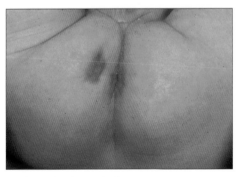

16.25 CGD. Buttock abscess.

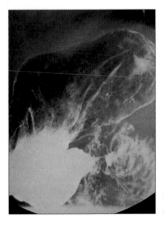

16.27 CGD. Gastric outlet obstruction.

TREATMENT

The mainstay of therapy is antibiotic and anti-fungal prophylaxis. Co-trimoxazole is the antibiotic of choice because of its anti-bacterial spectrum and concentration in the phagocyte. Itraconazole prophylaxis appears to have had an impact on the morbidity and mortality from *Aspergillus* infection. Interferon gamma has been shown to be useful both in preventing infection and as an adjunct to the treatment of deep-seated infections. Bone marrow transplantation has proved successful in a few cases.

PROGNOSIS

Steadily improving, with improved antibiotic and anti-fungal prophylaxis and bone marrow transplantation in selected cases.

HYPER IgE SYNDROME

Previously known as Job syndrome, this is characterized by recurrent staphylococcal infection, particularly of the skin and lung, and extremely high IgE levels.

PRESENTATION

Presentation is variable and infection may involve the skin, lungs, joints and other sites. Allergic symptoms include asthma, food allergy and eczema (16.28). Some patients have typically coarse facial features (16.29).

DIAGNOSIS

All patients have extremely high IgE levels which are dependent on the age at presentation. Patients presenting under one year may have levels >1000 IU/ml, whereas older patients may have IgE levels of 10,000–20,000 IU/l or higher. Patients with severe atopic disease alone may also have very high IgE levels. In atopic patients, specific IgE is directed against a multitude of food and environmental antigens. Other overall immunological findings *in vitro* are usually normal, although variable defects in humoral and cellular function, including neutrophils, have been described.

INHERITANCE

Autosomal dominant inheritance has been described in some families.

TREATMENT

The mainstay of therapy is antibiotic prophylaxis with an anti-staphylococcal agent. Cimetidine and ascorbic acid have both been used to improve neutrophil function. Immunoglobulin treatment might be attempted in selected cases. Bone marrow transplant has been described as curative, and immunosuppressive therapy has been used to control the symptoms.

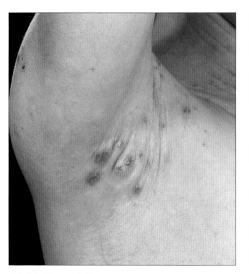

16.28 Hyper IgE syndrome. Axilla of an affected child showing site of recurrent infections with background chronic eczema.

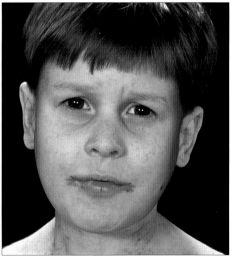

16.29 Hyper IgE syndrome. Face of an affected child showing coarse, pitted skin.

SEVERE COMBINED IMMUNODEFICIENCY (SCID)

SCID encompasses a group of inherited rare disorders characterized by the absence of functional T and B lymphocytes. SCID is clinically, immunologically and genetically heterogeneous (Table **16.1**).

INCIDENCE
Unknown, approximately 1 in 75,000 live births. X-chromosome linked and autosomal recessive (AR) variants.

PRESENTATION
Presentation is within the first year of life with failure to thrive, diarrhoea, severe infections (**16.30**) and opportunistic infections. In some infants an exanthematous skin rash due to graft versus host disease may be present (**16.31–16.33**).

DIAGNOSIS
Full blood count for total lymphocyte numbers. Phenotyping of lymphocyte subpopulations. Lymphocyte proliferation responses. Serum immunoglobulin levels. Further advanced and specific investigations.

PATHOLOGY
Lymphocyte development and function is severely impaired due to absence of essential membrane, cytoplasmic or nuclear proteins. Most infants with SCID have profound lymphocytopenia. However, normal lymphocyte numbers do not exclude SCID because lymphocytes may include only B cells, NK (natural killer) cells, non-functioning T cells or maternal T cells.

TREATMENT
Protective isolation and avoidance of live vaccines and non-irradiated and CMV (cytomegalovirus) positive blood products. Immunoglobulin replacement and anti-microbial prophylaxis, followed by allogeneic bone marrow transplantation.

PRENATAL DIAGNOSIS AND PROGNOSIS
Possible for a number of sub-types. Without treatment SCID is fatal in infancy and early childhood. After bone marrow transplantation 50–95% disease-free survival can be achieved, depending on donor tissue type matching and clinical condition at time of bone marrow transplantation.

Table 16.1 Some defined forms of SCID

Phenotype	Inheritance	Molecular defects
T– B+ NK–	X-linked	Common gamma chain*
T– B+ NK–	AR	Jak 3 deficiency
T– B– NK+ Omenn syndrome (T+ B– NK+)	AR	Rag1 and Rag2 deficiency
T– B– NK–	AR	Adenosine deaminase deficiency Purine nucleodside phosphorylase deficiency SCID with radiosensitivity
T– B+ NK+	AR	Interleukin 7 receptor **a** deficiency
CD8 deficiency	AR	ZAP70 deficiency
Low CD4, absent DR	AR	MHC class 2 deficiency

* Part of the multiple cytokine receptor
AR – Autosomal recessive
Jak – Janus- associated kinase
Rag – Recombinase activating genes
ZAP – T- cell-receptor Zeta-chain-associated tyrosine kinase
MHC – Major histocompatibility antigen

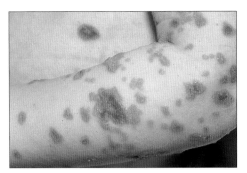

16.30 SCID. Lower arm of boy aged five months with SCID and skin lesions caused by *Varicella* virus contracted from his elder sister, with inadequate immune response mediated by maternally derived T lymphocytes.

OMENN SYNDROME (SCID VARIANT)

INCIDENCE
Unknown, very rare. Autosomal recessive.

AETIOLOGY
Mutations in the recombinase-activating genes 1 and 2 (RAG-1 and RAG-2) have been identified in a number of patients with this syndrome.

PRESENTATION
Within the first year of life, with failure to thrive, diarrhoea, severe infections and opportunistic infections. In addition, prominent generalized dermatitis (**16.34**), lymphadenopathy (**16.35**) and hepatosplenomegaly.

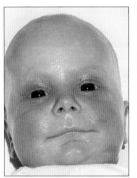
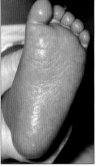

16.31 & 16.32 SCID. Face and plantar surface of left foot of boy aged four months with X-chromosome-linked SCID (common gamma chain deficiency). Exanthematous rash caused by Graft Versus Host Disease mediated by maternally acquired T cells.

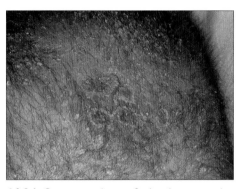

16.34 Omenn syndrome. Scalp of two-month-old girl, showing erythrosquamous exanthema and hair loss.

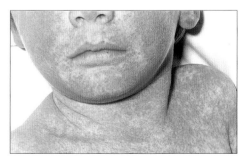

16.33 SCID. Lower part of face and upper part of chest of four-year-old boy with SCID due to purine nucleotide phosphorylase (PNP) deficiency. Exanthematous rash caused by Graft Versus Host Disease after transfusion with unirradiated platelets.

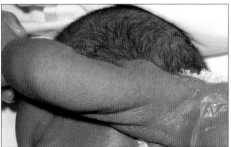

16.35 Omenn syndrome. Head and axilla of the same girl, showing erythrodermic rash and lymphadenopathy.

DIAGNOSIS

Full blood count for total lymphocyte numbers and eosinophils. Phenotyping of lymphocyte subpopulations and activation markers. Lymphocyte proliferation responses. Serum immunoglobulin levels including IgE level. Chimeric studies to exclude the presence of maternal or third-party lymphocytes.

PATHOLOGY

SCID with eosinophilia and lymphohistiocytosis. T cells may be present in normal numbers but the subset distribution, activation pattern and proliferative responses are abnormal. IgE levels may be increased. IgG, IgA and IgM levels are decreased. Omenn syndrome can occur in families with cases of autosomal recessive SCID lacking T and B cells, and both are caused by defects in the recombinase activating genes (RAG-1 and RAG-2).

TREATMENT

Avoidance of live vaccines and non-irradiated CMV (cytomegalovirus) -positive blood products. Immunoglobulin replacement and anti-microbial prophylaxis followed by allogeneic bone marrow transplantation.

PRENATAL DIAGNOSIS AND PROGNOSIS

If a mutation is identified in one of the RAG genes, prenatal diagnosis can be offered by DNA analysis of a chorionic villous sample. Otherwise, fetal blood sampling can be informative, although false positive and false negative test results may occur. Without treatment, the disorder is fatal in infancy and early childhood. After bone marrow transplantation 50–95% survival can be achieved, depending on donor tissue type match and clinical condition at time of bone marrow transplantation.

ADENOSINE DEAMINASE (ADA) DEFICIENCY (SCID)

INCIDENCE

Unknown, very rare, approximately 15% of patients with SCID. Autosomal recessive.

PRESENTATION

Usually in early infancy, with failure to thrive, diarrhoea, severe infections and opportunistic infections. Sometimes neurological symptoms and skeletal abnormalities are found. Milder variants, presenting later in childhood, may occur.

DIAGNOSIS

Full blood count for total lymphocyte numbers. Phenotyping of lymphocyte subpopulations. Lymphocyte proliferation responses. Serum immunoglobulin levels. Levels of ADA in red and/or white blood cells. Levels of toxic metabolites in plasma and urine.

PATHOLOGY

Absence of ADA results in accumulation of toxic metabolites which interferes with lymphocyte survival. ADA is variably expressed in all body tissues and therefore ADA deficiency may cause extra-lymphoid abnormalities (**16.36**).

TREATMENT

Avoidance of live vaccines and non-irradiated CMV-positive blood products. Immunoglobulin substitution and antimicrobial prophylaxis. Bovine PEG (polyethylene glycosylated) -ADA (intramuscular) may improve immune function in a subgroup of patients. Allogeneic bone marrow transplantation restores immune capacity permanently.

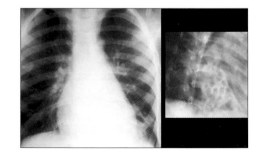

16.36 Chest x-ray of boy with SCID due to adenosine deaminase (ADA) deficiency who presented with tachypnoea, hypoxia and interstitial pneumonitis caused by *Pneumocystis carinii*. Note interstitial infiltration predominantly in the left upper lobe and absence of retrosternally located thymus shadow.

PRENATAL DIAGNOSIS AND PROGNOSIS

Possible by measuring ADA activity in chorion villus biopsy or fetal blood samples. The ADA gene is localized on chromosome 22q 13 and mutation analysis may allow for genetic prenatal diagnosis. Without treatment, the disorder is usually fatal in infancy and early childhood, although cases with milder phenotypes have been described. Continuous weekly treatment with PEG-ADA may improve survival. However, a subgroup of patients will not respond or will only respond transiently. After bone marrow transplantation (BMT) 50–95% survival can be achieved, dependent on donor tissue type match and clinical condition at the time of BMT.

MHC (MAJOR HISTOCOMPATIBILITY COMPLEX) CLASS II DEFICIENCY

Also known as bare lymphocyte syndrome.

INCIDENCE

Unknown, very rare. Autosomal recessive.

PRESENTATION

In infancy and early childhood, with failure to thrive (**16.37**), diarrhoea, severe infections and opportunistic infections (**16.38**).

DIAGNOSIS

Full blood count is usually normal. Investigation of lymphocyte sub-populations may show low CD4+ T-helper lymphocyte numbers. MHC class II (and sometimes class I) expression is absent or low. Serum immunoglobulin levels are low.

PATHOLOGY

Absence of MHC class II expression impairs appropriate antigen presentation, resulting in impaired T and B-cell function. Four distinct genetic subgroups are caused by different transacting gene defects interfering with MHC Class II gene expression.

TREATMENT

Protective isolation and avoidance of live vaccines and non-irradiated CMV-positive blood products. Immunoglobulin substitution and anti-microbial prophylaxis followed by allogeneic bone marrow transplantation.

PRENATAL DIAGNOSIS AND PROGNOSIS

Possible by investigation of MHC Class II expression on fetal blood cells. Without treatment the disorder is usually fatal in early childhood. After BMT 50–95% survival can be achieved, depending on the donor tissue type matching and clinical condition at the time of BMT.

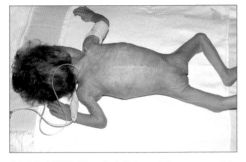

16.37 MHC Class II deficiency. Three-year-old girl with severe diarrhoea, dystrophy and failure to thrive.

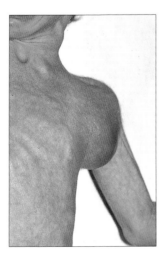

16.38 MHC Class II deficiency. Axilla of the same girl showing marked inflammation and abscess formation caused by BCG vaccination.

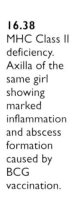

REFERENCES

CVI
Cunningham-Rundles C, Bodian C. Common variable immunodeficiency: clinical and immunologic features of 248 patients. *Clin Immunol* 1999; **92**(1): 34–48

Hypogammaglobulinemia with hyper-IgM
Levy J, Espanol-Boren T, Thomas C *et al.* Clinical spectrum of X-linked hyper-IgM syndrome. *J Pediatr* 1997; **131**(1 Pt 1): 47–54.

Wiskott-Aldrich syndrome
Ochs HD. The Wiskott-Aldrich syndrome. *Clin Rev Allergy Immunol.* 2001 Feb;**20**(1):61-86.
Sullivan KE, Mullen CA, Blaese RM, Winkelstein JA. A multi-institutional survey of the Wiskott-Aldrich syndrome. *J Pediatr* 1994; **125**: 876–885.

X-linked agammaglobulinemia (Bruton's disease)
Bruton OC. Agammaglobulinemia. *Paediatrics* 1952; **9**: 722–728.
Ochs HD, Smith CI. X-linked agammaglobulinemia. A clinical and molecular analysis. *Medicine* 1996; **75**(6): 287–299.
Stewart DM, Lian L, Nelson DL. The clinical spectrum of Bruton's agammaglobulinemia. *Curr Allergy Asthma Rep.* 2001 Nov;**1**(6):558-65.

X-linked lymphoproliferative disease
Gaspar HB, Sharifi R, Gilmour KC, Thrasher AJ. X-linked lymphoproliferative disease: clinical, diagnostic and molecular perspective. *Br J Haematol.* 2002 Dec;**119**(3):585-95.
Purtillo DT, Cassel CK, Yang YPS, Harper R. X-linked recessive progressive combined variable immunodeficiency (Duncan's disease). *Lancet* 1975; **1**: 935–940.

Chronic mucocutaneous candidiasis
Herrod HG. Chronic mucocutaneous candidiasis in childhood and complications of non-candida infections: a report of the paediatric immunodeficiency collaborative study group. *J Pediatr* 1990; **116**: 377–382.
Kalfa VC, Roberts RL, Stiehm ER. The syndrome of chronic mucocutaneous candidiasis with selective antibody deficiency. *Ann Allergy Asthma Immunol.* 2003 Feb;**90**(2):259-64.

Louis-Bar
Perlman S, Becker-Catania S, Gatti RA. Ataxia-telangiectasia: diagnosis and treatment. *Semin Pediatr Neurol.* 2003 Sep;**10**(3):173-82.

Chediak-Higashi syndrome
Ward DM, Shiflett SL, Kaplan J. Chediak-Higashi syndrome: a clinical and molecular view of a rare lysosomal storage disorder. *Curr Mol Med.* 2002 Aug;**2**(5):469-77.

Leucocyte adhesion defects
Inwald D, Davies EG, Klein N. Demystified...adhesion molecule deficiencies. *Mol Pathol.* 2001 Feb;**54**(1):1-7.

Di George syndrome
Hong R. The DiGeorge anomaly (CATCH 22, Di George/velocardiofacial syndrome). *Semin Haematol* 1998; **35**(4): 282–290.
Perez E, Sullivan KE. Chromosome 22q11.2 deletion syndrome (DiGeorge and velocardiofacial syndromes). *Curr Opin Pediatr.* 2002 Dec;**14**(6):678-83.

Chronic granulomatous disease (CGD)
Goldblatt D, Thrasher AJ. CGD: a review. *Clin Exp Imm* 2000; **122**: 1–9.
Heyworth PG, Cross AR, Curnutte JT. Chronic granulomatous disease. *Curr Opin Immunol.* 2003 Oct;**15**(5):578-84.

Hyper IgE syndrome
Buckley RH. The hyper-IgE syndrome. *Clin Rev Allergy Immunol.* 2001 Feb;**20**(1):139-54.
Geha RS, Leung DYM. Hyper Immunoglobulin E Syndrome. In: Rosen FS, Seligman M (eds). *Immunodeficiencies.* Switzerland: Harwood Academic Publishers, 1993: 571–583.
Grimbacher B, Holland SM, Gallin JI, Greenberg F, Hill SC, Malech HL, Miller JA, O'Connell AC, Puck JM. Hyper-IgE syndrome with recurrent infections--an autosomal dominant multisystem disorder. *N Engl J Med.* 1999 Mar 4;**340**(9):692-702.

Severe combined immunodeficiency (SCID)
Porta F, Friedrich W. Bone marrow transplantation in congenital immunodeficiency diseases. *Bone Marr Transpl* 1998; **21**(Suppl 2): S21–S23.

Omenn syndrome
Aleman K, Noordzij JG, de Groot R, van Dongen JJ, Hartwig NG. Reviewing Omenn syndrome. *Eur J Pediatr.* 2001 Dec;**160**(12):718-25.
Fischer A. Severe combined immunodeficiencies (SCID). *Clin Exp Immunol.* 2000 Nov;**122**(2):143-9.
Omenn GS. Familial reticuloendotheliosis with eosinophilia. N Engl J Med 1965; 273: 427–431.

Adenosine deaminase (ADA) deficiency
Hershfield MS. Adenosine deaminase deficiency: clinical expression, molecular basis, and therapy. *Semin Hematol.* 1998 Oct;**35**(4):291-8.

MHC (major histocompatibility complex) class II deficiency
Klein C, Lisowska-Grospierre B, LeDeist F *et al.* Major histocompatibility complex Class II deficiency: clinical manifestations, immunological features, and outcome. *J Paediatr* 1993; **123**: 921–928.

Rheumatology

Kevin Murray • Clarissa Pilkington Patricia Woo

JUVENILE IDIOPATHIC ARTHRITIS (JIA)

What was formerly termed juvenile chronic arthritis has now been determined to represent a heterogenous group of clinically and genetically distinct forms of chronic arthritis. These diseases are now grouped together under the term juvenile idiopathic arthritis (JIA) and are described below. The incidence of JIA overall is approximately 1 in 10,000, while the prevalence in children is 1 in 1,000 (15–20,000 children have JIA in the UK).

SYSTEMIC ONSET JIA

Incidence
1:100,000. Onset commonest between 1 and 5 years, but occurs throughout childhood and into adult years (adult onset Still's disease).

Diagnosis
Arthritis may be mild and remitting, or chronic, progressive and destructive (**17.1**). Growth failure is common, secondary to either disease or with use of corticosteroids. Inflammation of the pericardium, peritoneum (mimicking acute abdomen) and pleural surfaces may be a major feature. Daily spiking fevers (**17.2**) (once to

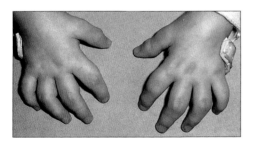

17.1 Symmetrical polyarthritis and tenosynovitis in a young child with systemic onset JIA.

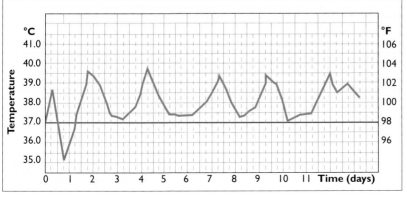

17.2 Typical swinging high fever chart in a child with systemic onset JIA.

thrice) and a typical rash, which is salmon pink, macular and evanescent (although erythematous, urticarial, or pruritic in some patients), persisting for more than two weeks (**17.3**).

Treatment
The disease can be steroid-dependent. NSAIDs (non-steroidal anti-inflammatory drugs) in high doses are frequently useful, but disease-modifying agents such as methotrexate or ciclosporin may be required. Biological agents, such as anti-tumour necrosis factor (TNF), may help. None of these therapies achieve remission in more than 30% of cases. Rehabilitation including physiotherapy and occupational therapy (e.g. splinting) are essential.

Prognosis
In approximately 50% of cases, the disease resolves in the first few years with or without permanent joint damage. In the other 50%, the disease is long-lasting with a risk of progressive joint destruction. Growth failure and osteoporosis occur in many patients and secondary amyloidosis in some patients.

POLYARTICULAR ONSET: RHEUMATOID FACTOR NEGATIVE JIA
Incidence
One in 25,000, with commonest onset <6 years of age; but seen throughout childhood

Diagnosis
Polyarticular JIA refers to five or more joints being affected at onset. It affects both large and small joints in either symmetrical or asymmetrical patterns. An early predilection for cervical spine and temperomandibular joint (TMJ) involvement (with resultant micrognathia) is common (**17.4**) but knee, ankle, wrist, hip and elbow involvement are commonest, and contractures are frequent if untreated (**17.5**). May be destructive in up to 30–40% of cases, especially if untreated. Up to 50% of patients are ANA positive with some risk of chronic anterior uveitis.

Treatment
NSAID therapy, joint injections with corticosteroids in most patients. Disease-modifying drugs such as methotrexate, are often required. Biological agents such as etanercept may be very useful for resistant disease. Physiotherapy and occupational therapy is mandatory and podiatry may be important.

Prognosis
Approximately 50% of patients go into remission between two and ten years after onset. The remainder continue with disease activity into adult years, with variable severity.

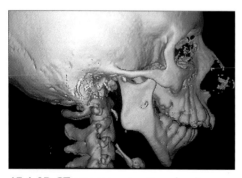

17.3 Typical 'salmon-pink' rash in the axilla and upper arm of a child with systemic onset JIA.

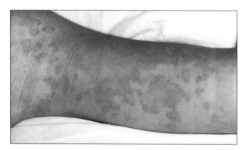

17.4 3D CT scan reconstruction, showing severe micrognathia in a 12-year-old boy with JIA.

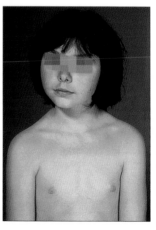

17.5 Torticollis due to cervical spine involvement in an eight-year-old girl with JIA.

POLYARTICULAR ONSET: RHEUMATOID FACTOR POSITIVE JIA

Incidence
Less than 1 in 100,000 in childhood.

Diagnosis
Childhood onset of the identical disease to adult onset 'seropositive' rheumatoid arthritis. Onset usually after eight years, most commonly in females. Associated with the presence of nodules, vasculitis and severe, progressive, destructive disease in many, if untreated. Symmetrical polyarthritis (**17.6**), typically involving proximal interphalangeal joints (PIPs), metocarpophalangeal joints (MCPs), wrists, knees and feet in early years, progressing to most joints later (**17.7**).

Treatment
As for rheumatoid factor negative polyarthritis, but earlier intervention with disease-modifying anti-rheumatic drugs (DMARDs) is usually mandatory. Steroids are required in a number of patients especially with vasculitis. Physiotherapy is mandatory to maintain joint function.

Prognosis
In some patients, the disease may remit in later teenage years, but it remains active in many. It is likely to be destructive unless treated early. In some patients, progression occurs despite treatment.

OLIGOARTICULAR ARTHRITIS

Incidence
This is the commonest type of JIA (60% of cases) occurring in 1 in 15,000 children. Commonest in young females, with onset typically between one and five years of age and a peak age of onset at three years.

Diagnosis
Oligoarticular JIA involves four or fewer joints. Patients are frequently anti-nuclear antibody positive ($\geq$75%) with a significant risk of anterior uveitis (approximately 25%), usually occurring in the first five years after onset of arthritis. Anterior uveitis is clinically silent and is diagnosed on slit lamp examination. Therefore three-monthly slit lamp examinations are recommended. The arthritis is usually asymmetric and affects the large joints and lower limbs including knees and ankles. In up to 25% of cases the disease may extend to multiple joints after the first six months and pursue a course identical to polyarticular JIA (extended oligoarthritis).

Treatment
Treatment of the arthritis is usually with NSAIDs and intermittent joint aspiration and corticosteroid injection. Eye disease is usually treated with topical steroids and mydriatics. Untreated uveitis can lead to visual impairment or blindness. Methotrexate may be useful for severe persistent disease.

Prognosis
Unless inflammation is suppressed, significant bony overgrowth may occur in the affected joints causing, for example, leg-length discrepancies and angular deformity which may

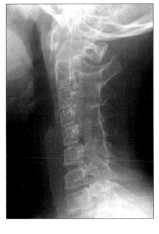

17.6 Symmetrical 'swan-neck' and 'boutonnière' deformities in a 15-year-old girl.

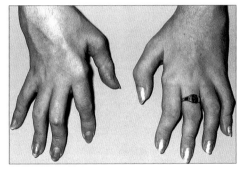

17.7 Cervical spine fusion and osteoporosis in a child with severe progressive JIA.

require surgery to correct (**17.8**, **17.9**). Between 10–20% of patients may go on to develop polyarticular (extended oligoarticular) arthritis, with greater risk for joint destruction and loss of function; ≥75% of patients tend to go into remission in late childhood, but the disease can persist or recur in adult years.

ENTHESITIS-RELATED ARTHRITIS

Formerly known as juvenile onset spondylo-arthropathy or juvenile ankylosing spondylitis.

INCIDENCE
One in 100,000 children per year. Usually occurs in males >8 years of age.

DIAGNOSIS
Predominantly lower limb, large joint, asymmetric arthritis (**17.10**). An acute, painful, anterior uveitis occurs, which rarely causes permanent visual loss if treated. Enthesitis (inflammation of ligament and tendon insertions) is typical and often very painful (**17.11**). Common sites of enthesitis include the Achilles tendon insertion or proximal plantar fascial insertion into the calcaneum, but patella tendon (quadriceps) insertion inflammation may occur also. Spinal and sacroiliac involvement (ankylosing spondylitis) is uncommon in childhood but may occur in later life in some patients. The arthritis may progress to involve the hip joints in adolescence and be very destructive. A family history of spondylo-arthropathy is common.

TREATMENT
As for oligoarticular arthritis, with NSAIDs, joint injections, and disease-modifying agents such as sulphasalazine and methotrexate for persistent or progressive arthritis. Anti-TNF therapy is particularly beneficial for spinal and sacral–iliac inflammation. Physiotherapy and occupational therapy input are critical.

PROGNOSIS
In many patients the disease persists or recurs intermittently into adult years. In some, remission occurs in late childhood.

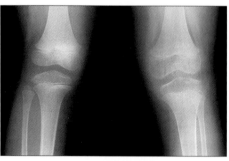

17.8 X-ray of a six-year-old boy with oligo-articular JIA of the left knee, showing medial overgrowth of the femoral and tibial condyles, osteoporosis and early valgus deformity.

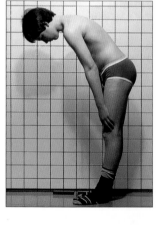

17.10 A 12-year-old boy with juvenile ankylosing spondylitis showing limited flexion of the lumbar spine and loss of lumbar lordosis.

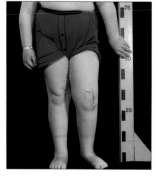

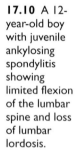

17.9 The child in 17.8, showing swelling and fixed flexion deformity of the left knee.

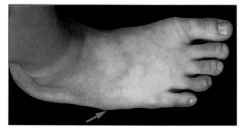

17.11 Enthesitis at the base of the right 5th metatarsal (arrow) in an eight-year-old girl with enthesitis-related arthritis.

PSORIATIC ARTHRITIS

INCIDENCE
Fewer than 1 in 100,000 children

DIAGNOSIS
Arthritis associated with psoriasis (**17.12**) may closely mimic oligoarticular or polyarticular JIA. Dactylitis (sausage fingers or toes) or swelling of the digits is characteristic (**17.13**). Nail pitting and the characteristic psoriatic rash (or a family history of this) are typical, although they may occur many years after the onset of arthritis and only be prominent in first-degree relatives. Joint destruction may occur in some patients. Some children get anterior uveitis.

TREATMENT
As for oligo/polyarticular JIA. Skin disease may respond to steroids or methotrexate.

PROGNOSIS
Remission may occur in late childhood, but the disease persists in a number of patients.

ARTHRITIS ASSOCIATED WITH OTHER CHRONIC DISEASES

INFLAMMATORY BOWEL DISEASE
Occurs in 10–20% of IBD patients with ulcerative colitis or Crohn's disease. Treatment of the underlying bowel disease may improve arthritis, but it can become progressive and destructive, requiring intensive anti-rheumatic therapy. Sulphasalazine is often useful. Arthritis and growth failure may precede clinical bowel disease (**17.14**).

CYSTIC FIBROSIS
Between 5 and 10% of patients may develop an inflammatory arthropathy. This is commonest in teenagers and young adults. It usually responds to NSAIDs and is rarely destructive. Hypertrophic osteoarthropathy with severe lung disease occurs and may require treatment.

IMMUNODEFICIENCY
Both humoral and cellular deficiency syndromes may be associated with inflammatory arthritis. This is rarely destructive or deforming, but often requires treatment with NSAIDs and physiotherapy.

ASSOCIATED SYNDROMES
Patients with Down and Turner syndromes and velocardiofacial (22q deletion) syndrome may all develop inflammatory arthritis requiring treatment.

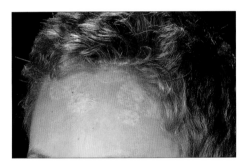

17.12 Scaly psoriatic plaques in a four-year-old boy who presented with arthritis of the knee.

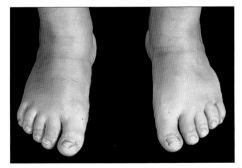

17.13 Dactylitis of multiple digits in the child in the previous picture.

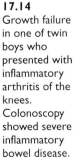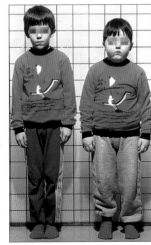

17.14 Growth failure in one of twin boys who presented with inflammatory arthritis of the knees. Colonoscopy showed severe inflammatory bowel disease.

SCLERODERMA

SYSTEMIC SCLEROSIS

Incidence
Fewer than 1 in 200,000 children per year. Systemic sclerosis is rare in childhood. It may occur as a progressive form with widespread skin and internal organ involvement, or in a limited form with oesophageal involvement and skin changes limited to more distal extremities. It may occur as part of overlap syndromes.

Diagnosis
Skin changes are typical on the face and limbs and include loss of subcutaneous tissues, hardening and tightening of the skin with telangiectasia and calcinosis. Joint contractures, particularly of the hand, are common (**17.15**). It is felt to be due to a vasculopathy with secondary changes in collagen and connective tissue. Involvement of the kidneys and lungs may be life-threatening.

Treatment
This consists of local skin-softening treatments and systemic treatment with steroids and immunosuppressives, though the disease may be unresponsive in some patients. Boseutan and ACE inhibitors, for cardiopulmonary and renal disease respectively, have improved the prognosis.

Prognosis
Mortality is 5–10% during childhood, but this is improved with early treatment of complications such as pulmonary hypertension and renal disease.

LOCALIZED SCLERODERMA (MORPHOEA)

Incidence
Rare: fewer than 1 in 200,000 children per year, though ten times more common than systemic sclerosis in childhood and rare in adults

Diagnosis
- Linear scleroderma – usually affecting one or more upper and/or lower limbs, or the face (*en coup de sabre*) or trunk.
- Morphoea – round or oval patches of indurated, hyper- or hypo-pigmented skin – may become widespread (diffuse form).

The *en coup de sabre* lesion may be associated with uveitis and cerebral involvement (seizures) (**17.16**). Involvement may be severe, with thickening of superficial skin, loss of subcutaneous tissue, deformity of long bones, and failure of limb growth (**17.17**). Contractures of joints are common.

Treatment
No definite therapy is successful but steroids, immunosuppressives (such as methotrexate) may lead to considerable improvement. Physical therapies are essential to improve function.

Prognosis
Active disease in many for five to six years then progress may stop. Treatment may prevent progress in some but in others it may be unrelenting.

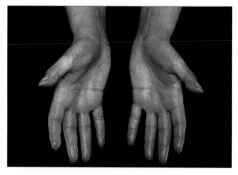

17.15 Severe sclerodactyly in a 15-year-old girl with systemic sclerosis.

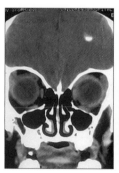

17.16 Intracerebral calcification shown on CT scan in five-year-old child with localized scleroderma of the face on the same side.

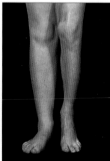

17.17 Severe localized scleroderma of the left leg in a six-year-old girl showing tissue atrophy and local growth failure.

DERMATOMYOSITIS

INCIDENCE

Rare: fewer than 1 in 200,000 children per year. Onset commonly between four and ten years of age. Later peak in adult years.

DIAGNOSIS

This is based on clinical features, muscle enzyme elevation (creatinine kinase – CK, aspartate aminotransferase – AST, alanine aminotransferase – ALT, LDH), abnormal electromyogram (EMG), magnetic resonance imaging (MRI) findings, and characteristic muscle biopsy appearances. Progressive proximal weakness of hip, shoulder, trunk and neck muscles, associated with painful, tender or swollen muscles and subcutaneous tissue, is typical. Most children have an erythematous, scaly rash affecting the eyelids, which may look 'bluish' (heliotrope) and be associated with periorbital oedema (**17.18**). The skin over the MCP and PIP joints and elbows and knees is typically involved, showing Gottron's papules. Palatal and oesophageal involvement causes dysphagia and dysphonia.

More generalized vasculopathy, with severe skin ulceration, gut involvement and other organ involvement, may occur in 5–10% (**17.19**). Respiratory muscle weakness may occur rarely, and may cause respiratory failure. Skin ulceration may also occur. Gastrointestinal vasculopathy with perforation may occur rarely. Disease activity is monitored clinically (muscle strength), biochemically and with MRI or ultrasound (**17.20**). Muscle enzymes may be helpful only in the early phases of the disease.

TREATMENT

Treatment is with high-dose steroids (initially intravenous then oral). Many require immunosuppressants such as methotrexate, ciclosporin or cyclophosphamide. Physio and occupational therapy with splinting is essential to prevent contractures. Hydroxychloroquine or mepacrine may be useful for a persistent severe rash.

PROGNOSIS

If untreated, muscle weakness may spread to thoracic muscles and lead to respiratory failure. Skin changes may be slow to resolve. Late treatment may be associated with permanent loss of muscle bulk and contractures. Calcinosis of the skin and subcutaneous tissues may occur, usually later in the disease, and be ulcerating and disfiguring. One third resolve within two to three years, one third resolve within six years, and one third persist longer. Mortality is 1–5% overall.

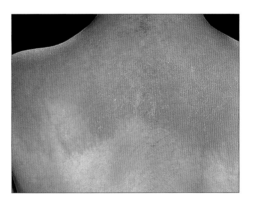

17.19 A photosensitive 'shawl' distribution rash in a 10-year-old girl with juvenile dermatomyositis.

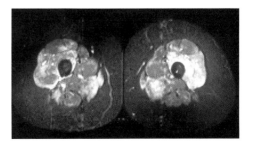

17.18 Typical heliotrope rash on the eyelids of a seven-year-old girl with juvenile dermatomyositis.

17.20 MRI of the thighs of an eight-year-old girl with juvenile dermatolmyositis showing widespread muscle oedema due to inflammation.

VASCULITIDES

KAWASAKI DISEASE

See also 'Emergency Medicine' (page 26) and 'Infectious Diseases' chapters.

Incidence

One in 33,500 in the UK. 1 in 700 in Japan.

Diagnosis

Kawasaki disease, distinct from infantile poly-arteritis nodosa, includes the classical features of fever, lymphadenopathy, conjunctival injection, oral mucosal/labial inflammation, together with distal extremity swelling, oedema and late desquamation of fingers and toes (**17.21–17.23**). Coronary artery involvement can occur in 10–25%, although early treatment usually prevents this. Arthritis, aseptic meningitis and other organ involvement may occur.

Treatment

Intravenous immunoglobulin in the first ten days, together with high-dose oral aspirin. Corticosteroids are used in relapsing cases.

Prognosis

Usually good with early treatment. Coronary artery involvement may lead to aneurysm, thrombosis or stenosis. Premature ischaemic heart disease can occur.

POLYARTERITIS NODOSA (PAN)

Incidence

Rare: fewer than 1 in 200,000. Commoner in males. Average onset at age five to seven years.

Diagnosis

The onset is at any time during childhood and can be insidious with malaise and fever of unknown origin. Common features are persistent fever, variable vasculitic skin lesions including livedo reticularis, purpura or ulcers, abdominal pain and arthritis (**17.24**). Renal involvement with proteinuria and haematuria is typical. Aneurysms of medium-size vessels (renal and gut) occur and are characteristic (**17.25**). Exclusive skin involvement is seen in cutaneous PAN, often post-infectious (streptococcal).

Treatment

Steroids and cyclophosphamide are necessary. Plasma exchange or prostaglandin analogues may be tried. Azathioprine and ciclosporin may be tried later.

Prognosis

The disease may be recurrent rather than monophasic and up to 20% mortality is seen.

OTHER VASCULITIDES

Microscopic polyangiitis, Wegener's granulomatosis, Takayasu's arteritis, cerebral angiitis, hypersensitivity angiitis (urticarial vasculitis) can occur in children, though all are rare and treatment usually involves steroids and/or immunosuppressive agents.

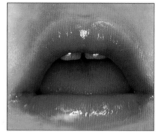

17.21 Oral changes in Kawasaki disease showing 'cherry-red' lips and 'strawberry' tongue.

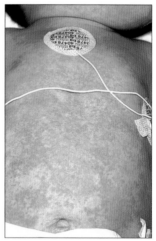

17.22 Characteristic pleomorphic maculopapular truncal rash.

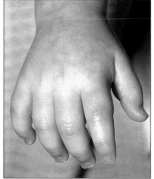

17.23 Polyarthritis of the wrist and hand with accompanying extremity oedema.

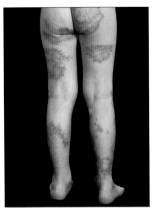

17.24 Superfical vasculitic rash in a 15-year-old boy with new-onset PAN.

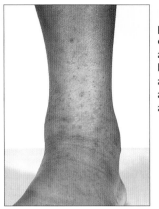

17.26 Palpable purpuric rash on the legs of a five-year-old boy with HSP, also showing arthritis of the ankles.

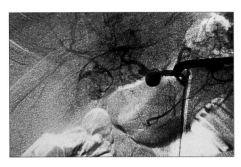

17.25 Angiogram demonstrating intrahepatic aneurysm formation in a 22-year-old with long-standing PAN.

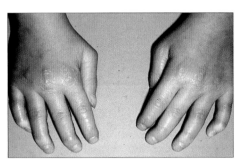

17.27 Polyarthritis, sclerodactyly and Gottrons papules in a 13-year-old boy with MCTD who is anti-RNP antibody positive.

HENOCH–SCHÖNLEIN PURPURA (HSP)

See also 'Renal Diseases' chapter.

INCIDENCE
Commonest vasculitis in childhood

DIAGNOSIS
Clinical diagnosis with typical palpable purpuric rash of lower limbs, buttocks, abdominal pain and glomerulonephritis (50%). Arthritis occurs in some patients but extremity oedema is more common (**17.26**). Chronic renal failure in less than 5%.

TREATMENT
Supportive, except steroids in severe abdominal pain or in Henoch-Schönlein nephritis (steroids and/or immunosuppressives).

PROGNOSIS
Usually good except if persistent nephritis when, in rare cases, end-stage renal failure develops.

MIXED CONNECTIVE TISSUE DISEASE (MCTD)

INCIDENCE
Uncommon: 1 in 50,000 children per year, mostly females.

DIAGNOSIS
Present with mixture of features of different connective tissue disorders, largely SLE, dermatomyositis and scleroderma. Generally, features are milder, with renal and CNS involvement being absent or late. Usually ANA positive and ENA positive with RNP antibodies characteristic (**17.27**).

TREATMENT AND PROGNOSIS
As for the underlying connective tissue disease, usually treatments used in SLE are appropriate.

SYSTEMIC LUPUS ERYTHEMATOSUS (SLE)

INCIDENCE
One in 3,000 to 10,000 children per year (Caucasians <Asians <Africans).

DIAGNOSIS
Occurs throughout childhood, though rare in children <5 years. Most common in females >12 years. Pathology is thought to be due to polyclonal B-cell activation and immune complex formation and deposition. Onset is commonly insidious, with fatigue, rash and polyarthritis, but it may be acute, with serositis, central nervous system or renal involvement. The typical rash is erythematous, scaling, photosensitive and occurs on the face in a malar distribution, and in sun-exposed sites. Elsewhere discoid lesions may occur (alone in some). SLE is an episodic, multisystem auto-immune disease with widespread inflammation of blood vessels and connective tissues. The skin involvement may result in malar rash, discoid rash, vasculitis and/or photosensitivity (**17.28, 17.29**) Arthritis is polyarticular and painful but rarely destructive.

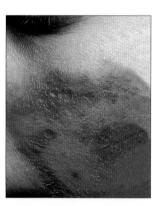

17.28 Typical malar rash in a 15-year-old showing some discoid lesions.

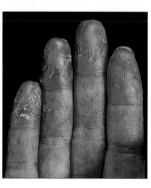

17.29 Severe vasculitis of the fingertips with scarring in a 13-year-old girl.

Suspected renal involvement can be defined by urinary albumin/creatinine ratio, serum creatinine GFR, and renal biopsy. Central nervous system involvement may manifest as seizures, chorea, depression or cognitive changes. CSF findings are non-specific. MRI findings may be supportive.

Antinuclear antibodies are found in virtually all patients, and in $\geq80\%$ antibodies to dsDNA. Anti-Smith antibodies, present in 20%, are very specific. Anticardiolipin (antiphospholipid) antibodies are present in more than 25% and are associated with risk of thrombosis. Patients with only anticardiolipin antibodies and throm-boses or recurrent abortions have the primary antiphospholipid syndrome.

TREATMENT
CNS and/or renal disease usually mandates immunosuppressive treatment with azathioprine or cyclophosphamide and high-dose steroids. Otherwise treatment with hydroxychloroquine, low dose steroids and NSAIDs is appropriate. Anti-platelet treatment with aspirin is required for antiphospholipid antibody positive patients. Patients with thrombosis require warfarin treatment.

PROGNOSIS
In patients with CNS and renal involvement significant morbidity may occur. In others, long periods of good disease control or remission can be seen.

OVERLAP CONNECTIVE TISSUE DISEASE (CTD)

INCIDENCE
Uncommon: 1 in 50,000 to 100,000, mostly females.

DIAGNOSIS
Some patients develop clinical features of two different connective tissue diseases at the same time or in progression, such as JIA and SLE, JIA and dermatomyositis (**17.30**), dermato-myositis and scleroderma. There are no specific antibodies but patients are often ANA positive. Occasionally, patients will have moderate fea-tures of a number of disorders, but insufficient to fulfil any diagnosis; often termed undifferen-tiated CTD.

TREATMENT AND PROGNOSIS
As for the underlying connective tissue disease.

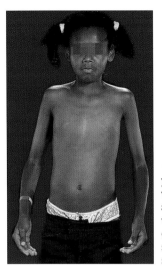

17.30 A 10-year-old girl with myositis, arthritis of wrists and elbows and scleroderma skin changes.

CHRONIC INFANTILE NEUROLOGICAL CUTANEOUS AND ARTICULAR SYNDROME (CINCA)

INCIDENCE
Very rare: fewer than 1 in 500,000

DIAGNOSIS
A triad of clinical symptoms, similar to systemic onset JIA, present neonatally:
- Non-pruritic persistent urticarial rash (75% of patients at birth) (**17.31**).
- Joint involvement (50% of patients in the first year).
- CNS involvement (aseptic meningitis, seizures, uveitis, papillitis, optic atrophy, low IQ, sensory anomalies).

Saddle nose deformity is seen early, with typical facies such as frontal bossing, and there may be progressive growth retardation (17.32). Abnormalities on x-ray include flared, irregular, cupped metaphyses and large, irregular, fragmented epiphyses.

Investigations show:
- Low haemoglobin.
- Raised white blood count.
- Raised erythrocyte sedimentation rate.
- Raised immunoglobulins.
- Raised CSF white cell count and/or protein.

Genetic testing reveals mutations in the CIAS1 gene in ≥50% of cases.

TREATMENT
NSAIDs help to deal with the pain. Steroids and immunosuppressants may help fever and pain but, in some, have little effect on skin lesions, joints or the central nervous system. This is now replaced by treatment with anakinra (IL-1 receptor antagonist).

PROGNOSIS
A chronic course, with frequent relapses. Fever, lymphadenopathy, enlarged spleen, severe developmental delay and significant mortality are seen.

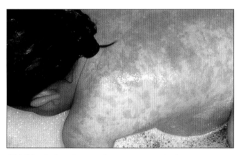

17.31 A fixed maculopapular rash from birth in a six-month-old child with uveitis and arthritis as part of CINCA syndrome.

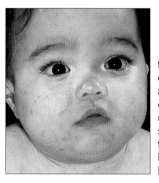

17.32 Typical facial features of CINCA in an the above child at 11 months, showing flattened nasal bridge and hydrocephalus.

CHRONIC RECURRENT MULTIFOCAL OSTEOMYELITIS (CRMO)

INCIDENCE
Rare: fewer than 1 in 200,000.

DIAGNOSIS
Presents with bone or joint pain, swelling, and fever. Pain is metaphyseal, joints are usually normal, with the tibia as the most common site. X-rays show osteolytic lesions in the metaphysis, osteitis and new bone formation (**17.33**). A bone scan is often helpful. Biopsy shows chronic inflammation consistent with osteomyelitis. Cultures are negative. May be related to or overlap with SAPHO.

TREATMENT
Antibiotics usually have no effect. NSAIDs may improve symptoms. Steroids may help resolve persistent lesions; other treatments experimental.

PROGNOSIS
Spontaneous remissions with periodic painful relapses. Bony overgrowth or loss of growth may cause leg length discrepancy or joint deformity. Occasionally, the patient has palmar plantar pustulosis and acne associated with arthritis and hyperostosis (SAPHO – synovitis, acne, pustulosis, hyperostosis and osteitis) (**17.34**).

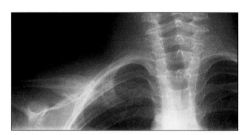

17.33 Clavicular osteitis in nine-year-old boy with CRMO.

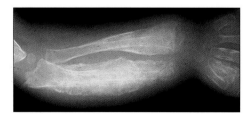

17.34 Extensive osteitis and new bone formation in an 11-month-old boy with SAPHO syndrome.

PERIODIC FEVER SYNDROMES

FAMILIAL MEDITERRANEAN FEVER
Incidence
Uncommon, except in Sephardic Jews (1 in 700 compared with fewer than 1 in 100,000 in other races), Turkish and Cypriot populations. Particularly seen in the Middle East and Mediterranean countries. The common gene mutations are now known.

Diagnosis
This is a genetic autosomal recessive condition. The defective gene (pyrin) has been identified on chromosome 16. Onset of the disease is usually between the ages of one and five years, with acute attacks of fever, peritonitis, arthritis and pleuritis. The attacks may occur frequently or irregularly with periods of remission. Rash, orchitis and pericarditis are seen less commonly. The arthritis may be chronic and destructive in some patients. Secondary amyloidosis occurs with significant morbidity and mortality.

Treatment
Colchicine for acute attacks and prevention of episodes and amyloidosis. NSAIDs and occasionally steroids may be required.

OTHER GENETIC PERIODIC FEVERS
TNF-receptor-associated periodic syndrome causes recurrent fever, rash (**17.35**) and arthritis from early childhood and is caused by an autosomal dominant mutation in the tumour necrosis factor receptor gene. A family history is common and amyloidosis may occur. Treatment with etanacept (a synthetic TNF receptor) is effective.

Hyper IgD syndrome causes recurrent fever, rash, abdominal pain and joint symptoms from early childhood, and is due to homozygocity for the autosomal recessive gene defect in mevalonate kinase enzyme. The prognosis is usually good but the frequent attacks in childhood may cause serious morbidty. Early reports of treatment with anakinra (IL-1 receptor antagonist) is promising.

17.35 Erythema multiforme rash in a seven-year-old girl with TNF-receptor-associated periodic syndrome.

CHRONIC PAIN SYNDROME

Both localized and diffuse chronic pain syndromes occur in childhood. More definable forms include reflex sympathetic dystrophy, fibromyalgia, myalgic encephalitis, chronic fatigue syndrome and post-viral fatigue syndrome. All of these conditions have major psychological components, which are either aetiological or result from the inciting illness. Psychological intervention and, usually, physiotherapy are mandatory in these conditions.

FIBROMYALGIA

INCIDENCE
Fewer than 1 in 10,000 children per year, but it is increasing (due largely to recognition), predominantly among adolescent females.

DIAGNOSIS
The patient complains of musculoskeletal problems, with generalized aching and stiffness in the back and peripheral muscles and joints (**17.36**). There are characteristic tender or trigger points in the back and shoulders. Non-restorative sleep, depressive symptoms and psychosocial factors are common and at least partly aetiological in this condition.

TREATMENT
Simple analgesia. Low- or higher-dose anti-depressants, intensive physiotherapy and hydrotherapy; psychological intervention is usually required and effective in many cases.

PROGNOSIS
Most improve with early intervention but chronic symptoms occur in many and in some are disabling.

REFLEX SYMPATHETIC DYSTROPHY (ALGODYSTROPHY)

INCIDENCE
Uncommon: $\leq 1{:}50{,}000$, predominantly in females over eight years of age.

DIAGNOSIS
RSD is a regionalized pain syndrome, thought to be an exaggerated response to minor trauma or other localized minor pathology, with psychosocial features. Alterations in skin temperature, soft tissue swelling, sweating, oedema and dysaesthesia occur, with pseudoparalysis, severe spontaneous pain, and pain on weight bearing. Atrophy of skin and bone may occur over time if untreated (**17.37**). Bone scans may show increased or reduced uptake; x-rays may show osteoporosis with long-standing disease.

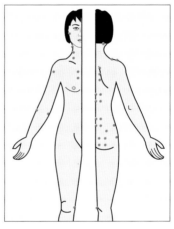

17.36 Sites of tender points in a young person with fibromyalgia.

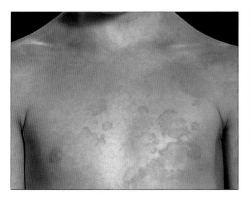

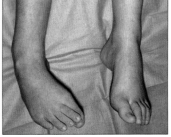

17.37 Long-standing reflex sympathetic dystrophy in a 13-year-old, showing skin colour changes and flexion posture of the left foot.

TREATMENT

Intensive physiotherapy and psychological input are considered essential. Inpatient treatment is often required. Sympathetic blocks rarely are required or useful in children.

PROGNOSIS

With early treatment most patients improve significantly, but recurrences do happen. Delay in diagnosis is associated with considerable prolonged morbidity and disability.

BENIGN JOINT HYPERMOBILITY SYNDROME

INCIDENCE

Common: children have a greater range of normal joint mobility than adults, but 5–10% have either localized or generalized hypermobility (up to 10% of which becomes symptomatic). Specific genetic syndromes, such as Marfan syndrome or Ehlers-Danlos syndrome, cause more severe joint problems.

DIAGNOSIS

The joints usually affected and symptomatic are knees, ankles, elbows and wrists (**17.38**).

Recurrent minor 'sprain' injuries, or more serious subluxation/dislocation, lead to recurrent arthralgias and occasional joint effusions. Growing pains are commonly related to hypermobility. Adolescents may present with back pain. Many persist with various symptoms into adults years. Psychosocial issues may predispose patients to chronicity, or poor response to treatment, and morbidity.

TREATMENT

Involves physiotherapy and/or hydrotherapy with specific muscle strengthening and joint protection measures (such as supportive shoes and insoles) anti-inflammatories and analgesics; activity modifications are often required.

PROGNOSIS

Generally good, many improving with age, function usually maintained.

REFERENCES

Madison PJ, Isenberg DA, Woo P, Glass DN (eds). *Oxford Textbook of Rheumatology* (2nd edn). Oxford: OUP, 1998.

Cassidy J, Petty R (eds). *Textbook of Paediatric Rheumatology* (4th edn). Philadelphia: Saunders, 2000.

Jacobs J. *Paediatric Rheumatology for the Practitioner*. New York: Springer Verlag, 1994.

Galon J, Aksentijevich I, McDermott MF, O'Shea JJ, Kastner DL. TNFRSF1A mutations and autoinflammatory syndromes. *Curr Opin Immunol* 2000; **12**(4): 479–486.

Frenkel J, Houten SM, Waterham HR *et al*. Clinical and molecular variability in childhood periodic fever with hyperimmunoglobulinaemia D. *Rheumatology* 2001; **40**(5): 579–584

Murray KJ, Woo P. Benign joint hypermobility in childhood. *Rheumatology* 2001; **40**(5): 489–491.

Murray CS, Cohen A, Perkins T, Davidson JE, Sills JA. Morbidity in reflex sympathetic dystrophy. *Arch Dis Child* 2000; **82**(3): 231–233.

Prieur AM, Griscelli C, Lampert F *et al*. A chronic, infantile, neurological, cutaneous and articular (CINCA) syndrome. A specific entity analysed in 30 patients. *Scand J Rheumatol* 1987; **66**(Suppl): 57–68.

Girschick HJ, Krauspe R, Tschammler A, Huppertz HI. Chronic recurrent osteomyelitis with clavicular involvement in children: diagnostic value of different imaging techniques and therapy with non-steroidal anti-inflammatory drugs. *Eur J Pediatr* 1998; **157**(1): 28–33.

Drenth JPH, Van Der Meer JWM. Hereditary periodic fever. *N Engl J Med* 2001; **345**(24): 1748–1757.

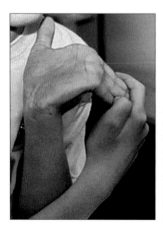

17.38 Hyperextension of the MCP joints of the hands demonstrated in a nine-year-old girl with benign joint hypermobility syndrome.

Speech and Language Therapy

Lesley Cavalli • Frances Cook • Michael Mars Jenny Nayak • Valerie Pereria • Katie Price Sheena Reilly • Martina Ryan • Debbie Sell Caroleen Shipster • Brian Sommerlad

INTRODUCTION

Speech and language therapists specialize in the management of developmental and acquired communication and feeding disorders and work within health and educational contexts (Kersner and Wright, 2001). The term 'developmental' refers to speech and language difficulties that are apparent usually from the initial stages of speech and language development. They are often idiopathic in origin or may have a multifactorial basis such as hearing, environmental or cognitive impairments. 'Acquired' disorders refers to a communication or feeding problem that arises as a result of neurological damage or structural changes to the vocal tract/feeding mechanism, and which follows after a period of normal communication or feeding development.

A distinction is drawn between disordered and delayed skills. Delay refers to the acquisition of speech and language and feeding skills that fits in with normal developmental patterns but at a slower rate. In contrast, disorder occurs when the normal developmental sequence is not followed.

Certain paediatric communication problems are by their nature 'disorders' (e.g. dyspraxia and dysarthria). Other problems require detailed assessment to distinguish delay versus deviancy/disorder.

Assessment requires consideration of multiple factors, including cognitive skills, anatomical, physical, psychological abilities and the child's social, language and cultural background. Assessment methods include parent/carer interview, structured observation and formal assessments. More recently, psycholinguistic principles have been adopted in assessment and management, during which there is a systematic hypothesis-testing approach to the investigation of each child's linguistic processing skills (Stackhouse and Wells 1997). Both assessment and treatment are usually best employed within the context of a multidisciplinary team. Therapy approaches combine impairment, participation and activity foci – depending on the nature, severity and time post-onset of disorders.

This chapter covers a selection of disorders commonly seen in tertiary care.

DEVELOPMENTAL DIFFICULTIES: SPEECH

CLINICAL PRESENTATION

The most obvious manifestation of speech difficulties is a reduction in intelligibility. A reduction in speech intelligibility can be caused by problems with articulation, prosody (intonation, stress, rhythm), voice, resonance, rate of speech and external environmental factors.

PHONETIC AND PHONOLOGICAL DIFFICULTIES

A child with a phonetic deviance or delay has difficulty in physically articulating certain sounds in the language. He/she is unable to, or does not, articulate certain sounds. In contrast, phonology is concerned with evaluating an individual's ability to signal differences in meaning – 'the organization and classification of speech sounds that occur as contrastive units within a language, as well as speech perception and production, cognitive and motor aspects of speech'. Therefore, phonetic or articulation difficulties refer to the peripheral motor activity, whereas phonology refers to the speaker's knowledge of the sound system and the rules that govern it.

DEVELOPMENTAL DYSARTHRIA

Developmental dysarthria may be caused by congenital neuromuscular disorders, such as myasthenia gravis and Moebius syndrome. It often accompanies physical handicap (e.g. cerebral palsy). For the child with developmental dysarthria, acquisition and development of speech can be greatly affected due to learned compensations, maladaptive patterns of speech and body posture, motor instability and altered mother-child interactions (see 'Acquired dysarthria' for clinical presentation).

DEVELOPMENTAL DYSPRAXIA

This is a motor speech disorder. Children with developmental dyspraxia have impaired motor planning skills. They make trial and error movements in producing sounds, leading to inconsistency of speech production. In doing so, they often appear to be 'groping' for articulatory precision. They may have one or more of the following:

- Inability to pronounce single consonants or vowels and/or organize and produce single words, multisyllabic words, phrases and sentences.
- Inability to control the prosodic features of speech.
- Associated language and learning problems, particularly in reading and spelling development.
- Current or previous feeding difficulties.

'Soft' neurological' signs such as clumsiness or delayed hand preference may be present.

ASSESSMENT

The initial aim of assessment is to differentiate between *disordered* and *delayed* speech patterns so that appropriate management can be implemented. Speech assessments involve imitation of single sounds, syllables, words and sentences, picture naming and description and spontaneous conversational speech. Formal tests are often used. Assessment of voice, prosody and oral structure and function are also carried out.

TREATMENT

The objective of intervention for all speech difficulties is to maximize the child's communicative ability.

Phonetic/articulation difficulties: This involves increasing the child's physical ability to produce consonant sounds.

Phonological difficulties: This involves providing the child with information about similarities and differences of sound classes so as to develop his/her knowledge and production of phonological contrasts with good self-monitoring skills.

Dyspraxia: This involves increasing the child's oral sensory awareness and teaching the child to make the correct oral movements for specific sounds and to sequence such sounds together through drill and repetition. Augmentative and/or alternative communication systems are often taught simultaneously, when dyspraxia is severely affecting intelligibility (see below).

Dysarthria: The child's physical and physiological limitations must be taken into account before therapy targets are set. Treatment is often multidisciplinary in nature, with communication and feeding usually incorporated as goals, using a functional approach. Treatment may involve improving the child's non-verbal skills. Often, alternative communication such as signing or communication aids are indicated.

PROGNOSIS

The prognosis differs according to the nature and severity of the problem, including the anatomical, physical, physiological and cognitive limitations, the child's motivation to communicate, the opportunities available for the child to communicate and the amount of support available. Developmental dyspraxia and dysarthria may persist throughout life. Phonological difficulties however usually resolve with maturation and treatment.

DEVELOPMENTAL DIFFICULTIES: LANGUAGE

CLINICAL PRESENTATION

Developmental language disorders include difficulties with receptive language, expressive language and/or pragmatics. Developmental language disorders can also be considered according to a linguistic model of Form, Content and Use. Often, a child presents with more than one type of difficulty – i.e. receptive, expressive and/or pragmatic difficulties (**Table 18.1**).

ASSESSMENT

A range of areas are examined dependent on the child's age and ability: attention and behaviour, pre-verbal skills (e.g. play, imitation), early vocabulary, receptive language, expressive language and pragmatic skills. The child's auditory perception (auditory discrimination, sequencing and memory) may also be assessed.

TREATMENT

In broad terms, the appropriate treatment is speech and language therapy when non-verbal cognitive skills are age-appropriate. Speech and language therapy can occur in the following settings; special schools, language units, child development centres, hospitals or the child's home, and is carried out individually or in groups, depending on the child's needs and abilities, taking advantage of a multidisciplinary setting wherever possible.

PROGNOSIS

The primary goal is to maximize the child's potential in terms of communication and language skills. The outcome of treatment is dependent on those factors outlined above in the developmental speech difficulties section.

Table 18.1 Language difficulties

Language area	Linguistic model*	Possible difficulties with:**
Receptive skills	Relates to content	• Receptive vocabulary • Concept formation • Information processing • Understanding of grammar
Expressive skills	Relates to form	• Speech–sound contrasts • Expressive vocabulary • Sentence building • Narratives • Word finding • Grammar
Pragmatic skills	Relates to use	• Non-verbal communication • Communicative intent • Organization of discourse • Pre-supposition

* Bloom and Lahey, 1978
** Lees and Urwin, 1992

ALTERNATIVE AND AUGMENTATIVE COMMUNICATION (AAC)

CLINICAL PRESENTATION

In children with severe dyspraxia or dysarthria and unintelligible speech and language, understanding levels can be much in advance of their abilities to express themselves. They communicate through eye pointing, vocalization, gesture and facial expression. Sometimes it is appropriate to teach a structured sign system such as Makaton in order to enhance expressive communication and reduce frustration. Some children may be able to use printed symbol material to further enhance their communication, or may benefit from microtechnology with recorded or synthesized voice output (**18.1**).

An assessment to determine appropriate AAC involves an appraisal of the child's general health, vision, hearing, appropriate seating and positioning, and switch use to allow an accurate assessment of communication skills. This is undertaken by an interdisciplinary team which includes a paediatrician, speech and language therapist, occupational therapist, rehabilitation engineer and psychologist. Following assessment, recommendations for appropriate equipment or strategies are made to the child's family, local therapy team and school staff.

SPEECH AND LANGUAGE THERAPY INVOLVEMENT

The speech and language therapist assesses communication skills including speech intelligibility, prognosis for the development of speech, language understanding and methods and functions of communication. The speech and language therapist contributes to the decision-making regarding equipment, and advises on its implementation in the classroom. In addition, the speech and language therapist needs to make clear to the child's listeners their role in enabling AAC users to become active and valued communicators. This will involve teaching that communicating without speech, through alternate means, is slower, less transparent, creative and flexible, and requires a good deal of input from the listener.

ACQUIRED NEUROLOGICAL SPEECH AND LANGUAGE DISORDERS

Causes of acquired communication disorders in children include traumatic head injuries, tumours, cerebrovascular accidents, degenerative conditions, infectious diseases, metabolic disorders and seizure disorders. The most common presenting communication disorders are listed below and can co-occur.

ACQUIRED CHILDHOOD APHASIA

Acquired childhood aphasia is an impairment of receptive and/or expressive language following neurological injury, after a period of normal language acquisition. Receptively, for example, there may be a difficulty in understanding the meanings of words and their grammatical relationship in sentences. Expressively, there may be problems accessing words, described as a word-finding difficulty or paraphasias where word confusions occur either by sound or meaning (e.g. 'door' for 'gate', or 'stable' for 'staple'). Other forms of language may also be affected, such as sign language, reading and/or writing and use of language may be disturbed, for example, understanding turn-taking.

ACQUIRED CHILDHOOD DYSARTHRIA

Dysarthria refers to a group of motor speech disorders characterized by paralysis, weakness and/or loss of control of the muscles of the speech mechanism and occurring as a result of damage to the central or peripheral nervous system. There are different types of speech presentation relating in part to the aetiology of the dysarthria. The muscles used in respiration, phonation, articulation, resonance and prosody, and ultimately intelligibility, may all be affected to varying degrees.

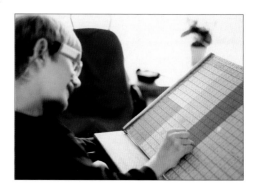

18.1 Communicating without speech, using symbols.

ACQUIRED CHILDHOOD ARTICULATORY DYSPRAXIA

Acquired dyspraxia is a disorder of motor speech programming, where voluntary control of the complex sequence of muscle movements for speech is affected by a cerebral lesion. This inability to perform voluntary articulatory movements occurs in the absence of abnormal muscle tone or 'hard' neurological signs. Articulatory errors, articulatory struggle behaviours and compensatory prosodic alterations combine to impact on intelligibility resulting in slow, laboured and imprecise speech. Articulatory dyspraxia may also combine with oral dyspraxia, affecting voluntary facial movements and more general fine motor movements, such as doing up buttons or holding a pen. It normally combines with a diagnosis of aphasia and/or dysarthria and the differential diagnosis of presentation is important for management.

Assessment

Assessment aims to provide a differential diagnosis of the components of the communication disorder (i.e. aphasia, dyspraxia and/or dysarthria). Structured observation, oral examination, parent/carer interview and informal assessments which must, where possible, include analysis of a spoken language sample, are supported by formal assessments (**18.2**). Some tests of developmental disorders can be adapted successfully, e.g. Clinical Evaluation of Language Fundamentals–Revised (CELF-R); Porch Index of Communicative Ability in Children (PICAC); and Test of Receptive Grammar (TROG). Others have been designed with both acquired and developmental disorders in mind, e.g. Paediatric Oral Skills Package (POSP). Certain adult tests can be used effectively when the child's premorbid abilities have been taken into consideration, e.g. Frenchay Dysarthria Assessment and some have produced childhood norms (The Boston Naming Test). Assessment of motor skills may include endoscopy and/or x–ray examination of the vocal tract.

Treatment

The treatment programme will be determined by the nature of the acquired disorder, its severity and time post onset as well as the child's other abilities. Speech and language therapy may combine direct work on language and speech skills, while at the same time considering environmental and augmentative/alternative means of communication. Environmental factors include minimizing background noise and increasing eye-to-eye contact between speaker and listener. Alternative and Augmentative systems of communication may be required (see previous section).

Prognosis

Although children can make a seemingly more rapid recovery from the effects of acquired aphasia than adults, the prognosis is often uncertain and determined by the type and severity of injury, as well as additional factors such as premorbid abilities. Children may make an apparent 'clinical recovery' but language difficulties can persist or come to light as educational demands increase with growing maturity. Many children who have acquired aphasia have difficulties with their education. Acquired dyspraxia appears to have a more rapid resolution than aphasia or dysarthria or its developmental counterpart, although there is scant research available.

As with acquired childhood aphasia, recovery from dysarthria appears to be greater in children than in adults but similarly guided by severity and type of lesion factors.

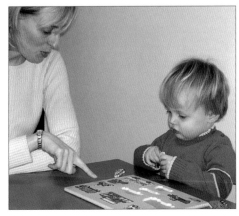

18.2 Informal assessment procedure designed to elicit a spoken language for analysis.

STAMMERING / STUTTERING DYSFLUENCY

Stammering is found in all parts of the world, in all cultures and in all races. It affects people of all ages, of all intelligence levels and of all socioeconomic groups. It has been recorded throughout history. It is characterized by an abnormally high frequency and/or duration of stoppages in the forward flow of speech. These stoppages may include repetitions, prolongations, or complete blocks in the airflow. As the problem persists, these dysfluencies may be accompanied by signs of physical tension and effort. Fears and avoidances may develop as well as considerable embarrassment, frustration and loss of self confidence.

PREVALENCE / INCIDENCE

Studies suggest that the prevalence of stammering is about 1%. While estimates of incidence have varied, most agree a figure of about 5%.

Like many developmental speech and language disorders, stammering has a higher incidence and prevalence in boys. Studies suggest a sex ratio of between 3:1 to 5:1.

AETIOLOGY / CLASSIFICATION

Most researchers now agree that stammering is the result of a complex interaction between neurophysiological, linguistic, psychological and environmental factors (**18.3**). It commonly begins in childhood between the ages of two and five years. It usually develops gradually, with cycles of fluency, but may start quite suddenly and severely. It is not usually associated with a particular incident or trauma.

ASSESSMENT

The speech and language therapist conducts a full assessment of the child's speech, language and fluency skills and elicits, through a structured case history, relevant physiological, linguistic, psychological and environmental information which may be influencing the current level of dysfluency.

TREATMENT OUTLINE

Recommendations for intervention are based on the findings of the assessment, the age of the child, the duration and severity of the dysfluency, his or her perceptions of the speech disorder and the effect it is having on his or her lifestyle. Therapy could include parent–child interaction therapy, direct therapy for fluency control, group intensive or non-intensive therapy with regular follow-up sessions as necessary.

PROGNOSIS

Research demonstrates that spontaneous remission is most likely to occur within the first six months. Where the problem persists it is important to refer the family to a speech and language therapist.

There is an increasing body of evidence which demonstrates the effectiveness of intervention for children between two and seven years of age. However the longer the problem has persisted, the more entrenched the difficulty becomes.

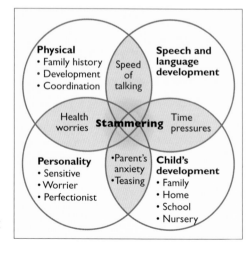

18.3 Framework for understanding stammering (Rustin et al 2001).

VOICE DISORDERS / DYSPHONIA

CLINICAL PRESENTATION
Dysphonia is a disruption of the quality, loudness and/or pitch of the voice. The voice deviates from those parameters appropriate for the child's age, sex, stature, language and culture. Dysphonia may be accompanied or signalled by reports of laryngeal discomfort, vocal fatigue or inconsistency of voice function. Onset may be gradual or sudden.

INCIDENCE
Studies suggest that 3–40% of school-age children present with hoarseness, most commonly in children aged between five and 11 years.

AETIOLOGY
Dysphonia may arise from either congenital or acquired laryngeal dysfunction and may co-occur with other speech and language problems. Dysphonia is classified according to the primary aetiology. For example, organic dysphonia refers to a primary organic aetiology, such as vocal fold palsy and papillomatosis. In contrast, a behavioural dysphonia arises directly from misuse, abuse and/or psychological factors. A behavioural dysphonia may present with or without pathology such as vocal fold nodules.

ESSENTIAL INVESTIGATIONS
The speech and language therapist requires a thorough ENT examination prior to intervention. This is offered ideally in a voice clinic where flexible and rigid fibreoptic endoscopy with stroboscopy is available for structural and dynamic laryngeal examination.

Sometimes an examination of the larynx and airway is performed under general anaesthetic, alongside other medical and physical evaluations. Perceptual analysis of voice tape-recordings and observation of voice production methods by the speech and language therapist is mandatory. Acoustic analysis is ideally undertaken using equipment such as electrolaryngography (**18.4**). This provides objective measures of pitch, irregularity of vocal fold vibration and intensity. A detailed case history is required to identify pertinent information from the medical, social, educational and psychological histories as well as the carer's and child's account of the voice problem, including remissions, recurrences, discomfort and other contributing factors.

TREATMENT OUTLINE
This may involve ENT medical and/or surgical management. Speech and language therapy provides pre- and post-operative advice to team members, parents and the patient. Voice therapy treatment may be appropriate to modify voicing patterns that may negatively influence post-operative recovery. In cases where the primary aetiology is behavioural, there is a need to adjust the aerodynamic muscular balance of voice production by learning optimal and restorative vocal techniques. This may address vocal hygiene and voice care, respiratory function for phonation, musculoskeletal relaxation techniques, vocal fold adduction techniques and intervention for any underlying psychological factors. Treatment incorporates the use of computerized biofeedback methods. Other professionals may be involved in therapy management such as osteopaths, physiotherapists, school teachers, special needs workers and psychologists.

PROGNOSIS
The primary goal is to restore the best possible voice for communication and educational and social demands. Where irreversible changes have occurred to the larynx or associated structures/systems, for example scarring, surgical modification of the larynx or neurological effects, return to normal voice function may be an unrealistic goal. Counselling will be an important role of the speech and language therapist.

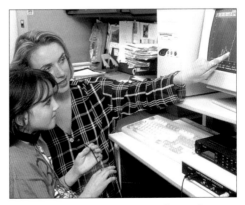

18.4 Instrumental assessment of voice forms part of the speech and language therapist's assessment.

TRACHEOSTOMY

CLINICAL PRESENTATION

Studies of communication skills in children with tracheostomy show that this population has a wide range of abilities with different pathologies. A tracheostomy can have an appreciable impact on the development of communication in young children, as well as affecting swallowing ability.

COMMUNICATION

The presence of a tracheostomy (**18.5**) can significantly affect the child's ability to vocalize. The voice may be completely absent (aphonia), or when present, of variable quality and efficiency and may not be adequate for oral communication. There are several reasons for this: an alteration in the oral-nasal airflow (in many cases this pathway is eliminated); reduced auditory/tactile feedback during attempted vocalization; significantly increased effort required to produce phonation; reduction in the number of syllables/words produced per breath.

The acquisition and development of speech and language may also be impaired as a consequence of the child's medical condition and/or exacerbated by long-term medical intervention. Aphonia is of particular concern in the infant or young child who is at a crucial stage in speech and language development. Early intervention by a speech and language therapist is essential.

SWALLOWING

A tracheostomy can affect swallowing, although oral feeding is possible even in very young babies. It is crucial to determine that oral feeding is safe, and that the oral and pharyngeal stages of swallowing are functional and able to support an adequate oral intake. The presence of a tracheostomy may additionally affect swallowing by restricting elevation of the larynx, which may reduce airway closure and possibly reduce cricopharyngeal relaxation.

Chronic air diversion through the tube is thought to desensitize the larynx and subsequently lead to depressed protective reflexes such as coughing. As the oral and nasal airways are being bypassed, uncoordinated swallowing may result. Any of the above may lead to aspiration and/or penetration of the airway during swallowing. Factors which require particular consideration are respiratory status and issues of fatigue, and history of prolonged intubation.

INCIDENCE

The incidence of tracheostomy in children is impossible to determine as estimations are specific to conditions. Chronic lung disease and subglottic stenosis are usually cited as the primary reasons for tracheostomy.

TREATMENT

Speech and language therapy involvement includes the management of swallowing problems and communication development with particular emphasis on advising on the suitability of 'speaking' valves and the assessment of suitability for alternative and augmentative communication, such as the sign language, Makaton.

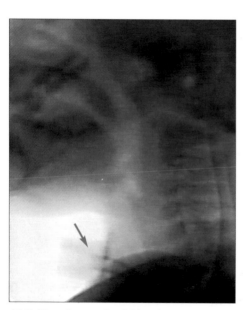

18.5 X-ray image of a child with a tracheostomy.

RESONANCE / AIRFLOW DISORDERS

CLINICAL PRESENTATION

Hypernasality is a disorder of tone resulting in an excessively nasal voice. This is frequently associated with excessive abnormal nasal airflow known as nasal emission or nasal turbulence. Nasal or facial grimace may be observed. Consonant production is often affected, in particular those requiring intraoral air pressure e.g. *pb*, *td*, *kg*, *fv*, *sz*, *sh*, *ch*, *ge*. Consonants may be weakened in their production. The place of articulation may be modified. For example, consonants usually produced in the oral cavity are produced further back in the mouth, often in the pharynx, glottis and nasopharynx below the level of the velopharyngeal sphincter. Patients with these characteristics may present with dysphonia, which is believed by many to develop as a compensatory behaviour for velopharyngeal dysfunction.

Another example of disordered tone is hyponasality. Its differential diagnosis with hypernasality is frequently difficult for the non-trained ear. Mixed hyper- and hyponasality may co-occur.

AETIOLOGY

Hypernasality and allied speech problems are usually associated with velopharyngeal dysfunction. This occurs when there is abnormal coupling of the nasal and oral cavities during speech: the soft palate and lateral pharyngeal walls do not effectively shut off the nasal cavity from the oral cavity during the production of oral consonants and vowels.

Historically, hypernasal speech has been managed by cleft lip and palate teams because of the association of nasal speech with cleft palate. Velopharyngeal dysfunction, however, may be the result of other conditions including overt or occult submucous cleft palate (**18.6**), postadenoidectomy (which may unmask a palate anomaly), or congenital 'box-shaped' pharynx, neurological disorders, severe hearing impairment, faulty learning, or a combination of these reasons. For example, velocardiofacial syndrome (VCF) is frequently associated with velopharyngeal dysfunction. Its aetiology is often multi-factorial including submucous cleft palate, pharyngeal hypotonia, and/or adenoidal hypoplasia.

ESSENTIAL INVESTIGATIONS

The perceptual assessment by the speech and language therapist is fundamental. Speech lies at the centre of the problem of velopharyngeal dysfunction and, indeed, the perceptual characteristics are the most important outcome measure of treatment. Objective measures using computerized aerodynamic and acoustic measures describe quantitatively the perceptual characteristics.

Direct visualization of the velopharyngeal mechanism is undertaken using nasopharyngoscopy and multiview videofluoroscopy (**18.7**), while the structure and function of the soft palate and lateral and posterior pharyngeal walls are examined during speech. The aim is to provide information on the anatomical and

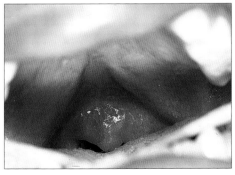

18.6 Oral view showing submucous cleft palate.

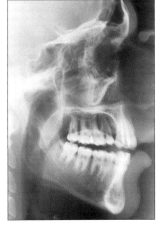

18.7 View of soft palate/ posterior pharyngeal wall: lateral videofluoroscopy.

functional characteristics, details about gap size, shape and location and the movements of the component parts of the velopharyngeal mechanism (**18.8, 18.9**). Both investigations are usually required since they give different information.

TREATMENT OUTLINE

Three modalities of treatment are possible: surgery, prosthetics, and speech and language therapy. Sometimes more than one treatment is required. Surgery is the commonest treatment method.

The generic description of surgery is pharyngoplasty, the exact nature of which is usually defined by the nature of the defect observed through nasopharyngoscopy and multiview videofluoroscopy. Many surgical techniques have been described, based on four different surgical principles: pharyngeal flap, muscle transfer or sphincter pharyngoplasty, palate repair or re-repair, and posterior pharyngeal wall augmentation.

Other treatment options include prosthetic appliances such as a palatal training appliance, palatal lift or speech bulb/obturator. Speech and language therapy is appropriate where an inconsistent pattern of velopharyngeal closure is found.

PROGNOSIS

Collaborative work between a surgeon, speech and language therapist and a prosthodontist/orthodontist in a specialist cleft lip and palate team is essential in the diagnosis and management of hypernasality and its associated speech problems.

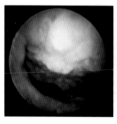

18.8 Endoscopic view of velopharynx during breathing.

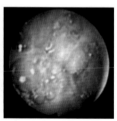

18.9 Endoscopic view of velopharynx during normal speech.

DYSPHAGIA

Oral and/or pharyngeal dysphagia (difficulty sucking, chewing or swallowing food or liquid) occurs in association with many syndromes and conditions (see **Table 18.2** below). Such problems may be congenital or acquired and structural or functional in nature. Any disruption of this highly complex process can result in impairment of the child's ability to feed safely and adequately.

CLINICAL PRESENTATION

Problems may present at birth and necessitate nasogastric tube feeding because of a poor or absent suck reflex. Oral stage involvement may be so severe that individuals are unable to move their tongue to manipulate, transfer or chew food. Drooling may be problematic. Pharyngeal stage problems include difficulty with swallow initiation, pharyngeal motility, crico-pharyngeal relaxation and incomplete clearance of the pharynx. Aspiration may occur because of an inability to protect the airway during feeding.

Table 18.2. Conditions commonly associated with oral and/or pharyngeal dysphagia in young children

Neurological	Cerebral palsy
	Neuromuscular disorders
	Bulbar palsy
	Tumour
	Stroke
	Head injury
	Syndromes – Riley-Day, Moebius
Metabolic	Acidaemias
Orofacial anomalies	Cleft lip and palate
	Micrognathia/Pierre Robin sequence
	Velocardiofacial syndrome
Dermatological	Epidermolysis bullosa
Gastrointestinal	Gastroesophageal reflux
Structural	Tracheoesophageal fistula
	Laryngomalacia
	Tracheostomy
	Laryngotracheal reconstruction
Respiratory/cardiac	Chronic lung disease
	Congenital heart disease

Oral-pharyngeal dysphagia can be life threatening as a result of aspiration and consequent impaired respiratory function. Children with dysphagia are at risk of growth retardation. Dysphagia can also create considerable stress for carers.

INCIDENCE
The prevalence of dysphagia in different conditions is unknown but clinicians have become increasingly aware that such problems are widespread. In preschool children with cerebral palsy for example, 90% have some degree of oral motor difficulty, approximately 60% of the most severely affected group are thought to be at risk of aspiration, and as many as 75% have been shown to have gastroesophageal reflux.

ESSENTIAL INVESTIGATIONS
Dysphagia management intersects many different disciplines, including speech and language therapy, occupational therapy, paediatrics, neurology, dietetics, gastroenterology, radiology and nursing. Diagnosis begins with detailed history taking and a comprehensive bedside evaluation or observation of the reported difficulty. Subsequent investigations when indicated include chest x-ray, pH monitoring, a videofluoroscopy swallow study (**18.10**) or barium swallow. Oral, pharyngeal, laryngeal and upper oesophageal function may be assessed in the latter.

The x-ray study includes lateral and/or anterior/posterior views, trialing a variety of textures and bolus size, modification of patient's position and adaptive equipment together with trialling of compensatory techniques.

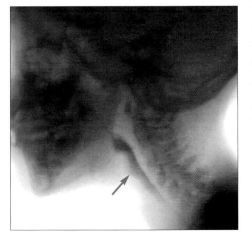

TREATMENT
Management strategies vary according to the age of the child and the duration and severity of the problem. The crucial decisions concern the presence/absence of aspiration, and achievement of adequate nutritional intake orally. Children with aspiration and/or inadequate oral intake may require nasogastric or gastrostomy feeding. Other options include modification of trunk and neck posture, alteration of textures, bolus size and pace of feeding, as well as a change in feeding equipment and utensils.

CRANIOFACIAL CONDITIONS

CLINICAL PRESENTATION
This group of disorders covers a broad spectrum of defects that affect the craniofacial complex and the oral structures.

SPEECH AND LANGUAGE THERAPY INVOLVEMENT
Many children with craniofacial anomalies have speech and language disorders as a result of deviant oral structures, hearing, visual and cognitive impairment. The psychosocial impact of the craniofacial dysmorphology may result in impaired social interaction and further adversely affect speech and language acquisition. In addition, many children with craniofacial conditions have oro-motor and feeding problems.

Evaluation of receptive and expressive language, speech, voice, resonance, oral motor and feeding skills, and pragmatic skills is carried out.

Multidisciplinary assessment is essential to meet the complex needs of this patient group. The speech and language therapist works closely with other members of the craniofacial team (neurosurgeon, ENT surgeon, plastic surgeon, audiologist, ophthalmologist, orthodontist, psychologist, geneticist and social worker).

TREATMENT
Preventative advice is given in the early stages but once areas of deficit have been identified, a course of speech and language therapy is instigated.

18.10 Lateral view of videofluoroscopy swallow study: child swallowing barium liquid.

PROGNOSIS

The primary goal is to ensure that each child achieves their optimal level of speech and language functioning. Outcome is highly dependent on a variety of factors, including the severity of the primary medical condition, the degree of hearing, visual and cognitive impairment, and other external factors such as the social environment of the child and the amount of therapeutic help that is available.

CLEFT LIP / PALATE

CLINICAL PRESENTATION

Clefts of the lip (CL) and/or the palate (CP) can occur separately or together (CLP) with very variable presentations – for example, bilateral cleft lip and palate (BCLP, **18.11**), unilateral cleft lip and palate (UCLP, **18.12**), clefts of the hard and soft palate (CP, **18.13**), and soft palate only. Submucous cleft palate occurs where the palatal muscle is defective but the mucosal cover appears to be intact. It is detected by abnormal speech, and is often associated with otitis media, and a positive history of nasal regurgitation.

INCIDENCE

CLP malformations are the most common congenital abnormalities in the craniofacial region (about 1 in 700 live births in the UK). Submucous cleft palate is an abnormality which occurs in about 1 in 1,200 births. Clefts may require multiple surgical procedures from birth to maturity and frequent outpatient attendance. Some patients suffer impaired facial growth, dental anomalies, speech disorder, poor hearing, difficulties in psychological wellbeing and social relationships. There are a significant number of associated syndromes, especially in isolated cleft palate, resulting in problems for cardiac, limb, ophthalmological and multiple other systems. This condition requires treatment by a large multidisciplinary team, including cleft surgeons, psychologists, orthodontists, clinical nurse specialists, audiologists, and speech and language therapists. Such treatment should take place in regional centres, in order to concentrate numbers of patients, permit audit and research and develop expertise.

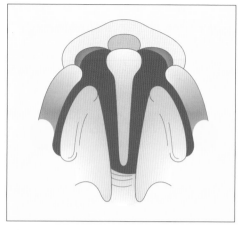

18.11 Bilateral cleft lip and palate (BCLP).

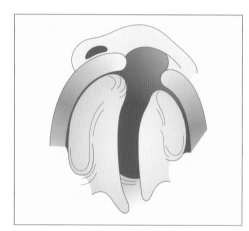

18.12 Unilateral cleft lip and palate (UCLP).

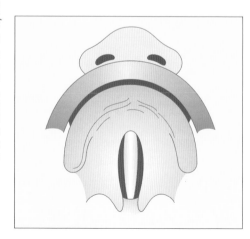

18.13 Cleft of the hard and soft palate (CP).

GENETICS

Three types of genetic risk are present: syndromic, familial and, by exclusion, sporadic. Over 400 syndromes are associated with clefting, so it is not a good pointer to diagnosis. More helpful is a family history of clefting or associated abnormalities. For example, in cleft palate with an autosomal dominant pattern, hearing difficulties and eye defects occur in Stickler syndrome, and lip pits are found in Van der Woude syndrome. Chromosomal abnormalities are increasingly recognized. In addition to trisomy 13 and 18, the gene deletion in the 22q11 region is associated with Di George and velocardiofacial syndromes. (See also 'Genetics' and 'Immunology' chapters.) Maternal steroids, anticonvulsants and a diet low in folic acid have also been implicated as causes.

Antenatal detection from 17 weeks is possible in up to 40% of those identified at birth. Other ultrasound abnormalities occur in a small percentage of all clefts detected antenatally. Counselling by the cleft team is offered.

If no other abnormality is found, the recurrence rate in siblings is 2% in isolated cleft palate, and in CLP 4%, ranging from 2–6% depending on severity. If two siblings or a parent and a child are affected, the risk is 1:10.

Antenatal counselling should take into account that not all abnormalities are detectable at that stage.

MANAGEMENT

This condition should be managed from birth to maturity by a specialist multidisciplinary team. Joint consultations should be undertaken, in order to maximize outcomes. The following clinicians need to be available to a multidisciplinary CLP team: paediatrician, plastic surgeon, oral and maxillofacial surgeon, otolaryngologist, audiologist, orthodontist, speech and language therapist, specialist nurse, clinical coordinator, psychologist, social worker and geneticist. The aims of treatment are to help in the development of a well-balanced and socially integrated individual whose appearance is acceptable to his peers, whose speech and hearing allow normal communication skills and whose dentition and facial development are acceptable.

There is much variation in treatment protocols and the following is a general guide to treatment principles and timing and is shown in abbreviated form in **Table 18.3**. Patients are visited within 24 hours of birth, usually by a cleft surgeon, and clinical nurse specialist.

Table 18.3 Broad timing of surgery and rehabilitation in cleft lip and palate in the UK*

Age	Surgery	Rehabilitation
Antenatal** or birth	–	Meet cleft lip and palate team, ± pre-surgical orthopaedics
0–3 months	Cleft lip repair	Nursing and feeding support
6–12 months	Cleft palate repair	Speech therapy monitoringand treatment to school age
Birth, 9 months, 18 months, 3 years	–	ENT/audiology monitoring and intervention through preschool years
3½–6 years	Pharygoplasty or secondary palate surgery if necessary	Assessment of nasal speech
4–6 years	Lip scar revision Nose revision	–
9 years	Alveolar bone grafting with repair of alveolar fistula	Pre- and post-orthodontic treatment
11–14 years	Repair alveolar fistula	Routine orthodontic treatment pre- and post-surgery
16–20 years	Maxillary osteotomy (if necessary)	Pre- and post-surgical orthodontic treatment; pre- and post-speech therapy assessment and, if indicated, treatment

Genetic counselling, psychology consultation or social worker offered at any stage
* precise timings vary between centres
** Antenatal diagnosis by ultrasound scanning is variously reported as being between 20 and 70%

Satisfactory feeding is usually achieved through a simple modification of the teat of a soft bottle. Breastfeeding is not usually possible, but, if achieved, it is rarely prolonged when the palate is cleft. Specialist feeding counselling should be available. Pre-surgical orthopaedics or feeding plates may be used depending on the team philosophy. This treatment is controversial. Lip repair is usual at 3 months (**18.14, 18.15**).

Palate closure is carried out between the ages of 6 and 18 months. Technique and timing are controversial. Grommet insertion may be combined with palate repair, depending on clinical indication and the team's protocols. Children with cleft palate are at increased risk of middle ear effusions.

Speech and language therapy, ENT monitoring and necessary intervention are imperative in the preschool and early school years. Children are at increased risk of speech and language problems: particular difficulties are consonant production and excessive nasal tone/nasal air escape. Velopharyngeal surgery for persistent nasal speech is usually based on investigations of velopharyngeal function, including nasopharyngoscopy and videofluoroscopy.

If required, lip and/or nose revision surgery may take place prior to schooling, at around 4 years of age.

When the tooth-bearing portion of the maxilla (the alveolar process) is cleft, alveolar bone grafting is undertaken between the ages of 9 and 11. This permits the creation of a normal alveolar architecture through which teeth can erupt. Pre- and postoperative orthodontics are undertaken (**18.16, 18.17**). Routine orthodontic treatment is undertaken between the ages of 11 and 14.

A proportion of patients will experience distorted mid-facial growth in later life, for which surgical advancement of the maxilla is required (**18.18**). Where indicated, further orthodontic treatment will be required prior to surgical correction of any skeletal discrepancy. This is managed through combined clinics, including the team psychologist, for orthognathic assessment where indicated.

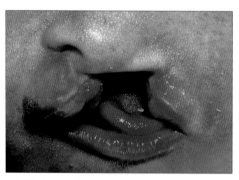

18.14 Before lip repair.

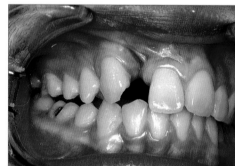

18.16 Before alveolar bone grafting.

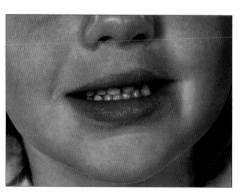

18.15 After lip repair.

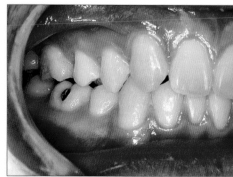

18.17 After alveolar bone grafting.

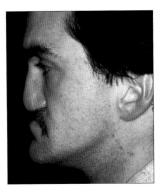

18.18
Distorted mid-facial growth, for which surgical advancement of the maxilla is required.

SPECIAL CONSIDERATIONS

Pierre Robin sequence: this may be associated with difficulty in breathing at birth due to the small mandible and posteriorly placed tongue, which may fall back through the U-shaped cleft of hard and soft palate, especially when lying supine (see also 'Respiratory Medicine' chapter). The prone position usually suffices to relieve this, otherwise a nasopharyngeal airway may be needed for a few weeks to overcome the obstruction and improve feeding. Rarely, tracheostomy is required. These babies are an exception to the recom-mended supine posture to reduce cot deaths.

Initial feeding difficulties may result in poor weight gain prior to surgery. Catch-up generally occurs by 2 years of age. In cases of apparently isolated cleft palate, it is specially important to monitor for short stature – a pointer to 22q11 deletion syndrome as well as growth hormone deficiency.

Psychological issues: counselling should be available to foster a positive approach within the family, and dealing with teasing and bullying at school if these should occur.

REFERENCES

Speech and language therapy
Enderby P. Outcome Measures in Speech Therapy: impairment, disability, handicap and distress. *Health Trends* 1992; **24**: 61–64.
Kersner M, Wright JA (eds). *Speech and Language Therapy: The Decision-making Process when Working with Children*. London: David Fulton, 2001.

Developmental difficulties
Bloom L, Lahey M. *Language Development and Language Disorders*. New York: Wiley, 1978.
Brown B, Margaret E. *Developmental Disorders of Language*. London, New Jersey: Whurr Publishers, 1989.
Grunwell P (ed.) *Developmental Speech Disorders*. Edinburgh: Churchill Livingstone, 1990.
Lees J, Urwin S. *Children with Language Disorders*. London, New Jersey: Whurr Publishers, 1992.

Stackhouse J, Wells B. *Children's Speech and Literacy Difficulties*. London: Whurr, 1997.
Stoel-Gammon C, Dunn C. *Normal and Disordered Phonology in Children*. Austin, Texas: PRO-ED, 1985.

Acquired neurological speech and language disorders
Murdoch B (ed). Acquired Neurological *Speech/Language Disorders in Childhood*. London: Taylor & Francis, 1990.

Alternative and augmentative communication (AAC)
Glennen SL, DeCoste DC. *Handbook of Augmentative and Alternative Communication*. San Diego: Singular Publishing, 1997.

Stammering/stuttering dysfluency
Bloodstein O. *A Handbook on Stuttering*. London: Chapman & Hall: 1995.
Rustin L, Cook F, Botterill W, Hughes C, Kelman E. *Stammering: A Practical Guide for Teachers and Other Professionals*. London: David Fulton, 2001.

Voice disorders/dysphonia
Greene M, Mathieson L. *The Voice and its Disorders* (5th edn). London, New Jersey: Whurr Publishers, 1989.

Tracheostomy
Bleile KM. *The Care of Children with Long-term Tracheostomies*. San Diego: Singular Publishing, 1993.

Resonance/airflow disorders
Watson ACR, Sell DA, Grunwell PG (eds). *Management of Cleft Lip and Palate*. London, New Jersey: Whurr Publishers, 2001.

Dysphagia
Sullivan PB, Rosenbloom L (eds). Feeding the Disabled Child. *Clinics in Developmental Medicine* (No. 140). London: MacKeith Press, 1996.

Craniofacial conditions
Shprintzen RJ. Genetics, *Syndromes and Communication Disorders*. San Diego: Singular Publishing, 1997.
Hayward R, Dunaway D, Evans R (eds). *Clinical Management of Craniosynostosis*. London: MacKeith Press, 2004.

Cleft lip/palate
Sell DA, Grunwell P. Speech Assessment and Therapy. In: Watson ACH (ed). *Management of Cleft Lip and Palate*. New Jersey: Whurr, 2001.
Sommerlad BC. Management of cleft lip and palate. *Curr Paed* 1994; **4**: 189–195.
Habel A, Sell D, Mars M. Cleft lip and palate: management of cleft lip and palate. *Arch Dis Child* 1995; **74**(4): 360–366.
Clinical Standards Advisory Group Report. *Cleft Lip and/or Palate*. London: Stationery Office, 1998.
Watson ACR, Sell DA, Grunwell PG (eds). *Management of Cleft Lip and Palate*. London, New Jersey: Whurr Publishers, 2001.

Neonatal and General Paediatric Surgery

Lewis Spitz

OESOPHAGEAL ATRESIA

INCIDENCE AND TYPES
One in 4,500 live births.
- Proximal atresia with distal tracheo-oesophageal fistula – 85%
- Isolated oesophageal atresia – 7%
- H-type tracheo-oesophageal fistula without atresia – 4%
- Atresia with proximal tracheo-oesophageal fistula –1%
- Atresia with proximal and distal fistula – 3%.

RISK CLASSIFICATION
The Waterston risk grouping (1962) has recently been superseded and an updated classification proposed as follows:
Group I: Infants with birthweight over 1,500g and no major congenital cardiac defect (96% survival).
Group II: Birthweight <1,500g or a major cardiac defect (60% survival).
Group III: Birthweight <1,500g and major cardiac defect (20% survival).

ASSOCIATED ANOMALIES
Congenital cardiac malformations are the single most common anomalies and are responsible for the majority of deaths. Cardiac defects occur in 25% of patients and, of these, ventricular septal defects and tetralogy of Fallot are the most common. The VATER association of defects is well-recognized (**V** = vertebral, **A** = anorectal, **TE** = tracheo-oesophageal, **R** = radial and/or renal anomalies) with the term 'VACTERL' used to denote also cardiac and limb defects.

PRENATAL DIAGNOSIS
The possibility of an oesophageal atresia is often heralded by the presence of polyhydramnios. The absence of a detectable stomach 'bubble' on prenatal ultrasound scan provides confirmatory evidence for the presence of an isolated atresia. In addition, the upper oesophageal pouch may be seen to be dilated and obstructed on the ultrasound scan.

POSTNATAL DIAGNOSIS
In the presence of polyhydramnios, all newborn infants should have a nasogastric tube passed. An oesophageal atresia (**19.1, 19.2**) should be suspected when the infant is 'excessively mucusy' at birth. The advent of coughing and cyanosis coinciding with the first feed is a consequence of delayed diagnosis.

DIAGNOSIS
Inability to advance a No.8–10F nasogastric tube beyond 10 cm from the lower gum margin and an x-ray showing the tip of the tube in the upper thorax provides confirmation of the diagnosis. The presence of gas within the gastrointestinal tract is indicative of a distal tracheo-oesophageal fistula.

TREATMENT
Optimal treatment is ligation of the tracheo-oesophageal fistula and primary oesophageal anastomosis. Occasionally, primary anastomosis is not possible and delayed repair is required. In rare circumstances, oesophageal replacement is necessary.

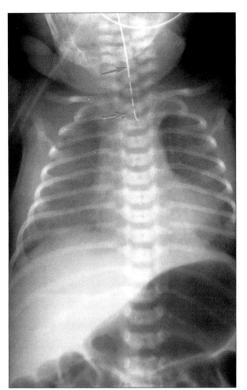

19.1 Oesophageal atresia with tracheo-oesophageal fistula. X-ray of chest and abdomen showing radio-opaque catheter in the upper blind oesophageal pouch and gas in the gastrointestinal tract.

CONGENITAL DIAPHRAGMATIC HERNIA

INCIDENCE

One in 4,500 live births, but probably as high as 1 in 2,500 gestations. The herniation of abdominal contents occurs through a defect in the pleuroperitoneal canal (Foramen of Bochdalek) which fails to close during intrauterine development.

PATHOPHYSIOLOGY

Herniation occurs more frequently on the left side (4:1) and causes compression of the ipsilateral developing lung and shift of the mediastinal structures to the opposite side. This is associated with hypoplasia of the ipsilateral and, to a lesser extent, of the contralateral lung. In addition, there is thickening of the musculature of the pulmonary arterioles with resultant pulmonary hypertension, which can lead to persistent foetal circulation with left-to-right shunting through the patent foramen ovale and arterial duct.

DIAGNOSIS

Detection of a diaphragmatic hernia can be made on prenatal scan (**19.3**) at around 20 weeks gestation. It is important to exclude lethal chromosomal defects at an early stage and to evaluate the heart for congenital cardiac anomalies. The first sign of a diaphragmatic hernia may be late in gestation, at birth or at any stage later on, even into adult life.

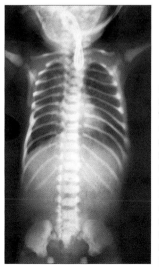

19.2 Pure oesophageal atresia without fistula. X-ray of chest and abdomen showing a radiographic catheter in the upper oesophagus and the complete absence of gas in the bowel.

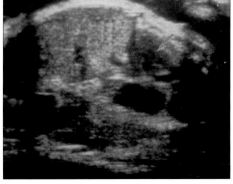

19.3 Congenital diaphragmatic hernia. Prenatal ultrasound scan showing the presence of a diaphragmatic hernia.

PRESENTATION

Respiratory distress is usually present at birth (with respiratory rate >40/min, heart rate >160/min, subcostal recession and cyanosis). There are decreased breath sounds on the ipsilateral side, the heart sounds are shifted to the contralateral side and the abdomen is flat or even scaphoid (**19.4**).

DIAGNOSIS

Plain chest and abdominal x-ray will reveal loops of intestine in the chest, shift of the mediastinal structures to the contralateral side and an absence of bowel gas shadows in the abdomen (**19.5**, **19.6**). In late presenting cases or when the diagnosis is doubtful, upper GI contrast studies will show contrast-filling intestinal loops within the pleural cavity.

TREATMENT

Emergency repair is no longer practised. The infant with respiratory distress requires urgent resuscitation and stabilization prior to surgery. This consists of endotracheal intubation, mechanical ventilation and elective sedation and paralysis. In refractory cases, oscillating ventilation, high frequency ventilation, nitric oxide and extracorporeal membrane oxygenation (ECMO) may be used. Operative repair consists of reduction of the herniated contents back into the abdomen and closure of the diaphragmatic defect with or without a prosthetic patch.

PROGNOSIS

The overall mortality for diaphragmatic hernia has not changed significantly over the past few decades. Survival rate remains around 50% but most infants succumb prenatally or prior to surgery, due to failure of stabilization of cardio-respiratory function.

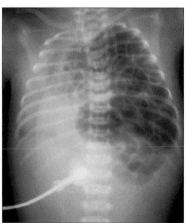

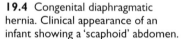

19.4 Congenital diaphragmatic hernia. Clinical appearance of an infant showing a 'scaphoid' abdomen.

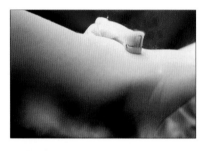

19.5 Congenital diaphragmatic hernia. X-ray of the chest and abdomen showing intestinal gas shadows in the left chest, a shift of the mediastinum to the right and absence of bowel in the abdomen.

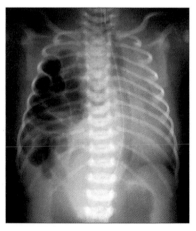

19.6 Congenital diaphragmatic hernia. X-ray of the chest and abdomen showing a right-sided diaphragmatic hernia, which is less common than left-sided hernia.

Table 19.1 Intestinal obstruction in the neonate (19.7, 19.8).

Mechanical

Intraluminal	– Meconium ileus
	– Meconium obstruction of the newborn
Intramural	– Atresia: duodenal, intestinal
	– Anorectal anomalies
	– Hirschsprung's disease
Extraluminal	– Malrotation
	– Duplication
	– Hernia
	– Cysts
	– Tumours

Paralytic ileus

Septicaemia
Necrotizing enterocolitis

Symptomatology
Bile-stained vomiting
Abdominal distension
Failure to pass meconium

Oedema and/or erythema of the anterior abdominal wall indicates peritonitis, perforation or gangrenous intestine.

NEONATAL INTESTINAL OBSTRUCTION

See **Table 19.1** for overview.

MECONIUM ILEUS

Incidence
One in 2,500.

Aetiology
Meconium ileus is a manifestation of cystic fibrosis, which is a genetic defect involving the long arm of chromosome 7, the commonest mutation being a single amino-acid substitution, $\Delta F508$ and is inherited as an autosomal recessive characteristic with 25% transmission. Meconium ileus occurs in 10–15% of infants with cystic fibrosis.

Pathophysiology
Due to the pancreatic exocrine deficiency, the meconium becomes tenacious and sticky and cannot be propelled by peristalsis through the gastrointestinal tract. The resultant intraluminal obstruction causes proximal dilatation which may culminate in volvulus with or without atresia, or perforation with or without meconium peritonitis.

Presentation
The infant is usually born with a distended abdomen (**19.9**). Bilious vomiting occurs soon after birth and it may be possible to palpate the distended loops of intestine impacted with meconium through the abdominal wall. No meconium will be passed and a small amount of mucus may follow rectal probing.

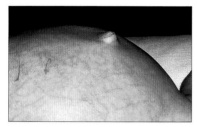

19.7 Neonatal intestinal obstruction. Infant with a distended abdomen.

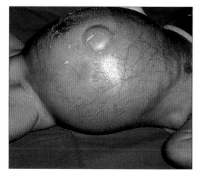

19.8 Neonatal intestinal obstruction. Oedema and erythema of the abdominal wall indicative of a perforation with peritonitis.

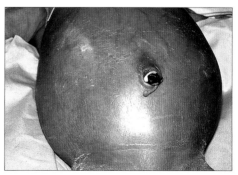

19.9 Meconium ileus. Infant with abdominal distension present at birth.

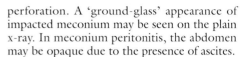

Diagnosis

The plain abdominal x-ray shows dilated loops of intestine of varying calibre (**19.10**) and, unless there is an atresia or volvulus, an absence of air-fluid levels (**19.11**). Calcification indicates the prior occurrence of an intestinal perforation. A 'ground-glass' appearance of impacted meconium may be seen on the plain x-ray. In meconium peritonitis, the abdomen may be opaque due to the presence of ascites.

Chromosomal analysis will reveal the ΔF508 defect in 90% of cases. Sweat test with pilocarpine iontophoresis is diagnostic when the volume of sweat obtained is over 100 g and the sodium and chloride content is in excess of 60 mEq/l.

Treatment

For uncomplicated meconium ileus, a carefully performed gastrografin enema may relieve the intraluminal obstruction. For complicated meconium ileus and when gastrografin enema fails to relieve the obstruction, surgery is required (**19.12**). The procedure consists of either enterotomy with washout of the obstructing meconium or resection and reanastomosis of the intestine.

Prognosis

The prognosis for meconium ileus is near 100% survival from the meconium obstruction. Lifelong replacement of pancreatic enzymes is required as is physiotherapy to improve the drainage of bronchial secretions and intensive antibiotic management of respiratory infections.

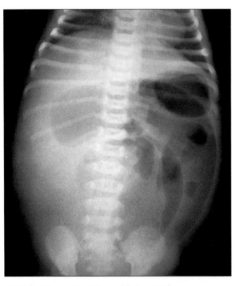

19.10 Meconium ileus. Abdominal x-ray showing dilated loops of intestine of varying calibre and an absence of air-fluid levels.

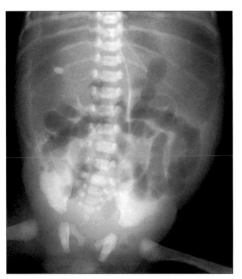

19.11 Meconium ileus. Abdominal x-ray of complicated meconium ileus showing free intraperitoneal gas and calcification.

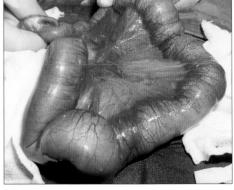

19.12 Meconium ileus. Operative appearance of the intestine showing dilated small intestine distended with impacted meconium.

DUODENAL ATRESIA

Incidence and type
One in 7,500
- Duodenal atresia – in continuity, with fibrous connection, or with gap.
- Duodenal web – perforated and/or windsock.
- Duodenal stenosis.

Associated anomalies
Down syndrome (30%), cardiac malformations, malrotation and atresias involving other parts of the alimentary canal, especially oesophageal atresia and anorectal anomalies.

Prenatal diagnosis
The presence of polyhydramnios should alert the clinician to the diagnosis of a proximal gastrointestinal obstruction. Prenatal ultrasound scan will show the typical 'double-bubble' of duodenal atresia.

Presentation
Bilious vomiting is the most prominent symptom when the obstruction is below the level of the ampulla of Vater (⅔ of cases). In higher obstructions, the vomitus is clear but persistent. There is usually upper abdominal distension and visible gastric peristalsis may be seen.

Diagnosis
Plain abdominal x-ray will reveal the 'double-bubble' diagnostic of duodenal atresia (**19.13**). In incomplete obstructions, a contrast study may be required to reveal the partial duodenal obstruction.

Treatment
Duodenoduodenostomy.

INTESTINAL ATRESIA

Incidence and types
One in 6,000.
- Type 1 – atresia in continuity.
- Type 2 – atresia with fibrous connection.
- Type 3 – atresia with gap in mesentery.
- Type 4 – multiple atresias.

Aetiology
Intrauterine vascular insufficiency to the involved segment of intestine (e.g. strangulation, intussusception, volvulus). Intestinal atresia is usually an isolated anomaly, although additional anomalies may be found in up to 10% of cases.

Prenatal diagnosis
The presence of an intestinal atresia may be suspected on prenatal ultrasound scan by the presence of dilated or echogenic bowel.

Presentation
Bilious vomiting is usually the first sign of an intestinal atresia. The degree of abdominal distension is proportional to the level of the obstruction, with massive distension sufficient to cause respiratory embarrassment occurring in low obstructions. A small amount of meconium may be passed but, in general, only mucus may be present in the rectum.

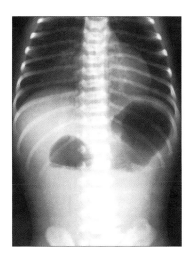

19.13 Duodenal atresia. Abdominal x-ray showing the typical 'double-bubble'.

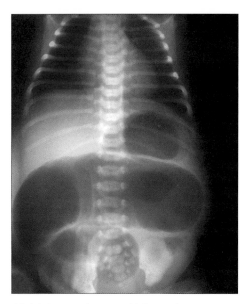

19.14 Intestinal atresia. Abdominal x-ray showing large dilated loops of obstructed proximal small intestine.

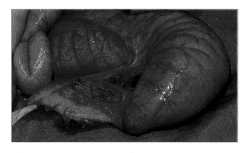

19.15 Intestinal atresia. Operative appearance, showing dilated proximal and collapsed distal bowel.

Table 19.2 Commonest anatomical varieties of anorectal anomalies

	High (supralevator)	Low (translevator)
MALE	Rectourethral fistula	Covered anus
FEMALE	Cloacal or recto-vaginal fistula	Ectopic anus or anovestibular fistula

Diagnosis

Plain abdominal x-ray shows dilated loops of proximal intestine with an absence of gas distally (**19.14**). It is not possible to differentiate small from large intestine on plain x-ray and occasionally it may be necessary to perform contrast studies to document the level of the obstruction.

Treatment

Surgical management consists of excising a portion of the grossly dilated proximal intestine and a small section of distal bowel and performing an end-to-end single-layer seromuscular intestinal anastomosis (**19.15**).

ANORECTAL ANOMALIES

Incidence

One in 3,000 live births. Anorectal anomalies arise out of failure to complete the final stages in the development of the hindgut.

Associated anomalies

Most frequent are anomalies of the urinary system (dysplastic kidney, hydronephrosis, vesico-ureteric reflux, neuropathic bladder) which occur in 66% of high anomalies and 33% of low lesions. Other commonly encountered associated anomalies include vertebral defects (particularly sacral), cardiac malformations, oesophageal atresia and limb deformities (VACTERL association).

Diagnosis

See **19.16** on next page.

Anatomical types

The number and variety of abnormalities is vast but a few basic principles in diagnosis and treatment should be adhered to (**Table 19.2**) (**19.17–19.22**).

Treatment

- High anomaly – colostomy followed later by posterior sagittal anorectoplasty.
- Low anomaly – local perineal procedure either as an anoplasty or limited posterior sagittal repair.

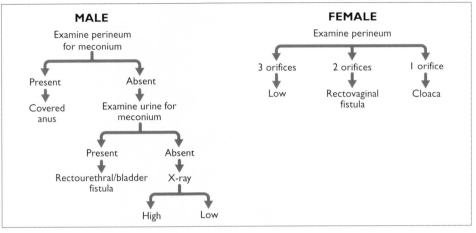

19.16 Diagnosis of anorectal anomalies.

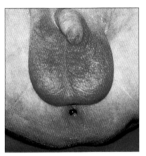

19.17 Low anorectal anomaly in a male infant, showing a spot of meconium on the perineum.

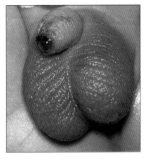

19.18 A high anorectal anomaly in a male infant, showing a 'flat' perineum and meconium in the urine.

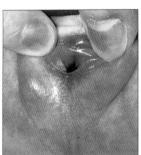

19.19 High anorectal anomaly in a female infant with a single opening on the perineum (a cloacal anomaly).

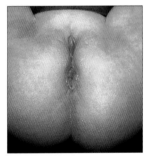

19.20 Low anterior ectopic anus, located immediately posterior to the fourchette, in a female infant.

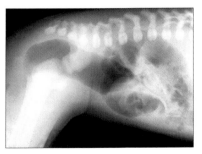

19.21 A low lesion shown by an invertogram, with bowel gas well below the pelvic muscles.

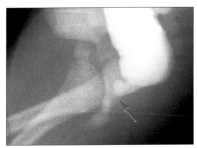

19.22 Rectourethral fistula. A cysto-urethrogram shows it arising in the region of the prostatic urethra.

HIRSCHSPRUNG'S DISEASE

Incidence
One in 5,000 live births. This condition is characterized by the absence of ganglion cells in the distal intestine. The anorectal region is always affected, with 75% of cases being confined to the rectosigmoid area and 10%, including the entire colon (total colonic aganglionosis), extending for a greater or lesser extent into the small bowel.

Genetics
There is a definite familial pattern of inheritance. Males are affected four times as frequently as females. There is a 25% risk of inheritance in total colonic aganglionosis where the male to female ratio is 1:1. One of the genes responsible for Hirschsprung's disease has been isolated on the RET proto oncogene.

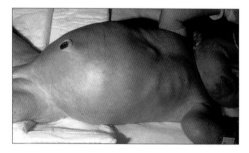

19.23 Hirschsprung's disease. Appearance of an infant showing a distended abdomen with dilated loops of bowel visible.

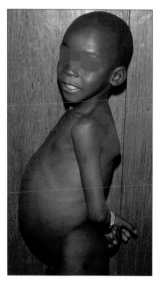

19.24 Hirschsprung's disease in an older child with a distended abdomen and thin limbs reflecting poor nutritional status.

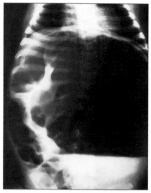

19.25 Hirschsprung's disease. Abdominal x-ray showing hugely distended loops of intestine.

Presentation
Delayed passage of meconium, in excess of 24 hours after birth, should arouse the suspicion of Hirschsprung's disease. There is usually abdominal distension (**19.23**) and bilious vomiting which may be relieved by rectal probing or washout, only for symptoms to recur shortly afterwards. Chronic intractable constipation may occur in later childhood (**19.24**).

Diagnosis
The plain abdominal x-ray shows dilated loops of intestine with an absence of gas in the rectum (**19.25**). A contrast enema may show a contracted rectum with dilated bowel proximally, but in the neonatal period this feature may be absent. Anorectal manometry reveals failure of relaxation of the internal anal sphincter in response to proximal distension. The definitive diagnosis is on histopathological examination of a rectal suction biopsy (**19.26, 19.27**). Typically, this will show an absence of ganglion cells with large nerve trunks present in the submucosa. Histochemistry shows a proliferation of acetylcholinesterase fibres in the submucosa and particularly in the lamina propria.

Treatment
Definitive treatment consists of either excising (Swenson) or bypassing (Duhamel, Soave) the aganglionic intestine. This may be carried out as a two- or three-stage procedure with an initial colostomy in normally ganglionic intestine or as a one-stage primary procedure.

Complications
The most feared complication is the development of enterocolitis which is characterized by profuse diarrhoea and toxicity in combination with gross abdominal distension and hypovolaemic shock.

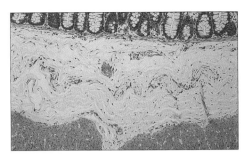

19.26 Hirschsprung's disease. Rectal biopsy (H&E) showing absence of ganglion cells and large nerve trunks in the submucosal layer.

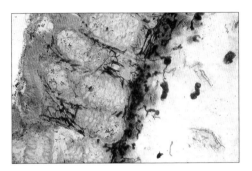

19.27 Hirschsprung's disease. Histochemistry of rectal biopsy showing increased acetyl-cholinesterase positive nerve fibres in the submucosa and in the lamina propria.

MALROTATION

Failure of the intestine (midgut) to rotate normally in the first 12 weeks of development results in an abnormally mobile midgut with a short narrow-based mesentery which has the propensity to twist, causing life-threatening midgut volvulus.

Prenatal diagnosis

The condition is not detectable on prenatal ultrasound scan unless complicated by intra-uterine volvulus.

Presentation

Bile-stained vomiting may be the only symptom (**19.28**). This alone should lead to investigations to confirm or refute the diagnosis of malrotation. In the presence of volvulus, there will be additional signs such as blood-stained nasogastric aspirate and/or bloody mucosy stools and hypovolaemic shock in cases with advanced intestinal necrosis.

In older children, malrotation may present with gastro-oesophageal reflux (see 'Gastro-enterology' chapter) with the occasional bilious vomit, symptoms suggestive of anorexia nervosa or recurrent abdominal pain.

Diagnosis

The diagnosis may be suspected on plain abdominal x-ray by the absence of intestinal gas in the presence of bilious vomiting, especially in the neonatal period. A contrast upper gastrointestinal (GI) study will reveal the abnormally rotated duodenum with a 'corkscrew' pattern in the case of midgut volvulus (**19.29**). An ultrasound scan may show abnormal orientation of the superior mesenteric vessels, with the artery anterior or lateral to the vein.

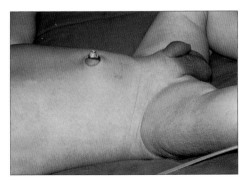

19.28 Malrotation. Clinical appearance of an infant showing an undistended abdomen in the presence of bile-stained vomiting.

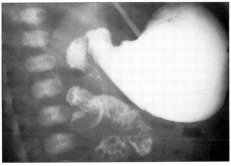

19.29 Malrotation. Lateral upper gastrointestinal contrast study showing 'corkscrew' appearance of the duodenum signifying a volvulus.

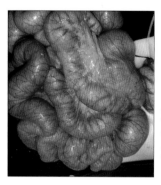

19.30
Malrotation.
Operative
appearance of
the twist in
the mesentery
of the midgut.
The intestine
is viable.

Treatment

Urgent surgical intervention is required to prevent volvulus. The procedure consists of straightening the duodenal loop, widening the base of mesentery of the small intestine by dividing fibrous adhesions and placing the intestines in a non-rotated position, with the small bowel on the right side and the caecum and large bowel on the left side of the abdomen (**19.30**). Where volvulus has already occurred, the intestines should be de-rotated and inspected for viability. In extreme cases (no viable bowel) it is advisable to resect frankly gangrenous intestine and to carry out a 'second-look' laparotomy 24 hours later. It may then be possible to salvage sufficient intestine for normal GI function.

DUPLICATIONS OF THE ALIMENTARY TRACT

Incidence

Duplications can occur anywhere in the alimentary tract, from the mouth to the anus. They most commonly occur in the small bowel mesentery. Duplications comprise a mucosal lining, frequently of an area remote from the site of duplication, and a muscular wall. They may be cystic or tubular in form.

Aetiology

The neurenteric canal theory of origin of duplication is generally accepted with failure of the canal to resorb totally.

Presentation

Cystic duplications (**19.31**) cause symptoms from pressure on the adjacent intestine. The most common clinical features are those of intestinal obstruction in association with a palpable mass. Tubular duplications (**19.32**) cause symptoms from peptic ulceration due to an acid-secreting mucosal lining. The ulceration develops in the adjacent normal intestine which is unable to resist acid-peptic digestion.

Diagnosis

An ultrasound scan will reveal the cystic nature of the mass. In tubular duplication, technetium pertechnetate scan may reveal the presence of ectopic gastric mucosa. The presence of split vertebra in the upper thoracic spine provides additional diagnostic support.

Treatment

Excision of the duplication with or without the adjacent intestine and end-to-end anastomosis is the treatment of choice. Where long lengths of intestine are involved or when the site of duplication is in a critical area (duodenum), stripping of the mucosal lining is the best option.

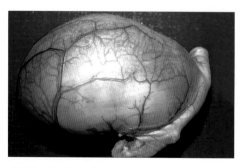

19.31 Cystic duplication.

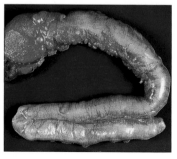

19.32 Tubal duplication.

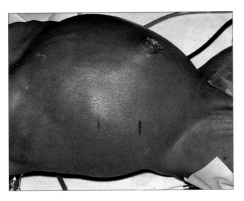

19.33 NEC. Premature infant with necrotizing enterocolitis, displaying a distended abdomen, with redness and oedema of the abdominal wall.

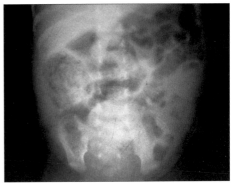

19.34 NEC. Plain x-ray showing pneumatosis intestinalis (gas in the bowel wall).

NECROTIZING ENTEROCOLITIS (NEC)

Incidence
Neonatal necrotizing enterocolitis occurs predominantly in the stressed premature infant and is currently one of the most common neonatal surgical emergency conditions.

Aetiology
Although not completely clear, it would appear that certain factors (e.g. prematurity, the presence of intraluminal substrate [breast milk is protective] and microorganisms [*Klebsiella*, *E coli*, *Clostridia*]) are commonly present. Other contributing factors, such as hypoxia, hypovolaemia, hyperviscosity, hypotension, and hypothermia, may be important. The most frequently affected parts of the GI tract are the terminal ileum and caecum and the splenic flexure of the colon. The final common pathway in the pathogenesis of the condition is an ischaemic process.

Pathology
The mesenteric ischaemia leads progressively from mucosal ulceration through to full-thickness necrosis and perforation with peritonitis.

Presentation
The first sign of the onset of NEC is reluctance of the infant to feed. This is followed rapidly by bilious vomiting or nasogastric aspirate, the passage of blood and mucus in the stool and abdominal distension (**19.33**). Erythema and/or oedema of the anterior abdominal wall is indicative of impending intestinal gangrene with perforation. In severe cases, the infant becomes shocked and hypovolaemic.

19.35 NEC. Plain x-ray showing pneumo-peritoneum indicative of a perforation.

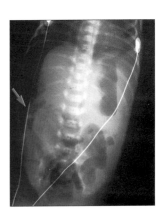

19.36 NEC. Plain x-ray showing portal venous gas.

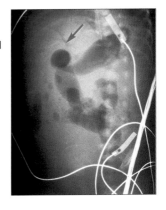

Diagnosis
The hallmark of the diagnosis is the finding of pneumatosis intestinalis on plain abdominal x-ray. Free air (pneumoperitoneum) is indicative of perforation. Gas in the portal venous system is a sign of advanced disease (**19.34–19.36**).

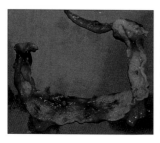

19.37 NEC. Operative specimen showing strictures in the colon – a late sequela of necrotizing enterocolitis.

Treatment

Immediate resuscitation in all cases. Conservative treatment consists of nasogastric aspiration, broad-spectrum antibiotics and complete GI rest for 7–10 days, during which total parenteral nutrition is administered.

Indications for surgery are intestinal perforation, intestinal obstruction or failure to respond to conservative measures. Late indication for surgery is stricture formation.

Operative procedures comprise resection with primary anastomosis or resection with stoma formation (**19.37**).

EXOMPHALOS

Incidence
One in 5,000 live births.

Aetiology
Failure of the physiological umbilical her fully reduce into the abdominal cavity 12th week of gestation.

Presentation
The infant is born with an obvious defect umbilicus. The anomaly can be detected in intrauterine life on ultrasound scan covering of the sac comprises an outer la amnion and an inner layer of peritoneum intervening layers of Wharton's jelly.
Exomphalos may be divided into two categ
- Minor – defect <5cm (**19.38**)
- Major – defect >5cm (**19.39**)
Major exomphalos is associated with a incidence of associated anomalies, e.g. ca gastrointestinal, genitourinary. Also chro mal anomaly, Beckwith syndrome (exomp gigantism, macroglossia and hypoglycaem

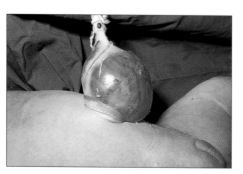

19.38 Minor exomphalos.

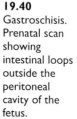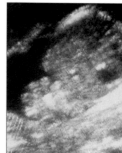

19.40 Gastroschisis. Prenatal scan showing intestinal loops outside the peritoneal cavity of the fetus.

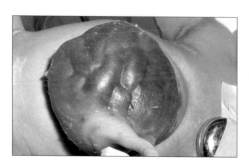

19.39 Major exomphalos, including liver.

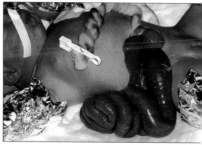

19.41 Gastroschisis. Appearance of the i at birth with a large amount of intestine extruding through a defect in the abdomin wall just to the right of the umbilical cord.

Investigations
Monitoring of blood glucose levels. Cardiac ECHO.

Management
Prenatal counselling, especially for larger exomphalos, including exclusion of a chromosomal anomaly; cardiac ECHO and detection of associated defects.

Immediately postnatal: covering the sac with plastic wrap to prevent excessive fluid and heat loss. Minor lesions are amenable to primary closure of the defect. Major lesions may be treated by surgical application of a silo, with gradual progressive reduction of the contents into the abdomen or application of an escharic agent.

Prognosis
Small lesions and larger exomphalos without associated anomalies have a good prognosis. Large exomphalos with other major associated anomalies have a poor prognosis.

GASTROSCHISIS
Incidence
One in 8,000 live births. The incidence appears to have increased in recent years. The term denotes an extrusion of part of the intestine through a defect to the right of an intact umbilicus.

Prenatal diagnosis
The lesion is usually recognized on routine antenatal scan (19.40). As it is not accompanied by any other major congenital anomaly, no further prenatal investigations are necessary.

Diagnosis
The diagnosis is self-evident at birth (19.41). The lesion with the extruded bowel, which may be grossly thickened and oedematous, should be covered with plastic wrap to prevent fluid and heat loss.

Treatment
Emergency repair of the defect should be undertaken as soon as possible after birth, when the bowel is generally pliable and easily reduced into the peritoneal cavity. If the extruded intestine is thickened and matted it will be necessary to place the bowel in a silo as a temporary measure.

Prognosis
Excellent, except in infants with associated intestinal atresia or short-bowel syndrome.

UMBILICAL HERNIA
Presentation
The hernia occurs through a defect in the umbilical cicatrix and usually contains omentum only (19.42). Umbilical hernia is extremely common in infancy and particularly in black infants. These hernias tend to resolve spontaneously by the time the children reach the age of five years. Incarceration is extremely unlikely except in the large truncated variety (19.43).

Treatment
Surgery is undertaken for large truncated hernias in infancy or following failure to close spontaneously after the age of five years. The operative procedure consists of closure of the neck of the hernial sac and repair of the fascia surrounding the defect.

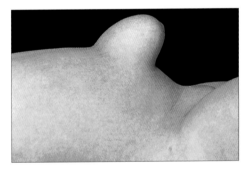

19.42 Umbilical hernia of moderate size.

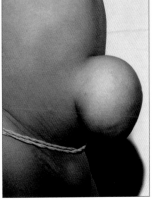

19.43 Umbilical hernia: large, truncated.

UMBILICAL ANOMALIES

INCIDENCE

A number of defects can occur at the umbilicus. Each requires precise diagnosis as their treatment differs considerably.

- Umbilical granuloma. This is due to failure of the umbilical cord to completely separate. Application of silver nitrate to the granulation tissue will result in its resolution (**19.44**).
- Umbilical polyp. This is due to the persistence of a remnant of the vitello–intestinal duct at the umbilicus. It is covered by mucosa requiring formal excision (**19.45**).
- Patent vitello-intestinal duct. There is a fistula at the umbilicus through which intestinal content is evacuated. There is a distinct risk of prolapse of the intestine through the fistula or volvulus around the 'band'. Urgent surgery is required to excise the fistula from the umbilicus to the ileum and restore intestinal continuity by end-to-end anastomosis (**19.46**).
- Patent urachus. This is a communication between the bladder dome and the umbilicus which may produce a persistent urinary leak. It is important to exclude a bladder outlet obstruction (e.g. posterior urethral valves) before attempting closure of the urachal remnant (**19.47**).

19.44
Umbilical granuloma. An infected remnant of the umbilical cord which has failed to separate completely.

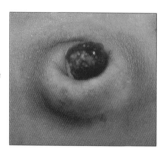

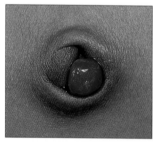

19.45
Umbilical polyp. Mucosal remnant of the vitello-intestinal duct at the umbilicus.

19.46
Patent vitello-intestinal duct due to persistence of the duct, which allows discharge of faeces.

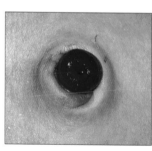

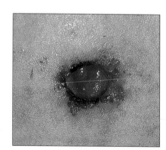

19.47 Patent urachus causing a urinary discharge from the orifice of the duct.

GASTROINTESTINAL HAEMORRHAGE

The presence of blood in the stool is an alarming symptom which is promptly brought to the attention of the doctor. It is important to determine the nature and quantity of blood loss and to search for additional physical signs such as hypovolaemic shock, anaemia or bilious vomiting.

DIAGNOSIS

The age of the patient may be an important determinant of the likely cause of haemorrhage:

- Age <2 years: volvulus, necrotizing enterocolitis, intussusception, Meckel's diverticulum.
- Age >2 years: oesophageal varices, peptic ulceration, colonic polyps, inflammatory bowel disease.

19.48 (below) shows a diagnostic scheme for children presenting with rectal bleeding.

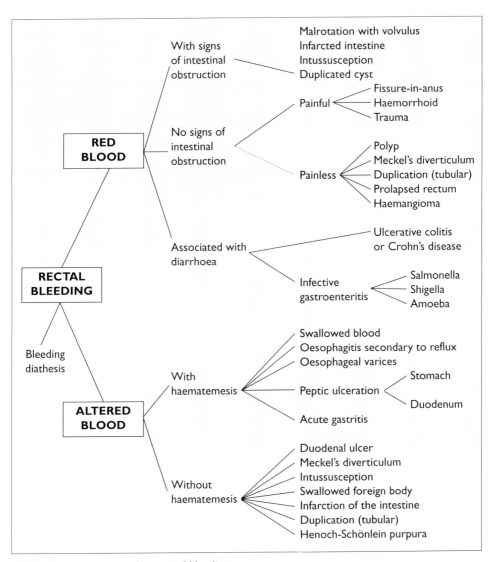

19.48 Diagnostic approach to rectal bleeding.

MECKEL'S DIVERTICULUM

INCIDENCE
Meckel's diverticulum represents persistence of the intestinal end of the vitello-intestinal duct. It is present in 2% of the population, is located two feet (60 cm) from the ileocaecal junction and may remain asymptomatic throughout life (**19.49**).

PRESENTATION
Symptoms arise out of complications with GI bleeding, due to the presence of ectopic gastric mucosa causing ulceration in the adjacent ileal mucosa. Haemorrhage can be significant and is dark red in colour (**19.50**). The most frequent age at which GI bleeding occurs is 6–24 months. Intestinal obstruction, due to kinking of the intestine by a fibrous band arising at the mesenteric attachment, or intussusception with the Meckel's diverticulum at its apex, or volvulus around a band connecting the Meckel's diverticulum to the umbilicus. Perforation of a peptic ulcer with resultant peritonitis. Diverticulitis can mimic acute appendicitis (**19.51**).

DIAGNOSIS
In the presence of ectopic gastric mucosa, the Meckel's scan will detect uptake of technetium, which localizes in the gastric mucosa (**19.52**).

TREATMENT
Operative management consists of resection of the Meckel's diverticulum together with a segment of the adjacent ileum and end-to-end anastomosis or wedge-resection and closure of the defect.

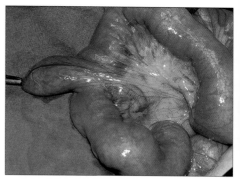

19.49 Meckel's diverticulum. Typical appearance of a Meckel's diverticulum originating on the antimesenteric border of the distal ileum.

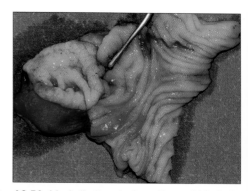

19.50 Meckel's diverticulum. Opened Meckel's diverticulum showing typical ectopic gastric mucosa leading to ulceration at the junction with the ileum. The ulcer may bleed or perforate.

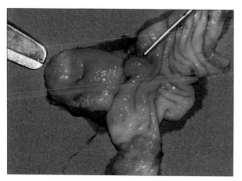

19.51 Diverticulitis of the Meckel's presents with acute abdominal pain indistinguishable from acute appendicitis.

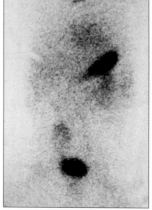

19.52 Meckel's diverticulum. Technetium (Tc99) isotope scan showing simultaneous appearance of isotope in the stomach, Meckel's diverticulum and bladder.

INTUSSUSCEPTION

INCIDENCE
One in 250 infants. An intussusception consists of invagination of one part of the intestine into the adjacent bowel. This causes an incomplete obstruction which, if unrelieved, leads to complete obstruction together with impairment of the vascularity to the invaginated (intussusceptum) bowel, initially venous congestion but ultimately ischaemic necrosis. The ileocaecal region is the most common site but any portion of the intestinal tract may be involved.

Peak incidence is six to nine months of age, with a seasonal variation, increased incidence in spring and early summer and again in midwinter.

PATHOPHYSIOLOGY
Over 95% of cases of intussusception in the age range three to 24 months do not have a recognizable leading pathological point and are assumed to occur as a result of an enlarged Peyer patch, secondary to an enteral infection. Leading points occur in 5% of cases and comprise polyps, Meckel's diverticulum, duplications, and tumours.

PRESENTATION
Colicky abdominal pain during which the infant draws up his/her legs and goes pale, vomiting (initially of food only but, as the obstructive element develops, becoming bilious and eventually faeculent) and the passage of 'redcurrant jelly'-like stools *per rectum* are the cardinal signs of intussusception. It may be possible to palpate a 'sausage-shaped' mass in the right upper quadrant of the abdomen.

DIAGNOSIS
Clinical examination. Diagnosis is by history and with investigations.

Plain abdominal x-ray: shows an absence of gas in the right iliac fossa and may show a soft tissue mass of the apex of the intussusception (**19.53**).

Ultrasonography: shows the intussusception with a 'doughnut' appearance.

Contrast radiography: shows the apex of the intussusception in the colon (meniscus sign) and seepage of contrast around the intussusception (coiled spring sign) (**19.54**).

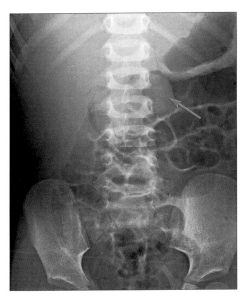

19.53 Intussusception. Plain abdominal x-ray showing obstructed small intestinal loops and an 'empty' right iliac fossa and flank. The arrow shows a soft tissue mass of the apex of the intussusception.

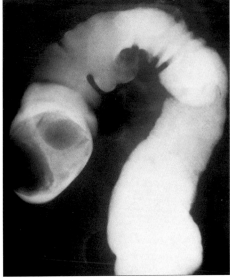

19.54 Intussusception. Barium enema showing an intraluminal obstruction in the right transverse colon.

TREATMENT

Resuscitation as required is an essential first priority. Non-operative reduction using air or contrast (hydrostatic) under fluoroscopic or ultrasound control. Contraindications for non-operative reduction are the presence of shock/toxicity, evidence of necrotic intestine, perforation.

Operative treatment consists of reduction of a viable intussusception or resection and primary anastomosis for necrotic intestine or to resect a pathological leading point (**19.55, 19.56**).

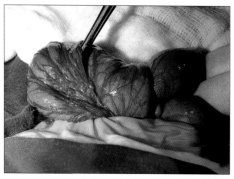

19.55 Intussusception. Operative appearance of an ileocolic intussusception.

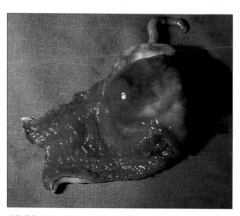

19.56 Intussusception with a duplication cyst as the leading point.

SACROCOCCYGEAL TERATOMA

INCIDENCE AND TYPES

One in 40,000 live births.
- Stage I: External sacrococcygeal mass (46%).
- Stage II; Mostly external but with presacral extension (35%).
- Stage III: Mostly presacral but with external element (9%).
- Stage IV: Entire presacral in location (10%).

The tumour consists of derivatives of all three germ-cell elements: ecto-, endo- and meso-derm.

PRENATAL DIAGNOSIS

The presence of a large sacrococcygeal teratoma can be detected on prenatal ultrasound scan. The mode of delivery may be dictated by the size of the lesion, with elective Caesarean section recommended for large lesions capable of causing dystocia or bleeding or rupture during delivery.

PRESENTATION

There may be a visible sacrococcygeal tumour at birth. Rectal examination will determine the extent of presacral extension (**19.57, 19.58**).

DIAGNOSIS

Plain x-ray may reveal calcification in the mass (**19.59**).

TREATMENT

Resection of the tumour *en bloc* with the coccyx soon after birth.
Incidence of malignancy:
- 1% at birth.
- 30% at six months of age.
- α-fetoprotein levels elevated in malignancy.

PROGNOSIS

Urinary and anorectal neuropathy may be present.

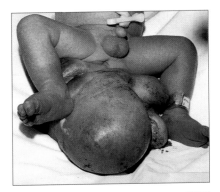

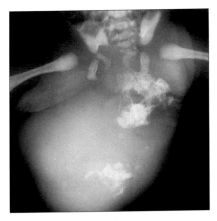

19.57 & 19.58 Sacrococcygeal teratoma. Clinical appearance of infants with massive sacrococcygeal teratomas.

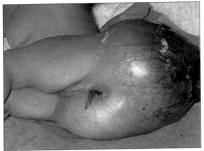

19.59 Sacrococcygeal teratoma. X-ray showing calcification in the mass.

19.60 Appendicitis. Plain abdominal x-ray showing a faecolith in the right iliac fossa (arrow).

APPENDICITIS

INCIDENCE
Appendicitis is one of the most common causes of acute abdominal pain in children.

CLINICAL PRESENTATION
The classical presentation is with acute onset of vague periumbilical pain which rapidly radiates and localizes in the right iliac fossa, where it is continuous in nature. The pain is invariably accompanied by anorexia and nausea, which usually culminates in vomiting. There is usually constipation, but diarrhoea may develop when there is pelvic appendicitis. Most children have a low-grade pyrexia of 38–39°C. Physical examination reveals localized tenderness in the right lower quadrant of the abdomen, ranging from pain on deep palpation in the earlier stages to guarding and rigidity later in the course of the disease. Rebound tenderness causes intense distress and should not be attempted.

DIAGNOSIS
Clinical features typical of appendicitis:
- Leukocytosis of $10–15 \times 10^9/l$.
- Plain x-ray of abdomen showing a faecolith (**19.60**).
- Ultrasound scan showing thickening of the wall of the appendix and free fluid in the right iliac fossa.
- Diagnostic laparoscopy.

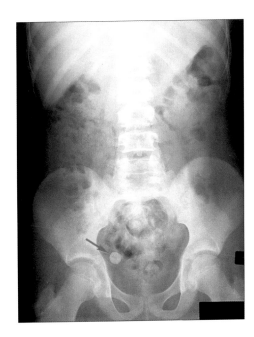

TREATMENT

For children in whom the diagnosis is not in doubt, the decision to proceed immediately to appendicectomy should be made (**19.61**). Where the diagnosis is in doubt, a period of active observation in hospital should be undertaken. The diagnosis of appendicitis will become clear within 24–48 hours.

In patients with perforated appendicitis and peritonitis, a period of active resuscitation with intravenous fluids, nasogastric decompression and intravenous antibiotics are essential prior to appendicectomy.

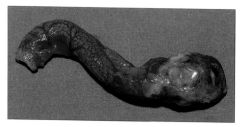

19.61 Appendicitis. Operative specimen of an acute appendicitis.

NECK LESIONS

During childhood, a variety of lesions occur in the neck. These are remnants of embryonic structures which have failed to resorb completely during development.

CYSTIC HYGROMA

Cystic hygroma are multicystic malformations of the lymphatic system and comprise innumerable small cystic spaces or larger single cysts.

Incidence

The majority of cystic hygromas are located in the neck, but they also occur in the axilla, abdomen, and groin. They appear as soft, cystic, discrete, non-tender masses which are transilluminable. They vary in size from a few centimetres in diameter to lesions which encase the entire neck (**19.62**, **19.63**). These latter lesions are particularly hazardous, in that rapid enlargement can develop as a result of inflammation; this can cause acute respiratory distress from compression of the airway, or dysphagia from compression of the oesophagus.

Diagnosis

Clinical examination followed by ultrasonography to confirm the cystic nature of the lesion and also the extent of involvement. CT or MRI will define the lesion more accurately and may be helpful in planning surgical excision.

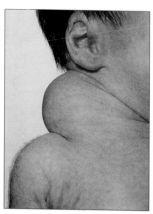

19.62 Cystic hygroma. Small, posterior, cervical cystic hygroma which is soft and fluctant and transilluminates brilliantly.

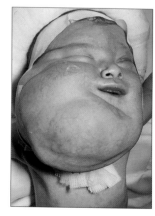

19.63 Massive cystic hygroma, extending from the temporal region across the parotid and cheek to cross the midline of the neck. The lesion caused respiratory embarrassment necessitating the tracheostomy.

Treatment
Spontaneous regression of the cystic hygroma is excessively rare. Injection sclerotherapy has been reported to be of benefit (e.g. hypertonic saline, bleomycin, OK-432). The mainstay of treatment remains surgical excision, which may prove difficult due to 'infiltration' of the cysts between vital structures (e.g. carotid artery, internal jugular vein, phrenic nerve, cranial nerves). It is important NOT to sacrifice vital structures but to accept that recurrences will occur which can then be treated on their merits.

BRANCHIAL SINUS / CYST
These arise out of failure of obliteration of the second pharyngeal pouch. Complete retention of the pouch leads to the development of a branchial fistula with an external opening in the lower one-third of the neck at the anterior border of the sternomastoid muscle (**19.64**).

The fistula extends from this tiny opening, which constantly produces mucus, through the subcutaneous tissue and platysma muscle, beneath the digastric muscle, over the hypoglossal and glossopharyngeal nerves and between the bifurcation of the carotid artery, to enter the lateral wall of the pharynx. Incomplete obliteration leaves remnants of the tract; these enlarge to form branchial cysts which are located deep to the sternomastoid muscle in the anterior triangle of the neck.

Treatment
Excision of the lesion and the associated tract.

PREAURICULAR SINUS
This occurs anterior to the tragus of the ear and may contain hair and other skin appendages (**19.65**). They may be asymptomatic but are prone to infection which will only respond to wide excision.

Treatment
Elective excision of uninfected sinuses is recommended.

DERMOID CYSTS
These occur at lines of embryonic fusion. The cyst wall contains sebaceous glands, hair follicles, connective tissue and papillae (**19.66**).

Diagnosis
The most common location is the lateral supraorbital region and in the midline of the neck. They must be differentiated from thyroglossal cysts which contains mucoid material – in contrast to the sebaceous content of dermoid cysts.

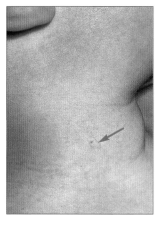

19.64
Branchial sinus. There is a tiny opening on the right side of the neck, anterior to the junction between the upper two-thirds and lower one-third of the sternomastoid muscles (arrow).

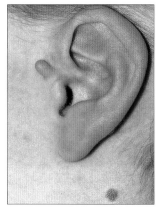

19.65 Pre-auricular sinus located anterior to the tragus of the ear. They may be marked with a remnant of cartilaginous tissue.

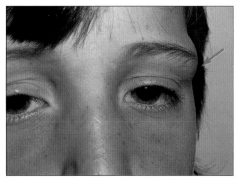

19.66 External angular dermoid cyst affecting the left lateral upper eyebrow.

THYROGLOSSAL CYSTS / FISTULAE

Thyroglossal cysts and fistulae arise out of remnants of the thyroglossal tract which fails to involute, following descent of the thyroid gland from the region of the foramen caecum of the tongue to its final position in the lower midline of the neck. Complete failure of migration leads to the development of a lingual thyroid. When the thyroid descends fully but remnants of the tract remain, a thyroglossal cysts may develop.

Diagnosis

The thyroglossal cyst is characteristically midline in location at approximately the level of the hyoid bone (**19.67, 19.68**) (see 'Otorhinolaryngology' chapter). The non-inflamed cyst is smooth and not tender and moves with swallowing and protrusion of the tongue. Inflammation results in a red, tender, well-localized swelling in the midline of the neck which, following drainage, produces a mucoid discharge.

Treatment

Excision of the cyst and the thyroglossal tract upwards to the base of the tongue, including the central portion of the hyoid bone.

INGUINAL HERNIA

INCIDENCE

One to two per 100 live births, but may be as high as 20–30% in premature infants. Male infants are four times more frequently affected than females and the right side twice as often as the left.

PRESENTATION

An inguinal hernia in a child comprises the protrusion of part of the intestine into the patent processus vaginalis. The hernia may be complete when it extends down into the scrotum or incomplete when it stops short in the groin. In infancy, the first presentation may be as an incarcerated hernia, but generally there is an intermittent swelling in the groin and/or scrotum which is noticed by the parents during bathing or changing of the nappy (**19.69, 19.70**). In female infants, there is a bulge in the groin which may extend into the labia and may contain an ovary (**19.71**).

DIAGNOSIS

Clinical presence of a hernia or a good history provided by the parents.

TREATMENT

In infancy there is a significant risk of irreducibility and urgent surgery is generally recommended. At all ages, a simple herniotomy is all that is required.

Irreducible hernias will usually reduce spontaneously or with 'taxis' following the administration of the analgesia. A strangulated hernia requires urgent resuscitation followed by surgical reduction of viable contents, resection of necrotic intestine, followed by herniotomy. The ipsilateral testis may be congested due to obstruction of the venous return.

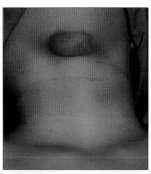

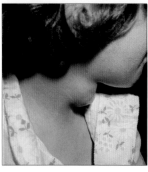

19.67, 19.68 Thyroglossal cysts, which are midline structures: the first is uncomplicated but the one below is infected.

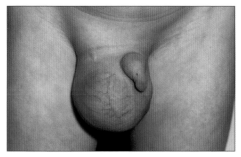

19.69 Uncomplicated right inguinal hernia.

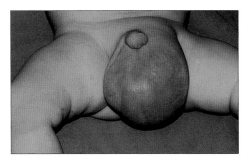

19.70 Incarcerated left inguinal hernia.

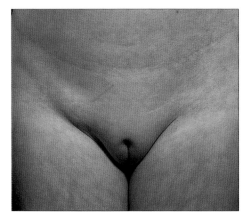

19.71 Right inguinal hernia in a girl (arrow).

HYDROCOELE

Failure of the processus vaginalis to undergo obliteration leads to the development of an inguinal hernia. When the communication between the peritoneal cavity is very narrow, the passage of peritoneal fluid only is possible and this results in the formation of a hydrocoele which may occupy the tunica vaginalis and surround the testis or may occur as a localized swelling anywhere along the cord.

PRESENTATION

A scrotal hydrocoele appears as a soft, non-tender, fluid-filled sac that is transilluminable. The swelling may fluctuate somewhat in size and it is possible to palpate a normal cord above the swelling. A hydrocoele of the cord presents as a well-circumscribed, fluid-filled mass in the inguinal region (**19.72, 19.73**).

TREATMENT

The majority of scrotal hydrocoeles regress spontaneously within the first two years of life. Operative correction is as for an inguinal hernia with ligation and division of the patent processus vaginalis and evacuation of fluid from the scrotum.

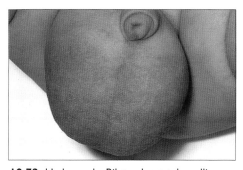

19.72 Hydrocoele. Bilateral scrotal swellings.

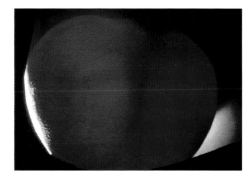

19.73 Hydrocoele. Transillumination depicting fluid in the scrotal sac.

UNDESCENDED TESTIS

The testes develop in the mesonephric ridge on the posterior abdominal wall. Descent occurs in two phases, both of which involve the gubernaculum:

- In the first phase (10–15 weeks) the gubernaculum enlarges and anchors the testis close to the inguinal region.
- In the second phase (28–35 weeks), the gubernaculum migrates out of the inguinal canal across the pubic region and into the scrotum. The processus vaginalis develops as a peritoneal out-pouching within the gubernaculum and creates a space into which the testis descends.

INCIDENCE

An 'empty' scrotum is present in 2–4% of mature newborn male infants and in 20–30% of premature infants (**19.74**). 'Spontaneous' descent can occur up to six months of age and by the age of one year the incidence is around 1%.

TYPES OF MALDESCENT

- Retractile testis is a normal testis which retracts into the inguinal canal by an actively contracting cremaster muscle. No surgery is required.
- Ectopic testis is a testis that has descended normally through the external inguinal ring and then taken an abnormal course – prepubic, perineal, femoral.
- Incompletely descended testis that has come to rest along a normal pathway of descent (e.g. intra-abdominal, at the internal ring or within the inguinal canal).

PRESENTATION

Absence of the testis at routine examination.

INDICATIONS FOR SURGERY

- To preserve spermatogenesis – degenerative changes occur around the age of one year.
- To treat an associated indirect inguinal hernia.
- To prevent torsion, which is more common in the undescended testis.
- To reduce the incidence of trauma.
- To reduce the risk of malignancy or at least to place the testis in a position where the diagnosis can be made early.
- For psychological reasons.

OPERATIVE PROCEDURE

Orchidopexy is the mobilization of the testis and spermatic cord and fixation of the testis within the scrotum. It is recommended that the optimal age for orchidopexy is between 6 and 24 months.

TORSION OF THE TESTIS

Testicular torsion occurs when the spermatic cord twists and occludes the blood supply to the testis and epididymis (**19.75**, **19.76**).

PRESENTATION

There are two common varieties.

- **Extravaginal**, due to twisting of the spermatic cord outside the tunica vaginalis secondary to inadequate fixation of the testis within the scrotum. This type usually occurs prenatally and the infant is born with an enlarged, non-tender testis. The testis is non-viable but it is vital to perform a contralateral orchidopexy as soon as possible to protect this testis.
- **Intravaginal**, due to abnormal suspension of the testis and epididymis within the tunica vaginalis ('bell-clapper anomaly'). The testis lies horizontally and the twist occurs towards the midline. Peak incidence in older children.

DIAGNOSIS

Acute onset of severe pain in the scrotum. The testis is swollen and acutely tender and is often elevated within the scrotum. There is frequently associated nausea and vomiting. Torsion of the testis can often be differentiated on clinical examination from torsion of a testicular appendage which appears as a tender nodule at the upper pole of the testis. Doppler ultrasound scan and/or radioisotope tests, if immediately available, may help to differentiate torsion from acute epididymo-orchitis. If in doubt it is best to treat as a torsion.

TREATMENT

Urgent surgical exploration with untwisting of the torsion. If viable, the testis is anchored within the scrotum whereas a necrotic testis should be excised. It is mandatory to anchor the contralateral testis.

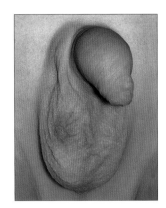

19.74 Right undescended testis with an empty right scrotum.

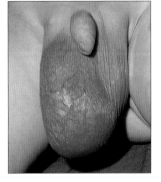

19.75 Torsion of the right testis showing a swollen, erythematous, right scrotal swelling.

19.76 Torsion of a testicular appendage which presents as a painful, tender nodule on the upper part of the scrotum above a normal testis. If the diagnosis is in doubt, it is safer to explore the scrotum.

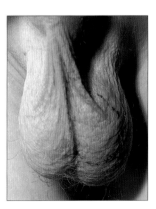

PHIMOSIS

Phimosis is scarring of the foreskin, which results in the inability to retract the foreskin over the glans.

PRESENTATION

True phimosis rarely occurs before the age of six years. The foreskin is scarred and whitish in appearance and the opening is severely narrowed resulting in non-retractability (**19.77**). During micturition there may be ballooning of the foreskin and dribbling may occur after voiding. Following an erection, the narrowed foreskin may remain around the glans, constricting its blood supply and culminate in a paraphimosis (**19.78**). The paraphimosis is an extremely painful swelling of the glans which requires emergency treatment either in reduction of the foreskin or a dorsal slit if reduction is not possible.

TREATMENT

True phimosis is an absolute indication for circumcision. Preputial adhesions are common in the first few years of life and normally resolve spontaneously – they do not constitute an indication for circumcision.

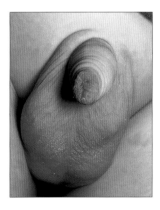

19.77 Non-retractable foreskin – a normal phenomenon.

19.78 Phimosis showing evidence of scarring of the foreskin resulting in non-retractability – a pathological condition.

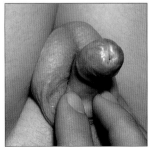

BILIARY ATRESIA

INCIDENCE
One in 12,000.

AETIOLOGY
Unknown but many theories have been postulated, including a genetic susceptibility, metabolic, infective and anatomical factors such as an abnormally long common channel at the junction of the biliary and pancreatic ducts.

PRESENTATION
Prolonged jaundice in the first few weeks of life. In addition, the stools are greyish in colour.

INVESTIGATIONS
Elevated conjugated serum bilirubin; hepatobiliary radionuclide imaging (DISIDA scan); ultrasound scan; endoscopic retrograde cholangiopancreatography (ERCP); laparoscopy; percutaneous liver biopsy; operative cholangiography.

DIFFERENTIAL DIAGNOSIS
Neonatal hepatitis, α-1-antitrypsin deficiency.

TYPES OF ANOMALIES
(**19.79**)
- **Type 1**: Atresia of the common bile duct which may be associated with a dilatation of the common hepatic duct at the porta hepatis (5%).
- **Type 2**: Atresia of the common hepatic duct with residual patency of the right and left hepatic ducts (3%).
- **Type 3**: Atresia of the whole of the extrahepatic biliary system (92%).

TREATMENT
Exploration of the extrahepatic biliary system and hepaticojejunostomy with a Roux-en-Y loop.

PROGNOSIS
The success rate is greatest when drainage of the biliary system is achieved within the first three months of life. Liver transplantation is a viable option for children who fail to respond to portoenterostomy or who develop intractable liver cirrhosis at a later age.

19.79 Three types of biliary atresia.

CHOLEDOCHAL CYST

A choledochal cyst is a dilatation of the biliary system, which may affect the extrahepatic and/or the intrahepatic bile ducts (**19.80, 19.81**).

CLASSIFICATION
- **Type I**: Cystic dilatation of the extrahepatic bile ducts with or without dilatation of the intrahepatic ducts.
- **Type II**: Fusiform dilatation of the extrahepatic ducts with or without dilatation of the intrahepatic ducts which are fusiformly dilated.
- **Type III**: Miscellaneous –
  - Diverticulum of common bile duct.
  - Intraduodenal choledochocele.
  - Intrahepatic dilatation alone (Caroli).

AETIOLOGY
Unknown, but two factors appear to be implicated :
- Weakness of the wall of the bile duct.
- Distal obstruction.

CLINICAL PRESENTATION
In infancy, obstructive jaundice with pale stools or a palpable mass in the right hypochondrium. **In older children**, mild jaundice which may be intermittent, abdominal pain, palpable mass. Rarely, ascending cholangitis or pancreatitis.

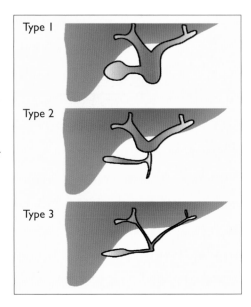

Type I

Type 2

Type 3

DIAGNOSIS

Abdominal ultrasonography; DISIDA scintigraphy; CT/MRI scan; barium meal examination; ERCP.

TREATMENT

The treatment of choice is excision of the cyst and Roux-en-Y hepaticojejunostomy. Internal drainage procedures, such as cystoduodenostomy and cystojejunostomy, carry a significant postoperative complication rate for cholangitis, pancreatitis and malignancy.

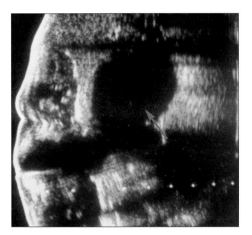

19.80 Choledochal cyst. Ultrasound scan revealing the cystic lesion inferior to the liver.

VASCULAR MALFORMATIONS

HAEMANGIOMA
Capillary haemangioma
Diagnosis

These are intradermal haemangiomas which vary in severity from 'salmon patch', which is a minor cosmetic deformity comprising a pinkish discoloration level with the surrounding skin surface and which blanches on pressure, to a 'port wine stain'. The port wine stain is dark purple in colour and is located most frequently on the face in the area of distribution of the fifth cranial nerve (**19.82**). There is no tendency for this type of haemangioma to regress spontaneously. Sturge-Weber syndrome is an occasional associated malformation. See also 'Dermatology' and 'Ophthalmology' chapters.

Treatment

Treatment is the judicious use of cosmetics to cover up the 'salmon patch', while laser therapy is currently the treatment of choice for 'port wine stains'.

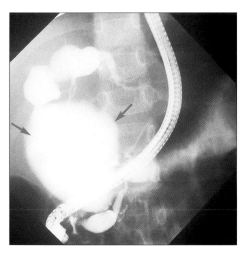

19.81 Choledochal cyst. Endoscopic retrograde cholangiogram showing the cystic dilatation of the common bile duct.

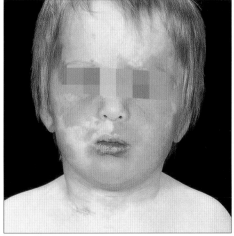

19.82 Capillary haemangioma (port wine stain) affecting the face.

Strawberry haemangioma

Presentation

These are the most common form of haemangioma. They appear initially as a tiny red spot in the first few days or weeks of life. This is followed by rapid growth for the next five to nine months, when the lesion becomes much more extensive, bright red in colour and raised above the surface of the surrounding skin with a well-defined margin (**19.83**, **19.84**).

Treatment

They tend to undergo spontaneous resolution over the next five years, during which there is gradual and progressive fading and contraction of the lesion. In most instances, specific treatment is not necessary but various modalities have been advocated in the past, such as intra-lesional injection of hypertonic saline, steroids or application of carbon dioxide snow, in an attempt to hasten resolution.

Associated complications

Large and extensive haemangiomas may occasionally be complicated by congestive cardiac failure due to shunting of blood via numerous arteriovenous fistulae within the lesion, or the development of Kasabach-Merritt syndrome with disseminated intravascular coagulation and bleeding due to platelet trapping within the haemangioma.

CONGENITAL VASCULAR MALFORMATIONS

Presentation

Usually involving the extremities or the head and neck region, these lesions appear as extensive spongy subcutaneous swellings with an overlying cutaneous capillary component (**19.85**).

Treatment

They are less prone to spontaneous resolution, which may be slow and prolonged and are more likely to continue to grow and produce major disfigurement. Attempts to induce resolution by systemic high-dose prednisolone gives variable results. Other treatments include intra-lesional injections of steroid or sclerosing agents or compression of the lesion if its position permits.

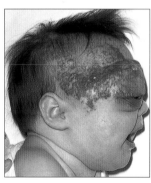

19.83 Extensive haemangioma involving the right eye and forehead.

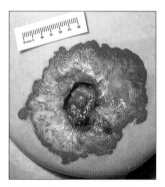

19.84 Haemangioma of the buttock with central ulceration and fading of the lesion in the immediate area of the ulcer.

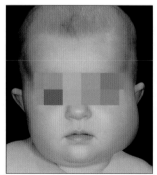

19.85 Haemangioma of the left parotid region – spontaneous resolution occurred.

KLIPPEL–TRENAUNAY SYNDROME

See also 'Dermatology' chapter.

Presentation

This syndrome affects one or more limbs and comprises haemangiomas, soft tissue hypertrophy, often to an alarming degree, bony overgrowth and varicosities on the surface (**19.86**). The bone overgrowth often produces inequality in leg length.

Treatment

Treatment is generally symptomatic and the use of a graduated elastic stocking may be of considerable benefit.

LYMPHOEDEMA

PRESENTATION

Due to a primary abnormality of the lymphatic (hypoplasia or aplasia), the condition almost exclusively affects the lower limb(s).

- **Lymphoedema** may be present at birth when it usually affects both feet and lower limbs and has a tendency to resolve spontaneously by the age of two years (**19.87**).
- **Lymphoedema praecox** appears in early adolescence and affects one or both legs. Girls are more commonly affected except in Milroy's congenital familial lymphoedema (2% of all cases) in which the sexes are equally affected.

DIAGNOSIS

The involved limb is swollen to a greater or lesser extent, the skin is thickened and there is non-pitting subcutaneous tissue oedema.

TREATMENT

Consists of prevention of infection by meticulous foot care and hygiene, elevation of the legs at night and the use of a graduated compression support stocking during the day. A sequential peristaltic pump applied to the leg overnight is extremely useful in reducing the swelling. Surgery is reserved for extreme cases.

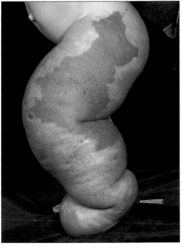

19.86 Klippel-Trenaunay malformation involving the lower extremity.

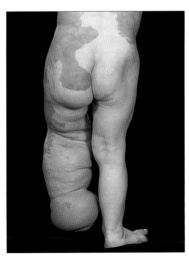

19.87 Lymphoedema involving the left lower limb.

SPINA BIFIDA

See also 'Neurology' and 'Orthopaedics and Fractures' chapters.

INCIDENCE

Varies greatly between regions but, in general, the overall incidence is continuing to decline from a peak of 3–4 per 1,000 births in 1970–80 to less than 1–2 per 1,000 births at the present time.

EMBRYOLOGY

Results from the failure of the neural groove to close fully by the end of the third week of intrauterine life.

AETIOLOGY

Multifactorial, with both genetic and environmental factors:

- **Genetic:** polygenetic inherited predisposition with the incidence in affected siblings being approximately ten times the incidence in the general population.
- **Environmental:** geographical (e.g. high incidence in South Wales and Northern Ireland compared with other regions in the UK); dietary factors (e.g. potato blight, folic acid deficiency, and higher incidence in social class 5 [unskilled labour]).

PRESENTATION

1 Local lesion, the extent of which varies:
   - Spina bifida occulta (**19.88**).
   - Skin-covered lesion such as lipoma of the cauda equina (**19.89**).
   - Meningocoele – lesion covered by meninges.
   - Myelomeningocoele – open lesion leaking cerebrospinal fusion (**19.90**).
   - Rachischisis – central canal open to the surface.

2 Hydrocephalus is present in over 80% of myelomeningocoele and 50% of meningocoele (**19.91**). The hydrocephalus occurs secondary to an Arnold Chiari malformation, which comprises caudal displacement of the cerebellar tonsils into the foramen magnum, obstructing the drainage of cerebrospinal fluid (CSF) out of the ventricles.
3 Musculo-skeletal effects. Partial or complete paralysis of the muscles below the lesion is almost invariable. In addition, deformities such as talipes equinovarus, dislocation of the hips and genu recurvatum are common.
4 Sensory disturbances occur in skin distal to the lesion and predispose to trophic effects on the ankles and heels.
5 Neuropathic bladder.
6 Anal sphincter dysfunction.

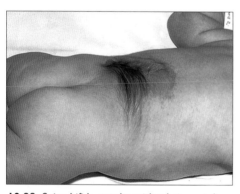

19.88 Spina bifida occulta with a hairy patch overlying the bony defect.

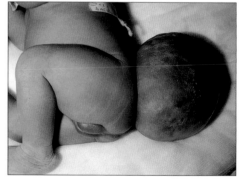

19.89 Skin-covered meningocoele in the lumbosacral region.

PREVENTION

Folate administration before and during pregnancy.

TREATMENT

Treatment includes surgical closure of the local lesion, management of the associated hydrocephalus and the neuropathic bladder, methods to improve bowel control and orthopaedic management of musculoskeletal deformities.

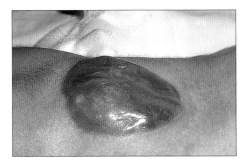

19.90 Myelomeningocoele showing the centrally exposed neural tissue.

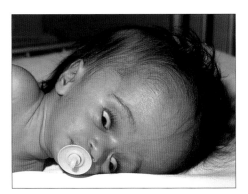

19.91 Hydrocephalus (untreated) showing the typical 'sunset' sign of the eyes.

REFERENCES

Oesophageal atresia
Beasley SW, Myers NA, Auldist A (eds). *Oesophageal Atresia* . London: Chapman and Hall, 1991.
Spitz L, Kiely EM, Morecroft JA, Drake DP. At risk groups in esophageal atresia. *J Pediatr Surg* 1994; **29:** 723–725.

Congenital diaphragmatic hernia
Azarow K, Messineo A, Pearl R. *J Pediatr Surg* 1997; **32:** 395
Puri P. Congenital Diaphragmatic Hernia. *Modern Problems in Pediatrics,* vol 24. Basel: Karger, 1989.
Wilson JM, Lund DP, Lillehai CW. Congenital diaphragmatic hernia – a tale of two cities. *J Pediatr Surg* 1997; **32:** 401

Meconium ileus
Murshed R, Spitz L, Kiely E, Drake D. Meconium Ileus, A ten-year review of thirty-six patients. *Eur J Pediatr Surg* 1996; **6:** 1–3.
Rescorla FJ, Grosfeld JL. Contemporary management of meconium ileus. *World J Surg* 1993; **17:** 318–325.

Duodenal atresia
Grosfeld JL, Rescorla J. Duodenal atresia and stenosis: reassessment of treatment and outcome based on antenatal diagnosis, pathological variance and long-term follow-up. *World J Surg* 1993; **17:** 301–309.
Murshed R, Nicholls G, Spitz L. Intrinsic duodenal obstruction: trends in management and outcome over 45 years (1951-1995) with relevance to prenatal counselling. *Br J Obs Gyn* 1999; **106:** 1197–1199.

Intestinal atresia
Louw JH, Barnard CN. Congenital intestinal atresia: observations on its origin. *Lancet* 1955; **2:** 1065.
Santulli TV, Blanc WA. Congenital atresia of the intestine: Pathogenesis and treatment. *Ann Surg* 1961; **154:** 939.

Anorectal anomalies
Pena A. *Atlas of Surgical Management of Anorectal Malformations.* New York: Springer Verlag, 1990.

Hirschsprung's disease
Holschneider AM. *Hirschsprung's Disease.* Stuttgart: Hipprokrates Verlag, 1982.

Malrotation
Skandalakes JE, Gray SW. *Embryology for Surgeons* (2nd edn). Baltimore: Williams and Wilkins, 1994.

Duplications of the alimentary tract
Stringer MD, Spitz L, Abel R *et al.* The management of alimentary tract duplications in children. *Br J Surg* 1995; **82:** 74–78.

Necrotizing enterocolitis (NEC)
Kliegman RM, Fanaroff AA. Necrotizing enterocolitis. *N Engl J Med* 1984; **310:** 1093.
Kosloske AM. Pathogenisis and prevention of necrotizing enterocolitis: a hypothesis based on personal observation and review of the literature. *Pediatrics* 1984; **74:** 1086–1092.

Gastroschisis
Glick PL, Harrison MR, Adzick NS *et al.* The missing link in the pathogenesis of gastroschisis. *J Pediat Surg* 1985; **20:** 406–409.

Umbilical hernia
Skinner MA, Grosfeld JL. Inguinal and umbilical hernia repair in infants and children. *Surg Clin N Am* 1993; **73**: 439–449.

Exomphalos
Grosfeld JL, Weber TR. Congenital abdominal wall defects: gastroschisis and omphalocele. *Curr Prob Surg* 1982; **19**: 159–213.
Langer JC. Fetal abdominal wall defects. *Sem Pediat Surg* 1993; **2**: 121–128.

Umbilical anomalies
Beasley SW. Vitellointestinal (omphalomesenteric) duct anomalies. In: Spitz L, Coran AG (eds). *Pediatric Surgery* (5th edn). London: Chapman and Hall, 1995.

Intussusception
Ravitch MM. *Intussusception in Infants and Children.* Springfield, Ill: Charles C Thomas, 1959.
Stringer DA, Ein SH. Pneumatic reduction : Advantages, risks and indications. *Pediatr Radiol* 1990; **20**: 475

Meckel's diverticulum
Beasley SW. Vitellointestinal (omphalomesenteric) duct anomalies. In: Spitz L, Coran AG (eds). *Pediatric Surgery* (5th edn). London: Chapman and Hall, 1995.

Sacrococcygeal teratoma
Altman RP, Randolph JG, Lilly JR. Sacrococcygeal teratoma. American Academy of Pediatrics, Surgical Section Survey. *J Pediat Surg* 1974; **9**: 389–398.
Rescorla FJ, Sawin RS, Coran AG, Dillon PW, Azizkhan RG. Long- term outcome for infants and children with sacrococcygeal teratoma: a report from the Childrens Cancer Group. *J Pediatr Surg* 1998;**33**: 171–6.

Appendicitis
O'Donnell B. *Abdominal Pain in Children.* Oxford: Blackwell, 1985.

Neck lesions
Skandalakis JE, Gray SW. *Embryology for Surgeons.* Baltimore : William and Wilkins, 1994.

Hiatus hernia
Grosfeld JL. Current concepts in inguinal hernia in infants and children. *World J Surg* 1989; **13**: 506–515.

Undescended testis
Hutson JM, Beasley SW. *Descent of the Testis.* London: Arnold, 1992.

Torsion of the testis
Clift VL, Hutson JM. The acute scrotum in childhood. *Pediat Surg Int* 1981; **4**: 185.

Phimosis
Gardner D. The fate of the foreskin. *BMJ* 1949; **ii**: 1433.

Biliary atresia
Howard ER. *Surgery of Liver Disease in Children.* Oxford: Butterworth-Heinemann, 1991.

Choledochal cyst
Alonso-Lej F, Rever WB Jr, Pessagno DJ. Congenital choledochal cysts, with a report of two and an analysis of 94 cases. *Int Abstr Surg* 1959; **108**: 1–30.

Lymphoedema
Milliken JB, Young AE. *Vascular Birthmarks: Hemangiomas and Malformations.* Philadelphia: Saunders, 1988.
Papendieck CM. *Colour Atlas of Angiodyoplasias in Pediatrics.* Buenos Aires: Editorial Medica Panamericana, 1988.

Spina bifida
Brocklehurst G. Spina Bifida for the Clinician. *Clinics in Developmental Medicine*, No 56. London: Heinemann, 1976.

Otorhinolaryngology
Murali Mahadevan
C Martin Bailey

OTITIS MEDIA WITH EFFUSION (OME, 'GLUE EAR')

DEFINITION
OME is defined as the presence of fluid (serous, mucoid or mucopurulent) in the middle ear cleft (**20.1, 20.2**).

INCIDENCE
The prevalence of OME in children between one and six years old in the normal population is 5–10% unilaterally and 20% bilaterally. It is more common in certain racial groups such as native Americans, Inuit, Aborigines and Maori, than in Caucasians and Afro-Caribbeans. The male to female ratio is 2:1.

AETIOLOGY
Aetiological factors may include eustachian tube dysfunction, viral and bacterial acute otitis media, craniofacial abnormalities and allergy. Other associated factors include adenoidal hypertrophy, dairy-product diet, bottle feeding, crèche attendance and passive smoking.

PRESENTATION
The most frequent presentation is with hearing loss, leading to speech and learning disability with behaviour problems. These symptoms may be associated with recurrent acute otitis media, or the child may be asymptomatic. Pneumatic otoscopy typically reveals a retracted tympanic membrane with reduced mobility. The membrane may be atrophic and draped over the ossicles.

DIAGNOSIS
Tympanometry is a sensitive test and will demonstrate fluid in the middle ear. A hearing loss can be demonstated by age-appropriate testing, and can be shown to be conductive in those children old enough to perform a pure tone audiogram (usually 4 years and over). A lateral skull x-ray will demonstrate the size of the adenoid pad. Occasionally, allergic or immunological investigation is required.

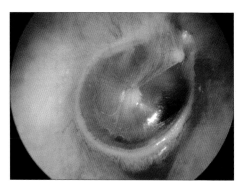

20.1 Normal tympanic membrane.

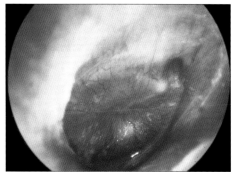

20.2 Otitis media with effusion (glue ear).

TREATMENT

A number of treatments are available, some well-established and researched and others less so. Decongestants and antihistamines are of no proven benefit, but intranasal steroid therapy may be effective when there is an underlying rhinitis. However, spontaneous resolution is common and a period of watchful waiting for at least three months should normally precede any surgical treatment. Hearing aids can be useful if conductive hearing loss is the only problem.

Grommet (ventilation tube) insertion (**20.3**) remains the most efficacious treatment for improving the hearing. Adenoidectomy has been shown to have an additive effect in resolution of otitis media with effusion when combined with grommets.

COMPLICATIONS

Local complications of otitis media with effusion include tympanosclerosis, perforation, ossicular erosion, retraction pocket formation and cholesteatoma. Tympanosclerosis (**20.4**) is the result of hyaline degeneration and dystrophic calcification and produces characteristic 'chalk patches' in the tympanic membrane: it may also occur with repeated grommet insertion and attacks of acute otitis media. Perforations are most commonly of the central type, but can be marginal and these are more likely to be associated with cholesteatoma. Tympanic membrane retraction pockets (**20.5**, **20.6**) can be of the pars tensa or flaccida and result from negative middle-ear pressures secondary to eustachian tube dysfunction. Ossicular erosion (most commonly affecting the long process of the incus) may result if the tympanic membrane becomes draped over the ossicles. Cholesteatoma may arise in a retraction pocket.

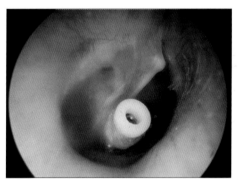

20.3 Grommet (ventilation tube) *in situ* in right tympanic membrane.

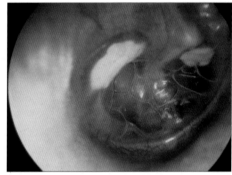

20.4 Tympanosclerotic plaque and otitis media with effusion.

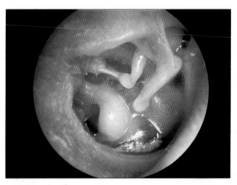

20.5 Retraction of the tympanic membrane onto the ossicles.

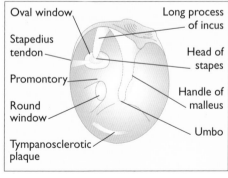

20.6 Line diagram demonstrating 20.5.

Oval window
Stapedius tendon
Promontory
Round window
Tympanosclerotic plaque
Long process of incus
Head of stapes
Handle of malleus
Umbo

ACUTE OTITIS MEDIA (AOM)

This is an acute infection of the middle ear cleft (**20.7**, **20.8**). It may be bacterial in origin with *Haemophilus influenzae*, *Streptococcus pneumoniae* and *Moraxella catarrhalis* being the commonest pathogens; often, however, it is of viral aetiology.

INCIDENCE

Fifty percent of children under five years of age will have at least one episode of acute otitis media, and 50% of episodes occur in those under five years of age. Males are affected more frequently than females, lower socioeconomic groups are more affected and the prevalence is higher in winter months. Other associated factors include adenoidal hypertrophy, allergy, immunodeficiency, cleft palate and some craniofacial syndromes.

DIAGNOSIS

Clinical features include systemic malaise, fever and otalgia. The tympanic membrane is erythematous and often bulging under pressure. The hyperaemia may extend onto the canal wall. If perforation has occurred, a microbiology swab should be taken.

TREATMENT

Analgesia should be given, and an antibiotic added if symptoms persist beyond 24 hours. Amoxicillin is the initial treatment of choice. In cases of incomplete resolution, the immunocompromised, or in the presence of a complication, myringotomy with grommet insertion is necessary, along with a culture for organisms.

COMPLICATIONS

- **Mastoiditis** is when the infection within the middle ear cleft involves the mastoid portion of the temporal bone where it may cause osteitis, erosion and suppuration. The features include fever and inflammatory swelling behind the ear with auricular protrusion (**20.9**). Treatment is with intravenous high-dose broad spectrum antibiotics with anti-pseudomonal and staphylococcal activity. Occasionally a cortical mastoidectomy is necessary.
- **Labyrinthitis** may occur due to infection extending into the labyrinth via the round or oval window. Vertigo and associated hearing loss can last weeks to months. Treatment is with antibiotics, steroids and labyrinthine sedatives.

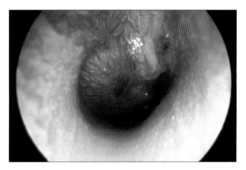

20.7 Early acute otitis media.

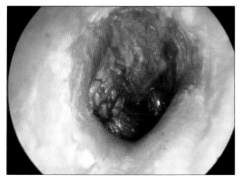

20.8 Acute otitis media with bulging of the tympanic membrane.

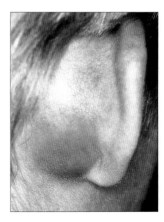

20.9 Acute mastoiditis showing postauricular swelling, erythema and protrusion of the pinna.

- **Sigmoid sinus thrombosis** is uncommon and results from thrombophlebitis developing adjacent to the middle ear cleft in the sigmoid sinus. The classical sign is a spiking 'picket-fence' pyrexia in a patient with acute otitis media or mastoiditis (without any evidence of an abscess elsewhere). The thrombus requires prompt evacuation via a cortical mastoidectomy.
- **Meningitis.** The spread of infection is usually haematogenous or via pre-existing anatomic dehiscences in the temporal bone. Early recognition and treatment is mandatory.
- **Brain abscess.** Abscesses of the temporal lobe are twice as common as cerebellar abscesses. Spread is mainly via venous channels and preformed anatomical pathways. Treatment requires neurosurgical drainage of the abscess together with a mastoidectomy, and appropriate antibiotic therapy. Brain abscess formation is estimated to occur in less than 1% of cases of AOM in the paediatric population. The incidence is increased in certain racial groups (e.g. American Indians, Australian aborigines, Maoris) and in lower socioeconomic groups.

CHOLESTEATOMA

PRESENTATION

Cholesteatoma is defined as the presence of keratinizing squamous epithelium within the middle ear or temporal bone. It may be congenital or acquired. Continuing desquamation causes the cholesteatoma to enlarge, with consequent erosion of bone and the risk of intracranial complications.

- **Congenital cholesteatoma** is characterized by the presence of keratinizing squamous epithelium behind an intact tympanic membrane (**20.10**) in a patient without a history of otitis media. These patients are often asymptomatic and present with a whitish mass seen on otoscopy behind the tympanic membrane, usually in the antero-superior quadrant (where a squamous epithelial cell rest may persist at the site of the primitive epidermoid body).
- **Acquired cholesteatoma** typically arises in a patient who has CSOM of the atticoantral type (see below). Tympanic membrane perforation or retraction with discharge is the characteristic presentation. Conductive hearing loss due to the perforation and ossicular erosion is usual; less commonly, vertigo may occur due to erosion of the horizontal semicircular canal and, rarely, facial nerve paralysis can develop due to pressure and inflammation from the cholesteatoma.

TREATMENT

Cholesteatoma requires surgical extirpation by means of a mastoidectomy. In children, the disease is often more aggressive than in adults` and so prompt surgery is required to reduce the long-term morbidity.

20.10 Congenital cholesteatoma behind an intact tympanic membrane.

CHRONIC SUPPURATIVE OTITIS MEDIA (CSOM)

PRESENTATION
CSOM is characterized by the presence of a tympanic membrane perforation with chronic inflammation of the middle ear and mastoid, resulting in discharge and hearing loss.

DIAGNOSIS
- **Tubotympanic ('safe') disease.** This is characterized by the presence of a central perforation (**20.11**) with conductive hearing loss and intermittent discharge. Discharge may be precipitated by an upper respiratory tract infection, or by water getting into the ear following bathing or swimming.
- **Atticoantral ('unsafe') disease.** This is characterized by the presence of a perforation or retraction pocket in the attic or in the posterior marginal segment of the tympanic membrane (**20.12**) with persistent malodorous discharge. This is often associated with the presence of cholesteatoma (**20.13**).

TREATMENT
Initial treatment should include microscopy and suction toilet of the ear, microbiological culture of the discharge and appropriate topical antibiotic ear drops. Audiometry should be done once the discharge has settled. Simple perforations can be repaired by myringoplasty; more advanced disease may require mastoidectomy, with or without tympanoplasty to reconstruct the tympanic membrane and ossicular chain.

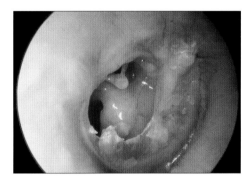

20.12 Chronic otitis media. Posterior marginal tympanic membrane perforation.

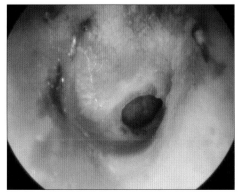

20.11 Chronic otitis media. Central tympanic membrane perforation.

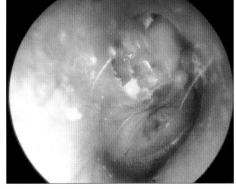

20.13 Acquired cholesteatoma arising from an attic retraction pocket.

OTITIS EXTERNA

PRESENTATION
This is an inflammatory condition of the external auditory canal skin (**20.14**), most commonly due to bacterial or fungal infection (**20.15**). Skin conditions such as dermatitis or psoriasis are less common aetiologies. Furunculosis may produce a particularly severe otitis externa (see below).

Acute otitis externa is the most common form, with many predisposing factors, including local trauma, irritants, meatal exostoses, a discharging perforation, dermatological conditions, and swimming (particularly in tropical waters, spas and hot pools).

DIAGNOSIS
The common organisms include *Pseudomonas aeruginosa*, *Staphylococcus aureus*, *Proteus* and *E coli*.

MANAGEMENT
This includes meticulous aural toilet, bacteriological swabs and, if necessary, the use of wicks with antibiotic/antifungal/steroid drops. If cellulitis spreads beyond the canal onto the auricle, systemic antibiotics are necessary. It is important to keep the ear dry and continue treatment for several days after the acute episode has settled.

Furunculosis is secondary to *S aureus* infection of the hair follicles located in the cartilaginous portion of the ear canal. In the typical case, there will be a short history of severe otalgia with a localized area of swelling, erythema and pus formation. Recurrent episodes are associated with staphylococcal carrier status. Treatment should include systemic antibiotics with incision and drainage.

AURAL POLYPS

Most polyps are benign (**20.16**) and consist of granulation tissue arising as a result of infection such as otitis media, otitis externa, or the presence of foreign material such as a grommet. Occasionally, there may be an underlying cholesteatoma. A differential diagnosis of rhabdomyosarcoma, glomus tumour or facial nerve neuroma should be considered. The decision to remove or biopsy the polyp will depend upon the history and the age of the patient. A CT scan will be useful in some cases. Treatment includes aural toilet, removal of the polyp and antibiotic ear drops.

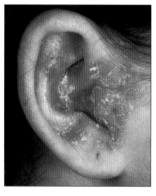

20.14 Bacterial otitis externa with involvement of the pinna.

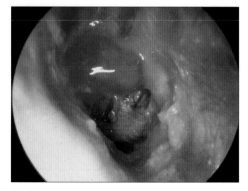

20.15 Fungal otitis externa.   **20.16** Benign aural polyp.

AURAL FOREIGN BODIES

PRESENTATION

Foreign bodies in the ear (**20.17**) are common in the 2–4 year age group. Inert foreign bodies may cause local pain as a result of secondary infection. Some foreign bodies, such as button batteries, vegetable material and insects produce an intense reaction with ulceration and otitis externa. There may be tympanic membrane perforation and, occasionally, ossicular disruption.

MANAGEMENT

Removal under a microscope is required, which frequently can only be achieved safely under general anaesthesia in children.

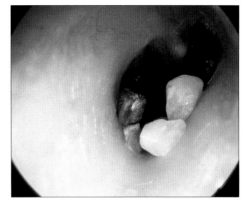

20.17 Multiple foreign bodies in the ear canal (stones).

CONGENITAL ANOMALIES OF THE EAR

PRE-AURICULAR SINUS AND ABSCESS

Presentation

Pre-auricular sinuses (**20.18**) arise from the inclusion of ectodermal elements between the six mesenchymal hillocks during embryological development of the pinna. They lie in close proximity to the anterior, ascending limb of the helix, running a tortuous branching course which is usually superficial to the temporalis fascia.

Treatment

These sinuses are often asymptomatic but can become infected and discharge, occasionally with abscess formation requiring incision and drainage. Interval surgical excision is then required.

EXTERNAL EAR

Presentation

These range from minor abnormalities such as bat ears, as a result of abnormal folding of the cartilage, through varying degrees of microtia (**20.19**), to complete absence of the pinna (anotia) with atresia of the external auditory meatus. Such anomalies can occur in isolation or in combination with other craniofacial or genetic syndromes, and there may be not only a cosmetic deformity but also a conductive hearing loss. The facial nerve may follow an abnormal course with these congenital ear anomalies.

Treatment

The pinna can be reconstructed by autologous tissue reconstruction or by a bone-anchored prosthesis from about the age of ten years.

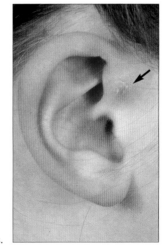

20.18 Infected pre-auricular sinus.

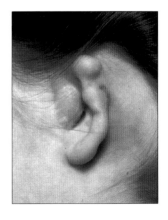

20.19 Microtia.

MIDDLE EAR ANOMALIES
Presentation
These vary from minor, isolated ossicular abnormalities to major deformities of the middle ear cleft associated with microtia and meatal atresia, and result in a conductive hearing loss. The results of attempted surgical correction for these anomalies are poor.

Treatment
If the problem is unilateral and the child has normal hearing on the opposite side, no treatment should be attempted. For bilateral cases, the treatment of choice is amplification via conventional air-conduction hearing aids if the external auditory meatuses are present, or a bone-conduction hearing aid if they are not. The bone-anchored hearing aid (BAHA) has proved to be a major advance in the long-term management of this latter group of children.

INNER EAR ANOMALIES
Presentation
Anomalies of the cochlea, vestibule, semi-circular canals, aqueducts and internal auditory meatus can occur in isolation or in combination with various syndromic and non-syndromic conditions. The usual presentation is one of severe bilateral sensori-neural hearing loss, which in some cases may be progressive.

Treatment
These children will need full audiological evaluation, appropriate amplification, speech and language therapy, support from a teacher of the deaf, and genetic counselling. Some are suitable for cochlear implantation, whereby the auditory nerve endings are electrically stimulated in response to sound.

NASAL POLYPS

Polyps are uncommon in children under the age of four. When present they are often associated with conditions such as cystic fibrosis (**20.20**), Young syndrome, Kartagener syndrome or immune deficiency syndromes.

PRESENTATION
Symptoms are nasal obstruction, discharge and anosmia. Many patients have a secondary sinusitis. The polyps arise from the ethmoid air cells and look like a bunch of pale, pearly grapes.

DIAGNOSIS
A CT scan will demonstrate the extent of disease if surgical treatment is planned. A sweat test, RAST test, serum immunoglobulins including IgG subclasses and ciliary function tests may be useful.

TREATMENT
The aim is to treat the underlying cause by medical means. Polyps are responsive to both topical nasal steroids and systemic steroids. Surgical treatment is reserved for those children who fail to respond to adequate medical treatment and comprises polypectomy with or without endoscopic intranasal ethmoidectomy. There is a high rate of recurrence despite total surgical clearance of polyps and medical treatment must be continued postoperatively.

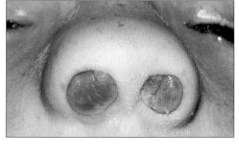

20.20 Cystic fibrosis. Bilateral nasal polyps in a child.

RHINOSINUSITIS

This is an inflammation of the nose and paranasal sinuses. The ethmoid sinuses are usually the primary site of infection. The ethmoid and maxillary sinus buds are present at birth: the frontal and sphenoid sinuses develop by the age of six and seven years respectively. The maxillary sinuses are fully developed by six years, the sphenoid sinuses by eight to ten years and the frontal sinuses by the age of 10 to 12 years.

AETIOLOGY

Causative bacteria include *Streptococcus pneumoniae*, *Haemophilus influenzae* and *Staphylococcus aureus*. Immunodeficiency, abnormal ciliary function, immunosuppression, malignancy, radiotherapy and anatomical abnormalities are all predisposing factors.

PRESENTATION

Symptoms of sinusitis include nasal obstruction, rhinorrhoea, anosmia, post-nasal drip, cough, facial pain, and headaches. Systemic symptoms of acute infection may be present.

DIAGNOSIS

Nasal swabs are of little value. Plain sinus x-rays are a useful screening investigation and may show opacification of the sinuses or air/fluid levels. However, a CT scan is the investigation of choice if complications develop or surgical treatment is contemplated.

TREATMENT

Acute rhinosinusitis should be treated with a combination of an antibiotic and a topical decongestant to facilitate drainage. When unusual organisms are suspected and a specimen for culture is needed, a maxillary sinus lavage ('antral washout') should be undertaken. Chronic rhinosinusitis is relatively uncommon in children and is usually associated with other medical problems. Treatment is complex but can involve endoscopic surgical clearance of disease from the ostiomeatal complex and ethmoids.

COMPLICATIONS

Acute rhinosinusitis may be complicated by periorbital cellulitis (**20.21**), subperiosteal abscess (**20.22**), orbital abscess, cavernous sinus thrombosis, cerebral abscess and optic neuritis. Treatment of these complications in children requires prompt referral to the paediatric otolaryngology team, a CT scan of the sinuses and brain, an ophthalmological and, if necessary, neurosurgical opinion.

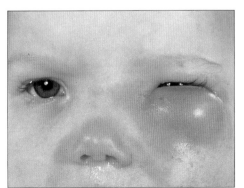

20.21 Periorbital cellulitis and subperiosteal abscess in a nine-month-old child.

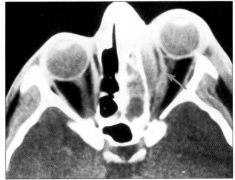

20.22 Periorbital cellulitis and subperiosteal abscess. Axial CT scan of the child in 20.21 demonstrating the subperiosteal abscess.

NASAL MASS

The differential diagnosis of a nasal mass is as shown in the chart below.

NASAL GLIOMA
Presentation

Nasal gliomas (**20.23**) account for approximately 5% of all congenital nasal swellings. They result from herniation of cerebral tissue through the anterior neuropore during foetal development, and present as a nasal mass.

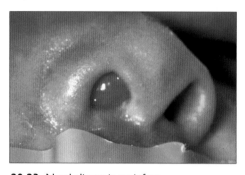

20.23 Nasal glioma in an infant.

Diagnosis

The differential diagnosis includes meningocoele, meningoencephalocoele and a simple nasal polyp. Any polypoid mass within the nose should raise the suspicion of a possible intracranial connection: simple excision may result in CSF leak or recurrence, and a CT or MRI scan is mandatory. A glioma does not increase in size with crying, straining or coughing (unlike a meningocoele). A glioma is a type of choristoma – 'normal tissue in an abnormal situation' – and as such it 'grows with the patient'.

Treatment

It usually requires a complete excision via an intranasal approach, lateral rhinotomy or bifrontal craniotomy. The prognosis is excellent.

POSTNASAL ANGIOFIBROMA
Incidence

This is a benign vascular neoplasm which affects young males: it arises in the region of the sphenopalatine foramen and expands into the pterygopalatine fossa and nasopharynx (**20.24**). Incidence is approximately 1 in 15,000 males, peaking at seven to 14 years of age.

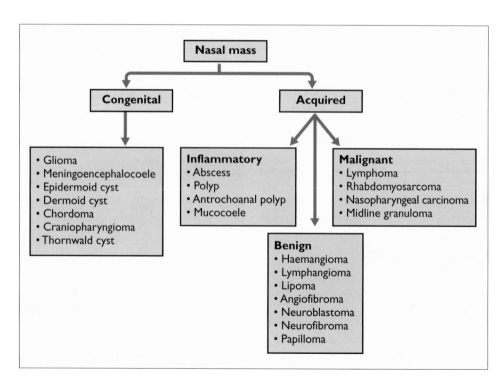

Nasal mass

Congenital

Acquired

- Glioma
- Meningoencephalocoele
- Epidermoid cyst
- Dermoid cyst
- Chordoma
- Craniopharyngioma
- Thornwald cyst

Inflammatory
- Abscess
- Polyp
- Antrochoanal polyp
- Mucocoele

Malignant
- Lymphoma
- Rhabdomyosarcoma
- Nasopharyngeal carcinoma
- Midline granuloma

Benign
- Haemangioma
- Lymphangioma
- Lipoma
- Angiofibroma
- Neuroblastoma
- Neurofibroma
- Papilloma

Presentation

Patients present with recurrent epistaxis and nasal obstruction. Examination reveals a mass in the nasopharynx. A CT scan with contrast or an MRI scan should be performed but biopsy should be avoided, as it may result in torrential haemorrhage.

Treatment

This includes selective preoperative embolization, followed by surgical resection via a lateral rhinotomy or mid-facial degloving approach. Prognosis is excellent when there is total microscopic clearance of tumour.

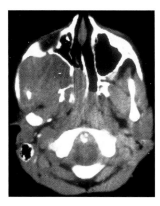

20.24 Large right postnasal angiofibroma. Axial CT scan.

NASAL FOREIGN BODIES

PRESENTATION

Nasal foreign bodies (**20.25**) are common in two- to five-year-old children, and present with a history of unilateral, purulent, malodorous discharge or with nasal obstruction. Button batteries may cause rapid ulceration. Foreign bodies may be multiple and bilateral.

DIFFERENTIAL DIAGNOSIS

The differential diagnosis includes rhinosinusitis, adenoiditis, sinonasal malignancy and unilateral choanal atresia.

TREATMENT

Retrieval using an angled hook, drawing the object from behind forwards under direct vision, is the most efficacious method of removal. The first attempt, under appropriate restraint, is generally the most successful because thereafter compliance is reduced. Inappropriate instrumentation, such as using forceps for retrieving a bead, may force the foreign body deeper into the nasal cavity or even into the lower airways. Foreign bodies can erode into the submucosa or become impacted under the turbinates, making clinical detection difficult. A CT scan may be required to detect the foreign body, followed by examination under general anaesthesia to remove it.

CHOANAL ATRESIA

INCIDENCE

This has been estimated at 1 in 8,000 live births, with females affected twice as often as males. Other congenital anomalies occur in over 50% of patients, and up to 30% may have the CHARGE association. The ratio of unilateral to bilateral cases is 2:1, and less than 10% are membranous, the rest being bony or mixed bony/membranous.

AETIOLOGY

Unknown.

PRESENTATION

Bilateral choanal atresia presents at birth as a result of incomplete breakdown of the buccopharyngeal membrane. The patient suffers from respiratory distress, as neonates are obligate nose breathers. Unilateral atresia often presents later with nasal obstruction and unilateral mucopurulent discharge. There is absence of air flow and inability to pass a size 8 French gauge nasal catheter beyond 5cm into the nose.

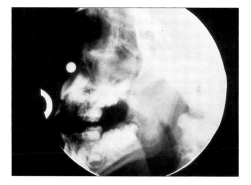

20.25 Ballbearing 'cannon ball' in the nose. Lateral neck x-ray demonstrating the position of this foreign body.

DIAGNOSIS

Contrast rhinography has long been replaced by the CT scan, which is diagnostic (**20.26**). Examination of the postnasal space under general anaesthetic confirms the diagnosis.

TREATMENT

Neonates with bilateral choanal atresia will require an oral airway and orogastric feeding tube until surgical correction is undertaken, usually within the first week of life. Surgery for unilateral atresia is performed electively when the diagnosis is made, usually at an older age. The repair is usually undertaken via a transnasal approach under endoscopic control (**20.27**), and the transpalatal approach has been largely abandoned. Stenting may be required for six to eight weeks and subsequent dilatations are often necessary.

PROGNOSIS

The outcome is excellent in almost all cases with normal growth, development and function of the nose.

TONSILLITIS (ACUTE, CHRONIC AND RECURRENT)

INCIDENCE

It is common for a child to have at least two episodes of tonsillitis during childhood, especially during the nursery or school-entry year.

AETIOLOGY

This may be viral – Epstein-Barr (EBV), adenovirus, respiratory syncytial (RSV) or bacterial (*Streptococcus pyogenes, Streptococcus pneumoniae, Staphylococcus aureus, Haemophilus influenzae*). The immunocompromised are more susceptible.

PRESENTATION

Acute tonsillitis (**20.28**) presents with a sore throat, fever, abdominal pain, dysphagia, otalgia, tender cervical lymphadenopathy, and is most frequently bilateral. Chronic tonsillitis is defined as lasting six weeks or more. Features associated with chronic tonsillitis include dysphagia, halitosis, tonsillar hypertrophy or fibrosis, debris-filled tonsillar crypts, persistent cervical lymphadenopathy and poor general health.

DIAGNOSIS

Throat swabs are helpful in prolonged/resistant infections, when an unusual organism is suspected or in the immunocompromised. A full blood count, monospot and EBV-titres may be useful. Differential diagnosis includes toxoplasmosis and infectious mononucleosis.

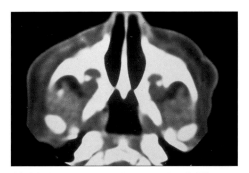

20.26 Bilateral choanal atresia. Axial CT scan.

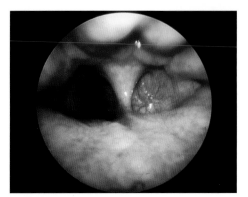

20.27 Unilateral choanal atresia – Nasopharyngeal endoscopic view.

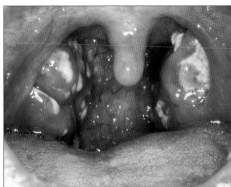

20.28 Acute follicular tonsillitis.

TREATMENT

Intravenous or oral penicillin for five days is the treatment of choice in acute infections (erythromycin in cases of penicillin sensitivity). For beta-lactamase-resistant infections, amoxicillin-clavulanate may be necessary. Rehydration, antipyretic and analgesic therapy is required. Tonsillectomy is recommended for recurrent, chronic or complicated tonsillitis. Recurrent tonsillitis may justify tonsillectomy if there are six or more episodes during a one-year period, four per year over two years, or three per year for three years or longer.

COMPLICATIONS

These include rheumatic fever, peritonsillar cellulitis or abscess, retropharyngeal or parapharyngeal abscess, septicaemia, and upper airway obstruction.

PERITONSILLAR ABSCESS (QUINSY)

PRESENTATION

This is a unilateral collection of pus outside the capsule of the tonsil, following an acute or acute-on-chronic infection. Quinsy should be suspected if there is fluctuating pyrexia, persistent unilateral sore throat and trismus following an adequate course of antibiotics in a child with tonsillitis.

TREATMENT

Incision and drainage, together with intravenous antibiotics are needed: usually this demands a general anaesthetic but needle aspiration under local anaesthesia may be sufficient in some older patients. Recurrent quinsy requires interval tonsillectomy, four to six weeks after the infection has resolved.

RETROPHARYNGEAL ABSCESS

PRESENTATION

This is an abscess arising in a retropharyngeal (prevertebral) lymph node, from which pus may track down inferiorly into the mediastinum. Causes include trauma secondary to a foreign body, tonsillitis, adenoiditis, cervical osteomyelitis or dental infection. Odynophagia, stiff neck and signs of upper airway obstruction are usual.

DIAGNOSIS

A lateral neck x-ray is the initial investigation of choice.

TREATMENT

Incision and drainage is performed under general anaesthesia with intravenous antibiotic cover.

OBSTRUCTIVE SLEEP APNOEA (OSA)

PRESENTATION

In children, this is usually the result of hypertrophy of the lymphoid tissues of Waldeyer's ring (**20.29**, **20.30**). It is deemed significant if apnoeas last for longer than ten seconds despite respiratory effort. Sleep apnoea syndrome is diagnosed when 30 or more apnoeic episodes occur during a seven-hour sleep period. Obstructive sleep apnoea can lead to daytime somnolence, physical and behavioural problems, and may ultimately result in cor pulmonale.

DIAGNOSIS

Polysomnography is required when the history is unclear or if central sleep apnoea is suspected. Symptoms of less severe upper airway obstruction include stertor/snoring, nasal obstruction and mouth-breathing.

TREATMENT

Adenotonsillectomy cures the vast majority of affected children, but not necessarily those with craniofacial abnormalities.

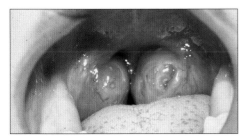

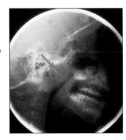

20.29 Tonsillar hypertrophy in a child with obstructive sleep apnoea.

20.30 Lateral neck x-ray showing adenoidal hypertrophy.

LARYNGOMALACIA

INCIDENCE
This is the commonest cause of stridor in neonates and infants, accounting for 35–40% of cases.

AETIOLOGY
It is thought to be due to laxity of the immature laryngeal tissue allowing collapse of the supraglottic structures on inspiration, but the exact cause is unknown.

PRESENTATION
Stridor is usually inspiratory and variable. Onset is generally a few days after birth and the stridor is worse with effort (e.g. when feeding or crying). Difficulty with feeds, reflux and vomiting are common; failure to thrive occurs in severe cases. Other signs include tachypnoea, subcostal recession, tracheal tug and pectus excavatum.

DIAGNOSIS
Examination of the larynx, either with a flexible fibreoptic nasendoscope or with a rigid laryngoscope, is necessary for all but the very mildest cases. On endoscopy, an omega-shaped epiglottis, short aryepiglottic folds, redundant arytenoid mucosa and collapse of supraglottic tissues into the laryngeal introitus with inspiration are diagnostic.

TREATMENT
Mild laryngomalacia can be observed and most cases will resolve by the age of 18–24 months. Those who show signs of failure to thrive should undergo endoscopic aryepiglottoplasty to trim the redundant supraglottic tissues.

RECURRENT RESPIRATORY PAPILLOMATOSIS

INCIDENCE
The incidence is 7 per million in the USA, with a bimodal age distribution; 66% of cases involve those under 16 years of age.

AETIOLOGY
This is a diffuse diathesis of respiratory mucosa, resulting in papillomatous proliferation characterized by benign non-keratinizing squamous epithelium. It can occur anywhere in the aerodigestive tract but especially in the larynx. It is caused by the human papilloma virus (HPV) types 6 and 11 (**20.31**).

PRESENTATION
The majority of children with recurrent respiratory papillomatosis present before the age of four years, with a hoarse voice, abnormal cry, stridor or respiratory distress, depending upon the location and severity of the disease. The younger the child, the more aggressive the clinical course. HPV 6 behaves more aggressively than HPV 11.

DIAGNOSIS
An initial biopsy is needed to confirm the diagnosis. Typing of HPV using the polymerase chain reaction (PCR) may be useful in the future.

TREATMENT
The aim is to maintain a good airway and adequate voice by 'debulking' the papillomas while awaiting spontaneous remission. CO_2 laser vaporization of the papillomas is the mainstay of treatment. Tracheostomy is occasionally necessary in severe cases, but may cause tracheobronchial spread of papillomas. Adjunctive interferon therapy may enable control of the airway to be maintained with the CO_2 laser and avoid tracheostomy.

PROGNOSIS
There is no effective systemic or surgical treatment to eradicate HPV. The disease can remit at any age, but 20% progress to adulthood. Malignant transformation is rare (<1%).

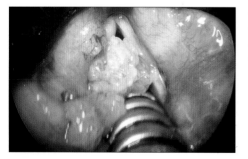

20.31 Recurrent respiratory papillomatosis of the supraglottis and glottis. Endoscopic view.

SUBGLOTTIC STENOSIS

INCIDENCE
The incidence is difficult to estimate but has reduced with increased awareness of the role of intubation: currently about 1–2% of intubated neonates develop an acquired subglottic stenosis. Approximately 7–8% of admissions for stridor are secondary to subglottic stenosis.

AETIOLOGY
The narrowest portion of a child's airway is the subglottis, where the airway immediately below the vocal cords is enclosed within the cricoid cartilage. Occasionally, subglottic stenosis is congenital, but more frequently it is acquired following prolonged or traumatic intubation (**20.32, 20.33**).

CLASSIFICATION
The severity of the stenosis can be measured from the outer diameter of a bronchoscope or endotracheal tube which will just pass. Current staging is based on the percentage of lumen occluded, in a system proposed by Cotton (**Table 20.1**).

PRESENTATION
Inspiratory stridor is the most common presenting symptom and may resemble recurrent croup. The child may present with failure to extubate following neonatal intubation and ventilation.

DIAGNOSIS
The investigation of choice is microlaryngoscopy and bronchoscopy.

TREATMENT
For the failed neonatal extubation a cricoid split procedure may be suitable, and is successful in 75% of appropriately-selected cases. Established Grade I stenosis may need no treatment, but more severe grades may require laryngotracheal reconstruction using a costal cartilage graft (with or without a covering tracheostomy).

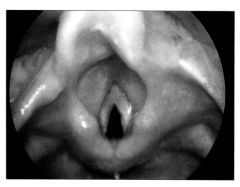

20.32 Normal larynx. Endoscopic view.

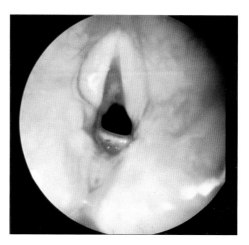

20.33 Acquired anterior and posterior subglottic stenosis. Endoscopic view.

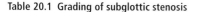

Table 20.1 Grading of subglottic stenosis

Grade	% of subglottic lumen occluded
I	0–50%
II	50–70%
III	70–99%
IV	>99%

LARYNGEAL AND TRACHEOBRONCHIAL FOREIGN BODIES

PRESENTATION

Inhaled foreign bodies are most common in toddlers. Objects tend to lodge at the carina or in the right main bronchus (**20.34**), as it branches off the trachea at a less acute angle than the left main bronchus. The inhalation may be witnessed; if not, coughing spasms, choking or respiratory obstruction may be evident. Occasionally, the episode may be asymptomatic, and these children may present with recurrent or chronic respiratory infections or with an irritable airway mimicking asthma.

DIAGNOSIS

Signs vary according to the site of the foreign body, with the general rule being inspiratory stridor when the foreign body is above the vocal cords, biphasic stridor at the level of vocal cords, and expiratory stridor below the cords. Classically with bronchial obstruction, there will be reduction of air entry to the affected lung segments with expiratory rhonchi.

The bronchial foreign body may have a ball-valve effect, causing air trapping and hyperinflation of the affected lung. Inspiratory and expiratory chest x-rays may give clues as to the location of a foreign body and show any hyperinflation, mediastinal shift (**20.35**) or atelectasis. Frequently, however, there may be little to suggest the presence of a bronchial foreign body after the initial episode of coughing/choking.

TREATMENT

With symptoms or signs of foreign body inhalation, bronchoscopy should be performed by an experienced surgical, anaesthetic and nursing team. Distal foreign bodies occasionally require flexible endoscopy for retrieval and, rarely, a thoracotomy is required.

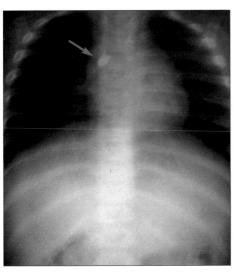

20.34 Peanut in the right main bronchus, demontrated by a chest x-ray.

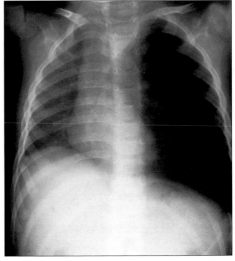

20.35 Hyperinflation of the left lung with mediastinal shift to the right due to air trapping by a foreign body in the left main bronchus.

BRANCHIAL SINUSES AND CYSTS

AETIOLOGY

These are rare embryological anomalies which arise from incomplete fusion of the branchial arches, resulting in a sinus, cyst or fistula. The commonest is a second branchial arch sinus, followed by first (IA and IB) and third. Fourth arch sinuses are very rare (fewer than eight reported cases in the literature). The details of these anomalies are shown in **Table 20.2**.

PRESENTATION

The sinus may intermittently discharge mucoid or mucopurulent fluid and, occasionally, an abscess may develop. Branchial cysts usually lie deep to the anterior border of the sterno-mastoid at the junction of its upper and middle thirds (**20.36**).

DIAGNOSIS

Ultrasound will give valuable information about the size and position of a cyst. To assess the sinus tract a sinogram or CT scan may be useful.

TREATMENT

Surgical excision of the entire tract is curative.

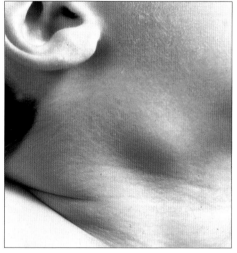

20.36 Second branchial arch cyst in an eight-year-old boy.

Table 20.2 Branchial sinuses and fistulae

Type	Internal opening	External opening	Pathway of tract
IA	Middle/external ear	Preauricular	Lateral to facial nerve
IB	Middle ear	Inferior to pinna, upper sternomastoid	Medial to facial nerve
II	Tonsillar fossa	Along anterior border of sternomastoid	Between external and internal carotid, above cranial nerves IX, X, and XII
III	Pyriform fossa	Mid/lower lateral neck	Medial to carotids above glossopharyngeal nerve, through thyrohyoid membrane
IV	Pyriform fossa	Over thyroid gland	Not established

PAEDIATRIC HEAD AND NECK MASSES

AETIOLOGY

Congenital masses are usually midline (except branchial cysts). Upper cervical swellings are often infective or congenital. Lower cervical lumps are often malignant. Malignant masses grow rapidly and are painless unless infected.

DIAGNOSIS

It is important to establish whether the lump is acute or chronic, rapid or slow growing, painful or painless, midline or lateral, solitary or multiple. Also to be determined are its size, shape, whether it is smooth or irregular, solid or cystic, its mobility (i.e. fixation to skin or underlying tissue), any change in colour of the overlying skin, any functional disability, whether it transilluminates, and any other local or systemic features. Consideration of the above should lead to the appropriate differential diagnosis.

Ultrasound will give information regarding tissue density, size, location, depth and often diagnosis. CT and MRI scans can give additional information but require a general anaesthetic in most small children. Serology, FBC, Mantoux test, thyroid function tests and chest x-ray may be contributory. An otolaryngological opinion should be obtained as soon as possible. Fine needle aspiration cytology (FNA) is often diagnostic but needs general anaesthesia in small children; open biopsy is usually preferable.

THYROGLOSSAL DUCT CYST

EMBRYOLOGY

During development, the thyroid descends from the level of the floor of the primitive pharynx at the foramen caecum into the lower neck. The tract usually disappears after descent, but a remnant may persist anywhere along its course, enlarge and present as a cyst. The tract has an intimate relationship with the body of the hyoid bone.

INCIDENCE

This affects males and females equally. Seventy percent of cysts lie below the hyoid and 98% are midline.

PRESENTATION

The solitary midline cystic swelling (**20.37**) may be of variable size and may become infected to form an abscess. The cyst lifts with protrusion of the tongue and can be attached to the hyoid.

DIAGNOSIS

Thyroid ultrasound to demonstrate the cyst and ascertain the presence of normal thyroid tissue is mandatory – a thyroglossal cyst may very rarely contain the only functioning thyroid tissue.

TREATMENT

Excision is advisable because of the risk of infection and abscess formation, and because of the rare possibility of papillary thyroid carcinoma arising from a thyroglossal cyst. An abscess requires incision and drainage, followed by excision of the cyst when the infection has completely resolved. Definitive excision of the tract should consist of Sistrunk's procedure to remove the cyst, tract, body of the hyoid, and a core of tissue leading towards the foramen caecum at the tongue base. Tissue should be histologically sectioned to look for columnar epithelium.

PROGNOSIS

Incomplete excision carries an 80% risk of recurrence.

20.37 Thyroglossal duct cyst in a seven-year-old boy.

OROPHARYNGEAL AND OESOPHAGEAL FOREIGN BODIES

INCIDENCE
These can occur in any paediatric age group. Fish, lamb and chicken bones are common foreign bodies. Small objects such as fish bones tend to lodge in the oropharynx, particularly in the tonsil, base of tongue and the valleculae. Larger foreign bodies such as coins are typically found at the cricopharyngeal level.

DIAGNOSIS
Older children may be able to localize a foreign body above the cricopharyngeus. Younger children present with drooling, dysphagia or irritability. Examination may reveal cricoid tenderness and, occasionally, surgical emphysema is present. A normal lateral neck x-ray does not exclude a foreign body. The x-ray may demonstrate a radio-opaque foreign body (**20.38**), prevertebral soft tissue swelling, retropharyngeal or mediastinal air. Further imaging with a contrast swallow or CT may be helpful.

TREATMENT
If there is suspicion of an ingested or inhaled foreign body, an urgent otolaryngological opinion should be obtained. Surgeons should have a low threshold for endoscopy to exclude an ingested foreign body. A spiking temperature ('picket fence' type) should suggest the possibility of complications such as a retropharyngeal abscess, perforated viscus, mediastinitis, or septicaemia.

If such a complication is suspected, the child should be placed nil-by-mouth, blood cultures obtained, and a contrast swallow or CT scan considered. The child should be placed on high-dose systemic antibiotics with anaerobic and gram-negative cover.

FURTHER READING

Stool SE, Berg AO, Berman S *et al*. *Otitis media with effusion in young children*. Clinical practice guideline. Number 12. Rockville, Maryland: Agency for health care policy and research, Public Health Services, US Department of Health and Human Services, 1994.

Cantekin EI, Bluestone CD, Fria TJ *et al*. Identification of otitis media with effusion in children. *Ann Otol Rhinol Laryngol* 1980; **89**: 190–195.

Rosenfeld RM, Post JC. Meta-analysis of antibiotics for the treatment of otitis media with effusion. *Otol Head & Neck Surg* 1992: **106**: 378–386.

Hendley JO, Otitis Media (Clinical Practice). *N Engl J Med* 2002: **347(15)**: 1169–1174.

Cotton RT, Myer CM *et al*. *Practical pediatric otolaryngology*. Philadelphia: Lippincott-Raven, 1999.

Rosenfeld RM, Kay D. Natural history of untreated otitis media. *Laryngoscope* 2003; **113(10)**: 1645–1657.

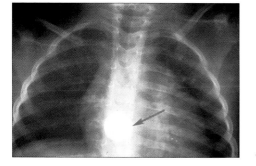

20.38 Chest x-ray demonstrating a radio-opaque foreign body (coin).

Oral and Dental Surgery
Graham Roberts

DENTAL FLUOROSIS

INCIDENCE
Varies with the level of fluoride intake from water and/or fluoridated toothpaste. Where the level of fluoride is 1mg per litre of water (1 ppm), fewer than 10% of children have mild to trivial white flecks. In parts of Africa, where the fluoride in the water supply is up to 53 mg per litre (53 ppm), up to 50% of the population have severe to moderate brown mottling.

PRESENTATION
Dental enamel with a range of appearances from lustreless, opaque white patches to brown mottled discoloration of varying intensity; distribution is symmetrical. It occurs if there is excessive dietary intake of fluoride at the time of enamel formation (**21.1, 21.2**).

DIAGNOSIS
Clinical appearance and a history of living in an area where fluoride levels in the water supply are known to be higher. In recent times, some children thought to be swallowing toothpaste have clinically discernible levels of fluorosis.

PROPHYLAXIS
Use a measure of toothpaste only the size of a small pea on the toothbrush. Fluoride in the water supply at 1 ppm is associated with a 50% reduction in dental caries. Fluoride toothpaste brings a reduction of approximately 35%.

TREATMENT
Microabrasion of the surface brings about dramatic improvement. If required, porcelain veneers can be used. These give an excellent result but are fragile and require lifelong attention by a dentist.

GINGIVAL INFLAMMATION

INCIDENCE
Some degree of gingivitis somewhere in the mouth affects virtually every child and adult in the world. The severity and extent varies with oral hygiene competence. Periodontal disease, which progresses from gingivitis, is the single greatest cause of tooth loss across the world.

PRESENTATION
Large deposits of bacterial dental plaque due to poor oral hygiene (**21.3**). Associated with this is the development of an area of chronic gingival inflammation.

DIAGNOSIS
Visual examination of attached gingivae. Minimal signs are mild erythema of the gingival margin. Established gingivitis involves a greater width and breadth of attached gingivae, as shown.

TREATMENT
The establishment of a high standard of oral hygiene. This does not come naturally and requires one-to-one tuition and regular review from a health care professional such as a dental hygienist.

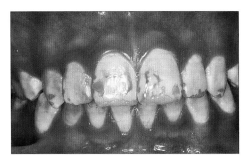

21.1 Dental fluorosis.

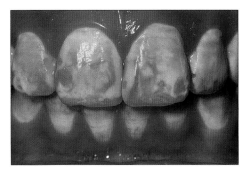

21.2 Dental fluorosis.

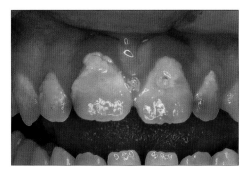

21.3 Gingival inflammation adjacent to the two upper central incisors.

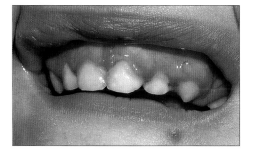

21.4 Herpetic gingivostomatitis.

HERPETIC GINGIVOSTOMATITIS

PRESENTATION

The primary attack occurs in infants and children unprotected by circulating antibodies. The mouth is painful, with a widespread appearance of yellowish fluid-filled vesicles on the tongue and lips (**21.4**). These quickly rupture to form painful, greyish ulcers surrounded by an erythematous margin. The gingivae develop widespread inflammation.

CLINICAL PROGRESS

The ulceration and inflammation lead to a very sore mouth, dysphagia, malaise, irritability, regional lymphadenopathy and pyrexia. The severity of these signs and symptoms varies considerably. Dehydration may occur due to dysphagia. On rare occasions, it is necessary to admit a child for intravenous fluids. A rare complication is viral encephalitis.

TREATMENT

The disease is usually well-established by the time a diagnosis can be made, so the associated viraemia has passed. For practical purposes, therapy with aciclovir is rarely of value, as by the time the diagnosis is made it is too late. Oral or intravenous aciclovir is used prophylactically during the period of severe immunosuppression that occurs during treatment for leukaemia.

TETRACYCLINE STAINING

INCIDENCE
Almost all children who have ingested tetracycline during the period of enamel growth develop tetracycline staining. It is now rare in the UK, as prescribing practices have changed and tetracycline is rarely used in children under 12 years of age. The discoloration is still common in countries where tetracycline can be bought over the counter, because it is an inexpensive antibiotic.

PRESENTATION
Linear bands of grey to deep-brown discoloration. The banding is closely correlated to the incremental growth lines in enamel (**21.5**).

DIAGNOSIS
Clinical presentation and confirmatory history of tetracycline usage. For forensic purposes, an exfoliated tooth can be used to prepare semi-thin ground sectors. The tetracycline fluoresces yellow/green under ultraviolet light.

TREATMENT
It is necessary to use porcelain veneers or full porcelain crowns. These give an excellent aesthetic result (**21.6**).

FISSURE SEALANT

PRESENTATION
The occlusal surfaces of the first permanent molars are the most caries-prone surfaces in the human dentition (**21.7**). These teeth are also important in the establishment and maintenance of occlusal stability.

TECHNIQUE
A permanent tooth is identified as caries-free and then:
- It is isolated to prevent saliva contaminating the occlusal surface.
- The occlusal surface is carefully cleaned and polished with a mild abrasive toothpaste.
- The occlusal table is washed and dried.
- A weak acid (30% w/v orthophosphoric acid) is applied to the occlusal surface for 30 seconds.
- The occlusal surface is then rewashed and carefully dried until the enamel looks like frosted glass.
- The dental resin is flowed gently on the occlusal surface and made to polymerize by shining a blue spectrum light for 60 seconds.

EFFICACY
The glass-like resin seals the fissure and is over 90% effective in preventing occlusal caries.

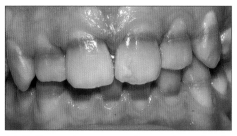

21.5 Tetracycline staining showing linear bands of discoloration.

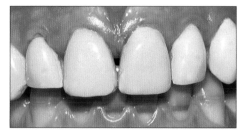

21.6 Tetracycline staining after treatment with porcelain veneers.

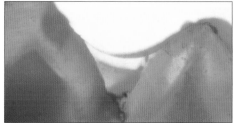

21.7 Fissure sealant.

RETAINED DECIDUOUS INCISORS

INCIDENCE
Between 0.5% and 1% of UK children experience delayed eruption.

PRESENTATION
A single (or multiple) deciduous upper incisor is retained beyond the normal time for exfoliation (21.8).

- The upper right central incisor is present, although the upper left central incisor is unerupted. The upper left deciduous central incisor is retained and is also grossly discoloured.
- The radiograph (21.9) shows the presence of the permanent successors which have probably been prevented from erupting by the retained deciduous and lateral incisors.

DIAGNOSIS
This is based on the clinical appearance and the radiographic findings.

TREATMENT
Extraction of the retained deciduous teeth is usually sufficient to encourage the permanent teeth to erupt spontaneously. Unusually, the delay may be so extensive that surgical exposure and the placement of orthodontic brackets with chains for traction may be advisable.

PROGNOSIS
The results of treatment are almost always highly successful.

UNERUPTED (DISPLACED) UPPER LEFT CENTRAL INCISOR

INCIDENCE
The condition is not uncommon, affecting approximately 1% of all children in varying degrees of severity.

PRESENTATION
A single (sometimes multiple) tooth is seen clinically or radiographically to be in an inappropriate position. In 21.10 the tooth is high in the labial sulcus, slightly across the midline and partly rotated.

MANAGEMENT
The tooth may be uncovered surgically (if required) and an orthodontic bracket placed on the tooth. A removable orthodontic appliance is used to apply traction to the tooth to pull it down and into its correct position in the arch.

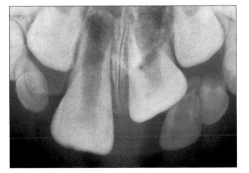

21.8 Retained deciduous incisor.

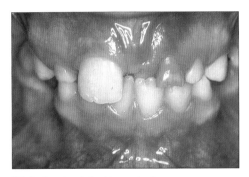

21.9 Retained deciduous incisors. The radiograph shows the presence of the permanent successors.

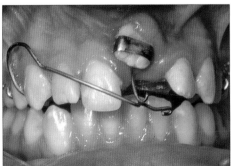

21.10 Unerupted (displaced) upper left central incisor.

DENTIGEROUS CYST

INCIDENCE
Impacted third molars occur in about 10–20% of the population. Of these, approximately 37% show signs of a circumcoronal radiolucency of sufficient magnitude to be regarded as a dentigerous cyst.

PRESENTATION
The failure of eruption of a permanent tooth, usually a third molar, and the presence of a rounded eminence over the presumed site of the tooth is usually the presenting complaint.

CLINICAL FEATURES
The gum is enlarged at the site of the cyst. An intra-oral or panoramic radiograph shows the expansion of the bone above and around the crown (**21.11**). Although rare, this enlargement of the coronal part of the dental follicle can lead to considerable enlargement, bony destruction, and even hollowing out of the ramus of the mandible.

TREATMENT
The size of the lesion usually dictates surgical management. Smaller cysts can be removed in their entirety. Larger cysts, which involve gross destruction of bone, can be decompressed by placement of a surgical drain.

PROGNOSIS
There is a risk of spontaneous infection so such cysts should not be ignored. A small proportion may go on to become an ameloblastoma. This is a form of odontogenic tumour.

ODONTODYSPLASIA

INCIDENCE
The condition is rare; a specialist paediatric dentist may see only five cases in a full professional lifetime.

PRESENTATION
The teeth appear to be crumbled and of poor form when they erupt. The eruption is usually associated with severe pain. This is sometimes the presenting symptom. At other times, a tooth of abnormal form appears and concern about its appearance is the reason for the patient to visit the dentist.

DIAGNOSIS
The radiographic appearance is universally referred to as 'ghost teeth' (**21.12**). The sporadic absence of mineralized tissue, coupled with abnormal form, confers the ghost-like quality. When the radiograph is taken, it is usual to see several teeth in the affected quadrant affected with the same condition. This sometimes leads to the teeth being called 'regional odontodysplasia'.

The ground section (**21.13**) demonstrates clearly the grossly hypoplastic appearance, with the dentine displaying increased areas of interglobular dentine. There is a large area of dystrophic calcification where the pulp should be present.

TREATMENT
Unless the condition is very mild, the only suitable form of treatment is extraction. This results in severe localized dento-alveolar damage, which will need orthodontic and/or prosthetic management.

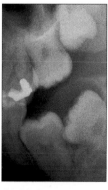
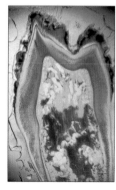

21.11 Dentigerous cyst.

21.12 Odontodysplasia. Radiographic view showing 'ghost teeth' appearance.

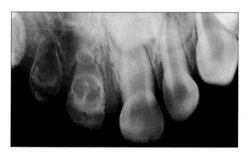

21.13 Odontodysplasia. Ground section showing hypoplastic appearance.

AUTOTRANSPLANTATION

PRESENTATION
An occasional presentation is an unsaveable first permanent molar (**21.14**). Such infected roots need to be removed. The space created may allow the teeth behind the extraction to tilt into the space, creating a risk of periodontal pocketing.

TREATMENT
The tooth needs to be replaced. In the case shown, the damaged roots have been extracted (**21.15**). The lower right third molar has been removed and the tooth placed in the lower left first molar socket. The tooth is held gently by a 'criss-cross' suture and antibiotics are prescribed.

PROGNOSIS
Such teeth usually exhibit only very limited further growth. Nevertheless they provide normal form and function for many years. This prevents the need for potentially damaging prosthetic appliances or crown and bridges.

COMPLEX PERIODONTITIS

INCIDENCE
The major difference between children and adults is that, generally, children suffer from gingivitis (inflammation of the attached gingivae) and adults suffer from periodontitis (inflammation of the gingivae coupled with breakdown of the tissues attaching the teeth to the bony support). In adolescence, there is a small degree of crossover although gingivitis predominates. True periodontitis in children is rare.

PRESENTATION
A child with glycogen storage disease Type IIb presented with extensive gingival inflammation involving all erupted teeth (**21.16**). Gentle probing revealed 4–6 mm pockets around several of the teeth. Radiographs confirmed early destruction of bony tissue. The underlying metabolic defect is the principle aetiological factor. Even small amounts of bacterial dental plaque can cause widespread inflammation.

TREATMENT
Careful and thorough scaling and polishing coupled with chlorhexidine gluconate 0.2% as the chemical antiplaque agent. The mouth should be rinsed carefully with this for two minutes daily.

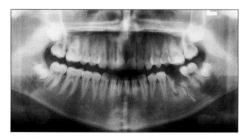

21.14 Autotransplantation. An unsaveable first permanent molar (lower left first molar).

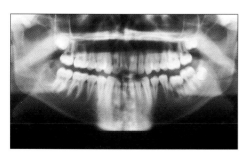

21.15 Autotransplantation. The damaged roots have been extracted.

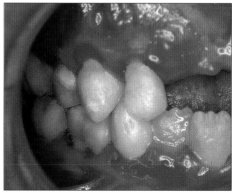

21.16 Complex periodontitis with extensive gingival inflammation.

ENAMEL HYPOPLASIA

DIAGNOSIS

The term applies to any macroscopic defect occurring during the growth of enamel. The term is most commonly applied to enamel hypoplasia caused by a systemic upset such as a febrile illness.

PRESENTATION

The essential characteristic is involvement of all enamel forming at the time of systemic upset (e.g. severe febrile illness). Clinically, contra-lateral pairs of teeth are affected in an identical pattern (**21.17**). The upper permanent central incisors have a band of hypoplasia across the middle of the crown of the tooth. The pattern on the lower permanent central and lateral incisors is similar. The upper permanent lateral incisors are affected closer to the incisal edge, as the development of these teeth is 4–6 months later than that of the other incisors.

The main complaint from the patient is the poor appearance of the teeth. This can be easily masked by the use of enamel bonding and composite tooth-coloured restorative materials. Occasionally, coupled with poor toothbrushing, the hypoplastic areas become decayed and require more careful cleaning.

DENTINOGENESIS IMPERFECTA

INCIDENCE

Approximately 1 in 8,000 births.

AETIOLOGY

The condition is a rare autosomal dominant pattern of inheritance.

PRESENTATION

As teeth erupt, it is usually abundantly clear that they have a distinct brown and opalescent appearance (**21.18**).

DIAGNOSIS

As time progresses and the teeth come into occlusal contact, the enamel flakes away, exposing the dentine. This leads to severe attrition and consequent loss of tooth structure (**21.19**).

The radiological appearance of the teeth is pathognomic, with accelerated pulpal and root canal obliteration. In addition, the roots are short and narrower than normal. The crowns are also reduced in size but not as much as the roots. This gives a characteristic appearance of 'tulip teeth' (**21.20**). Occasionally, pathological fractures of the root are apparent.

TREATMENT

The course of the condition is varied. Some children's teeth wear very little and no intervention is needed. In others, the enamel flakes off very easily because of poor attachment via the amelo-dentinal junction. As a consequence, semi-permanent crowns are required to prevent excessive wear during childhood and adolescence. During late adolescence and young adult life, the whole dentition may need extensive crowning.

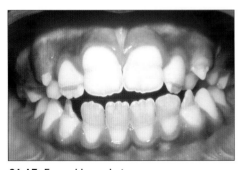

21.17 Enamel hypoplasia.

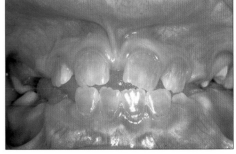

21.18 Dentinogenesis imperfecta. Opalescent appearance of teeth.

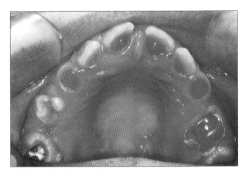

21.19 Dentinogenesis imperfecta. Exposure of dentine and loss of tooth structure.

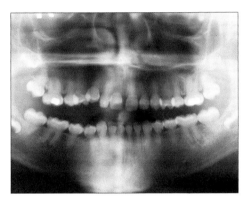

21.20 Dentinogenesis imperfecta. Characteristic 'tulip teeth' appearance.

AMELOGENESIS IMPERFECTA (HYPOPLASTIC VARIETY)

INCIDENCE
Approximately 1 in 15,000 births.

AETIOLOGY
The condition is inherited.

PRESENTATION
A variety of presentations, depending upon the precise pattern of inheritance. There is hypoplasia with pigmentation. The absence of enamel makes the teeth look small and leads to significant spacing between the teeth. (**21.21**)

DIAGNOSIS
Radiographically, the teeth are normal in appearance except that little or no enamel appears to be present.

TREATMENT
The patient's main complaint is the poor appearance. This is managed in childhood by temporary composite restorations on the anterior teeth (**21.22**) and bonded onlay for posterior teeth. As with dentinogenesis imperfecta, little is done for the primary teeth, the main effort being directed at preserving the patient's cooperation until they are much older when extensive treatment can be carried out.

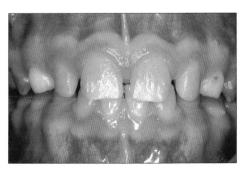

21.21 Amelogenesis imperfecta.

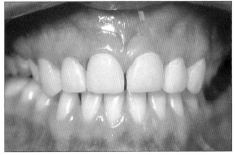

21.22 Amelogenesis imperfecta. Composite restorations.

AMELOGENESIS IMPERFECTA (HYPOMINERALIZED VARIETY)

INCIDENCE
Approximately 1 in 14,000 children.

AETIOLOGY
The inheritance is varied and this coincides with variations in the subtypes for the condition.

PRESENTATION
As with the hypoplastic variety, the defect is immediately apparent when the teeth erupt. The teeth have a normal amount of enamel, but during maturation a large proportion of the matrix remains in the enamel, causing significant discoloration. A further problem is chipping and loss of some enamel under occlusal stress (**21.23**).

DIAGNOSIS
Radiologically the teeth appear relatively normal, except for the enamel (less radiopaque).

MANAGEMENT
Apart from the appearance, there are no significant problems with the teeth. As the patients become older, the need to use aesthetic restorations becomes compelling (i.e. composite veneers in early adolescence, followed by porcelain veneers later).

INFECTED TOOTH GERM

INCIDENCE
This is a rare condition, especially when one considers that over 30% of children develop dento-alveolar abscesses on deciduous molars.

AETIOLOGY
A non-vital primary tooth, usually a molar, has infection that spreads through the apex of the tooth roots into the permanent tooth germ, which develops in very close physical association with the primary tooth.

PRESENTATION
Usually with the presence of a bout of severe pain, swelling, and pus formation in the jaw, in the position of a permanent successor. The primary tooth has usually been lost and its eruption delayed.

DIAGNOSIS
There is a large area of radiolucency completely surrounding the permanent tooth germ. The occlusal view clearly shows the radiolucency isolating the tooth germ (**21.24**). In this case, it is the second premolar.

TREATMENT
Surgical drainage of the abscess surrounding the tooth germ followed by surgical exploration of the area. This usually reveals the slightly discoloured coronal element of the tooth 'floating' free. It should be removed, as it is also non-vital.

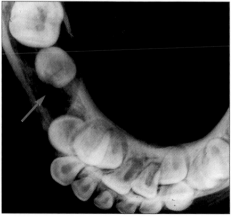

21.24 Infected tooth germ showing radiolucency surrounding the permanent germ.

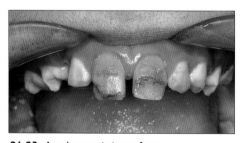

21.23 Amelogenesis imperfecta.

FACIAL ABSCESS

AETIOLOGY
The cause is almost always an abscessed tooth that has been neglected. The infection transfers from within the tooth to the surrounding dento-alveolar bone; this leads to the infection boring through the alveolar bone into the surrounding soft tissues. The path taken is determined by the local anatomy of muscle insertions and fascial planes.

PRESENTATION
The patient usually complains of severe pain, fever, and swelling (**21.25**).

DIAGNOSIS
Radiographically, there is invariably a carious and non-vital tooth with a medium to large periapical area of radiolucency.

TREATMENT
The surgical drainage of the abscess is essential. This is usually achieved by administering a general anaesthetic, removing the focus of the abscess (the infected tooth), establishing intra-oral drainage of the soft tissue infection by blunt dissection and prescribing systemic antibiotics as an adjunct.

DENS INVAGINATUS

INCIDENCE
This varies between 0.25–5% of incisor teeth. The difference is partly ethnic but also due to a wide variation in the diagnostic criteria used.

AETIOLOGY
There is a genetic element. During development there is an infolding of the enamel organ. This is usually incomplete, resulting in a break in the enamel surface which leads to bacteria passing through the tooth and causing infection.

PRESENTATION
This is most often a chance finding during a clinical examination, or from radiographs taken as a screening process during orthodontic assessment. Even less frequently, the patient develops a darkening of the tooth followed by a dento-alveolar abscess. On close examination, there is a small invagination on the palatal surface of the tooth concerned. This is most commonly the upper lateral incisor(s).

DIAGNOSIS
Radiologically (**21.26**) the appearance varies from a small inverted enamel pearl within the tooth to the appearance of a 'tooth within a tooth'– hence the synonym 'dens in dente'.

TREATMENT
Depending on the severity and whether or not the tooth has been caught early, the invagination may be sealed with a fissure sealant. (see **21.7**). If the tooth is non-vital, it will be necessary to attempt root-canal filling. Frequently, the configuration of the invagination is such that the tooth has to be extracted.

21.25 Facial abscess.

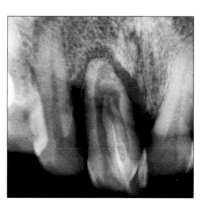

21.26 Dens invaginatus.

HYPODONTIA

INCIDENCE
The pattern of missing teeth in isolated hypo-
dontia varies, but the most commonly absent
teeth in descending order are :
- Third permanent molars (35%).
- Lower second premolars (23%).
- Upper permanent lateral incisors (22%).

All other permanent teeth can be missing but
to a much lesser extent.

AETIOLOGY
There is usually a hereditary pattern. It is also
common for missing teeth to be part of the
syndromic presentation of other conditions,
such as ectodermal dysplasia.

PRESENTATION
This is a common condition of the teeth and
is manifest as absent teeth or 'failure to erupt'
(**21.27**). Radiographic examination confirms
the absence of teeth (**21.28**).

MANAGEMENT
The condition requires careful monitoring from
a very early age. As the child grows, it may be
necessary to use a variety of restorative techniques so that the position and appearance of
the teeth can be maintained.

PROGNOSIS
Refinements in the use of enamel bonding are
leading to the use of a number of tooth-gentle
bridging techniques. In addition, the use of
titanium implants to replace missing teeth is
showing great promise.

CAVERNOUS HAEMANGIOMA OF THE TONGUE

AETIOLOGY
This is a developmental defect.

PRESENTATION
A discrete developmental lesion which is
harmatomatous. The lesion is clearly delineated
and is blue-purple in colour, with a thin
epithelial covering (**21.29**).

TREATMENT
Usually no special treatment is required. If the
lesion is sufficiently large to be a nuisance or
there is a risk of damage, it should be treated
with appropriate surgical procedures, such as
sclerosing agents, cryosurgery or laser therapy.

PREVENTION
During the child's early years, care must be
taken to avoid injury to the haemangioma by
trauma. This can occur if the child carries an
object, such as a colouring pencil, in the mouth
when learning to walk. In the event of a fall, the
pencil may cause a penetrating wound in the
mouth which, if it involves the haemangioma,
can cause severe bleeding.

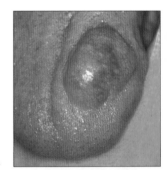

21.29
Cavernous
haemangioma
of the tongue.

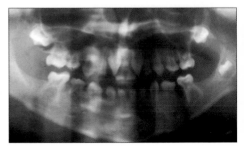

21.27 Hypodontia. There are two conical
incisors and several retained primary teeth.

21.28 Hypodontia. Radiography confirms the
absence of teeth.

CERVICO-FACIAL LYMPHADENITIS

INCIDENCE
Relatively infrequent but no precise figures are available.

AETIOLOGY
Inflammation from the upper face and/or the intra-oral soft tissues (e.g. gingivitis), which drains through the facial lymph node.

PRESENTATION
A small (1–1.5cm), painful swollen lymph gland (**21.30**).

TREATMENT
It is important to remember that the facial lymph node is closely associate with a branch of the facial nerve. Therefore it is important that the lymph node is NOT surgically drained.

PROGNOSIS
This is very good with the use of systemic antibiotics.

EOSINOPHILIC GRANULOMA

PREVALENCE
Fewer than 1 in 150,000 of the population.

AETIOLOGY
Not known.

PRESENTATION
This example presented with a small and painless enlargement on the lower border of the mandible (**21.31**).

DIAGNOSIS / TREATMENT
The child was investigated under general anaesthesia as he would not cooperate for radiography. The oblique lateral jaw view was taken and developed immediately before waking up the child. This shows a lesion breaking through the lower border of the mandible in the region of the canine (**21.32**). There is a clearly defined radiolucency approximately 2 cm in diameter. The lesion was also biopsied.

PROGNOSIS
This is usually very good, as the act of biopsy coupled with surgical curettage initiates the healing process and within a few months the bone is healed.

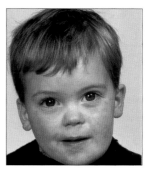

21.31 Eosinophilic granuloma.

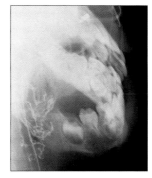

21.32 Eosinophilic granuloma. Radiology shows a lesion breaking through the lower border of the mandible.

21.30 Cervico-facial lymphadenitis.

CONGENITAL EPULIS

AETIOLOGY
This is not known but it has been suggested that the lesion is a form of embryonic hamartoma. Histologically, there are numerous epithelial inclusions which are reminiscent of fragments of the dental lamina.

PRESENTATION
The tumour is present at birth and is usually a discrete, pedunculated soft tissue mass attached to the alveolus. Although the lesion in **21.33** is attached to the mandible, it is more common in the maxilla.

TREATMENT
It is usually recommended that the lesion is excised surgically under local anaesthesia. A painless and simpler alternative is to 'lasso' the lesion with a silk suture, then tie the suture very tight so that the blood vessels entering the epulis are strangulated and the lesion drops away spontaneously.

PROGNOSIS
The congenital epulis, once removed, rarely recurs.

PYOGENIC GRANULOMA

AETIOLOGY
This is probably a response of the oral tissues to a non-specific infection usually by *Staphylococcus*. This infection arises as a result of minor trauma followed by bacterial ingress and infection.

PRESENTATION
Usually seen as a discrete enlargement of granulation tissue attached to the gingival margin (**21.34**), although it may also affect the tongue, or cheeks. It may develop rapidly and then remains static for considerable periods of time.

TREATMENT
The pyogenic granuloma should be treated by surgical excision under local anaesthesia. Recrudescence may occur, as it is difficult to identify the precise borders of the lesion. It is important to ensure that there are no niduses of infection (e.g. calculus on the adjacent teeth).

PROGNOSIS
Usually very good, although there can be a recurrence, mostly due to inadequate cleaning of the adjacent tooth surface.

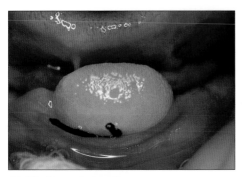

21.33 Congenital epulis.

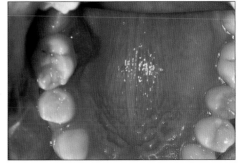

21.34 Pyogenic granuloma.

SEVERE GINGIVITIS

AETIOLOGY
The underlying cause in this case was a neutrophil malfunction due to glycogen storage disease.

PRESENTATION
Soon after eruption of the teeth, the gingivae appear bright red with widespread inflammation (**21.35**).

TREATMENT
The basic principles of a high standard of oral hygiene (tooth brushing and dental flossing) are paramount. This can be supplemented with twice-daily use of chlorhexidine gluconate (0.2%).

PROGNOSIS
This is unfortunately poor, as the underlying metabolic disease will lead inevitably to a severe periodontal breakdown and, eventually, loss of teeth.

BENIGN MIGRATORY GLOSSITIS (GEOGRAPHIC TONGUE)

AETIOLOGY
Unknown. Microbial factors, anaemia, drugs, and diet have all been postulated, without any good supporting evidence to justify the claims.

PRESENTATION
This presents as single or multiple areas of desquamation of the filiform papillae in irregular but rounded areas. The major part of the central portion of the lesion is thinned and reddish and the borders are usually outlined by a thin white line (**21.36**). The areas of filiform thinning and desquamation remain for a few days in one location, heal and re-appear in another location.

TREATMENT
The condition is benign, so treatment is limited to simple advice such as dietary changes; for example, the avoidance of acidic foods.

PROGNOSIS
This is good, as the condition rarely causes more than mild irritation to the patient.

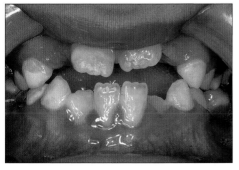

21.35 Severe gingivitis.

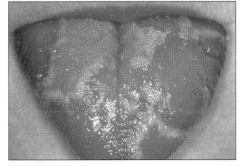

21.36 Benign migratory glossitis (geographic tongue).

MUCOUS CYST

AETIOLOGY
Obstruction of the duct of a minor salivary gland as a result of trauma (e.g. biting or squashing of the lip).

PRESENTATION
Usually as a small (2–6 mm) swelling on the lips, most commonly on the lower lip (**21.37**). It may occur on any mucosal surface, particularly where there is mild trauma.

TREATMENT
The lesion is removed surgically under local anaesthesia.

PROGNOSIS
Because the minor salivary glands from which this lesion develops are numerous in this part of the mouth, the surgical procedure to remove the lesion may damage other glands and lead to the development of a further cyst. For this reason, the recurrence rate is of the order of 40%.

CANDIDIASIS AND RADIATION MUCOSITIS

PRESENTATION
Following extensive radiation for cancer therapy, the mucosal tissues in the line of the beam demonstrate considerable damage (**21.38**). The cell turnover is severely disrupted, causing thinning and even ulceration of the mucosa. Damage to the minor salivary glands leads to poor mucosal immunity, resulting in the development of candidal infection.

TREATMENT
The patient should be given symptom care in the form of mouthwashes, with chlorhexidine gluconate 0.2% twice daily and a fluoride mouthwash in the form of 0.05% sodium fluoride once daily.

PROGNOSIS
As the patient's health returns to normal, so the severity of the lesion reduces and, in time, may be difficult to delineate.

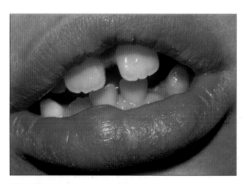

21.37 Mucous cyst.

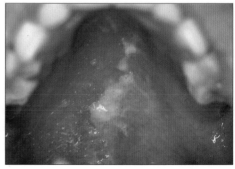

21.38 Candidiasis and radiation mucositis.

HERPES LABIALIS (RECURRENT HERPES)

AETIOLOGY

Herpes (cold sore) lesions are always secondary to a primary infection that usually occurs in childhood. The virus remains latent in the nerve tissue serving the oral tissues. Following some irritant stimulus (e.g. constant rubbing and blowing of the nose associated with a cold, sunburn, or even mild trauma following a visit to the dentist) the vesicle may erupt. In immunocompromised patients, the lesions may develop spontaneously.

PRESENTATION

The patient will report a burning lesion prior to the eruption of small aggregates of vesicles (**21.39**). These may coalesce to form a larger vesicle and, if damaged, lead to crusting over of the lesion.

TREATMENT

If the premonitory tingling is recognized early, Aciclovir cream can be applied and will often abort the development of vesicles.

PROGNOSIS

Usually good, although recurrent bouts can be troublesome and may be an early indication of systemic debilitation.

SUGGESTED READING

Cawson RA (ed), *Lucas's pathology of tumours of the oral tissues* (5th edition). London: Churchill Livingston 1998.

Shafer WG, Hine MK, Levy B. *A textbook of oral pathology* (4th edition). Philadelphia: WB Saunders Company 1983.

Whaites E. *Essentials of dental radiology* (3rd edition). London: Churchill Livingston 2003.

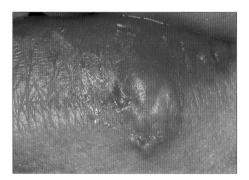

21.39 Herpes labialis (recurrent herpes).

Orthopaedics and Fractures

Victor J Woolf John A Fixsen
Robert A Hill David HA Jones

INTRODUCTION

This chapter aims to develop a methodology for approaching paediatric orthopaedic and fracture challenges. It emphasizes normal ranges and the differences between adults and children, and stresses the importance of thinking in terms of 'associations'. Some of the conditions covered are common, others rare. They are not intended to be exhaustive but illustrative of the spectrum of conditions encountered and the principles of diagnosis and management.

COMMON NORMAL VARIANTS

A knowledge of natural history and normal ranges is very useful in allaying anxieties and in distinguishing normal variants from pathological conditions.

> **Assess under the categories of the 5 S's:**
> - **S**ymmetry
> - **S**tiffness
> - **S**ymptoms
> - **S**keletal dysplasia
> - **S**ystemic disorder

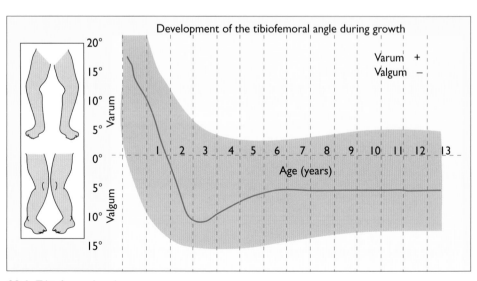

22.1 Tibiofemoral angles.

TIBIOFEMORAL ANGLE (22.1)
Knock knees (genu valgum) and bow legs (genu varum) are a common cause of concern. Most normal babies have bow legs associated with internal tibial torsion until about two years of age. Knock knees are common between two-and-a-half and four years.

Intermalleolar and intercondylar distances are useful clinical monitors and save on radiation exposure (22.2). An intermalleolar distance of up to 10 cm is considered normal.

TORSIONAL DEFORMITY
- Foot progression angle (22.3).
  Mean = +10°, range = −3° to +20°.

- Hip rotation (next page, 22.4).
  Male: internal = 15° to 65°;
  external = 25° to 65°.
  Female: internal = 15° to 60°;
  external = 25° to 65°.
  (Best assessed in extension, lying prone.)
- Thigh/foot angle (22.5). Mean = +10°.

FLAT FEET
In infants and toddlers, the longitudinal arch has not yet developed, therefore flat feet can be a normal finding until the age of three. (22.6)

GROWTH CHARTS
See 22.7 (overleaf) for an example.

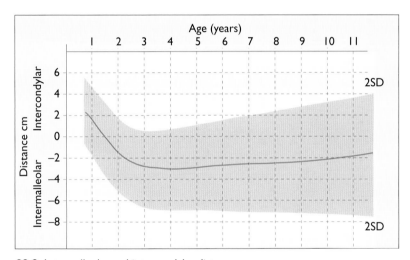

22.2 Intermalleolar and intercondylar distances.

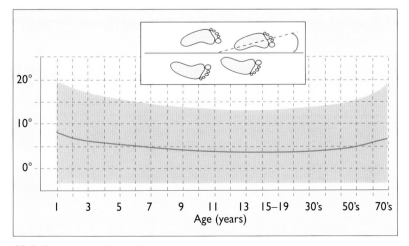

22.3 Foot progression angle.

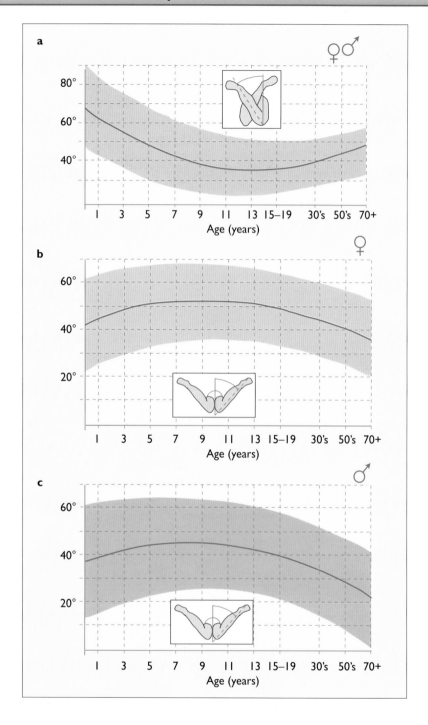

22.4 Hip rotation: **a)** normal ranges for lateral hip rotation in males and females, **b)** normal ranges for medial hip rotation in females, **c)** normal ranges for medial hip rotation in males.

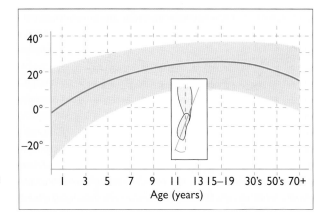

22.5 Thigh–foot angle (measure of tibial hindfoot rotation).

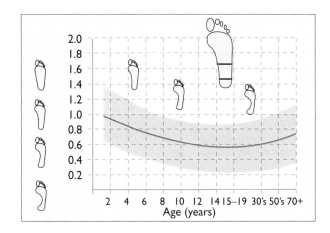

22.6 Flat feet. Development of the longitudinal arch.

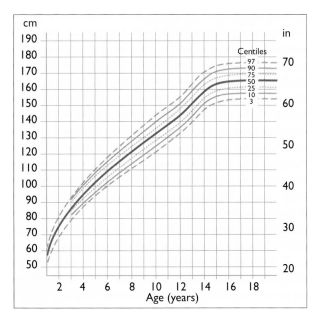

22.7 Example of growth chart (separate ones are available for males and females of different ages).

LOWER LIMB ANOMALIES

FLAT FEET

Incidence
The incidence of mobile flat feet is 30–40%. There are strong familial and racial connections, and association with generalized joint laxity. Rigid, painful flat feet are rare.

Presentation
Flat feet present clinically (**22.8**) but be aware that they can be a normal finding in children under 3 years of age (see normal variants, **22.6**). There are two main types:
- **Mobile and usually pain free.**
  The severity is variable but, at the worst end of the spectrum, the heel is in valgus and patients may develop discomfort over the insertion of tibialis posterior into the navicular. It can occur as part of generalized joint laxity, Down syndrome (Trisomy 21) and cerebral palsy. It is important to exclude tight tendo Achilles.
- **Rigid and usually painful.**
  Tarsal coalition, congenital vertical talus (approximately 50% have associated neurological problems) (**22.9, 22.10**) and juvenile idiopathic arthritis.

Diagnosis
The important clinical features are assessment of whether the foot is pain-free, has normal mobility and muscle power and corrects on standing on tip toe or when the great toe is dorsiflexed by the examiner (Jack test).

Radiological assessment can help exclude underlying bony abnormalities. Standing dorsiplantar and lateral views are required to assess the talocalcaneal angle (normal range is 15–35°). Computerized tomography (CT) scans are usually helpful in diagnosing tarsal coalitions. Congenital vertical talus requires a plantarflexion stress lateral radiograph to show the navicular remaining dorsally dislocated on the talus.

Treatment
Mobile pain-free flat feet require reassurance. Mobile painful or severe cases may benefit from an arch support or heel cup. Rigid flat feet may require soft tissue or bone surgery.

Prognosis
Flexible flat feet normally have an excellent prognosis. In the rest, the outlook and requirement for treatment depends on the underlying pathology.

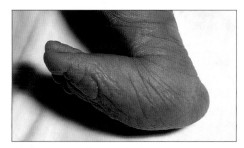

22.8 Flat feet.

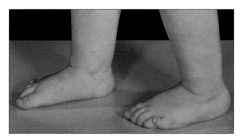

22.9 Congenital vertical talus.

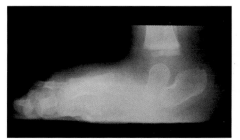

22.10 Congenital vertical talus.

PES CAVUS

Presentation

A high-arched foot (**22.11**) which is frequently associated with claw toes. The hindfoot is usually calcaneous and in varus, but may be valgus in paralytic neurological cases.

Associations

Underlying conditions include muscular dystrophy, peripheral neuropathy from hereditary motor and sensory neuropathy, polyneuritis, sciatic nerve injury, spinal cord lesions such as poliomyelitis, myelomeningocoele, diastematomyelia, spinocerebellar tract disease (such as Friedreich's ataxia, Roussy-Levy syndrome), and cortical defects as in cerebral palsy and dystonia musculorum deformans.

Diagnosis

Clinical examination and neurological assessment are essential. Coleman's block test, in which a block is placed under the heel and lateral border of the foot, is used to assess hindfoot flexibility: once the forefoot is in plantarflexion, a flexible hindfoot goes in to normal valgus. Spinal radiographs, MRI scans and electrophysiological studies may be indicated.

Treatment

Non-operative treatment with suitable footwear, metatarsal supports and braces can be worthwhile.

Stripping of the plantar ligaments and intrinsic muscles from the calcaneum (Steindler) to decrease the longitudinal arch is sometimes beneficial. If the block test is positive, a more radical medial release (Coleman) may be warranted, to elevate the pronated forefoot and correct the cavovarus. The toe clawing can be improved by flexor to extensor tendon transfer (Girdlestone). The big toe deformity may benefit from transfer of extensor hallucis longus to the neck of the first metatarsal with tenodesis or arthrodesis of the interphalangeal joint (Robert Jones).

Calcaneal osteotomy may be worth considering. Triple arthrodesis (after 12 years of age) can give relief, but long term results may be disappointing.

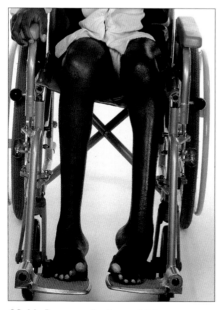

22.11 Pes cavus (poliomyelitis).

GENU VALGUM AND GENU VARUM
Presentation
A knowledge of the normal range and development is essential in distinguishing normal variants from pathological conditions (see 22.1).

Diagnosis
Pathological genu varum (22.12) or genu valgum (22.13) should be suspected if the measurements are outside the normal ranges or the deformity is unilateral. A family history of deformity and previous trauma is relevant. Examination should include measurement of the patient's height and weight and exclude deformity elsewhere.

Treatment
Physiological genu varum is maximum at 18 months and valgum at 3–4 years. The majority are 'normal' by 9–10 years (22.1). Consider hemiepiphysiodesis or stapling when outside the normal range.

Pathological genu varum is seen in Blount's disease (22.15, 22.16) which is genu varum due to growth disturbance of the medial portion of proximal tibial physis; this may occur in infantile and adolescent forms and is treated by proximal tibial osteotomy. It is also associated with rickets (22.17) (dietary or renal 1,25-dihydroxycholecalciferol [DHCC] deficiency) and usually corrects with treatment of the underlying condition but some may need surgery.

Congenital posteromedial bowing of tibia normally corrects spontaneously albeit with shortening.

Anterolateral bowing of tibia is likely to be pathological and is associated with pseudarthrosis (22.14). Fifty percent of pseudarthrosis patients have neurofibromatosis and bowing occurs in 10% of those patients. Osteogenesis imperfecta and congenital short tibia/absent or hypoplastic fibula should be excluded. Treatment depends on the underlying condition: options are internal fixation, vascularized bone graft, bone transport, or amputation/prosthesis.

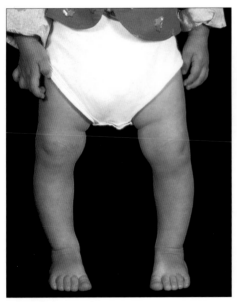

22.12 Genu varum.

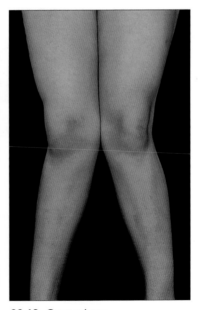

22.13 Genu valgum.

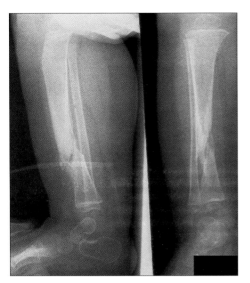

22.14 Anterolateral bowing with pseudarthrosis.

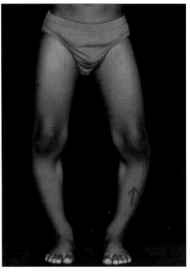

22.15 Blount's disease. Pathological demonstration genu varum.

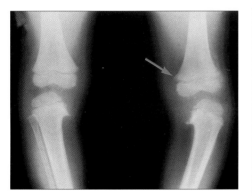

22.16 Blount's disease showing medial tibial plate partial growth arrest.

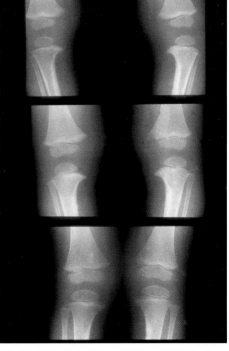

22.17 Rickets showing osteopenia and lipping of the physes.

IN-TOE / OUT-TOE GAIT

Incidence

Symmetrical in-toe or out-toe gait is common. Asymmetry warrants follow-up or further investigation.

Aetiology

At the foot, metatarsus varum or adductus (**22.18**) can be responsible. Tibial torsion can contribute. Femoral neck anteversion (**22.19**–**22.21**) (hip internal rotation greater than external rotation) or retroversion (the converse) may be present.

Presentation

There is a normal range of foot alignment (see **22.2**–**22.5**). This reflects angulations from hip to foot.

Treatment

The majority correct sufficiently not to require osteotomy. There is no substantiated role for orthoses.

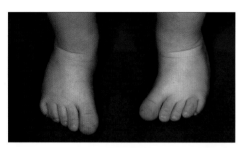

22.18 Metatarsus adductus.

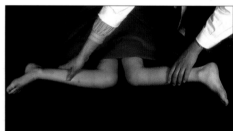

22.19 Femoral neck anteversion.

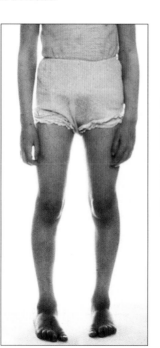

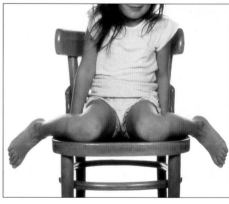

22.20 & 22.21 Femoral neck anteversion.

CLUB FOOT (CONGENITAL TALIPES EQUINOVARUM)

Incidence

This is a relatively common condition, with an incidence of 1.5–3 in 1,000 births. It is 2.5 times more common in males. Fifty percent of cases are bilateral. There is a 2–6% risk in subsequent siblings and a 25% risk in subsequent offspring.

Aetiology

Club foot is usually idiopathic or primary. It is important to look for secondary causes. These may be neuromuscular (e.g. spinal dysraphism or congenital myopathy); localized (e.g. constriction ring or tibial dysplasia); chromosomal (e.g. trisomy 13); or syndromic (e.g. diastrophic dwarfism, arthrogryposis, or Larsen syndrome). Hand anomalies can be present in association.

Presentation

Club foot is usually noticed at birth. It is defined as forefoot adduction and supination; hindfoot varus and equinus with calf wasting (**22.22**).

Diagnosis

Diagnosis is mainly clinical. Imaging is helpful in confirming the presence of normal bony elements and may be indicated when the presentation is atypical or other abnormalities are present. Spinal imaging to exclude spinal dysraphism may be appropriate. Neurophysiological assessment and muscle biopsy may be warranted.

Treatment

Primary treatment consists of manipulation and strapping or serial plasters. Resolution rates are 90% with non-surgical treatment, if there is no fixed deformity or it corrects to neutral, but only 45% if less than 20° equinus/varum and only 10% if more than 20°. Surgical release of soft tissues is indicated for failure.

Secondary treatment entails revision, soft tissue release and consideration of tendon transfer, and bone surgery such as wedge resection or application of Ilizarov technique.

Over-correction can occur and is difficult to treat.

One must be aware of aiming to achieve a functional, pain-free, plantargrade foot while maintaining as much mobility as possible. The calf usually remains wasted.

22.22 Club foot.

DEVELOPMENTAL DYSPLASIA OF THE HIP (DDH)

Incidence
The overall incidence is 1 in 400, of which 85% are female. The left hip accounts for 60%, and 20% are bilateral. Sixty percent are firstborn children, 30% are breech and there is a positive family history in 20%. This condition was previously known as congenital dislocation of the hip, or CDH.

Risk factors
Oligohydramnios and breech presentation are risk factors. The risk to a subsequent sibling if the patient is male is 1%, compared to 11% if female. If a parent is affected, the risk to a male is 6%, wheras to a female it is 17%.

Associations
There is an association with torticollis and calcaneovalgus.

Developmental dysplasia of the hip can feature in Down, Ehler-Danlos and Larsen syndromes, also spinal dysraphism, sacral agenesis and arthrogryposis.

Presentation
Early detection by screening clinically and by ultrasound examination. Late presentation is with asymmetry, restricted hip movement or shortening. After walking, children may present with a limp. There is a spectrum ranging from neonatal instability to painful dysplasia in adolescence or adult life.

Diagnosis
Clinical examination consists of the Ortolani reduction manoeuvre and Barlow provocation test in the neonatal period; decreased abduction and femoral shortening (late). Asymmetric skin folds are noteworthy but unreliable.

Imaging with ultrasound is valuable in the first 6 months. Plain radiographs are informative from about 3 months (**22.23**). Arthrography is often definitive (**22.24**).

Treatment
The aim is to achieve and maintain early concentric reduction. If diagnosed early, this may be achieved by splintage (e.g. with Pavlik harness). Reduction must be confirmed clinically and with imaging. There is a risk of avascular necrosis.

The value of traction is debatable, but some surgeons use it prior to surgery.

Failure of non-operative treatment or late presentation necessitate open reduction with or without femoral or acetabular realignment. Persistent acetabular dysplasia may require further realignment or acetabular augmentation.

Prognosis
The outlook is good with early, stable reduction. Late degenerative changes are likely in the presence of avascular necrosis, failure of concentric reduction, or persistent acetabular dysplasia.

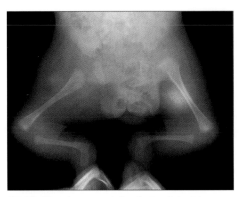

22.23 Developmental dysplasia of the hip.

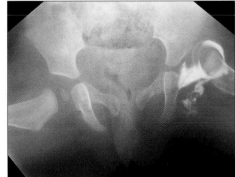

22.24 DDH: Arthrogram.

LIMB LENGTH DISCREPANCY

Aetiology

Limb length discrepancies arise from congenital bone deficiencies, vascular malformations, neurofibromatosis, acquired growth plate arrest secondary to trauma, infection or radiotherapy and diaphyseal fracture. Neurological conditions such as spina bifida, spinal dysraphism, polio and cerebral palsy can also underlie.

Presentation

This is usually clinical (**22.25**).

Diagnosis

Clinical measurement with tape and blocks. Further radiological investigation to establish the details of the deformity.

Treatment

Predictive charts (e.g. Anderson) are useful in planning treatment. Options range from shoe raise or orthosis, to amputation and prosthesis. Equalization can be achieved by shortening through epiphysiodesis before maturity or bony excision after maturity, or lengthening by circumferential periosteal release, callus distraction (**22.26**) or physeal distraction.

Prognosis

Complications, especially infection, contractures, joint displacement and malunion, are common with limb-lengthening procedures.

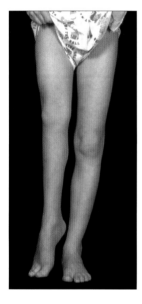

22.25 Limb length discrepancy.

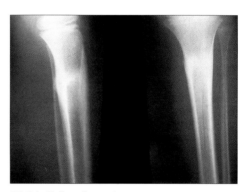

22.26 Callus distraction.

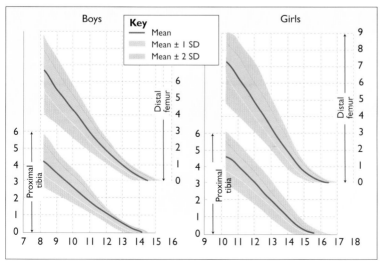

22.27 Growth remaining chart (SD = standard deviation).

PROXIMAL FEMORAL FOCAL DEFICIENCY

Incidence
One in 50,000.

Classification
The early appearance of the acetabulum and proximal femur are predictive of the subsequent joint development (**22.28**).

Presentation
This condition presents clinically, associated with knee instability and fibular hypoplasia as well as upper limb defects and abnormal facies.

Diagnosis
X-ray gives anatomical detail of the defect (**22.29**).

Treatment
There are a range of options depending on severity, such as external prosthesis, extension surgery to facilitate prosthetic fitting, and reconstruction operations, including lengthening and rotationplasty.

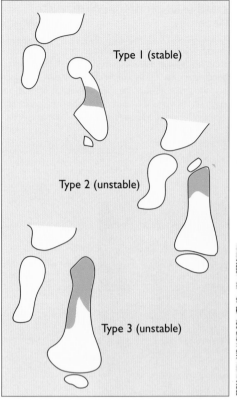

Type 1 (stable)

Type 2 (unstable)

Type 3 (unstable)

22.28 Proximal femoral focal deficiency.

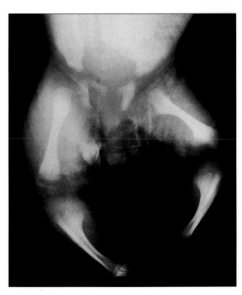

22.29 X-ray of proximal femoral focal deficiency.

CONGENITAL TIBIAL DEFICIENCY

Incidence
One in 1,000,000.

Classification
The three types are shown in **22.30**.

Presentation
This presents clinically with equinovarum deformity of the foot and varum of the knee. There may be associated polydactyly in hands and feet.

Diagnosis
Diagnosis is by clinical suspicion (**22.31**) and x-ray (**22.32**).

Treatment
Amputation through the knee is often appropriate, but the Ilizarov technique may enable salvage in certain cases.

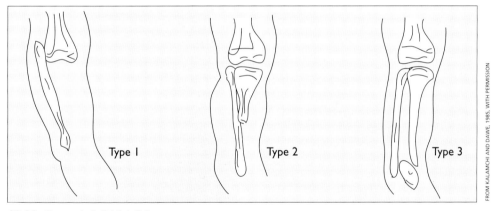

Type 1   Type 2   Type 3

FROM KALAMCHI AND DAWE, 1985, WITH PERMISSION

22.30 Congenital tibial deficiency.

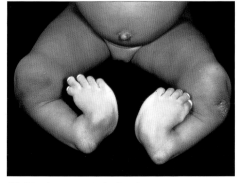

22.31 Congenital tibial deficiency.

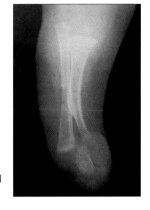

22.32 Congenital tibial deficiency.

CONGENITAL FIBULAR DEFICIENCY

Incidence
One in 25–30,000.

Classification
The patterns of fibular defiiency are shown in **22.33**.

Presentation
A short lower leg, with anterior bowing of the tibia, and absent foot x-ray(s). The knee is in valgus and the femur is usually hypoplastic.

Diagnosis
Diagnosis is by clinical assessment (**22.34**) and radiological evaluation.

Treatment
Depending on severity, the options are provision of extension prosthesis, lengthening with Ilizarov technique, or amputation and prosthesis.

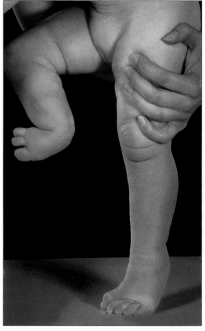

22.34 Congenital fibular deficiency.

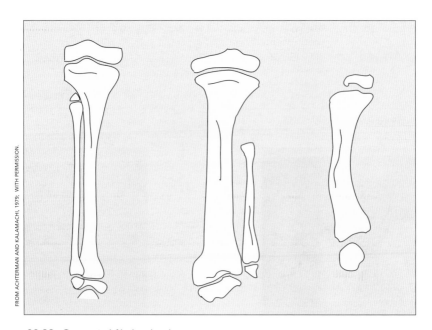

FROM ACHTERMAN AND KALAMACHI, 1979; WITH PERMISSION.

22.33 Congenital fibular dysplasia.

PAINFUL LIMP

Presentation

The child presenting with a limp or unwillingness to bear weight needs careful assessment.

Incidence

This is common.

Differential diagnoses

A wide range of conditions can present this way, including special childhood orthopaedic problems and medical conditions. They are:

- Trauma.
- Reactive, transient synovitis, 'irritable hip'.
- Septic arthritis.
- Osteomyelitis (**22.35**).
- Slipped upper femoral epiphysis (SUFE) (**22.36**).
- Perthes disease (**22.37**).
- Tumours: benign/malignant, of bone, cartilage, synovium.
- Juvenile arthritis.
- Coagulopathy.
- Henoch-Schönlein purpura.

They are distinguished by clinical examination, including temperature recording. Laboratory investigations should include: full blood count (FBC), sickle test, erythrocyte sedimentation rate (ESR), 'C'-reactive protein (CRP), anti-streptolysin O (ASO) titre, blood culture, rheumatoid screen and thyroid function tests. Ultrasound is useful in seeking joint effusions. Plain x-ray changes are often late. Isotope scanning can help in localization and seeking multifocal lesions. Magnetic resonance imaging (MRI) is sensitive to early vascular changes and is good for defining tissue planes, but is not a first-line investigation.

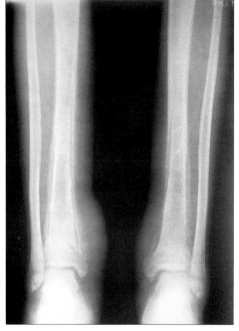

22.35 Osteomyelitis.

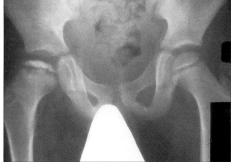

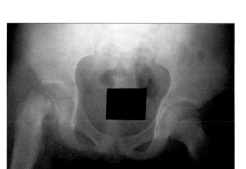

22.36 Slipped upper femoral epiphysis.

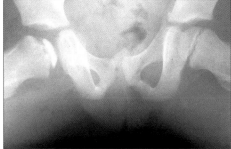

22.37 Perthes disease.

Treatment

Symptomatic treatment for pain and pyrexia should be given. The underlying condition needs specific treatment, often urgently. Septic arthritis needs urgent drainage and antibiotics. In osteomyelitis, consider a trial of antibiotics if the history is short (e.g. less than 24 hours), otherwise, or if no response, drainage should be undertaken. Slipped upper femoral epiphysis needs urgent stabilization. Perthes disease may benefit from containment of the femoral head. Trauma is treated on its merits. Tumours need biopsy, staging and appropriate treatment. Juvenile idiopathic arthritis (**22.38**, **22.39**) needs recognition and predominantly medical management (see 'Rheumatology' chapter). Irritable hip needs appreciation of its natural history and symptomatic treatment: it is a diagnosis reached by exclusion.

DIGITAL ANOMALIES

SYNDACTYLY

Syndactyly is incomplete differentiation of digital rays.

Incidence

The incidence is 1 in 2,000, and 20% have a genetic basis. (Presenting alone, it is transmitted by a dominant gene with partial penetrance).

Diagnosis

This is by clinical observation (**22.40**) and selective investigation of the tissues, as the spectrum ranges from an incomplete skin bridge to complex conjoined bone, tendon, and neurovascular involvement.

It may occur as part of syndromes (e.g. craniofacial, Poland and Apert – see also 'Genetics' chapter); and in association with other anomalies (e.g. ulnar dysplasia).

Treatment

This requires planning based upon definition of the defect, which may not be achievable for several months. Deficiency of skin requires planning of z-plasties and grafts.

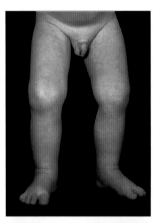

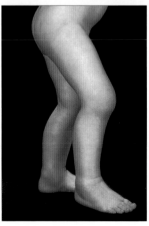

22.38 & 22.39 Juvenile arthritis.

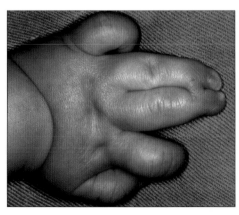

22.40 Syndactyly.

POLYDACTYLY

Incidence
About 1 in 2,000.

Diagnosis
This is clinical (**22.41**, **22.42**) but requires definition of the anomaly and assessment of function. Duplication of the little finger is usually autosomal recessive and syndromic in contrast to the thumb.

The Wassel classification (although strictly relating to the thumb) outlines the types of duplications encountered (**22.43**). Type IV is the commonest.

Treatment
A balance between salvage and utilization of discardable tissues is required. Early surgery should be considered to prevent increasing deformity of the usable elements.

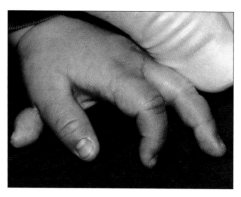

22.41 Accessory digit.

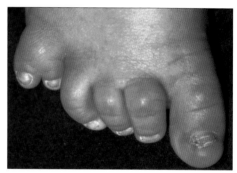

22.42 Polydactyly.

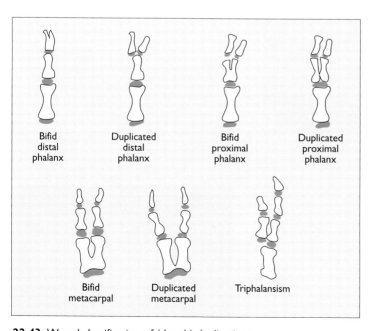

Bifid distal phalanx

Duplicated distal phalanx

Bifid proximal phalanx

Duplicated proximal phalanx

Bifid metacarpal

Duplicated metacarpal

Triphalansism

22.43 Wassel classification of (thumb) duplications.

UPPER LIMB ANOMALIES

PSEUDARTHROSIS OF THE CLAVICLE

Presentation
This is a rare condition in which the right side is affected (except in dextrocardia). It presents clinically as a non-tender lump (**22.44**) or may be mistaken for a fracture (**22.45**).

Treatment
Where there are no symptoms, the lump can be accepted. Operative possibilities are: re-section of the pseudoarthrosis with suture of the periosteum, fixation and bone grafting, excision of the outer end of the medial portion of the clavicle.

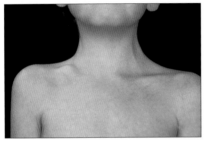

22.44 Congenital pseudarthrosis of the right clavicle.

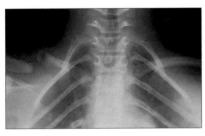

22.45 Fracture of the clavicle.

SPRENGEL'S CONGENITAL SCAPULAR ELEVATION

Incidence
Rare. More common in girls.

Presentation
The child presents with a high, small scapula, the superior angle of which is rotated upwards and forwards with restriction of abduction and external rotation. Associated abnormalities are common, including cervical ribs, vertebral anomalies, and hypoplasia of the clavicle and humerus.

Diagnosis
Radiological confirmation should be obtained.

Treatment
Function is not usually impaired and operations are mainly for improvement of appearance. Consideration should be given to resection of the superomedial angle of scapula for cosmesis or a combination of soft tissue releases and bony procedures to reposition the scapula.

CONGENITAL DISLOCATION OF RADIAL HEAD

Incidence
Rare.

Presentation
There is a painless restriction of flexion with anterior dislocation and extension with posterior dislocation. Abnormal bony morphology is apparent on radiography (**22.46**). The defect in isolation is often autosomal dominant, but it occurs in association with various syndromes. The condition is often bilateral.

Treatment
Attempts at reconstruction are ineffective. Excision of the radial head after skeletal maturity should be considered.

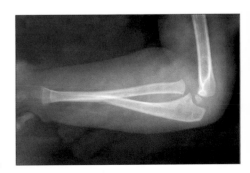

22.46 Congenital dislocation of radial head.

RADIOULNAR SYNOSTOSIS

Incidence

Rare and not usually associated with other malformations.

Presentation

It presents with restriction of pronation and supination and is confirmed radiologically (22.47). It is bilateral in 60% of cases.

Treatment

Osteotomy may be considered to facilitate activities of daily living. If the forearm is fixed in pronation, osteotomy may be undertaken to bring the hand to the more functional neutral position.

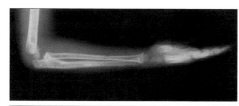

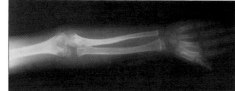

22.47 Radioulnar synostosis.

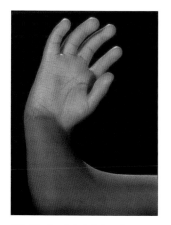

22.48 Radial club hand.

MADELUNG'S DEFORMITY

Presentation

Prominence of the distal ulna, radial deviation of the hand and restriction of range of movement, which is confirmed radiologically. It is associated with other skeletal dysplasias (mostly dyschondrosteosis) and may occur after epiphyseal trauma or infection.

Treatment

Options are: distal ulna resection for cosmesis, osteotomies at skeletal maturity, or resection of a tether between radius and lunate.

RADIAL CLUB HAND

Incidence

About 1 in 30,000.

Diagnosis

It is diagnosed clinically and confirmed radiologically (22.48). It is associated with cardiac, gastrointestinal and haematological disorders (especially Fanconi anaemia, with its genetic implications). Other upper extremity muscles may be affected.

Treatment

Function is usually surprisingly good but centralization and pollicization of index finger can be considered.

ULNAR DEFICIENCY

Incidence

Rare.

Diagnosis

It is diagnosed clinically and radiologically (22.49). Other limb abnormalities occur in association with it.

Treatment

Options include excision of the cartilaginous band, release of syndactyly if present, or fusion of radius and ulna for stability.

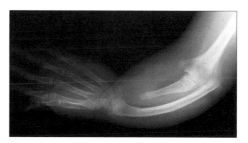

22.49 Ulnar deficiency.

FLEXED THUMB

Incidence
Common.

Presentation
This is often noticed during the first few months of life. Trigger thumb presents as painless loss of passive movement at the interphalangeal joint, with or without a nodule (22.50). It should be differentiated from congenital clasped thumb which affects the metacarpophalangeal joint.

Treatment
Persistence of trigger thumb beyond first year warrants surgical release by division of the flexor sheath at its proximal entrance.

Supple clasped thumb should be splinted initially and then consideration given to tendon transfer. Complex clasped thumb requires extensive release and reconstruction.

SPINAL PROBLEMS

SCOLIOSIS

Incidence
Six percent of normal children have structural scoliosis, and 1 in 200 have deformity of more than 20°.

Presentation
Scoliosis is a lateral curvature; kyphosis is a deformity in the sagittal plane. Diagnosis is by observation and a screening programme.

Associations
Eighty-five percent are idiopathic. In the infantile type, the recurrence risk for siblings or children is approximately 2.6%. In the adolescent type, the recurrence risk for siblings or children is about 11%.
The remainder are:
- Congenital, due to failure of bone formation and/or segmentation and are seen in association with myelodysplasia, diastomatomyelia, spina bifida, cord lesions (30%), renal tract abnormalities (15%), and cardiac defects (5%).
- Neuromuscular, with underlying cerebral palsy, polio, syringomyelia (increased index of suspicion if abdominal reflexes absent), muscular dystrophy, Friedrich's ataxia, or spinal muscular atrophy.
- Related to neurofibromatosis (autosomal dominant).
- Mesenchymal – e.g. Marfan and Ehler-Danlos syndromes, osteogenesis imperfecta, mucopolysaccharidoses.
- Due to Scheuermann's osteochondritis of vertebral end plates.
- Trauma.
- Tumour, which can be benign or malignant (primary or secondary).
- Infection, either from pyogenic organisms or tuberculosis.
- Compensatory – e.g. limb length inequality.

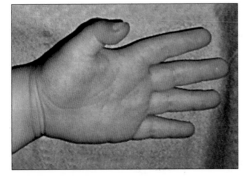

22.50 Trigger thumb.

Diagnosis

Forty degrees of kyphosis as measured by the Cobb technique (**22.51**) is normal, while 0° to 40° is defined as hypokyphosis. More than 40° is hyperkyphosis. The Cobb angle measures scoliosis (**22.51a, b**). The rib/vertebra angle difference measures infantile scoliosis (**22.51c**).

Diagnosis is by clinical assessment (**22.52**) and imaging (**22.53**): anteroposterior and lateral x-ray of the whole spine with pulled and lateral flexion views if necessary; and CT or MRI if a structural abnormality or tether is suspected.

22.51 Cobb angle measurement.
a) Identify the limits of the primary curve by drawing tangents to the bodies and noting where the disc spaces begin to become widened on the concavity of the curve.
b) Erect perpendiculars from the vertebrae forming the limits of the curve. Note the angle between them. This measures the primary curve.
c) Rib angle measurement at the apex of the curve in infantile scoliosis.

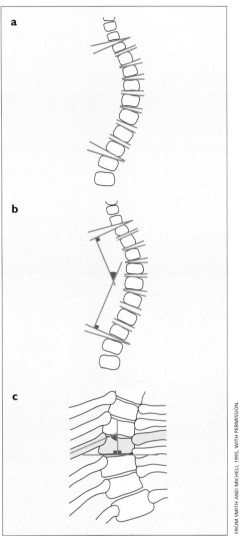

a

b

c

FROM SMITH AND MICHELI, 1995, WITH PERMISSION.

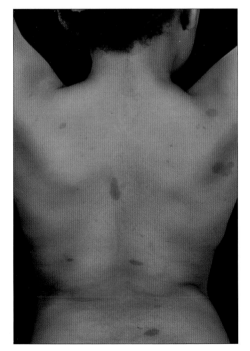

22.52 Scoliosis (neurofibromatosis). Note typical pigmentation of neurofibromatosis.

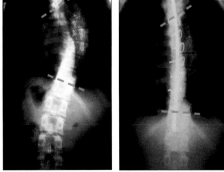

22.53 Scoliosis.

Treatment

Treatment depends on extent and progression. Generally, curves greater than 50° deteriorate. Progression is associated with increasing visible deformity, worsening cardiopulmonary compromise and pain (which may be early, from impingement of ribs on iliac crest, or late, from degenerative changes in the spine).

In neuromuscular patients, pulmonary compromise and early death occur and there are progressive seating and nursing difficulties. In the congenital type, with unsegmented bar and/or hemi-vertebra, progression is inevitable.

Bracing has a role if the curve is 25–50° and vertebral growth potential is still present. It is of little value in congenital types.

Fusion (with or without instrumentation) (**22.54**, **22.55**) is indicated if the curve is more than 50°, if growth potential remains, in neuromuscular types of curve and if a congenital curve is showing any progression at any age. The dangers are infection 2%, implant failure 2%, and neurological injury less than 1% (except greater risk in syringomyelia).

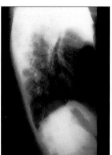
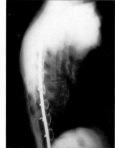

22.54 Scoliosis.

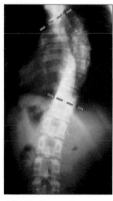
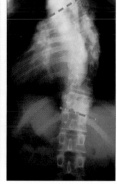

22.55 Scoliosis.

BACK PAIN

Presentation

This is an unusual complaint in children but frequently due to significant pathology such as tumours (especially osteoid osteoma), infection, spondylolysis/spondylolisthesis, urinary tract problems, and trauma.

Diagnosis

In the history, significant clues are night pain with tumours, and relief in osteoma with non-steroidals. Spondylolisthesis may cause nerve root tension signs, loss of abdominal reflexes or clonus.

Useful investigations are bone scan and selective use of MRI or CT.

Treatment

This is of the underlying cause. Spondylolysis/spondylolisthesis: usually responds to a conservative regimen with possible bracing but deterioration warrants posterior fusion.

SPINA BIFIDA

See also 'Neurology' and 'Neonatal and General Paediatric Surgery' chapters.

Incidence

One in 1,000, but increases to 1 in 20 if one sibling is affected, or 1 in 2 if two siblings are affected. There are associations with Arnold-Chiari malformation, hydrocephalus, cerebellar hypoplasia, syringomyelia, diastomatomyelia, and hydromyelia. Orthopaedic implications are contractures, kyphoscoliosis, neuropathic ulcers and pathological fractures.

Presentation

This can range from complete myelomeningocoele (**22.56**) to occult with skin stigmata such as a pit or hairy patch. It can be detected antenatally by alpha-fetoprotein assay and ultrasound scans.

Diagnosis

This is clinical and radiological by plain x-ray and MRI to look for cord tethers or syrinx.

Treatment

This requires a team approach to optimize function: orthotics, and surgery to balance muscles and correct deformities.

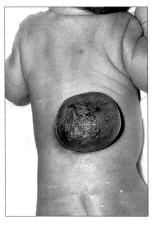

22.56 Large thoraco-lumbar myelo-meningocoele.

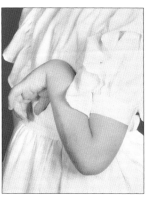

22.57 Brachial plexus injury.

BRACHIAL PLEXUS INJURIES

PRESENTATION

Clinically (**22.57**) with arm palsy and possible Horner syndrome (meiosis, anhydrosis and ptosis). Risk factors are macrosomia, forceps deliveries, breech presentations and prolonged labour.

DIAGNOSIS

This is made by clinical assessment. It is worth considering a myelogram for traumatic pseudo-meningocoele in preganglionic lesions, the histamine axon reflex test (normal triple response in preganglionic lesion but wheal without flare in postganglionic lesions) and neurophysiological investigations.

TREATMENT

A lack of clinical/neurophysiological recovery of biceps function by three months is an indication for exploration with a view to repair (**22.58**). Residual deformities may benefit from tendon transfers and/or osteotomies (e.g. intervention in troublesome medial rotation contracture of shoulder to prevent posterior dislocation and facilitate function).

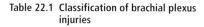

Table 22.1 Classification of brachial plexus injuries

I
- C5, C6: paralysis of shoulder and elbow flexors
- Erb-Duchenne, 'waiter's tip position'
- 90% spontaneous recovery

II
- C5, C6, C7: paralysis of shoulder, elbow flexion, pronation/supination, wrist drop and altered hand sensation
- 60% spontaneous recovery

III
- C5, C6, C7, C8, T1: total paralysis
- 40% spontaneous recovery
- Nerve repair/muscle transfers mitigate disability

IV
- Severe damage and sympathetic injury
- Klumpke's, claw hand
- Full spontaneous recovery not seen
- Surgery to attempt to mitigate situation

From Gilbert A and Tassin JL.
Classification of Brachial Plexus Injuries.

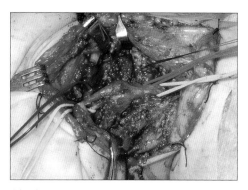

22.58 Brachial plexus injury exposed at operation.

TORTICOLLIS

PRESENTATION
Clinical (**22.59**), with head tilt and rotatory deformity of head and neck. This is common but there are some rare differentials to consider (**Table 22.2**).

DIAGNOSIS
Clinical and by x-ray of the cervical spine.

TREATMENT
Directed to the underlying cause. The majority respond to non-surgical treatment within one year. Surgical release or lengthening of sternocleido-mastoid can be offered when appropriate.

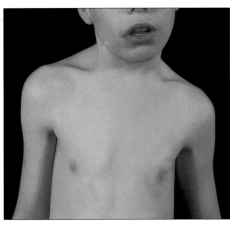

22.59 Torticollis.

Table 22.2 Torticollis – associations

- Congenital
- Klippel-Feil syndrome
- Morquio syndrome
- Down syndrome
- Sandifer syndrome
- Cervical lymphadenitis
- Retropharyngeal abscess
- Juvenile idiopathic arthritis
- Spontaneous atlanto-axial rotatory subluxation following acute pharyngitis
- Acute calcification of cervical disc
- Trauma
- Bone dysplasias
- Neurological tumours (especially posterior fossa)
- Ocular torticollis

CEREBRAL PALSY

See also 'Neurology' chapter.

INCIDENCE
A non-progressive neuromuscular disorder due to damage to the immature brain. The incidence is 1 in 400 children of school age.

ASSOCIATIONS
Epilepsy, neurodevelopmental delay, speech disorders, and visual impairment.

DIAGNOSIS
This is clinical and by exclusion of metabolic disorders and cord tethering. Advice from a paediatric neurologist should be sought.

CLASSIFICATION
This is divided into spastic (hemiplegia, diplegia, quadriplegia), athetotic, ataxic, and mixed types.

TREATMENT
A multidisciplinary approach, commencing as early as possible, is desirable.
Surgery is aimed at enhancing function and posture, and to prevent disabling deformity. Orthopaedic intervention should generally only be considered in the spastic type of cerebral palsy for:
- Control of spinal deformity: bracing, instrumentation.
- Control of hip displacement: splintage, soft tissue and/or bony reconstruction.
- Control of muscle balance/contractures: tendon lengthening, tendon transfers.

Appliances such as various orthoses, customized wheelchairs, and communication aids can contribute significantly.

ARTHROGRYPOSIS

INCIDENCE

A heterogeneous group of conditions resulting in multiple rigid joint deformities with defective muscles, normal sensation and lack of skin creases (**22.60**). There is an association with maternal myasthenia gravis and myotonic dystrophy. Recurrence risk is virtually nil for sporadic cases but 50% for dominantly inherited forms. The incidence is 1 in 10,000.

ASSOCIATIONS

These are cryptorchidism, hernias, gastroschisis, bowel atresia, and neuromuscular and connective tissue disorders.

DIAGNOSIS

As this is a descriptive 'diagnosis', radiology, chromosome analysis, creatinine kinase (CK) assay, electromyogram (EMG) studies and muscle/nerve biopsies may be useful in establishing the underlying diagnosis and prognosis.

TREATMENT

This consists of early physiotherapy to mobilize joints, and splintage (especially for hands to maintain correction). Corrective surgery aims to place joints in position for optimal function.

BRITTLE BONES (OSTEOGENESIS IMPERFECTA)

INCIDENCE

One in 20,000. Inheritance can be autosomal dominant (mainly via mutation), autosomal recessive or occasionally gonadal mosaicism.

PRESENTATION

This is with fractures (**22.61**).

CLASSIFICATION

See **Table 22.3**.

DIAGNOSIS

Clinical, paying attention to any family history. Radiography shows osteoporosis, slender bones, thin cortices and 'wormian' bones on lateral skull x-ray. Beware misdiagnosis of non-accidental injury (especially in type IV). Densitometry and collagen analyses may be required.

TREATMENT

This is symptomatic with analgesics and splintage. Correction of deformities, especially by intramedullary rodding techniques and protection with orthoses, aims to break the cycle: fracture → immobilization → disuse porosis → fracture → immobilization.

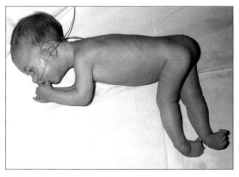

22.60 Arthrogryposis.

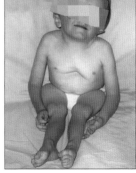

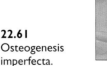

22.61 Osteogenesis imperfecta.

Table 22.3 Classification of brittle bones

I Autosomal dominant, blue sclerae, preschool age (tarda), hearing loss;
 a = with dentinogenesis imperfecta, **b** = without dentinogenesis imperfecta.

II Autosomal recessive, blue sclerae, lethal.

III Autosomal recessive, fractures at birth, progressive deformity and short stature.

IV Autosomal dominant, normal hearing; **a** = with dentinogenesis imperfecta, **b** = without dentinogenesis imperfecta.

All have ligamentous laxity and capillary fragility.

From: Sillence DO, Osteogenesis imperfecta *Clin Orth* 1981; **159** (11)

FRACTURES

GENERAL PRINCIPLES OF TREATMENT

Children's fractures heal faster and have a greater potential for remodelling than those of adults. Children's ligaments are stronger than their bones so avulsion fractures are commoner. Greenstick 'buckle' fractures occur, as paediatric bone is more 'plastic'. Growth plate injuries are unique to children (see also 'Child Protection' chapter).

Presentation

As with adult fractures, one needs to consider the five R's:

- **R**esuscitation
- **R**eduction
- **R**est
- **R**elief of pain
- **R**ehabilitation

Diagnosis

General assessment includes looking for other injuries and conditions, enquiring about medication and allergies and assessing fluid requirements.

Local assessment entails attention to the soft tissues (skin, vessels, nerves and compartments) and to the fracture 'personality'.

Radiography of the contralateral area for comparison can be helpful, as can arthrography for cartilaginous elements. CT (**22.62**) or MRI may be required.

Treatment

First aid should be given with attention to the airway, breathing, and circulation; dressing of any wounds; temporary splintage of fractures; and analgesia.

Urgent debridement of wounds should be undertaken.

Reduction of fractures and dislocations is obtained by closed, percutaneous or open manoeuvres, and stabilized by splintage, percutaneous K-wiring, external fixation or internal fixation. Avoidance of additional iatrogenic damage, particularly to the growth plate, is important.

Indications for fixation are similar to those for adults: failed non-surgical treatment, multiple injuries, associated head injury, fractures in ipsilateral limb, complicated fractures (open, neurovascular damage), articular fractures, pathological fractures and associated conditions (e.g. spasm in cerebral palsy).

Early mobilization and rehabilitation are the goals, but are rarely as problematical as in adults.

Planning the timing of removal of internal fixation devices is a further consideration.

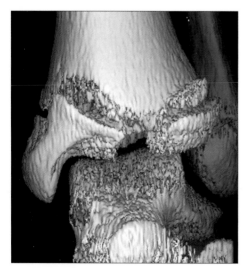

22.62 CT reconstruction of a triplanar fracture of the ankle.

GROWTH PLATE INJURIES
Classification
According to Salter-Harris, as shown in **22.63**.

Treatment
The relevance is in relation to risks of growth disturbance. Prompt, accurate reduction and appropriate maintenance with splintage/K-wires/screws offers the best chance of avoiding complications.

22.63 Salter-Harris classification of growth plate injuries.
Type I: shear through physeal plate.
Type II: partial shear through physeal plate and partial metaphyseal fracture (commonest injury – around 70%).
Type III: partial physeal separation with an intra-articular epiphyseal fracture.
Type IV: plane passes from joint surface through physis and metaphysis.
Type V: compression of articular surface and impaction of epiphyseal bone into metaphyseal bone.

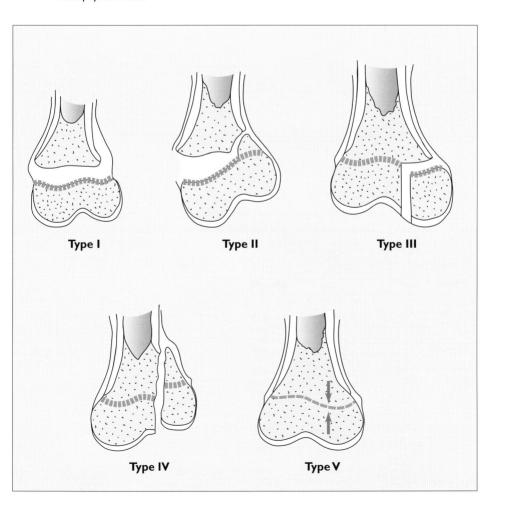

Type I   Type II   Type III

Type IV   Type V

REMODELLING
Presentation
If angulation is in the plane of joint motion, the fracture is close to the epiphysis, and there is at least a couple of years of growth potential, the outlook for remodelling is favourable. (**Table 22.4** and figure **22.64**).

Treatment
Rotational deformities, displaced intra-articular fractures and fractures through the growth plate do not remodel well.

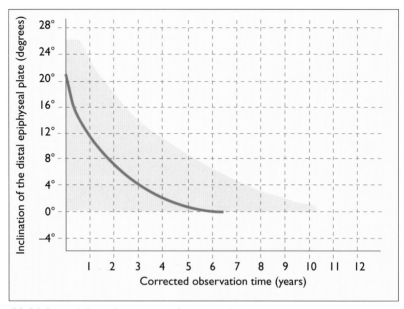

22.64 Remodelling of angulation of distal epiphyseal plate.

Table 22.4 Guidelines for acceptable alignment of forearm shaft fractures

Age <9 years
Complete displacement
Angulation 15°
Malrotation 45°

Age 9–14 years (girls) or 9–16 years (boys)
Distal shaft
    Complete displacement
    Angulation 15°
    Malrotation 30°
Proximal shaft
    Complete displacement
    Angulation 10°
    Malrotation 30°

Reproduced with permission from: Letts RM. *Management of Paediatric Fractures.* London: Churchill Livingstone, 1994: 329

'SPECIAL' PAEDIATRIC FRACTURES

SUPRACONDYLAR FRACTURE OF THE HUMERUS

Classification

This is according to the mechanism of injury:

- In extension, with or without displacement (90%) (22.65).
- In flexion, with or without displacement (10%) (22.66).

Presentation

The particular risks with these injuries are: immediate vascular (compartment syndrome), or neurological damage; and late, entailing stiffness of the elbow, fibrotic contracture (Volkmann's), cubitus varus (22.67), and myositis ossificans.

Treatment

This is by reduction, which may be closed or open, and stabilization with either a sling or backslab, traction (22.68) or (percutaneous) K-wire fixation.

Emergency neurovascular decompression/reconstruction may be needed.

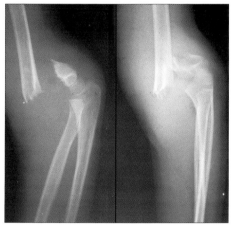

22.65 Supracondylar fracture of humerus.

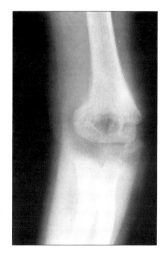

22.66 Supracondylar fracture of humerus.

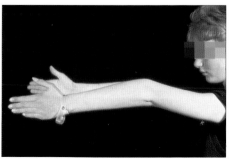

22.67 Cubitus varus.

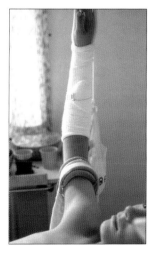

22.68 Traction.

(EPI)CONDYLAR FRACTURE OF HUMERUS

Presentation

Medial epicondylar fracture is common and associated with posterior dislocation of the elbow. Lateral condylar fracture (**22.69**) is also common and has a significant non-union rate (i.e. usually requires fixation). Medial condylar fracture is rare. Classifications by Salter-Harris and Milch are shown in **22.70.**

Diagnosis

- It is important not to miss the fracture because the secondary ossification centre is not yet present.
- A high index of suspicion is required with the information from clinical assessment.
- Consideration must be given to obtaining an arthrogram to delineate 'capsize' of fragment into the joint or incongruence of joint surfaces.
- Ulnar palsy can occur as an acute or tardy complication.

Treatment

This is by accurate reduction and maintenance with screw or K-wire fixation.

RADIAL NECK FRACTURE

A typical radial neck fracture is shown in **22.71**. The radial head epiphysis may not be visible before three to five years of age. With index of suspicion, imaging with ultrasound or arthrography is required.

Treatment

This can usually be manipulated into an acceptable position. Consideration should be given to using a percutaneous wire as a temporary lever. If unstable, a K-wire can be introduced but transcondylar placement should be avoided. Alternatively, a lag screw can be inserted via a proximal Henry approach (vascular supply of fragment obtained from lateral tissues).

Beware of associated distal fracture/interosseous membrane disruption, risk of avascular necrosis and physeal overgrowth or arrest. Beware of posterior interosseous nerve injury.

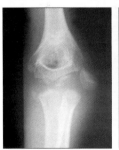 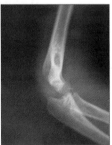

22.69 Lateral condylar fracture.

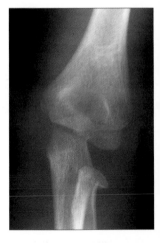

22.71 Radial neck fracture.

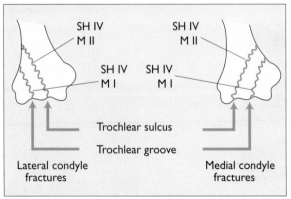

22.70 Salter-Harris (SH) and Milch (M) classifications of condylar fractures. The Milch classification is based on the position of the fracture line. In Type I injury, the fracture line runs through the trochlear groove; in Type II, it runs through the trochlea sulcus.

FOREARM FRACTURES
See **22.72** and **22.73**.

Particular pitfalls
- Monteggia: ulna fracture with radial head subluxation.
- Gallaezzi: radial fracture with distal radioulnar subluxation.

(These are less likely to be overlooked if one always x-rays the whole forearm.)

- Malrotation of mid forearm bones, as there is poor potential for remodelling and this can result in impaired pronation or supination.
- There is a risk of cross-union if plating both bones through single approach. Consider using K-wires or flexible intramedullary (Nancy) nails to stabilize fractures.

FEMORAL FRACTURES
Presentation
- Femoral neck fractures are rare and subject to avascular necrosis, non-union, coxa vara and growth arrest. They need accurate reduction and internal fixation. Undisplaced fractures in young children can sometimes be managed in a spica.
- Mid-femoral fractures (**22.74**) are prone to overgrowth. Gallows traction is appropriate for children under two years of age; balanced traction (**22.75** and **22.76**) or spica cast is suitable for older children, especially as override usually remodels satisfactorily. Occasionally, external fixation plating or intramedullary rodding is necessary.

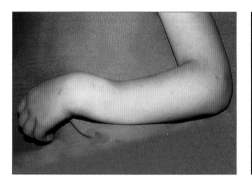

22.72 Distal forearm fracture.

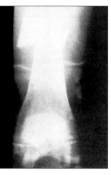

22.74 Femoral fracture.

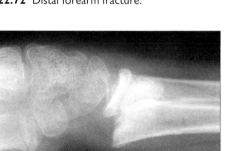

22.73 Forearm fracture (Salter II).

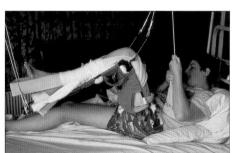

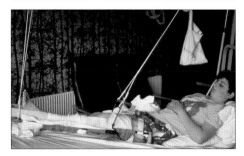

22.75 & 2.76 Traction.

PATELLAR FRACTURES
Diagnosis
Beware bipartite patella (**22.77**), which is a normal variant: it is differentiated from a fracture by history and examination, especially without haemarthrosis and maintenance of extensor mechanism integrity.

Treatment
This is by tension band wiring of displaced fractures. Marginal or osteochondral fragments may warrant arthroscopic removal.

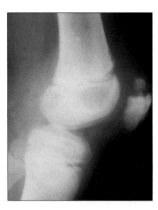

22.77 Bipartite patella.

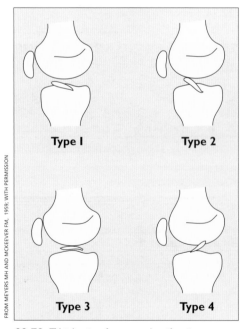

FROM MEYERS MH AND MCKEEVER FM, 1959, WITH PERMISSION

Type 1   **Type 2**

Type 3   **Type 4**

22.78 Tibial spine fracture classification.

PROXIMAL TIBIAL FRACTURES
Diagnosis
Classification of tibial spine fractures is shown in **22.78**.

Treatment
In a cylinder cast in extension if undisplaced (type 1); if type 2 fully reduces in extension, otherwise open reduction and lag screw (**22.79**) or tunnelled reattachment is required.

TRACTION INJURIES AND STRESS FRACTURES
Presentation
- Osgood-Schlatter disease (tibial tubercle apophysitis) (**22.80**): true avulsion is unusual and resolution with conservative treatment is the norm.
- Stress fractures (**22.81**): usually heal without operative intervention.

NON-ACCIDENTAL FRACTURES
Diagnosis
(See 'Child Protection' chapter). Suspicious features:
- History is inappropriate or inconsistent.
- Presentation is delayed.
- Child is not yet walking.
- Parents with inappropriate demeanour.
- Child with various ages of bruises/injuries, subconjunctival haemorrhages, rib fractures, skull fractures or metaphyseal fractures.

Differential diagnosis
Vigilance is required to avoid overlooking the following differential diagnoses:
- Haemophilia
- Osteogenesis imperfecta.
- Leukaemia.
- Copper deficiency.
- Congenital pseudarthrosis (clavicle, tibia).
- Neuropathic limb.
- Osteoporosis.

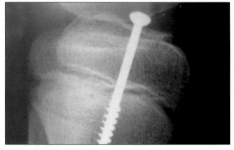

22.79 Tibial spine fracture.

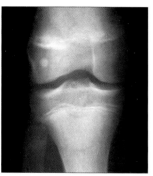

22.80 Osgood-Schlatter disease.

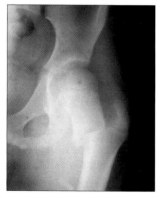

22.81 Stress fracture.

PATHOLOGICAL FRACTURES
Presentation
These may present as:

- Birth fractures in osteogenesis imperfecta, hypophosphatasia, Silverman syndrome, arthrogryposis or from birth trauma.
- Childhood fractures in generalized conditions (e.g. fibrous dysplasia, liver failure, iatrogenic immunosuppression, hyperparathyroidism, leukaemias, malnutrition or copper deficiency).
- Localized conditions (e.g. polio, spina bifida, cerebral palsy, arthritis, post-irradiation or congenital pain insensitivity).
- Localized bony lesions (e.g. benign bone cyst, tumour (benign, or malignant [primary or secondary]) or stress fracture. (**22.82–22.85**)

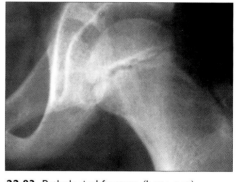

22.82 Pathological fracture.

22.83 Pathological fracture (bone cyst).

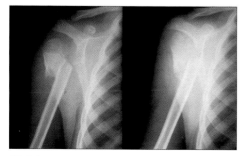

22.84 Pathological fracture.

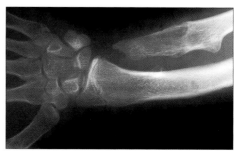

22.85 Pathological fracture (enchondroma).

TREATMENT OF LATE DEFORMITIES

DIAGNOSIS

Detailed assessment, clinical and with plain radiographs, tomograms (computerized) and MRI is essential.

TREATMENT

The techniques available are: physiolysis with or without fat interposition, transphyseal distraction, completion of partial physiodesis, calodistraction and osteotomy.

REFERENCES

General references

Benson MKD, Fixsen JA, Macnicol MF. *Children's Orthopaedics and Fractures*. Churchill Livingstone, 1994.

Fixsen JA. Minor Orthopaedic Problems in Children. In: *ABC of 1 to 7*. Br Med J, 1981: 283.

Jones KL. *Smith's Recognisable Patterns of Human Malformation* (5th edn). Philadelphia: Saunders, 1997.

Rang M. *Children's Fractures* (2nd edn). Lippincott, 1983.

Rockwood CA, Wilkins KE, Beaty JH. *Fractures in Children* (4th edn). Lippincott, 1996.

Staheli LT. *Fundamentals of Pediatric Orthopedics*. Raven Press, 1992.

Tachdjian MO. *Paediatric Orthopaedics* (2nd edn). Saunders, 1990.

Tibiofemoral angle

Salenius P, Vanka E. The development of tibiofemoral angle in children. *J Bone Joint Surg* 1975; **57**(A): 259–261.

Heath CH, Staheli LT. Normal limits of knee angle in white children – *genu varum* and *genu valgum*. *J Paed Orthopaed* 1993; **13**(2): 259–262.

Torsional deformity

Kling TF, Hensinger RN. Angular and torsional deformities of the limbs in children. *Clin Orthopaed Rel Res* 1983; **186:** 136–142.

Staheli LT, Corbett M, Wyss C, King H. Lower extremity rotational problems in children: normal values to guide management. *J Bone Joint Surg* 1985; **67**(A):39–47.

Flat feet

Staheli LT, Chew DE, Corbett M. The longitudinal arch: asurvey of 882 fet in normal children and adults. *J Bone Joint Surg* 1987; **69**(A): 426–428.

Growth charts

Anderson MS, Messner MB, Gteen WT. Distribution of lengths of the normal femur and tibia in children from 1 to 18 years of age. *J Bone Joint Surg* 1964; **57**(A): 259–261.

Tanner JM, Whitehouse RH, Takaishi M. Standards from birth to maturity for height, weight, height velocity and weight velocity: British children. *Arch Dis Child* 1966; **41:** 454–471, 613–635.

In-toe/out-toe gait

Fixsen JA. Borderline orthopaedic abnormalities in children. *Hospital Update* April 1977:185–188.

Club foot (congenital talipes equinovarum)

Harrold AJ, Walker CJ. Treatment and prognosis in congenital club foot. *J Bone Joint Surg* 1983; **65**(B): 8.

Developmental dysplasia of the hip (DDH)

Anderson MS, Messner MB, Green WT. Growth Remaining Chart. *J Bone Joint Surg* 1964; **46**(A): 1197–1202.

Mackenzie IG, Wilson JG. Problems encountered in the early diagnosis and management of congenital dislocation of the hip. *J Bone Joint Surg* 1981; **63**(B) 38–42.

Limb length discrepancy
Saleh M. Technique selection in leg lengthening: the Sheffield experience. *Sem Orthopaed* 1992; 7(3):137–151.

Proximal femoral focal deficiency
Fixsen JA, Lloyd-Roberts GC. The natural history and early treatment of proximal femoral dysplasia. *J Bone Joint Surg* 1974; **56**(B): 86–95.

Congenital tibial dysplasia
Kalamchi A, Dawe RB. Congenital deficiency of the tibia. *J Bone Joint Surg* 1985; **67**(B): 581–584.

Congenital fibular dysplasia
Achterman C, Kalamachi A. Congenital absence of the fibula. *J Bone Joint Surg* 1979; **61**(B):133–137.

Painful limp
Hill RA, Fixsen JA. Investigation and management of the painful hip in childhood. *Br J Hosp Med* 1994; **51**(6): 270–274.

Polydactyly
Wassel HD. Wassel classification of (thumb) dysplasia. *Clin Orth Rel Res* 1969; **64**: 175–193.

Kyphoscoliosis
Cobb JR. Outline for the Study of Scoliosis. *Am Acad Orthoped Surg Instruct Course Lect* 1948; **5**: 261.
Mehta MH. The rib vertebral angle in the early diagnosis between resolving and progressive infantile scoliosis. J Bone Joint Surg 1972; **54**(B): 230–243.
Smith RM, Micheli LJ. The Spine. In: Harris NH, Birch R (eds). *Postgraduate Textbook of Clinical Orthopaedics* (2nd edn). Oxford: Blackwell, 1995.
Lonstein JE, Bradford DS, Winter R, Ogilvie JW. *Moe's Textbook of Scoliosis and Other Spinal Deformities.* Philadelphia: Saunders, 1995.

Spina bifida
Feiwell E. Spina bifida (myelomeningocele). *Orth Clin N Am* 1981; **12**: 101–106.

Brachial plexus injuries
Gilbert A, Tassin JL. Classification of brachial plexus injuries. In: Reparation chirurgicale du plexus brachial dans la paralysie obstetricale chirugie.

Cerebral palsy
Fixsen JA. The role of orthopaedic surgery in cerebral palsy. Sem Orthopaed 1989; **4**: 215–219.
Rang M, Wright J. What have 30 years of medical progress done for cerebral palsy? *Clin Orthopad Rel Res* 1989; **247**: 55–60.

Joint deformities (arthrogryposis)
Thomsen GH, Bilenker RM. Comprehensive management of arthrogryposis multiplex congenita. *Clin Orthopaed* 1985; **194**: 6–14.

Brittle bones (osteogenesis imperfecta)
Sillence DO. Classification of brittle bones. In: Osteogenesis imperfecta: an expanding panorama of variants. *Clin Orthopaed* 1981; **159**: 11.
Smith R, Francis MJO, Houghton GR. *The Brittle Bone Syndrome. Osteogenesis Imperfecta.* Oxford: Butterworth, 1983.

Growth plate injuries
Salter RB, Harris WR. Salter-Harris classification of growth plate injuries. *J Bone Joint Surg* 1963; 45(A):587–622.

Remodelling
Friberg KSI. Remodelling after distal forearm fractures in children II. The Final orientation of the distal and proximal epiphyseal plates of the radius. *Acta Orthopaed Scand* 1979; **50**: 731–739.
Letts RM. Guidelines for Acceptable Alignment of Forearm Shaft Fractures. In: *Management of Paediatric Fractures.* Edinburgh: Livingstone, 1994: 329.

(Epi)condylar fracture of humerus
Milch J. Milch classification of condylar fractures. In: Fractures and fracture dislocations of humeral condyles. *J Trauma* 1964; **4**: 592–607.

Proximal tibial fractures
Meyers MH, McKeever FM. Meyers and McKeever classification of tibial spine fractures. In: Fracture of the intercondylar eminence of the tibia. *J Bone Joint Surg* 1959; **41**(A):209–222.

Urology
John M Hodapp
Pierre DE Mouriquand

MULTICYSTIC DYSPLASTIC KIDNEY

INCIDENCE
One in 5000 births, with males and females being equally affected.

AETIOLOGY
Failure of renal development, which may be due to abnormal interaction between ureteric bud and metanephric blastema; ipsilateral ureter absent or atretic; contralateral upper tract anomalies in 20% of cases (pelviureteric junction obstruction; megaureter; vesicoureteric reflux).

DIAGNOSIS
Most are diagnosed on antenatal ultrasound. May present as an abdominal mass in an infant. Rarely presents as urinary tract infection or hypertension. Ultrasound will show multiple cysts of varying sizes and no normal renal parenchyma (**23.1**). Isotope scans will demonstrate no function.

TREATMENT
Most of these kidneys will involute and disappear. Large, persistent multicystic dysplastic kidneys should be removed (**23.2**).

PROGNOSIS
Should be excellent. Contralateral kidney needs to be carefully assessed. Association with hypertension controversial.

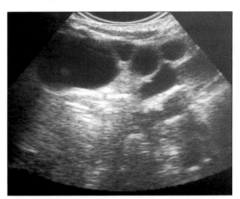

23.1 Multicystic dysplastic kidney. Typical ultrasound appearance. No normal renal parenchyma can be found.

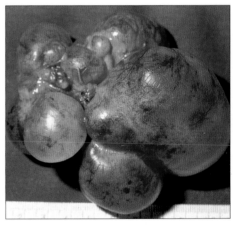

23.2 Multicystic dysplastic kidney. Gross specimen. No normal parenchyma can be seen.

NEUROPATHIC VOIDING DYSFUNCTION AND INCONTINENCE

INCIDENCE

Neuropathic voiding dysfunction is the rule when spinal cord or anorectal anomalies are present. It can occur in the absence of proven neurologic pathology but much less commonly.

DIAGNOSIS

Physical examination may reveal overt lower extremity neurological deficit (the lower spine may show signs of spina bifida occulta – hairy patch, skin dimple or skin tag). Ultrasound should be carried out to assess upper tract dilatation, thick-walled bladder and incomplete bladder emptying. A plain abdominal x-ray (**23.3**) will show spinal and sacral abnormalities as well as demonstrating whether constipation is present. A micturition cystourethrogram (MCUG) needs to be done to diagnose vesico-ureteric reflux. An isotope scan will assess kidney function (usually DMSA – dimercapto-succinic acid) and drainage (MAG-3). Urodynamic studies will document whether the bladder stores urine at high pressures (and is likely to lead to renal damage) or low; see **Table 23.1**.

TREATMENT

The first goal is to protect the kidneys from deterioration by achieving low-pressure storage of urine. The second goal is to provide urinary continence and protect against infection. Both of these are achieved by clean intermittent catheterization of the urethra. If the urethra is unavailable or the child is non-compliant, then the appendix can be used to create a catheterizable stoma on the abdominal wall (Mitrofanoff procedure). Anticholinergics such as oxybutynin are extremely valuable in lowering bladder storage pressures. If those measures fail then the bladder is augmented with bowel (ileocystoplasty, colocystoplasty).

PROGNOSIS

Generally quite good, but requires a high degree of patient compliance. All children must have very close monitoring and undergo frequent assessment of renal tract with ultrasound scans and DMSA imaging.

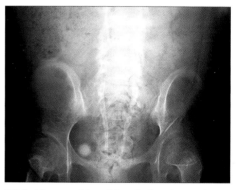

23.3 Neuropathic voiding dysfunction and incontinence. Plain abdominal film of patient with neurogenic voiding dysfunction. Note spinal dysraphism, V-P shunt, faecal loading and bladder stone.

Table 23.1 Categories of bladder dysfunction

Problem	Clinical manifestation	Treatment
Bladder is primary problem		
Failure to store	Incontinence, high pressure storage	Anticholinergics, clean intermittent catheterization, bladder augmentation in those refractory to medical treatment
Failure to empty	Usually continent, low pressure storage	Clean intermittent catheterization
Sphincter/bladder neck is primary problem		
Failure to store	Incontinence, low leak pressure	Clean intermittent catheterization, bladder neck reconstruction, artificial urinary sphincter, consider urinary diversion
Failure to empty	Usually continent, storage pressures variable	Clean intermittent catheterization

EXSTROPHY / EPISPADIAS COMPLEX

INCIDENCE
Classic exstrophy occurs in 1:30,000 live births, with a male to female ratio of 5:1(the risk of recurrence in a given family is 1:100). Pure epispadias occurs in 1:120,000 males. Females can be born with pure epispadias but it is much less common. Cloacal exstrophy occurs in1:300,000 live births, with a male to female ratio of 2:1.

PRESENTATION
A continuum of anomalies, ranging from mild glandular epispadias of the penis through classic bladder exstrophy, to cloacal exstrophy, which is the most severe form (**23.4–23.7**).

DIAGNOSIS
This is usually evident on physical examination.
- **Exstrophy/epispadias.** The bladder is open on the anterior abdominal wall. In both sexes there is a widened pubic symphysis (**23.8**), a short, broad perineum, and an anteriorly placed anus. In the male, the phallus is short and broad with the opened urethral plate visible on the dorsal surface. Testes are usually descended. In the female, the labia are divergent and the clitoris is bifid. The vagina is single. The bladder of both sexes often has abnormal histology, but the upper urinary tracts are usually normal. There is bilateral vesicoureteric reflux in nearly 100% of cases, with bilateral inguinal hernias commonly present.
- **Cloacal exstrophy.** As above, plus omphalocoele with prolapse of terminal ileum. In the male, the penis is usually of very poor quality. In the female, the vagina is bifid. Hindgut usually short. Thirty percent have spinal dysraphism, 25% have lower extremity deformities.

TREATMENT
Bladder closure at birth, usually with pelvic osteotomies to take the tension off the soft tissues. Epispadias repair in boys between six and 12 months of age. Bladder-neck reconstruction in older children may be required for continence. Augmentation cystoplasty is often needed. Cloacal exstrophy also requires hindgut reconstruction and some of these children will have permanent ileostomies or colostomies.

PROGNOSIS
Generally good, in terms of overall health, with classic bladder exstrophy and epispadias. Urinary continence (greater than four hours without leakage) is only achieved in 50–60% of patients. Most children undergo multiple operations. Fertility has been reported but is lower than normal controls. Females often develop uterine prolapse as adults. Males may have retrograde ejaculation. Renal tracts are most often preserved. Cloacal exstrophy carries a worse prognosis. Fertility has not been reported in cloacal exstrophy.

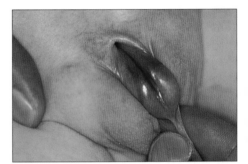

23.4 Epispadias without exstrophy.

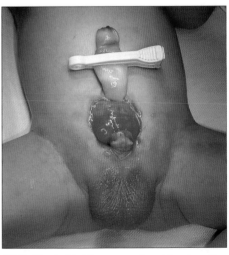

23.5 Classic bladder exstrophy with epispadias in a male.

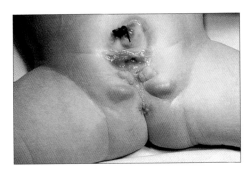

23.6 Classic bladder exstrophy in the female.

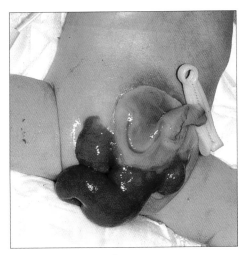

23.7 Cloacal exstrophy.

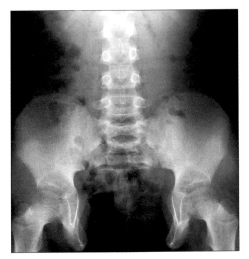

23.8 Widened symphysis pubis.

TESTICULAR TUMOURS

INCIDENCE
Uncommon: 1–2% of all paediatric tumours. Usually present within first two years of life. Yolk sac tumour is the most common testicular tumour in children. Teratoma is the next most common (it does not metastasize). Four percent of patients with Burkitt's lymphoma and 25% of patients with ALL have testicular involvement. Metastases, when they occur, are typically to the retroperitoneal lymph nodes.

DIAGNOSIS
Painless scrotal swelling (**23.9**). The mass is firm and does not transilluminate. A secondary hydrocoele may be present. A scrotal ultrasound will identify the mass and allow examination of the contralateral testis. Serum alpha-fetoprotein (AFP) is often greatly elevated with a yolk sac tumour, although 10% of these will have a normal AFP 9 and it is not a prognostic indicator (see 'Solid Tumours and Histiocytosis' chapter). Serum beta-hCG is elevated with most chorio-carcinomas, embryonal carcinomas and 10% of seminomas. A CT scan will evaluate the retroperitoneum for adenopathy. All testicular masses need to be surgically explored through an inguinal incision.

TREATMENT
Inguinal orchidectomy in all cases. There should be close surveillance of serum AFP and serial CT scans if the surgical specimen shows disease confined to the testis. Chemotherapy is necessary for metastatic disease (cisplatin, etoposide, bleomycin). A residual retroperitoneal mass or a serum AFP that does not return to normal after treatment may require a retroperitoneal lymph node dissection (RPLND).

PROGNOSIS
90% survival.

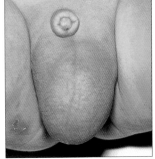

23.9 Testicular tumours. Scrotal mass caused by tumour.

HYPOSPADIAS

INCIDENCE
One in 300 live male births.

PRESENTATION
Hooded foreskin that is deficient ventrally (not a constant feature). Ectopic ventral urethral meatus (**23.10**). Possible ventral curvature (chordee) (**23.11**). Ambiguous genitalia. Possible penoscrotal transposition. Atresia of ventral penile tissues (skin and corpus spongiosum). May also have cryptorchidism and inguinal hernia.

DIAGNOSIS
Physical examination.

TREATMENT
The first step is the correction of chordee. The second step is urethroplasty. The final step is obtaining penile skin cover and performing glanduloplasty.

PROGNOSIS
A cosmetically acceptable result should be attainable. Between 5% and 15% of patients will develop a urethrocutaneous fistula. One to 5% of patients will develop urethral or meatal strictures. Fertility should not be impaired. Long-term follow-up for voiding efficiency and penile cosmesis is recommended.

WILMS' TUMOUR (23.12–23.15)

See also 'Solid Tumours and Histiocytosis' chapter.

INCIDENCE
One in 10,000 children. It is the most common solid abdominal mass and the most common abdominal cancer in children. May be associated with a deletion of chromosome 11p13 (WT 1).

PRESENTATION
Abdominal mass (sole presenting sign in 50% of patients). Other presentations include anorexia, vomiting, anaemia and abdominal pain (with infarction of tumour). May be accompanied by hemihypertrophy, aniridia, macroglossia, abdominal wall defects, neonatal hypoglycaemia (Beckwith-Weidemann syndrome) and ambiguous genitalia with renal failure (Drash syndrome). It is a well-encapsulated, tan-coloured tumour with areas of infarction. The tumour may have areas of 'unfavourable histology' such as anaplasia that impart a worse prognosis. Metastases tend to involve regional nodes, lung and liver.

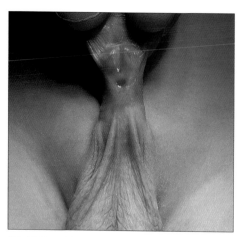

23.10 Distal hypospadias.

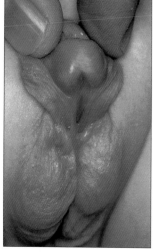

23.11 Severe hypospadias with chordee.

DIAGNOSIS

Ultrasound will show renal mass that may be calcified. A CT scan is the best method of evaluating the tumour. The mass tends to be well- encapsulated, splaying the kidney apart (a normal kidney is not often identifiable). Heterogeneous appearance common with central necrosis. True-cut biopsy may be performed when preoperative chemotherapy is planned.

TREATMENT

Surgical excision combined with chemotherapy. Preoperative chemotherapy is useful for surgically unresectable tumours and metastatic tumours. Actinomycin D and vincristine are the agents of choice, with adriamycin being added for unfavourable histology or metastatic disease. Radiation therapy is also used to manage metastatic sites.

PROGNOSIS

The most important factor is presence or absence of unfavourable histology. Four-year disease free rates: with a favourable histology, 80–90%; with an unfavourable histology, 50–60%. In short, the majority of Wilms' tumours encountered are favourable histology, but the vast majority of deaths are in the unfavourable histology group: histology is more predictive of survival than stage.

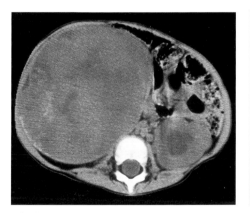

23.12 Wilms' tumour. Typical CT appearance.

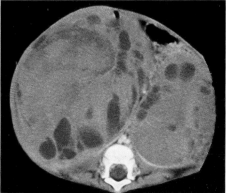

23.13 Bilateral Wilms' tumours. Note that tumours are not homogeneous.

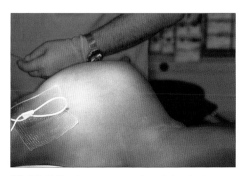

23.14 Wilms' tumour causing abdominal mass.

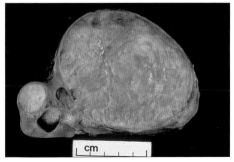

23.15 Wilms' tumour: cut surface of specimen.

UROGENITAL RHABDOMYOSARCOMA

INCIDENCE
Four in 1,000,000 white children (less common in black children). Accounts for 5% of all malignancies in children. 50% of all childhood sarcomas are rhabdomyosarcomas. Most usual sites in the genitourinary system are bladder (**23.16**), prostate, and vagina.

PRESENTATION
Gross haematuria. Bladder outlet obstruction, dysuria, interlabial mass in the female.

DIAGNOSIS
Vaginal tumours are often visible on physical examination. Ultrasound may show a bladder or prostatic mass. A CT scan will define the extent of disease but a biopsy is essential. The tumour often has a botryoid or polypoid appearance. Electron microscopy will show cross-striations characteristic of skeletal muscle. Tumours often invade locally in an aggressive manner. Frequent sites of metastases are lung, bone, liver and bone marrow.

TREATMENT
Combination radiotherapy, chemotherapy and surgery.

PROGNOSIS
Varies with site of primary, clinical stage and histological grade. Vaginal rhabdomyosarcoma has excellent long-term survival. Bladder rhabdomyosarcoma has an 80% survival, with 60% of patients retaining their bladders. Twenty percent of patients treated with radiation will have radiation cystitis. Impotence in the male can result from pelvic exenteration or radiation.

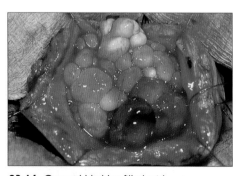

23.16 Opened bladder filled with rhabdomyosarcoma.

PRUNE-BELLY SYNDROME

INCIDENCE
Rare. Occurs only in males.

PRESENTATION
Antenatal ultrasound demonstrates dilated renal pelvis and ureter. The patient has a lax, wrinkled abdominal wall with redundant skin (**23.17**). Triad of absence of abdominal muscles, undescended testes and general dysplasia of the urinary tract. Azoospermia, gastrointestinal and musculo-skeletal abnormalities are often present.

DIAGNOSIS
Physical examination demonstrates the absence of abdominal muscles and cryptorchidism. Ultrasound will demonstrate bilateral dilatation of renal pelvis and ureter. MCUG often shows vesicoureteric reflux.

TREATMENT
Conservative management is the rule unless there is documented obstruction of the kidneys (unusual). If the patient cannot empty the bladder efficiently, then clean intermittent catheterization is an excellent option. Bilateral orchidopexies (usually carried out as two-stage procedures). Prophylactic antibiotics if recurrent urinary tract infection is a problem. Abdominoplasty may be useful.

PROGNOSIS
Depends on the degree of renal dysplasia. Infertility is likely.

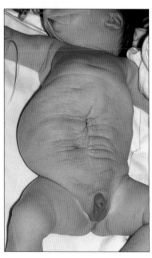

23.17 Appearance of abdominal wall in prune-belly syndrome.

CONGENITAL ABNORMALITIES OF URINE FLOW (PELVIURETERIC AND VESICOURETERIC ANOMALIES)

INCIDENCE
Antenatal ultrasound screening has led to detection of urinary tract dilatation in 1:800 to 1:1,500 pregnancies. Half of the babies with antenatal dilatation will have persistent postnatal dilatation.

PRESENTATION
The majority of patients present with antenatally diagnosed urinary tract dilatation. The postnatal presentation of previously undiagnosed obstruction is an abdominal mass, urinary tract infection, loin pain or, less commonly, haematuria, hypertension and failure to thrive.

DIAGNOSIS
Ultrasound will assess dilatation of the upper tracts. Isotopic studies will document differential renal function as well as assess renal drainage. MCUG needs to be performed to rule out vesicoureteric reflux as a cause of dilatation and posterior urethral valve pathology in males (**23.18–23.21**).

TREATMENT
Spontaneous resolution is common, when the renal pelvic anteroposterior diameter is less than 20 mm. Pyeloplasty (Anderson-Hynes procedure) or ureteral reimplantation are required if renal function deteriorates, there are bilateral anomalies, urine flow impairment is symptomatic or the renal pelvic diameter increases.

PROGNOSIS
Excellent if the problem is unilateral. Variable if it is bilateral. Pyeloplasty is a safe procedure with excellent long-term results. Reimplantation of an obstructed megaureter (UVJ obstruction) carries a higher complication rate than reimplantation for other reasons. It is still a highly successful operation. Long term follow-up is essential until nuclear scans show adequate drainage.

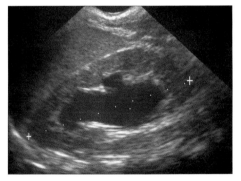

23.18 Typical ultrasound of dilated renal pelvis.

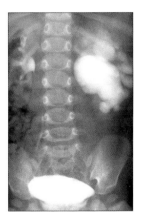

23.19 IVU demonstrating massive dilatation of left renal pelvis and calyces.

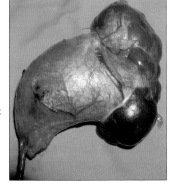

23.20 Pelviureteric junction (PUJ) obstruction: Gross pathology.

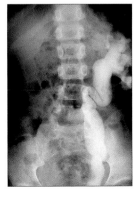

23.21 IVU of a solitary kidney with an obstructed megaureter.

UROLITHIASIS

INCIDENCE
Children are not as susceptible to stone disease as adults, but it is not uncommon. Urine stasis caused by an anatomically abnormal urinary tract is commonly associated with stone formation. A history of recurrent urinary tract infection is often present and can be causative of the stones. In the absence of urine stasis or recurrent infection, stones are uncommon and point to a metabolic disturbance.

PRESENTATION
Renal colic, persistent or recurrent urinary tract infection, haematuria and dysuria (with bladder stones). Primary urolithiasis is seen in primary hyperoxaluria, hyperuricosuria, renal tubular disorders such as renal tubular acidosis, cystinuria and hypercalcaemic states as in hyperparathyroidism or prolonged immobilization (because of calcium reabsorption from bones). Idiopathic calcium oxalate urolithiasis is also commonly seen. Secondary urolithiasis is seen in urinary stasis (PUJ obstruction, neuropathic bladders) and chronic infection (bladder stones, staghorn calculi). Even children with an obvious cause of secondary urolithiasis need full metabolic investigations.

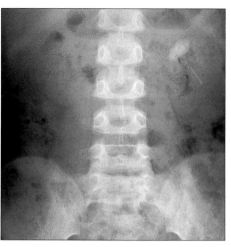

23.22 Abdominal plain film. Large calculus in left kidney.

DIAGNOSIS
There may be a family history of stones, a history of recurrent UTI or an abnormal fluid intake pattern. Urinalysis will assess haematuria, pyuria, crystalluria and pH. Twenty four-hour urine biochemistry for creatinine, calcium, oxalate, phosphate, citrate and uric acid (best done after stones removed). Serum chemistry for electrolytes, urea, creatinine, bicarbonate, calcium, magnesium, phosphate, albumin, ALP and uric acid (can be done while stones still in the patient). Ninety percent of stones are radiopaque on plain abdominal x-ray (KUB) (**23.22**, **23.23**). Ultrasound will show stones that are in the bladder and renal pelvis as hyperechoic areas with shadowing, but it does not visualize ureteral stones well. Intravenous urography (IVU) will demonstrate stones as well as give information regarding anatomy and urinary obstruction. A CT scan without contrast (**23.24**) is the most sensitive scan for stones (especially ureteral stones) and all stones appear as calcific densities. A DMSA scan will demonstrate differential function and scarring.

The ultimate diagnosis depends on the chemical analysis of stones retrieved from the patient.

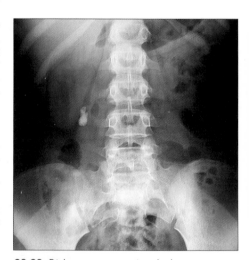

23.23 Right upper ureteric calculus.

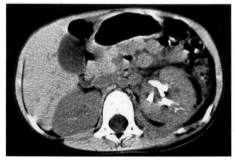

23.24 Non-contrast CT showing staghorn calculus filling left renal pelvis.

TREATMENT

A high fluid intake is essential. Dietary modification is less successful. Thiazide diuretics may help patients with hypercalciuria or hyperoxaluria. The majority of stones can be managed without open surgery. Extracorporeal shock wave lithotripsy is very successful in children. Endoscopic electrohydraulic or laser lithotripsy can be used for bladder or ureteral stones. Percutaneous nephrostolithotomy is another minimally invasive yet highly successful technique. A minority of stones will require open removal.

PROGNOSIS

Generally good, although, in patients with primary urolithiasis, stones often recur throughout life (**23.25**). Staghorn calculi (usually made of magnesium ammonium phosphate) can fill the renal pelvis and lead to xanthogranulomatous pyelonephritis and total loss of kidney function.

POSTERIOR URETHRAL VALVES

INCIDENCE

One in 5,000 males.

PRESENTATION

Antenatal diagnosis is becoming more common with the severe cases. They may present with bilateral hydronephrosis *in utero* with oligohydramnios and pulmonary hypoplasia. Up to 70% present in first year of life (with up to 50% as neonates). May present as a poor urinary stream in the older boy. There is a thin membrane in the posterior urethra, just distal to verumontanum. Renal dysplasia is common. There is vesicoureteric reflux in 50% of patients (**23.26–23.28**).

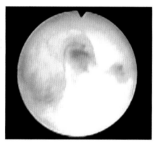

23.26 Endoscopic view of posterior urethral valve filling urethral lumen.

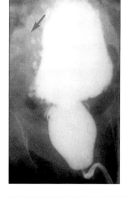

23.27 MCUG showing dilated posterior urethra and multiple bladder diverticula.

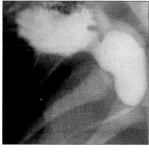

23.28 MCUG. Note massively dilated posterior urethra and small, trabeculated bladder.

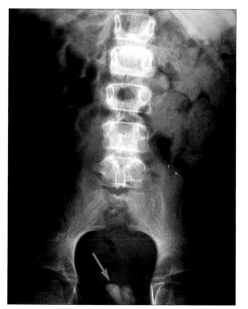

23.25 Bladder stone in a patient with sacral agenesis and a neuropathic bladder.

DIAGNOSIS

Antenatal ultrasound diagnosis of renal pelvic and ureteric dilatation with a thick-walled bladder. Postnatally, may present with renal failure and/or sepsis/urinary tract infection. MCUG is the gold standard and will show a dilated posterior urethra with a narrowing near the external sphincter and vesicoureteric reflux. If present, ultrasound may demonstrate a dilated posterior urethra but is more helpful in showing failure of bladder emptying and a thick bladder wall. Ultrasound will also assess upper tract dilatation and renal parenchyma. Radionuclide scans (DMSA or MAG-3) will assess relative renal function and drainage.

TREATMENT

Prompt bladder drainage is essential if there is infection or evidence of compromised renal function. Suprapubic drainage is preferred in infants. Correction of electrolyte and fluid imbalances must be prompt. Endoscopic trans-urethral valve ablation is the definitive treatment. In infants too small or ill to undergo valve ablation, a suprapubic vesicostomy may provide temporary drainage but should not be thought of as primary treatment for most infants. Infants with severe sepsis may require upper tract drainage in the form of cutaneous ureterostomies.

PROGNOSIS

Should be considered as guarded. Impairment of renal function is found in 30–50% of patients. With treatment of the valves, 30–50% of patients will have resolution of reflux. Dysfunctional voiding due to detrusor decompensation in the bladder is very common in childhood. Boys with valves often gain urinary continence (especially at night) much later than those without. Urodynamic abnormalities are seen in 75% of patients. Ultrasound evidence of renal pelvic dilatation, as well as radionuclide scan evidence of poor drainage, may persist throughout childhood. Close urological and nephrological follow-up is mandatory. Valve patients represent 15–20% of patients progressing to renal transplantation. Those with the worst bladder function may need bladder augmentation with bowel and lifelong intermittent bladder catheterization to obtain continence and protect renal function.

CRYPTORCHIDISM

INCIDENCE

Thirty-three percent of premature infants, 3% of term infants, 1% of one-year-olds. Testes that have failed to descend by the age of one are unlikely to do so.

PRESENTATION

Undescended testes (**23.29**) are testes not in the scrotum but found along the path of normal descent. Ectopic testes are not found along the path of normal descent (most will be in a superficial inguinal pouch, but they may be in the thigh, at the base of the penis or in the perineum). Intra-abdominal testes have failed to enter the inguinal canal. Vanishing testes occur when evidence is present that a testis existed at some time (i.e. vas and spermatic vessels are present) but no testis is found on exploration. Retractile testes are capable of being drawn down manually into the scrotum but subsequently are drawn back into the inguinal canal by the cremasteric reflex.

Undescended testes will show germ cell hypoplasia or aplasia (poor spermatogenic potential) and Leydig cell hyperplasia. 'Normal' descended testes will often show some degree of poor germ cell development if the contralateral testis is cryptorchid. Many undescended testes will have an abnormal vas or epididymis. Inguinal hernia is often associated with a cryptorchid testis. The risk of developing a germ cell tumour in a cryptorchid testis is 5–10 times higher than in a normally descended testis. Ten percent of all germ cell tumours of testes arise in undescended testes.

DIAGNOSIS

Physical examination, with laparoscopy to assess impalpable testes. With bilateral impalpable testes, an hCG stimulation test may point to the presence or absence of functioning testicular tissue by assessing a testosterone surge. Asymptomatic boys with isolated undescended testes do not need screening of the upper urinary tracts.

TREATMENT

Retractile testes do not require therapy. Impalpable testes are best evaluated with laparoscopy. Orchidopexy is the treatment of choice for all palpable testes.

Spermatic vessels may be ligated (Fowler-Stevens technique) as long as the collateral vessels to the testis (vasal and cremasteric) are intact. Treatment ideally is before the age of two years.

PROGNOSIS

Only 25% of men with bilateral cryptorchidism will be fertile. Seventy-five percent of men with unilateral cryptorchidism will be fertile. Early orchidopexy may lead to better spermatogenic function in cryptorchid testes but this is not proven. Orchidopexy does not decrease the risk of malignant degeneration but it allows the testis to be examined by palpation. Orchidopexy helps to alleviate the psychological problems caused by the empty scrotum.

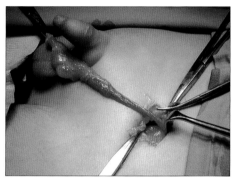

23.29 Undescended testis being brought down into scrotum at surgery.

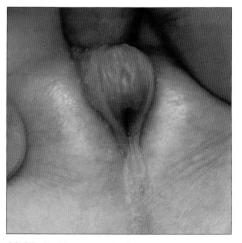

23.30 Ambiguous genitalia.

AMBIGUOUS GENITALIA

See also 'Endocrinology' chapter.

CLASSIFICATION
- The undervirilized male.
- The virilized female (congenital adrenal hyperplasia).
- True hermaphroditism.
- Gonadal dysgenesis.

INCIDENCE
Congenital adrenal hyperplasia is common (most common intersex disorder). Mixed gonadal dysgenesis is uncommon. Undervirilization in the male (androgen insensitivity) is uncommon. True hermaphroditism (where both testicular and ovarian tissue are present) is extremely rare.

PRESENTATION
Ambiguous genitalia (**23.30**) may present with clitoromegaly/fused labia, penoscrotal hypospadias with impalpable gonad and circulatory collapse (salt wasting in congenital adrenal hyperplasia). Females may present with inguinal hernia (hernia sac may contain a testis) and primary amenorrhoea (in an undervirilized male that is phenotypically female). Pathology is highly variable and depends on the diagnosis and degree of intersexuality.

DIAGNOSIS
Investigations include karyotype, serum levels of progesterone and androstenedione and urine 17-keto steroids (elevated in congenital adrenal hyperplasia). Genitogram will define the anatomy and assess for vagina and uterus. A gonadal biopsy is often needed for definitive diagnosis.

TREATMENT
Depends on gender assignment. Feminizing genitoplasty in congenital adrenal hyperplasia. Repair of hypospadias and removal of dysgenetic gonads. May require hormone replacement as child grows. Endocrine referral essential.

PROGNOSIS
Generally good if gender assignment is done early and properly. Girls with congenital adrenal hyperplasia are usually fertile. All others are typically infertile or subfertile.

ANOMALIES OF KIDNEY POSITION AND NUMBER

INCIDENCE
- Unilateral renal agenesis 1:1,200 births.
- Horseshoe kidney 1:700 births.
- Simple ectopia 1:1,000 births.
- Crossed ectopia 1:7,000 births.

PRESENTATION
Virtually all anomalies of kidney position and number are incidental findings:
- Bilateral renal agenesis is incompatible with life.
- Unilateral renal agenesis leads to a solitary kidney.
- Horseshoe kidneys (**23.31**) occur when kidneys are connected across the midline by a fibrous band or functioning parenchyma.
- Simple renal ectopia occurs when a kidney is on the same side of the body as the insertion of its ureter into the bladder, but not in the proper place (usually found in pelvis) (**23.32**).
- Crossed renal ectopia occurs when a kidney lies on contralateral side to the insertion of its ureter into the bladder (may be fused to contralateral kidney) (**23.33**).

DIAGNOSIS
Ultrasound or IVU will usually define the anatomy clearly. Non-visualization of a kidney on IVU should prompt an ultrasound of the renal fossa for diagnosis (e.g. absent kidney, non-functioning kidney, multicystic kidney).

These conditions are typically asymptomatic. Horseshoe kidneys have a higher incidence of pelviureteric junction obstruction and urolithiasis. Ectopic kidneys may be associated with vesicoureteric reflux. Absent kidney often associated with absent ipsilateral vas deferens in males.

TREATMENT
If asymptomatic then none is indicated. Some horseshoe kidneys may require pyeloplasty. Stones are treated with standard techniques if they arise.

PROGNOSIS
These conditions should not affect the long-term health of the patient. They typically do not interfere with renal function.

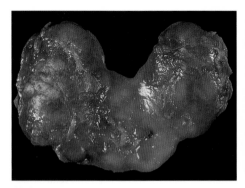

23.31 Horseshoe kidney.

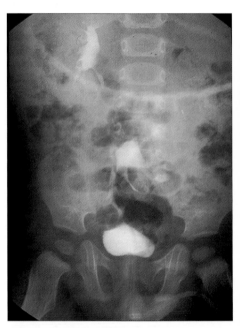

23.32 IVU demonstrating a pelvic kidney overlying the sacrum.

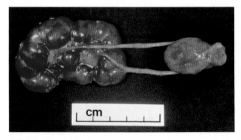

23.33 Fused kidneys.

URETERAL DUPLICATION

INCIDENCE
Partial and complete duplication without ectopia of the ureters is common. Complete duplication with ectopia is much less so.

PRESENTATION
Partial duplication occurs when two separate ureters from one kidney join prior to entering the bladder. Complete duplication occurs when there are two separate ureters draining one kidney as well as two separate ureteral orifices on that side. It is often asymptomatic and discovered incidentally. Urinary infection can be seen with complete duplication and a refluxing lower pole or an obstructed upper pole. Ectopic duplicated ureters can lead to continuous urinary dribbling in girls (when they terminate in the vagina) but not in boys.

The upper pole ureter will enter the bladder medial and inferior to the lower pole ureter. In girls, ectopic ureters may enter into the vagina or urethra causing continuous urinary incontinence.

In boys, ectopic ureters may enter into the posterior urethra or seminal vesicles but will always terminate proximal to external urinary sphincter. Upper pole ureters tend to obstruct. Lower pole ureters tend to reflux. The upper pole segment may be dysplastic or non-functioning. Commonly seen on antenatal ultrasound scans when there is hydronephrosis. May also present with urinary tract infection.

DIAGNOSIS (23.34–23.38)
Ultrasound may show abnormal orientation of calyces, suggesting duplication. IVU will define anatomy more clearly with direct visualization of the duplicated ureters. A duplex kidney with a non-functioning upper pole will manifest

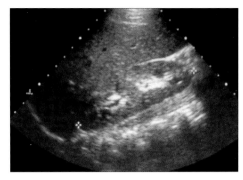

23.35 Ultrasound appearance of duplex kidney.

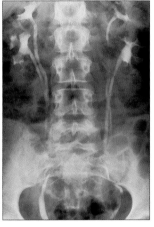

23.36 IVU demonstrating bilateral duplex kidneys.

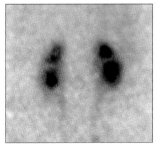

23.37 MAG-3 scan of bilateral duplex kidneys.

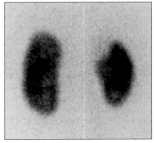

23.38 DMSA demonstrating a non-functioning upper-pole moiety of a duplex right kidney.

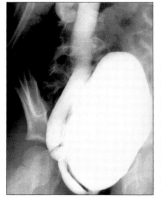

23.34 MCUG demonstrating reflux into a ureter from the upper pole of a duplex kidney that enters ectopically into the urethra.

itself on IVU as lateral and inferior rotation of the lower pole calyces ('drooping lily' sign). Non-functioning systems may require retrograde pyelography for diagnosis.

TREATMENT

No treatment is indicated for partially duplicated ureters or incidentally discovered completely duplicated ureters. If antireflux surgery is required, ureters are reimplanted as a single system (double-barrel reimplant). Non-functioning renal segments associated with duplicated ureters may need to be removed if they are a source of infection.

PROGNOSIS

Generally quite good. Remember that most ureteral duplication is a variation of normal. Prognosis ultimately depends on the amount of kidney damage from reflux or obstruction (if present).

VESICOURETERIC REFLUX

INCIDENCE

Less than 1% of healthy children. Appears to be more common in white children than in black children. It is much more common in girls.

PRESENTATION

Two groups of patients are typically seen. The first are those seen to have hydronephrosis on antenatal ultrasound (these are usually the male patients); the second group are diagnosed after recurrent urinary tract infections in childhood (these are usually the female patients). There may be a primary anomaly of the vesicoureteric junction consisting of an abnormal insertion of the ureter into the bladder. More commonly it is the result of lower urinary tract dysfunction (e.g. posterior urethral valves, neuropathic bladder, subtle bladder dysfunction).

DIAGNOSIS (23.39–23.42)

MCUG is the gold standard. MAG-3 renal scan with an indirect isotope cystogram is helpful in assessing renal function and scarring as well as to follow reflux once diagnosed. The indirect isotope cystogram (or direct cystogram if the bladder is catheterized and filled with isotope) entails less radiation.

TREATMENT

Conservative therapy with prophylactic antibiotics is the mainstay of therapy as long as renal function remains stable and there are no breakthrough infections. Reflux of sterile urine does not harm the kidney. Surgery may be required in the setting of falling renal function, new onset renal scars or breakthrough infections. Surgery can be carried out either through

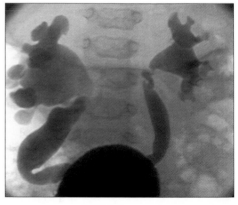

23.39 MCUG. Bilateral vesicoureteric reflux.

open techniques (ureteric reimplantation), which are most common, or endoscopically.

PROGNOSIS

One-third of antenatally diagnosed boys and two-thirds of antenatally diagnosed girls will have spontaneous resolution of their reflux. If renal damage is present, 10 to 30% of patients may develop hypertension. Ten percent of patients awaiting renal transplantation have a history of reflux. Close nephrological and urological follow-up is essential.

URETEROCOELE

INCIDENCE

One in 500 autopsies. Less common clinically. Commonly associated with upper pole of duplex kidney. Sixty percent associated with ectopic ureter. Ten percent bilateral. More common in girls.

PRESENTATION

Antenatal ultrasound shows renal pelvic dilatation and/or ureterocoele seen in the bladder (**23.43**). Postnatal presentation with urinary tract infection/sepsis, bladder outlet obstruction, dysuria or interlabial mass.

The pathogenesis is unclear. Ureterocoele represents cystic dilatation of the intramural ureter. There is a 50% incidence of ipsilateral lower pole vesicoureteric reflux and a 25% incidence of contralateral vesicoureteric reflux. Ureterocoele typically obstructs the renal segment it drains. It may prolapse into the urethra and obstruct bladder outflow (**23.44**).

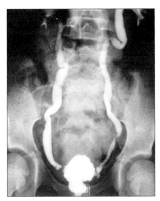

23.40 MCUG. Bilateral vesico-ureteric reflux.

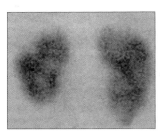

23.41 DMSA scan showing bilateral renal scarring in vesico-ureteric reflux.

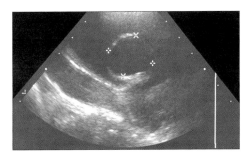

23.43 Bladder ultrasound demonstrating a ureterocoele.

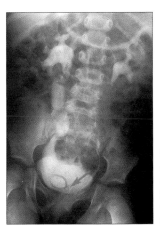

23.42 IVU showing ureterocoele in the bladder that contains a stone.

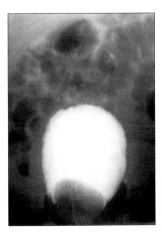

23.44 Ureterocoele obstructing bladder outlet.

DIAGNOSIS

Ultrasound of bladder shows cystic mass with overlying membrane. Ultrasound of kidneys may show a duplex collecting system. MCUG may show a filling defect in bladder. Isotope scan often shows non-function of upper pole.

TREATMENT

Depends on age of patient, presentation and function of kidney. Transurethral incision is often the first line of treatment, especially in babies diagnosed antenatally. It is curative in 90% of intravesical ureterocoeles and in 50% of ectopic ureterocoeles. If the upper pole is non-functioning then heminephroureterectomy is the procedure of choice. Ten to 20% of patients who undergo upper-pole heminephroureterectomy alone eventually require subsequent reconstructive bladder surgery for the removal of the residual ureteral stump or reimplantation of the refluxing ureters. Bladder reconstruction in infants and small children is inadvisable.

PROGNOSIS

The long-term prognosis is excellent. Voiding dysfunction may result from reconstructive bladder surgery in the infant or small child.

REFERENCES

Multicystic dysplastic kidney
Menster, M. Mahan J, Koff S et al. Multicystic dysplastic kidney. Ped Nephrol 1994; **8**(1): 113–115.

Neuropathic voiding dysfunction and incontinence
Fernandez E, Reinberg Y, Vernier R, Gonzalez R. Neurogenic voiding dysfunction in children: a review of pathophysiology and current management. J Ped 1994; **124**(1): 1–7.

Exstrophy/epispadias complex
Langer JC. Fetal abdominal wall defects. Semin Ped Surg 1993; **2**(2): 121–128.

Testicular tumours
Levy DA, Kay R, Elder JS. Neonatal testis tumors: a review of the prepubertal testis. Tumor Registry. J Urol 1994; **151**(3): 715–717.

Hypospadias
Mouriquand PD, Persad R, Sharma S et al. Hypospadias repair: current principles and procedures. Br J Urol 1995; **76**(Suppl): 9–22.

Wilms' tumour
National Wilms' Tumor Study Group. The treatment of Wilms' tumor – results of the National Wilms' Tumor Study. Hematol Oncol Clin N Am 1995; **9**(6): 1267–1274.

Urogenital rhabdomyosarcoma
Shapiro E, Strother D. Pediatric genitourinary rhabdomyosarcoma. J Urol 1992; **148**: 1761–1768.

Prune-belly syndrome
Skoog S. Prune-belly Syndrome in Clinical Pediatric Urology. In: Kelalis P, King R, Belman A (eds). Clinical Pediatric Urology (4th edn). Philadelphia, Saunders, 2000.

Congenital abnormalities of urine flow (PUJ and UVJ anomalies)
King L. Hydronephrosis. When is obstruction not obstruction? Urol Clin N Am 1995; **22**(1): 31–42.

Urolithiasis
Harman E, Faerber GJ. Pediatric urolithiasis. Curr Opin Urol 2001; **11**: 385–389.

Posterior urethral valves
Churchill BM. Emergency treatment and long-term follow-up of posterior urethral valves. Urol Clin N Am 1990; **17**(2): 343–360.

Cryptorchidism
Fonkaisrud E. Testicular undescent and torsion. Ped Clin N Am 1987; **34**(5): 1305–1318.

Ambiguous genitalia
Hughes I, Mouriquand P. Ambiguous genitalia in the newborn. Surgery 1995; **13**(12): 265–271.

Anomalies of kidney position and number
Churchill BM, Abaro EO, McLorie GA et al. Ureteral duplication, ectopy and ureteroceles. Ped Clin N Am 1987; **34**(5): 1273–1290.

Ureteral duplication
Churchill BM, Abaro EO, McLorie GA et al. Ureteral duplication, ectopy and ureteroceles. Ped Clin N Am 1987; **34**(5): 1273–1290.

Vesicoureteric reflux
Belman AB. A perspective on vesicoureteral reflux. Urol Clin N Am 1995; **22**(1): 139–150.

Ureterocele
Coplen C, Duckett J. The modern approach to ureteroceles. J Urol 1995; **153**: 166–171.

Heart and Lung Transplantation

Bruce F Whitehead
Jackson YW Wong

HEART TRANSPLANTATION: ENDOMYOCARDIAL BIOPSY

RATIONALE

Biopsy forceps are introduced through an intravenous sheath in the internal jugular vein.

Endomyocardial biopsies are taken from the right ventricle (**24.1**). These are examined histologically for evidence of acute rejection. Other investigations performed include ECG, echocardiography and chest x-ray.

COMPLICATIONS / INCIDENCE

Pneumothorax and haemothorax can develop from the cannulation of the internal jugular vein. Myocardial puncture may occur resulting in haemopericardium. These are, in fact, rare. Overall incidence of complications is less than 1%.

MONITORING / OTHER TREATMENT

If acute rejection is diagnosed, then this is treated with augmentation of the immuno-suppression therapy. This may include high dose intravenous methylprednisolone and/or anti-lymphocyte globulin.

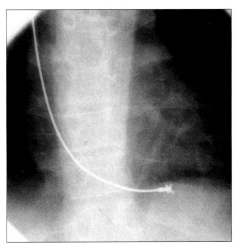

24.1 Fluoroscopic appearance of the position of forceps to obtain an endomyocardial biopsy in a heart transplant recipient. The forceps are introduced through an intravenous sheath, which has been inserted into the right internal jugular vein. Biopsies are taken routinely to observe for evidence of acute rejection and therefore modify immunosuppressive therapy.

HEART AND LUNG TRANSPLANTATION

RATIONALE

For end stage respiratory disease, e.g. associated with cystic fibrosis.

CLINICAL PRESENTATION

Figure **24.2** shows the chest x-ray appearance of a 14-year-old girl with severe cystic fibrosis pulmonary disease before and after combined heart and lung transplantation. Note the hyperinflation ('horizontal' ribs, depressed diaphragm), ring shadows and generalized increased bronchial wall markings before, with complete resolution of abnormalities after transplant.

COMPLICATIONS / SURVIVAL

This is a high-risk procedure. One-year survival is approximately 70–80%; three-year survival is approximately 50–60%. Complications such as rejection and infection may occur and require specific therapy.

MONITORING / OTHER TREATMENT

Radiology, formal pulmonary function testing and bronchoscopy/transbronchial biopsy may be indicated. If rejection is identified, then high dose intravenous methylprednisolone may be required.

LUNG FUNCTION MONITORING

RATIONALE

Daily home monitoring of pulmonary function is a useful aid in the monitoring of the lung transplant recipient (**24.3**). Any deviation in pulmonary function may indicate an episode of rejection and/or infection.

COMPLICATIONS / INCIDENCE

As shown on the lung function graph (**24.8**, page 621), there are episodes of rejection and infection which punctuate the post-transplant course. Falls in lung function may prompt further investigation such as radiology, bronchoscopy and transbronchial biopsy.

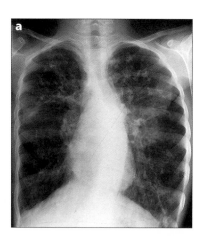

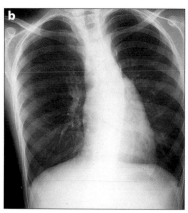

24.2 Chest radiographs of a 14-year-old cystic fibrosis patient with severe pulmonary disease **(a)** before and **(b)** after combined heart and lung transplantation.

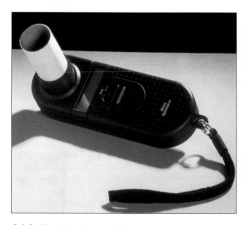

24.3 Hand-held portable spirometer (Microspirometer, Micromedical, Kent) used to measured FEV$_1$ and FVC in children following heart–lung transplantation.

TRANSBRONCHIAL BIOPSY

RATIONALE

Transbronchial biopsy (**24.4–24.7**) is used for the diagnosis of rejection and infection following lung transplantation. It is also used in immunosuppressed and immunocompetent patients with non-specific lung infiltrates.

COMPLICATIONS

Pneumothorax (incidence approximately 3–5%). Haemorrhage (less than 1%).

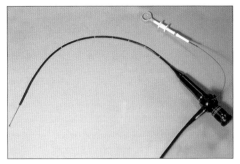

24.4 A 4.9 mm flexible fibreoptic bronchoscope (Olympus, Japan) with alligator-head transbronchial biopsy forceps inserted through the suction channel. Used for monitoring of pulmonary allografts.

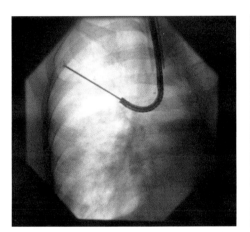

24.5 Fluoroscopic appearance of position of transbronchial biopsy forceps through the flexible fibreoptic bronchoscope.

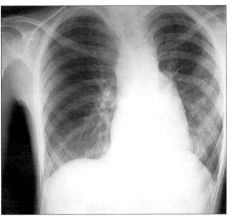

24.6 Chest radiograph from a heart–lung transplant recipient who presented with fever, dyspnoea, cough, sputum and crackles on auscultation. This shows bilateral, lower zone reticular shadowing, suggestive of acute rejection or a pneumonitis due to an opportunistic organism.

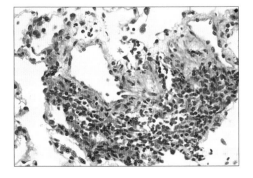

24.7 Photomicrograph of a section of a transbronchial biopsy from the same patient showing a perivascular infiltration of mononuclear cells – pathognomonic of acute allograft rejection.

ACUTE ALLOGRAFT REJECTION

This is common after lung transplant and always signifies a sense of urgency that necessitates aggressive diagnosis and therapy. The goal of therapy is to terminate an accelerating process of immune-mediated cell injury that may result in progressive tissue damage and acute deterioration in lung function. Clinical suspicion is prompted by a $\geq 15\%$ fall in spirometry (FEV_1 or FVC) with or without clinical manifestations: feeling generally unwell, shortness of breath, fatigue, pyrexia, the new onset of inspiratory crackles on auscultation, hypoxia and new interstitial infiltrates and/or pleural effusion on chest radiograph. It has been reported that 70% or more of lung transplant patients experience at least one episode of acute rejection within the first 90 postoperative days. Concordance of clinical suspicion and histological findings are poor (48% false rate) during the first 6 months.

The majority of verified episodes of acute rejection occur in the first months after transplantation. The natural history of silent rejection is unknown but is potentially worrying in relation to chronic allograft dysfunction. Endomyocardial biopsies are usually unnecessary in heart–lung transplant patients, since the lung is the more vulnerable of the two organs to immunologic discovery and attack. Hyperacute rejection and humoral rejection are not discussed in detail here. In essence, ABO mismatch and the presence of pre-existing HLA antibodies in the recipient are important risk factors. This section will concentrate on acute cellular rejection.

PATHOPHYSIOLOGY

Acute rejection is cell-mediated, predominantly by CD4+ helper T cells (T_H), CD8+ cytotoxic T cells (T_C) and macrophages, which mediate DTH responses. Recognition of donor *MHC* (major histocompatiblility complex) molecules by recipient T cells can be direct (CD8+ and CD4+) or indirect (CD4+), as processed allopeptides presented by recipient antigen presenting cells. CD4/CD8-mediated adhesion is restricted to either *MHC* class II/*MHC* class I molecules respectively. Binding of *MHC* molecules or epitopes to recipient T-cell receptor (TCR)/CD3 complex is reinforced by cell surface adhesion molecules and ligands (e.g. CD28/B7-1 and 2). Activation of Th1 CD4+ T_H cells triggers a host of intracytoplasmic enzymes and signalling that result in the transcription of inflammatory cytokines such as IL-2 and INF-γ. They, in turn, promote activation and proliferation of the CD4+ cells, CD8+ T_C activation and clonal differentiation, antibody production, DTH responses and upregulation of donor cell expression of MHC molecules. This process is counterbalanced by Th2 CD4+ TH cells related anti-inflammatory cytokine production (IL-4, IL-10 and IL-13) that facilitates anergy (non-responsiveness of activated T cells). When a CD8+ TC cell is activated, intracellular contents of granzyme and perforin increase in anticipation, and kill donor cells upon contact.

DIAGNOSIS

All suspected episodes of acute rejection should be confirmed by transbronchial biopsies (TBB), whenever possible. A minimum of six pieces of biopsy are required for accuracy. Specificity and sensitivity >90% were reported by experienced centres. Since the vascular endothelium is the primary front line of donor-recipient immune interface, histological acute rejection is typified by mononuclear cell infiltration around small blood vessels. Extension of these cells to the alveolar, peribronchiolar tissue and interstitium is seen in high-grade rejection. About 72% of clinically indicated TBB will show evidence of clinically significant acute rejection ($\geq$A2/mild rejection). Around 25% of surveillance TBB will be positive in those who are clinically well during the first 4–6 post-transplant months. After 2–4 years post-transplantation, the yield of annual surveillance TBB diminishes progressively. Complication rate of TBB is small in competent hands: <10% of cases have pneumothorax or bleeding, mostly non-problematic, and fatality is exceptional.

INVESTIGATIONS

Clinical, radiological, and physiological criteria do not differentiate acute rejection from infection and they can coexist. Bronchoscopy, BAL and TBB are essential both at diagnosis and on follow-up, as histological acute rejection has been found in 40% of patients after treatment, in one large study. Children who are too small for TBB and too young for spirometry test are particularly challenging. Eosinophilia found in BAL and peripheral blood samples could be helpful pointers of acute rejection if other causes can be excluded. Open lung biopsy could be considered as a last resort when an accurate diagnosis is deemed imperative.

TREATMENT

High-dose daily IV methyprenisolone (10–15 mg/kg/day) given for 3–5 consecutive days has a 90–95% success rate in most centres. Cytolytic therapy (ALG/ATG/OKT3) should be considered after two failed pulse steroid treatments. Anaphylaxis, cytokine storm, neutropenia, thrombocytopenia and increased infection risks are possible adverse effects. Recurrent low-grade acute rejections warrants augmentation of baseline immunosuppressants: increasing oral steroids, adding inhaled steroids/cyclosporin or low-dose oral methotrexate, and switching to tacrolimus and/or mycophenoate mofetil. A six-week course of once weekly methotrexate (0.1–0.25 mg/kg) has also been used in some centres. Some have reported the use of total lymphoid irradiation against recalcitrant acute rejection with success. Rapamycin and leflunomide are being evaluated in experimental settings.

PROGNOSIS

Although previously reported rejection related mortality rates were 5–30%, current mortality rates of treated acute rejection is likely to be around 1–2%. While pulses of intravenous prednisolone are often effective, the impact on the development of bronchiolitis obliterans syndrome appears to be limited (**24.8**). Attention has been drawn to preventative treatments (inductive chimeric/humanized monoclonal IL-2 receptor blockers), development of tolerance strategies (clonal deletion, mixed chimerism) and blocking co-stimulation pathways (e.g. CTLA4Ig).

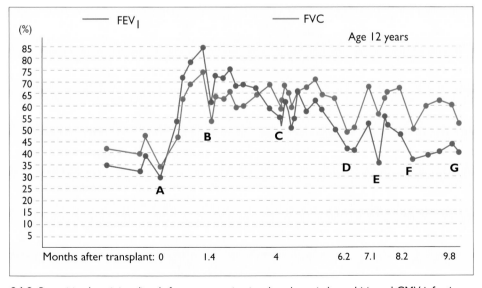

24.8 Repetitive lung injury/insult from acute rejection, lymphocytic bronchitis and CMV infection leading to a gradual fall in baseline FEV_1 and eventual bronchiolitis obliterans syndrome. Aggressive therapy with each injury restored lung function at least briefly and may have slowed lung function losses. A = heart–lung transplantation for CF; B = CMV infection; C, D & F = acute rejection; E = lymphocytic bronchitis; G = bronchiolitis obliterans syndrome.

BRONCHIOLITIS OBLITERANS SYNDROME (BOS)

This denotes irreversible post-transplant graft deterioration secondary to progressive small airway disease for which there is no other cause. It is a major cause of allograft dysfunction in lung and heart–lung transplant recipients. It is likely, though unproven, that this is a manifestation of chronic rejection. Histologic confirmation is not sensitive or required and may not reflect the clinical activity monitored by pulmonary function test. The term 'bronchiolitis obliterans' (BO) is used when a histological diagnosis is available. Cumulative risk of BO is from 32–90% 5 years post transplantation. Allo-immunologic injury against the airway epithelium and non-alloimmunologic inflammatory conditions, including viral infections or ischaemic injury, are likely to play a role in BO. Risk factors are summarized in **Table 24.1**.

Table 24.1 BOS risk factors

Risk factors
- Acute rejection*
- Lymphocytic bronchitis/bronchiolitis (Ross *et al*) (**24.9**)*
- Non-compliance to medication

Potential risk factors
- CMV pneumonitis* (**24.10**)
- Bacterial/fungal/CMV and non-CMV viral infection
- Donor (>40 years) and recipient age (3–20 years)
- Graft ischaemic time
- Cytokine gene polymorphisms

* Transbronchial lung biopsies required

PATHOPHYSIOLOGY

BO is a cicatrical process affecting the allograft small airways. It progresses through a sequence of lymphocytic infiltration of the submucosa to the airway epithelium, followed by necrosis of epithelial cells and mucosal denudation. Proliferation of fibroblasts and myofibroblasts into the luminal exudate leads to intraluminal granulation polyp formation. Fibrous plaque formation in the wall of the airway (**24.11**) and intraluminal granulation tissues may completely obliterate the lumen, reducing the small airway passages to stenotic cords of scar tissue. Various cytokines and growth factors are implicated and underlying cytokine gene polymorphisms of TNFα, IFγ, IL-10, IL-6 or TGF-β genes are potentially important.

DIAGNOSIS

Symptoms range from none to cough, wheeze, and dyspnoea. A diagnosis of BOS should only be made after evaluation of other conditions (e.g. acute rejection, infection, stenosis of the airway anastomosis and bronchial hyper-responsiveness) that may alter graft function and treatment of these conditions, when found. Spirometric measurements are essential for diagnosis. A sustained decline in FEV_1 ≥20% from previous stable baseline is diagnostic. The International Society of Heart–Lung Transplantation has recently updated the diagnostic criteria of BOS. Young children who cannot perform pulmonary function reliably, and are suspected of developing BO, should undergo bronchoscopic examination of the airway and transbronchial biopsy when possible. Open lung biopsy may be indicated in those present with obscuring clinical pathology.

INVESTIGATIONS

Although transbronchial lung biopsies can be normal even in the presence of advanced BO, they are essential for exclusion of confounding conditions and identifying treatable risk factors. The presence of air trapping on expiratory CT scans is suggestive of the diagnosis (**24.12**). Other indicators of BO include broncho-alveolar lavage neutrophilia, diffuse heterogeneous defects on ventilation perfusion scan, airway hyperreactivity, raised exhaled nitric oxide, and abnormalities in indices of ventilation distribution, using inert gases single-breath washout technique. Specificity of these surrogate markers of BO is likely to be low. High values of reported specificity are likely, due to selection bias.

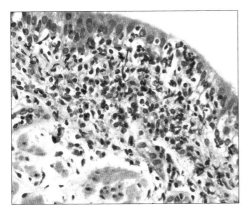

24.9 Lymphocytic bronchitis. The bronchiole wall shows a mixed inflammatory cell infiltrate which extends around the smooth muscle and into the superficial epithelium.

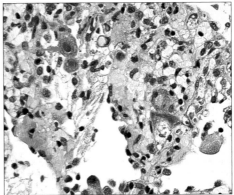

24.10 CMV (cytomegalovirus) pneumonitis. Histological section of transplanted lung, showing a moderate interstitial inflammatory infiltrate and prominent CMV viral inclusions (arrow) in alveolar lining cells.

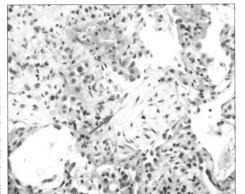

24.11 Bronchiolitis obliterans. A "plug" of loose fibrous tissue is seen in the central airway.

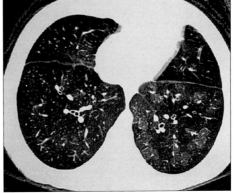

24.12 High resolution chest CT image through the lower lobes, right middle lobe and the lingular, showing variable lung attenuation and bronchial wall thickening. The low density areas represent foci of air trapping, and this was more conspicuous on expiratory images.

TREATMENT

Fibrous obliteration of the bronchioles is likely to be irreversible in BO. However, heterogeneous histologic lesions are often present, with some small airways showing lymphocytic infiltration that are potentially amenable to treatment. As BO is often diagnosed following bouts of acute allograft rejection and/or infection, adequate treatment of these conditions may modulate the rate of deterioration (**24.13**). Augmentation of immunosuppression may be worthwhile in patients diagnosed with BO within 18 months of transplantation. BO with onset many years post-transplantation is unlikely to benefit from such treatment. Supportive treatment such as controlling intercurrent infections, physiotherapy and oxygen therapy could be helpful in selected patients. One-year survival rate after retransplantation for BO is only 45%. Recently, the use of rapamycin appears to have beneficial fibrinolytic effects in animal BO models. Multicentre trials of its use in lung transplant patients are currently underway.

PROGNOSIS

The mortality rate of BO is around 50%. Median survival after diagnosis is approximately 2.5–3 years. The rate of deterioration varies greatly among patients. Recurrent lower respiratory infections are common; *Pseudomonas aeruginosa* is a particularly common pathogen. Because patients and families often are under tremendous stress after a diagnosis of BO, emotional support is crucial. Most transplant centres do not consider retransplantation for patients with end-stage BO.

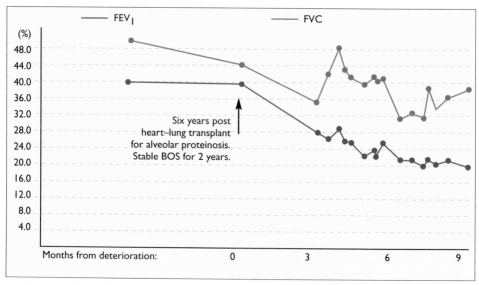

24.13 A significant fall in lung function was due to recurrent bacterial chest infections and *Aspergillus* bronchitis. Aggresive antimicrobial therapy and bronchoscopic clearance of mucus had stabilized lung function and sustained exercise tolerance (NYHA Class I).

REFERENCES

Endomyocardial biopsy of transplanted heart
Caves PK, Stinson EB, Billingham ME, Shumway NE. Serial transvenous biopsy of the transplanted human heart. Improved management of acute rejection episodes. *Lancet* 1974; **1**: 821–826.

Heart and lung transplantation
Whitehead BF, Rees PG, Sorensen K *et al.* Results of heart-lung transplantation in children with cystic fibrosis. *Eur J Cardio-Thorac Surg* 1995; **9**: 1–6.

Lung transplantation
Theodore J. Physiology of the lung in human heart-lung transplantation. *Cardiovasc Clin* 1990; **20**: 57–69.

Transbronchial biopsy (TBBx)
Whitehead B, Scott JP, Helms P *et al.* Technique and use of transbronchial biopsy in children and adolescents. *Ped Pulmonol* 1992; **12**: 240–246.

Acute allograft rejection
Griffith BP, Hardesty RL, Armitage JM *et al.* Acute rejection of lung allografts with various immunosuppressive protocols. *Ann Thor Surg* 1992;**54(5)**: 846–851.

Guilinger RA, Paradis IL, Dauber JH *et al.* The importance of bronchoscopy with transbronchial biopsy and bronchoalveolar lavage in the management of lung transplant recipients. *Am J Resp Crit Care Med* 1995; **152**: 2037–2043.

Higenbottam T, Hutter JA, Stewart S, Wallwork J. Transbronchial biopsy has eliminated the need for endomyocardial biopsy in heart-lung recipients. *J Heart Transplant* 1988; 7(**6**): 435–439.

Kesten SD, Chamberlain D, Maurer J. Yield of surveillance transbronchial biopsies performed beyond two years after lung transplantation. *J Heart Lung Transplant* 1996; **15**: 384–388.

Scott JP, Fradet G, Smyth RL *et al.* Prospective study of transbronchial biopsies in the management of heart-lung and single lung transplant patients. *J Heart Lung Transplant* 1991; **10(5 Pt 1)**: 626–636.

Trulock EP, Ettinger NA, Brunt EM *et al.* The role of transbronchial lung biopsy in the treatment of lung transplant recipients. An analysis of 200 consecutive procedures. *Chest* 1992; **102**: 1049–1054.

Yousem SA, Berry GJ, Cagle PT *et al.*. Revision of the 1990 working formulation for the classification of pulmonary allograft rejection: Lung Rejection Study Group. *J Heart Lung Transplant* 1996; **15(1 Pt 1)**: 1–15.

Bronchiolitis obliterans syndrome (BOS)
Boucek MM, Faro A, Novick RJ *et al.* The Registry of the International Society for Heart and Lung Transplantation: Fourth Official Pediatric Report – 2000. *J Heart Lung Transplant* 2001; **20(1)**: 39–52.

Estenne M, Maurer JR, Boehler A *et al* Bronchiolitis obliterans syndrome 2001: an update of the diagnostic criteria. *J Heart Lung Transplant* 2002; **21(3)**: 297–310.

Husain AN, Siddiqui MT, Holmes EW *et al.* Analysis of risk factors for the development of bronchiolitis obliterans syndrome. *Am J Respir Critical Care Med* 1999; **159(3)**: 829–833.

Novick RJ, Stitt LW, Al Kattan K *et al.* Pulmonary retransplantation: predictors of graft function and survival in 230 patients. *Pulmonary Retransplant Registry. Ann Thorac Surg* 1998; **65(1)**: 227–234.

Ross DJ, Marchevsky A, Kramer M, Kass RM. 'Refractoriness' of airflow obstruction associated with isolated lymphocytic bronchiolitis/bronchitis in pulmonary allografts. *J Heart Lung Transplant* 1997; **16(8)**: 832–838.

Snell GI, Esmore DS, Williams TJ. Cytolytic therapy for the bronchiolitis obliterans syndrome complicating lung transplantation. *Chest* 1996; **109(4)**: 874–878.

Valentine VG, Robbins RC, Berry GJ *et al.* Actuarial survival of heart-lung and bilateral sequential lung transplant recipients with obliterative bronchiolitis. *J Heart Lung Transplant* 1996; **15(4)**: 371–383.

ACE	angiotensin-converting enzyme
ACTH	adrenocorticotrophin hormone
ADA	adenosine deaminase
ADHD	attention deficit hyperactivity disorder
AFB	acid-fast bacilli
AIDS	acquired immunodeficiency syndrome
ALCAPA	anomalous origin of the left coronary artery from the pulmonary artery
ALD	adrenoleukodystrophy
ALL	acute lymphoblastic leukaemia
ALS	advanced life support
AML	acute myeloid leukaemia
ANA	antinuclear antibodies
ANCA	antineutrophil cytoplasmic antibodies
ANLL	acute non-lymphoblastic leukaemia
APLS	advanced paediatric life support
ASD	atrial septal defect
ASO	antistreptolysin O
AT	α-1-antitrypsin
A-V	atrioventricular
BAL	bronchioalveolar lavage
BCG	bacille Calmette-Guèrin
BMT	bone marrow transplantation
BOS	bronchiolitis obliterans syndrome
BP	blood pressure
CAA	coronary artery aneurysm
CCAM	congenital cystic adenomatoid malformation
CF	cystic fibrosis
CFTR	cystic fibrosis transmembrane conductance regulatory protein
CGD	chronic granulomatous disease
CINCA	chronic, infantile, neurological, cutaneous and articular syndrome
CK	creatine kinase
CHRPE	congenital hypertrophy of the retinal pigment epithelium
CLE	congenital lobar emphysema
CMV	cytomegalovirus
CNS	central nervous system

CPAP	continuous positive airway pressure
CPK	creatine phosphokinase
CPP	cerebral perfusion pressure
CRH	corticotrophin-releasing hormone
CRP	C-reactive protein
CSE	convulsive status epilepticus
CSF	cerebrospinal fluid
CT (scan)	computed tomography
CT	congenital toxoplasmosis
CTD	connective tissue disease
CVP	central venous pressure
DDH	developmental dysplasia of the hip
DIC	disseminated intravascular coagulation
DIOS	distal intestinal obstruction syndrome
DKA	diabetic ketoacidosis
DNA	deoxyribonucleic acid
2,3 DPG	2,3 diphosphoglycerate
EB	epidermolysis bullosa
EBS	epidermolysis bullosa simplex
EBV	Epstein-Barr virus
ECG	electrocardiogram
ECMO	extracorporeal membrane oxygenation
EEG	electroencephalogram
ELISA	enzyme-linked immunosorbent assay
ENT	ear, nose and throat
ERCP	endoscopic retrograde cholangiopancreatogram
ESR	erythrocyte sedimentation rate
FBC	full blood count
FEV1	forced expiratory volume in one second
FSH	follicle stimulating hormone
FVC	forced vital capacity
G6PD	glucose-6-phosphate dehydrogenase
GABA	gamma-aminobutyric acid
GAGs	glycoylsaminoglycans
GCS	Glasgow coma score
GH	growth hormone

GnRH	gonadotrophin-releasing hormone
GSD	glycogen storage disease
HAART	highly active anti-retroviral therapy
Hb	haemoglobin
HbF	fetal haemoglobin
hCG	human chorionic gonadotrophin
HCV	hepatitis C virus
HES	hypereosinophilic syndrome
HHV	human herpes virus
HIV	human immunodeficiency virus
HLA	human leucocyte antigen
HPV	human papilloma virus
HR	heart rate
HSP	Henoch-Schönlein purpura
HSV	herpes simplex virus
IBD	inflammatory bowel disease
ICP	intracranial pressure
IgA/E/G/M/D	immunoglobulin A/E/G/M/D
IGF	insulin-like growth factor
ITP	idiopathic thrombocytopenic purpura
IVU	intravenous urogram
JEB	junctional epidermolysis bullosa
JIA	juvenile idiopathic arthritis
JML	juvenile myelomonocytic leukaemia
LAD	leukocyte adhesion deficiency
LCH	Langerhans' cell histiocytosis
LFT	liver function tests
LIP	lymphocytic interstitial pneumonitis
MCAD	medium chain acyl Co-A dehydrogenase
MCP	metacarpophalangeal
MCUG	micturating cystourethrogram
MHC	major histocompatibility complex
MODY	maturity onset diabetes of the young
MPS	mucopolysaccharidoses
MRI	magnetic resonance imaging
MSU	midstream urine specimen
NHL	non-Hodgkin's lymphoma
NRTI	nucleoside reverse transcriptase inhibitors
NSAIDs	non-steroidal anti-inflammatory drugs
NTBC	2-(2-nitro-4-trifluoromethyl-benzoyl)-1,3-cyclohexanedione
OME	otitis media with effusion
OTC	ornithine transcarbamylase
PAD	patent arterial duct
PAN	polyarteritis nodosa
PAS	periodic acid Schiff
pCO2	partial pressure of carbon dioxide
PCP	*Pneumocystis carinii* pneumonia
PCR	polymerase chain reaction
PCV	packed cell volume
PEEP	positive end expiratory pressure
PEFR	peak expiratory flow rate
PET	positron emission tomogram
PICU	paediatric intensive care unit
PK	pyruvate kinase
PKU	phenylketonuria
PUO	pyrexia of unknown origin
PUVA	psoralen ultraviolet A (therapy)
RAD	reflex anal dilatation
RAG	recombinase activating gene
RAST	radioallergosorbent test
rhGH	recombinant human growth hormone
ROP	retinopathy of prematurity
RR	respiratory rate
RSD	reflex sympathetic dystrophy
RSV	respiratory syncytial virus
SAPHO	synovitis, acne, pustulosis, hyperostosis and osteitis
SCID	severe combined immunodeficiency
SLE	systemic lupus erythematosus
SPT	skin prick test
STD	sexually transmitted disease
SUFE	slipped upper femoral epiphysis
SVT	supraventricular tachycardia
TAR	thrombocytopenia with absent radius
TB	tuberculosis
TBB	transbronchial biopsy
TNF	tumour necrosis factor
ToF	tetralogy of Fallot
TS	tuberous sclerosis
TSH	thyroid stimulating hormone
TSS	toxic shock syndrome
VLCFA	very long chain fatty acids
VSD	ventricular septal defect
VUR	vesico-ureteric reflux
VWD	von Willebrand's disease
VZV	varicella zoster virus
WCC	white cell count